Drug Delivery Systems in Cancer Therapy

Drug Delivery Systems in Cancer Therapy

Edited by

Dennis M. Brown

ChemGenex Therapeutics, Inc.
Menlo Park, CA

Humana Press ✳ Totowa, New Jersey

© 2004 Humana Press Inc.
999 Riverview Drive, Suite 208
Totowa, New Jersey 07512
www.humanapress.com

For additional copies, pricing for bulk purchases, and/or information about other Humana titles, contact Humana at the above address or at any of the following numbers: Tel.: 973-256-1699; Fax: 973-256-8341; E-mail: humana@humanapr.com or visit our Website: http://humanapress.com

Due diligence has been taken by the publishers, editors, and authors of this book to ensure the accuracy of the information published and to describe generally accepted practices. The contributors herein have carefully checked to ensure that the drug selections and dosages set forth in this text are accurate in accord with the standards accepted at the time of publication. Notwithstanding, as new research, changes in government regulations, and knowledge from clinical experience relating to drug therapy and drug reactions constantly occurs, the reader is advised to check the product information provided by the manufacturer of each drug for any change in dosages or for additional warnings and contraindications. This is of utmost importance when the recommended drug herein is a new or infrequently used drug. It is the responsibility of the health care provider to ascertain the Food and Drug Administration status of each drug or device used in their clinical practice. The publisher, editors, and authors are not responsible for errors or omissions or for any consequences from the application of the information presented in this book and make no warranty, express or implied, with respect to the contents in this publication.

Production Editor: Mark J. Breaugh.

Cover illustration:Hollow and porous microparticles of PLAGA prepared using ethyl acetate and poly(vinyl alcohol) at a magnification of ×1250. (See Fig. 3 on page 120.) Microscopic images of PLAGA microparticles containing 5-fluorouracil after 21 days of degradation in phosphate buffered saline. (See Fig. 8 on page 128.)

Cover design by Patricia F. Cleary.

This publication is printed on acid-free paper. ∞
ANSI Z39.48-1984 (American National Standards Institute) Permanence of Paper for Printed Library Materials.

Printed in the United States of America. 10 9 8 7 6 5 4 3 2 1

E-ISBN:1-59259-427-1

Library of Congress Cataloging-in-Publication Data

Drug delivery systems in cancer therapy / edited by Dennis M. Brown.
      p. ; cm. -- (Cancer drug discovery and development)
   Includes bibliographical references and index.
   ISBN 0-89603-888-2 (alk. paper)
    1. Antineoplastic agents--Administration. 2. Drug delivery systems. I. Brown, Dennis
M., 1949– II. Series.
    [DNLM: 1. Drug Delivery Systems--methods. 2. Neoplasms--drug therapy. 3.
Antineoplastic Agents--administration & dosage. 4. Drug Delivery Systems--trends. QZ
267 D7932 2003]
RS431.A64D78 2003
616.99'4061--dc21
                                                                                2003042321

Preface

The use of drug delivery systems to improve the efficacy of cancer chemotherapy remains an important strategy for achieving progress against this disease. Over the past 20 years, the number of novel therapeutic approaches has expanded from traditional small chemical medicinals to a wide variety of biomolecules, including peptide/protein- and nucleic acid-based therapeutics. All of these therapies require the administration of stable dosage forms in adequate concentrations and exposure periods to realize their potential. For the treatment of many forms of cancer, the presentation and maintenance of adequate drug concentrations to the target disease tissues without overexposure to drug-sensitive normal tissues is the major limitation for successful chemotherapy.

The purpose of *Drug Delivery Systems in Cancer Therapy* is to provide a general overview of the drug delivery technologies available for research oncologists looking to improve the potential utility of their novel lead candidates. This text focuses on a number of important topics critical for successful cancer chemotherapy development. Pharmacological considerations of conventional and non-conventional routes of drug administration are reviewed and opportunities for product development are identified. The use of novel formulation technologies, including synthetic polymers and biomaterials for prolonged or sustained drug release to achieve potentially greater therapeutic indices, is outlined and discussed. The technologies described have resulted in a number of approved and late-stage clinical products. These are profiled as well.

The intent of this book is to serve as a springboard for a scientist, not necessarily affiliated with this field, to become "comfortable" to explore a broader platform of formulation and delivery system strategies during the preclinical phases of development. It is hoped that the subjects covered and referenced in this volume would help expand the pharmaceutical potential for a new agent. In addition, for formulation scientists, experimental pharmacologists, and medicinal chemists, chapters are devoted to new therapeutic areas where their expertise may be needed to help secure a successful product outcome.

In *Drug Delivery Systems in Cancer Therapy* the focus has primarily been on small molecule delivery. However, many of the technologies described can be applied to larger biomolecules. We are fortunate to have assembled leading experts in the fields of cancer medicine, experimental therapeutics, pharmacology, biomaterials and formulation design to provide a broad view of this exciting and fruitful field of cancer research.

I wish to thank all the contributors to this volume for their time and patience. I would also like to thank Beverly A. Teicher, the series editor, for her guidance, and Andrea Dorey for editorial assistance and Shawnya Michaels in the organization and development of this volume.

Dennis M. Brown

Contents

Contributors

NAMJIN BAEK, PhD • *Departments of Pharmaceutics and Biomedical Engineering, Purdue University, West Lafayette, IN*

MICHAEL BENTLEY, PhD • *Research and Development Department, Shearwater Polymers Inc., Huntsville, AL*

CHRISTOPHER C. BENZ, PhD • *Program of Cancer and Developmental Therapeutics, Buck Institute for Age Research, Novato, CA*

DUANE T. BIRNBAUM, PhD • *Biogel Technology Inc., Indianapolis, IN*

LISA BRANNON-PEPPAS, PhD • *Department of Biomedical Engineering, The University of Texas at Austin, TX*

HENRY BREM, MD • *Department of Neurosurgery and Oncology, Johns Hopkins University School of Medicine, Baltimore, MD*

STANLEY T. CROOKE, MD, PhD • *ISIS Pharmaceuticals Inc., Carlsbad, CA*

FRANCESCO DIMECO, MD • *Department of Neurosurgery, Istituto Nazionale Neurologico C. Besta, Milan, Italy*

DARYL C. DRUMMOND, PhD • *California Pacific Medical Center Research Institute, San Francisco, CA*

ARDITH W. EL-KAREH, PhD • *Arizona Research Laboratories, Microcirculation Division, University of Arizona, Tucson, AZ*

LYNNE W. ELMORE, PhD • *Department of Pathology, Medical College of Virginia at Virginia Commonwealth University, Richmond, VA*

REGINALD B. EWESUEDO, MD, MSC • *Department of Experimental Medicine, AstraZeneca, Wilmington, DE; Department of Pediatrics, Ohio State University, Columbus, OH*

WOLFGANG FRIESS, PhD • *Department of Pharmacy, Pharmaceutical Technology and Biopharmaceutics, Ludwig-Maximilian University, Munich, Germany*

SHAWN E. HOLT, PhD • *Department of Pathology, Department of Human Genetics, Department of Pharmacology and Toxicology, Massey Cancer Center, Medical College of Virginia at Virginia Commonwealth University, Richmond, VA*

KEELUNG HONG, PhD • *Hermes Biosciences Inc., San Francisco, CA*

STEPHEN B. HOWELL, MD • *University of California at San Diego, San Diego, CA*

SUNG-JOO HWANG, PhD • *Pharmaceutics and Biomedical Engineering, Purdue University, West Lafayette, IN*

DMITRI KIRPOTIN, PhD • *California Pacific Medical Center Research Institute, San Francisco, CA*

SANKARAM B. MANTRIPRAGADA, PhD • *SkyePharma Inc., San Diego, CA*

FRANCESCO M. MARINCOLA, MD • *Immunogenetics Laboratory, Department of Transfusion Medicine, Clinical Center, National Institutes of Health, Bethesda, MD*

MAURIE MARKMAN, MD • *The Cleveland Clinic Taussig Cancer Center; Department of Hematology/Medical Oncology, The Cleveland Clinic Foundation, Cleveland, OH*

ALESSANDRO OLIVI, MD • *Department of Neurosurgery, Johns Hopkins University School of Medicine, Baltimore, MD*

ELAINE K. ORENBERG, PhD • *Orenberg-Anderson Biopharmaceutical Consultants, Stanford, CA*

SUSANNE OSANTO, MD, PhD • *Department of Clinical Oncology, LUMC Leiden University Medical Center, Leiden, The Netherlands*

HAESUN PARK, PhD • *Pharmaceutics and Biomedical Engineering, Purdue University, West Lafayette, IN*

JOHN W. PARK, MD • *Division of Hematology/Oncology, Department of Medicine, University of California at San Francisco, San Francisco, CA*

KINAM PARK, PhD • *School of Pharmacy, Purdue University, West Lafayette, IN*

RICHARD PARKER, PhD • *Vanderbilt University Center for Lung Research, Nashville, TN*

MARK J. RATAIN, MD • *Department of Medicine, University of Chicago, IL*

TIMOTHY W. SECOMB, PhD • *Department of Physiology, University of Arizona, Tucson, AZ*

ROBERT G. L. SHORR, PhD • *United Therapeutics, Inc., Silver Spring, MD*

S. ESMAIL TABIBI, PhD • *Avicenna Pharmaceuticals, Rockville, MD*

JON D. WEINGART, MD • *Department of Neurosurgery, Johns Hopkins University School of Medicine, Baltimore, MD*

BRENDAN WHITTLE, PhD • *William Harvey Research Institute, St. Bartholomew's and Royal London School of Medicine, Charterhouse Square, London, UK*

SIMON ZHSAO, PhD • *Research and Development Department, Shearwater Polymers Inc., Huntsville, AL*

I

PHARMACOLOGICAL CONSIDERATIONS FOR DRUG DELIVERY SYSTEMS IN CANCER MEDICINE

1

Systemically Administered Drugs

Reginald B. Ewesuedo, MD, MSc
and Mark J. Ratain, MD

1. INTRODUCTION

Although the use of drugs in the management of cancer has made a significant impact on the outcome of most types of malignancies, one of the lingering challenges in cancer therapeutics is how to influence the outcome of cancer treatment by optimal and careful application of anticancer drugs. Addressing this challenge requires the adoption of treatment strategies that employ sound pharmacologic principles in the use of anticancer agents.

The majority of drugs used in cancer treatment are administered systemically, orally, or loco-regionally (Table 1). Of these, only loco-regional delivery presumes restriction of an administered drug to the site or location of the tumor. Thus, because the concentration of the antineoplastic agent at the tumor site is enhanced, systemic exposure is avoided or significantly minimized. Consequently, it is assumed that the therapeutic benefits as well as therapeutic window of the drug are improved upon. However, these assumptions are not always true because the loco-regional delivery of drugs could present unique and/or similar adverse events in comparison to systemically administered antineoplastics *(1–4)*.

Systemic delivery of cytotoxic anticancer drugs has and will continue to play a crucial role in cancer therapeutics, however, one of the major problems with this form of drug delivery is the exposure of normal tissues/organs to the administered drug. Clearly, any new strategy to enhance systemic delivery of anticancer drugs should be intended to ameliorate this problem.

2. RATIONALE AND TYPES OF SYSTEMIC DRUG DELIVERY

The systemic delivery of anticancer drugs provides a unique opportunity for the treatment of micrometastatic disease as well as assisting in local control of a malig-

From: *Drug Delivery Systems in Cancer Therapy*
Edited by: D. M. Brown © Humana Press Inc., Totowa, NJ

Table 1
Methods of Drug Delivery for Commonly Used Antineoplastics

Drugs	Mode of action	Potential uses	Route of drug delivery
Nitrogen mustards			
Cyclophosphamide	Crosslinking DNA	Leukemia, lymphoma, sarcomas, Ca breast, ovary, cervix and lung, multiple myeloma, retinoblastoma, mycosis fungoides	intravenous, oral
Ifosfamide	Crosslinking DNA	Germ cell testicular Ca, sarcomas, pediatric solid tumors resistant to cyclophosphamide, lymphoma	intravenous
Melphalan	Crosslinking DNA	Multiple myeloma, ovarian Ca, sarcomas, ALL, amyloidosis, lymphoma, breast Ca, neuroblastoma	intravenous
Chlorambucil	Crosslinking DNA	Chronic lymphocytic leukemia, Waldenstrom's macroglobulinemia, lymphoma, Ca of breast, testis, ovary, and choricarcinoma, nephrosis	oral
Mechlorethamine	Crosslinking DNA	Lymphoma, cutaneous histiocytosis	intravenous
Nitrosoureas			
Carmustine (BCNU)	Crosslinking DNA	Brain tumors lymphoma, melanoma, GI tumors	intravenous, loco-regional (intracranial)
Lomustine (CCNU)	Similar to CCNU	Melanoma, brain tumors, colon Ca, lymphoma	oral
Fotemustine	Crosslinking DNA	Brain tumors, lung Ca, melanoma	intravenous
Streptozocin	Inhibition of DNA synthesis by methylation of DNA	Carcinoid tumors, pancreatic islet cell Ca	intravenous
Ethyleneimine			
Thiotepa	Crosslinking DNA	Ca breast, ovary, brain tumors lymphoma, Ewing's sarcoma (?), leptomeningeal metastases	intravenous, loco-regional (intracavity)
Hexamethylamine	Crosslinking DNA	Ovarian carcinoma	intravenous
Alkane sulfonates			
Busulfan	Crosslinking DNA	Chronic myelogenous leukemia	oral, intravenous (investigational)
Treosulfan	Crosslinking DNA	Ovarian carcinoma	intravenous

4

Drug	Mechanism	Indications	Route
Tetrazine			
Temozolomide	Crosslinking DNA	Brain tumors, melanoma	oral
Dacarbazine	Multifactorial, but includes DNA alkylation	Melanoma, lymphoma, brain tumors, sarcomas	intravenous, oral
Procarbazine	Crosslinking DNA	Lymphoma, glioma, melanoma	oral
Mitomycin C	Alkylation of DNA	Anal squamous cell carcinoma, Ca of breast, prostate and lungq	intravenous
Platinum compounds			
Cisplatin	Inhibits DNA precursors	Most adult solid tumors and osteosarcoma, brain, tumors neuroblastoma in pediatrics	intravenous, loco-regional (intracavity)
Carboplatin	Similar to cisplatin	Similar to cisplatin	similar to cisplation
Pyrimidine analogs			
5-Fluorouracil	Inhibits DNA and RNA synthesis by: incorporation of active metabolites, 5-FUTP into RNA and inhibition of thymidylate synthase	Head/neck, colorectal, breast, pancreatic GI cancers liver,	intravenous
Capecitabine	similar to 5-FU after activation by tumor cells	Similar to 5-FU	oral
Gemcitabine	Inhibits DNA synthesis by: termination of DNA chain, elongation through competitive inhibition by GEM-TP and GEM-DP	Locally advanced and metastatic pancreatic cancer, head- and neckcancer, lymphoma	intravenous
Cytosine arabinoside	Inhibits DNA synthesis by direct inhibition of DNA polymerase	Leukemia, lymphoma	intravenous, intrathecal

5

(Continued)

Table 1 (*Continued*)

Drugs	Mode of action	Potential uses	Route of drug delivery
Purine analogs			
6-Mercaptopurine	Inhibits DNA synthesis by blockade of purine synthesis, through incorporation of 6-TGN into DNA and RNA templates	Leukemia	oral
6-thioguanine			oral
Fludarabine	Inhibits purine synthesis by inhibiting DNA polymerase and ribonucleotide reductase enzymes	Chronic leukemia	intravenous, oral
Pentostatin	Inhibits purine synthesis by inhibiting adenosine deaminase	Hairy cell leukemia	intravenous
Other antimetabolites			
Cladribine	Inhibition of DNA synthesis by formation of DNA breaks, NAD and ATP depletion	Hairy cell leukemia AML, CLL, lymphoma, Waldenstrom's macroglobinemia	intravenous
Hydroxyurea	Inhibits DNA synthesis and repair	CML, acute leukemia with hyperleukocytosis, sickle hemoglobinopathy, essential thrombocytosis, polycythemia vera	oral
Folate analogs			
Methotrexate	Inhibition of purine and thymidylate synthesis by inhibiting DHFR enzyme	Sarcomas, Ca of breast, head/neck, colon, ovarian bladder and lung, leukemia, lymphoma	intravenous, subcutaneous, oral intrathecal
Trimetrexate	Similar to methotrexate	Brainstem gliomas, neuroblastoma, renal cell Ca	oral
Anthracyclines			
Doxorubicin	Inhibition of DNA/RNA synthesis, by intercalating DANN	Breast Ca, sarcomas	intravenous
Daunorubicin	Inhibition of DNA synthesis	Acute leukemia, sarcomas, melanoma	intravenous
Epirubicin	Similar to doxorubicin	Breast cancer, bladder Ca	intravenous
Idarubicin	Same as daunorubicin	acute leukemia	intravenous
Mitoxantrone	Inhibition of DNA synthesis by topo II inhibition and intercalating DNA	Acute leukemia, lymphoma	intravenous

6

Drug	Mechanism	Indication	Route
Taxanes			
Taxol	Inhibits DNA synthesis by stabilizing microtubule assembly	Ca breast, ovary, cervix, prostate NSCLC, gastric carcinoma, lymphoma	intravenous
Taxotere	Similar to taxol	Sarcomas, head and neck Ca, ovarian, breast and pancreatic cancer	intravenous
Vinca alkaloids			
Vincristine	Inhibit DNA synthesis by blockade of tubulin assembly	Leukemia, lymphoma, brain tumors, Ca of Breast, lung, liver and multiple myeloma	intravenous
Vinblastine	Similar to vincristine	Prostate carcinoma	intravenous
Topoisomerase (topo) I inhibitors			
Irinotecan (CPT-11)	Inhibition of DNA synthesis by inhibiting topo I enzyme	5-FU refractory colorectal carcinoma	intravenous
Topotecan	Similar to irinotecan	Cisplatin refractory ovarian carcinoma	intravenous
Topoisomerase (topo) II inhibitors			
Etoposide (VP-16)	Inhibition of DNA synthesis by inhibiting topo II enzyme	Leukemia, lymphoma, Kaposi's sarcoma, cancer of lung, testis	intravenous, oral
Teniposide	Similar to etoposide	Refractory leukemia	intravenous
Other anticancer drugs			
Hormonal agents			
Tamoxifen	Inhibition of estradiol binding to estrogen receptor	Metastatic (estrogen) receptor positive breast cancer	oral
Anastrozole	aromatase inhibitor	Breast cancer	oral
Flutamide	inhibition of androgen binding to cytosolic DHT receptors	Metastaic prostate cancer	oral
Bicalutamide	similar to flutamide	Similar to flutamide	oral
Enzyme			
L-Asparaginase	depletion of L-asparagine in tumor cells	Leukemia	intramuscular
Bleomycin	single-strand scission of DNA	Germ cell tumors, Hodgkin's disease Non-Hodgkin's lymphoma	intravenous, intramuscular, subcutaneous, loco-regional (intra-cavity)

nancy. It is therefore imperative that strategies aimed at improving the efficacy of systemically delivered drugs are undertaken. In this regard, different strategies, including
modification in administration schedules and/or infusion regimens (bolus, intermittent,
or continuous infusion), are being used to administer antineoplastics. Several investigators have demonstrated that the efficacy of some anticancer drugs, including
antimetabolites and anthracyclines, are schedule-dependent (5). Also, some cytotoxics
are thought to be effective against tumor cells that are in a specific phase of the cell
cycle. Therefore it is conceivable that the type of infusion schedule used in the systemic delivery of anticancer drugs could play a significant role in determining optimal
efficacy. Of the commonly employed regimens for systemic drug delivery, continuous
infusion would appear to present the best opportunity for a tumor cell to be exposed to
an antineoplastic agent at a specific phase of the cell cycle. Carlson (5) reviewed some
of the factors that predicted superiority of continuous infusion chemotherapy over
other forms of systemic drug delivery. Nevertheless, it should be noted that some antineoplastics are cell cycle nonspecific in tumor cell kill; as a result, modifying infusion
schedules for anticancer drugs will not be a panacea for improving the efficacy of all
antineoplastics.

Furthermore, there are other factors that could also influence the dosing schedule of
a drug. One such factor is the systemic clearance of the drug. A drug that is slowly
eliminated from the body might not be required to be given as a continuous infusion
because there is the likelihood of therapeutic blood concentrations being maintained at
a tumor site over a longer period of time. In contrast, a drug with high systemic clearance will probably need to be administered either on a more frequent basis or as continuous infusion therapy in situations where desired pharmacodynamic effects require
prolonged exposure to the drug. Notwithstanding, high systemic clearance does not
preclude a drug from being administered as a once-a-day infusion over a short period
of time. It is obvious that irrespective of infusion schedules and the clearance of an
anticancer drug, in the majority of cases it is the intracellular concentration of an anticancer agent that determines antitumor effect. Interestingly, because there are clear evi-
dences linking drug administration modalities and pharmacokinetics to desired
pharmacodynamic endpoints, it is not clearly understood how the different forms of
systemic delivery of an anticancer drug affect intracellular drug concentration with
some classes of drugs (6–8).

Another consideration in designing strategies for the systemic delivery of drugs is
the mechanism of action of an anticancer agent. Most antineoplastic agents bring about
cell death by an interruption or aberration of cell kinetics through intermediate mechanisms. In a few instances, as with some alkylating agents, such mechanisms have been
demonstrated to be greatly enhanced by the presence or coadministration of other compounds or biochemical modulators (9). In situations like these, the schedule for the systemic delivery of an anticancer drug should be in relation to deriving optimal benefit
from the presence of the biochemical modulator(s). Although the various modalities of
drug delivery are intended to improve the efficacy of administered anticancer agents,
toxicities associated with individual drugs continue to be a problem in cancer therapeutics. This complication has remained the bane of cancer therapeutics and necessitates
the need for drug delivery strategies that will allow only selective drug delivery to a
tumor cell or target organ, or ensure maximum protection for normal tissues from the
administered antineoplastic agent. Such strategies will lead to improved efficacy by

increasing the therapeutic window of an anticancer agent while minimizing the chances of any systemic drug-related toxicity. These considerations have, so far, led to the use of novel drug formulations or delivery systems including controlled-release biodegradable polymers, polymeric microsphere carriers, or liposomes in the systemic delivery of anticancer drugs, as well as the coadministration of cytoprotective agent(s) with antineoplastics *(10–15)*. Some of these strategies have been shown to result in favorable outcomes. Presant et al. *(16)* observed minimal toxicity and significant anti-tumor activity when liposomal preparations of doxorubicin were used to treat patients with doxorubicin-resistant Kaposi's sarcoma. However, although some of these drug delivery strategies have been shown to result in favorable outcomes, more studies are needed; some of the vehicles for delivery of water-soluble drugs into cell cytoplasm have been demonstrated to be limited by a rapid uptake from circulation by the reticuloendothelial system *(17)*.

As our knowledge of cancer biology continues to expand, our understanding of the unique characteristics of individual tumor types should allow for systemic drug delivery techniques that will take advantage of this new knowledge. For example, the long scheduling of intravenous 5-fluorouracil in the treatment of cancer is usually done to optimize the effect of the drug in the presence of leucovorin. In this instance, leucovorin increases cellular levels of reduced folates, thereby increasing the stability of a ternary complex formed from the association of fluorodeoxyuridine monophosphate (FdUMP), thymidylate synthetase, and reduced folate *(18)*. Another scenario involves adopting a strategy to overcome drug resistance secondary to unique tumor characteristics. Thus, knowing that a significant expression of thymidylate synthase confers drug resistance in patients with gastric carcinoma *(19)* presents an opportunity for designing drug delivery strategies that utilize prodrugs that are activated only at the tumor site. This approach provides for selective exposure of the tumor to a high concentration of the antineoplastic agent. In this regard, capecitabine, an oral analog of 5-fluorouracil, which is activated within the tumor, has been used to increase efficacy and decrease systemic toxicity owing to the drug *(20)*. Alternatively, compounds that are known to modulate repair proteins unique to, or overexpressed by, a particular tumor are being coadministered with systemically delivered anticancer agent as a way to increase efficacy *(21,22)*.

Though resistance by tumor cells to anticancer drugs is through various mechanisms *(23)*, there are data to suggest that the concentration of a drug at the tumor site plays a significant role in tumor cell kill *(24)*. Therefore, for systemically delivered antineoplastics to be more efficacious, ways of increasing the therapeutic window must be explored. Such strategies currently include the use of high doses of drug in combination with supportive measures such as the use of colony-stimulating factors, hematopoietic transplantation to ameliorate the toxicity of a drug, and coadministration of compounds that protect normal tissues from the anticancer agent(s). However, because the practice of combining systemic high-dose chemotherapy with hematopoietic transplantation has been used for selected chemosensitive tumors to improve the efficacy of cytotoxic drugs, this approach, though successful in some types of malignancies, has not proven to be useful in some types of cancer such as glioblastoma multiforme *(25)*.

Another consideration for the systemic delivery of anticancer drugs is related to the location of a tumor. In situations where a tumor is inaccessible for surgery or locoregional therapy, any chance of effective therapy can only be realized by either parenteral or oral delivery of anticancer drug(s). Because anticancer agents delivered

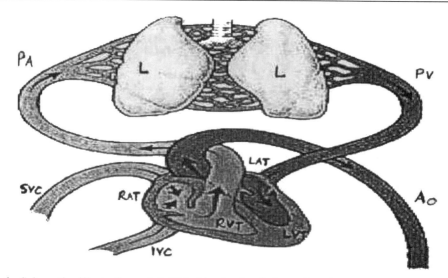

Fig. 1. Schematic illustration of initial (drug) circulation after intravenous Administration. (IVC/SVC *(infusion)* → RAT → RVT → PA → L *(pulmonary circulation)* → PV → LAT → LVT → AO *("Systemic exposure/distribution")*. AO: aorta; IVC: inferior vena cava; SVC: superior vena cava; L: lung; LAT: left atrium; LVT: left ventricle; PA: pulmonary artery; PV: pulmonary vein; RAT: right atrium; RVT: right ventricle.

systemically are not subject to an initial hepatic first-pass metabolism, the use of this form of drug delivery in the foregoing cases potentially ensures the delivery of a significant amount of drug to the tumor site. The flipside of this phenomenon, however, is that normal tissues/organs are also likely to be exposed to the same high drug concentrations as the tumor mass. This exposure will account significantly for the disparity in observed adverse effects between the different drug delivery modalities.

Notwithstanding, it should be noted, as illustrated in Fig. 1, that with the probable exclusion of lung tumors, a drug delivered systemically would have to circulate through the pulmonary system before being distributed to the tumor site. It is worth noting that the lungs also have been shown to function as a metabolic organ *(26,27)*. The implication, therefore, is that systemically delivered drugs could potentially be subject to significant metabolism in this organ system.

The efficacy of systemically delivered drugs relies also on factors such as the physicochemical properties of the drug, the characteristics of a biological membrane, and the perfusion of the tumor bed/locale. For example, using the systemic route for drug delivery of therapy for malignant brain tumors implies that the efficacy of the administered drug will be determined to a large degree by the extent of passive diffusion of the drug through an interface, namely the blood–brain barrier (BBB). However, many systemically delivered chemotherapeutic agents are precluded from penetrating the BBB because they are large, water soluble, charged, or excessively protein-bound. To address the problem of drug diffusion across the BBB, it is clear that "membrane modifiers" will have to be considered where appropriate. An illustration of this strategy is the use of compounds that disrupt the BBB by osmosis (e.g., mannitol [28,29]) or that selectively increase permeability of the BBB (e.g., bradykinin analog, RMP7 [30]). When used in combination with systemically delivered chemotherapeutic agents for treatment of brain tumors, these compounds have proven very useful. It should be noted also that although the use of hyperosmotic solutions usually resulted in exposure of normal brain tissue to the administered drug(s), RMP7 delivery was significantly tumor-specific while sparing normal brain tissue.

3. ADVANTAGES AND DISADVANTAGES

3.1. Advantages

Systemic delivery of antineoplastics presents unique advantages. In cases of advanced or disseminated cancer, this form of drug delivery provides an opportunity to ensure optimal exposure of tumor masses to administered anticancer agent(s). The systemic delivery of anticancer drugs is therefore an assured way of effectively treating micrometastatic disease as well as assisting in local control of a malignancy. Thus, this form of delivery of antineoplastic agents will continue to be a major and important route for drug administration in cancer treatment.

Although the oral route of drug delivery should potentially assure systemic exposure to an antineoplastic, this form of drug delivery is often compromised by problems such as hepatic first-pass metabolism and the need for proper formulation of the drug *(31)*. Most anticancer drugs are not usually administered orally because of the lack of suitable oral formulations. In addition, oral drug delivery presents such problems as the following: lack of bioequivalence of oral formulations, low patient compliance, poor drug absorption, variability in achievable plasma/tissue concentrations owing to inter- and intraindividual differences in drug absorption and disposition, and drug–drug interactions because most cancer patients are also using other medications. On the contrary, systemic delivery of anticancer drugs obviates some of these problems, thereby, providing an opportunity for optimizing the therapeutic benefits of anticancer agents.

Another recognized advantage of systemic delivery of anticancer drugs is the ease with which it can be done in an outpatient setting, and with minimal expertise required. Also, schedule variations can be carried out as required. In contrast, loco-regional drug delivery involves highly technical procedures that cannot be routinely done in outpatient settings, frequently requiring the use of sophisticated materials (e.g., microspheres, programmable infusion pumps), and patients cannot be exposed to this therapy frequently.

3.2. Disadvantages

Given the fact that drugs delivered systemically also interact with normal tissue, systemic toxicity from these agents continues to be the major problem plaguing this form of drug delivery. Undisputedly, minimizing toxicity will greatly impact the overall outcome of chemotherapeutic management of cancer. Toxicity is usually generalized or organ-specific. Although loco-regional therapy is designed to minimize systemic toxicity of cancer drugs, this has not been found to be universal *(32)*.

Nevertheless, there are studies examining ways of alleviating this problem, including strategies for minimizing toxicity of systemically delivered drugs by the use of systemic neutralizing agents. One example is the systemic administration of leucovorin to permit prolonged exposure of tumor tissues to methotrexate, given the cell cycle phase-specificity of the drug. Other investigators are studying the use of gene therapy to manipulate stem cells to be resistant to known pharmacodynamic endpoints of a drug *(33)*, and others have used cytoprotective agents to minimize the adverse effects of anticancer agents *(18,19)*. In contrast, loco-regional or tumor-specific drug delivery usually results in minimal toxicity. Thus, this form of drug delivery provides a unique opportunity to increase the therapeutic window of an antineoplastic and does not require the use of supportive measures such as hematopoietic transplantation or hematopoietic growth factors. Compared to oral means of drug delivery, systemic delivery is invasive, and often requires the use of a secured catheter in a major blood vessel. Another disadvantage of systemic delivery of anticancer drugs is the cost in comparison with that of the oral route of delivery. This could be significant in situations where effective oral cytotoxics are available.

4. COMPLICATIONS AND TREATMENT
4.1. Local

Because systemic delivery of drugs requires the use of veins, either peripheral or central, this method of therapy can expose a patient to local complications. Phlebitis is a common local complication that results from the use of peripheral veins for systemic drug delivery. It does not usually result in a severe complication. Most of the dangers in the administration of systemic therapy arise as a result of extravasation of a drug leading to vesicant/tissue damage at the local site. Common examples are vinca alkaloids and anthracyclines. In the case of the vinca alkaloids, treatment involves the immediate application of heat to the affected area, several times a day for 3–5 d, and injection of hyaluronidase solution subcutaneously through six clockwise injections into the infiltrated area. For the anthracyclines, management includes application of ice immediately to the affected area for up to 60 min, then every 15 min for a day, and elevation of the extremity for up to 48 h. If symptoms or signs of extravasation persist for greater than 48 h, the patient is usually seen by a surgeon for possible debridement surgery. Clearly, in the systemic delivery of anticancer drugs, careful consideration is required in ensuring that a drug is infused directly into a vein to avoid any local complication(s).

4.2. Systemic

Systemic complications arising from this form of drug delivery are usually secondary to hypersensitivity reactions, coagulopathy, and organ damage—especially pulmonary damage. Management of such cases usually depends on the drug(s) in question. For drugs that are well-characterized in clinical studies to result in systemic complications, preventive measures are usually instituted before, during, and after infusions of such compounds. However, some of the adverse events may be anaphylactoid in nature and this renders it usually difficult to predict which patients will manifest any untoward reactions. For the prevention of hypersensitivity reactions because of the delivery vehicle used in the formulation of the anticancer drug (e.g., Cremophor® EL in 50% ethanol, for paclitaxel formulation), premedications consisting of corticosteroids and histamine blockers have been found to be useful.

5. CONCLUSION

Systemic delivery of anticancer drugs is highly desirable in cancer therapeutics. However, because this mode of delivery of anticancer drugs continues to be a major way to administer these agents, it is now more important than ever before, for implementation of strategies to improve this form of drug delivery. To do so would require strategies that channel systemically administered antineoplastics to tumor sites only, thereby minimizing the toxicity of cancer agents to normal tissues, or the use of supportive measures including growth factors or hematopoietic stem cell transplantation to ameliorate toxicities. In addition, drug administration schedules could be formulated to potentially target molecular characteristics of a specific tumor.

It is clear that, apart from the presence of a drug at the tumor site, factors unique to a tumor might dictate the degree of activity of an antineoplastic agent. This is particularly true if a drug has to be converted by enzymes significantly expressed by the tumor type in question. Such a situation is well characterized by the use of 5-florouracil analogs, where intratumoral biotransformation of a prodrug, and not the route of administration, determines the extent of tumor cell kill.

Finally, it is obvious that, while systemic toxicity continues to be a major problem with systemically delivered drugs, other modalities for antineoplastic delivery have not been clearly demonstrated to be significantly devoid of fewer undesirable events. Future strategies aimed at developing more selective agents are needed to decrease the need for regional delivery of anticancer agents.

REFERENCES

1. Glass LF, Jaroszeski M, Gilbert R, Reintgen DS, Heller R. Intralesional bleomycin-mediated electrochemotherapy in 20 patients with basal cell carcinoma. *J Am Acad Dermatol* 1997; 37:596–599.
2. Gagliano RG, Costanzi II. Paraplegia following intrathecal methotrexate. Report of a case and review of the literature. *Cancer* 1976; 37:1663–1668.
3. Siegal T, Melamed E, Sandbank U, Cantane R. Early and delayed neurotoxicity of mitoxantrone and doxorubicin following subarachnoid injection. *J Neurooncol* 1988; 6:135–140.
4. Didolkar MS, Jackson AJ, Lesko LJ, et al. Pharmacokinetics of dacarbazine in the regional perfusion of extremities with melanoma. *J Surg Oncol* 1996; 63:148–158.
5. Carlson RW. Continuous intravenous infusion chemotherapy, in *The Chemotherapy Source Book* (Perry MC, ed). Williams & Wilkins, Baltimore, MD, 1996, pp 225–251.
6. Derendorf H, Hochhaus G, Meibohm E, Mollmann H, Earth J. Pharmacokinetics and pharmacodynamics of inhaled corticosteroids. *J Allergy Clin Immunol* 1998; 101(4 Pt. 2):8440–8446.
7. Suri A, Estes KS, Geisslinger G, Derendorf H. Pharmacokinetic-pharmacodynamic relationships for analgesics. *Int J Clin Pharmacol Ther* 1997; 35(8):307–323.
8. Muller M, Rohde B, Kovar A, Georgopoulos A, Eichler HG, Derendorf H. Relationship between serum and free interstitial concentrations of cefodizime and cefpirome in muscle and subcutaneous adipose tissue of healthy volunteers measured by microdialysis. *J Clin Pharmacol* 1997; 37(12):1108–1113.
9. Dolan ME, Mitchell RB, Mummert C, Moschel RC, Pegg AB. Effect of 06-benzylguanine analogues on sensitivity of human tumor cells to the cytotoxic effects of alkylating agents. *Cancer Res* 1991; 51:3367–3372.
10. Kumanohoso T, Natsugoe S, Shimada M, Aikou T. Enhancement of therapeutic efficacy of bleomycin by incorporation into biodegradable poly-d,I-lactic acid. *Cancer Chemother Pharmacol* 1997; 40:112–116.
11. Sipos EP, Tyler B, Piantadosi S, Burger PC, Brem H. Optimizing interstitial delivery of BCNU from controlled release polymers for the treatment of brain tumors. *Cancer Chemother Pharmacol* 1997; 39:383–389.
12. Sharma D, Chelvi TP, Kaur J, et al. Novel Taxol formulation: polyvinylpyrrolidone nanoparticle-encapsulated Taxol for drug delivery in cancer therapy. *Oncology Res* 1996; 8(8–9):281–286.
13. Chonn A, Cullis PR. Recent advances in liposomal drug-delivery systems. Curr. opinion in *Biotechnology* 1995; 6(6):698–708.
14. Schiller JH, Storer B, Berlin J, et al. Amifostine, Cisplatin, and Vinblastine in metastatic non-small-cell lung cancer: a report of high response rates and prolonged survival. *J Clin Oncol* 1996; 14:1913–1921.
15. Kemp G, Rose P, Lurain I, et al. Amifostine pretreatment for protection against cyclophosphamide-induced and cisplatin-induced toxicities: results of a randomized control trial in patients with advanced ovarian cancer. *J Clin Oncol* 1996; 14:2101–2112.

16. Presant CA, Scolaro M, Kennedy P, et al. Liposomal daunorubicin treatment of mv-associated Kaposi's sarcoma. *Lancet* 1993; 341:1242–1243.
17. Slepushkin VA, Simoes S, Dazin P, et al. Sterically stabilized pH-sensitive liposomes. Intracellular delivery of aqueous contents and prolonged circulation in vivo. *J Biological Chem* 1997; 272(4):2382–2388.
18. Mini E, Trave F, Rustum YM, Bertino JR. Enhancement of the antitumor effects of 5-fluorouracil by folinic acid. *Pharmacol Ther* 1990; 47:1–19.
19. Yeh K-H, Shun C-T, Chen C-L, et al. High expression of thymidylate synthase is associated with the drug resistance of gastric carcinoma to high dose 5-fluorouracil-based systemic chemotherapy. *Cancer* 1998; 82:1626–31.
20. Belanich M, Pastor M, Randall T, et al. Retrospective study of the correlation between the DNA repair protein alkyltransferase and survival of brain tumor patients treated with carmustine. *Cancer Res* 1996; 56:783–788.
21. Bajetta E, Camaghi C, Somma L, Stampino CG. A pilot safety study of capecitabine, a new oral fluoropyrimidine, in patients with advanced neoplastic disease. *Tumori* 1996; 82:450–452.
22. Dolan ME, Pegg AB. 06-benzylguanine and its role in chemotherapy. *Clin Cancer Res* 1997; 3:837–847.
23. Goldie JH, Coldman AJ. The genetic origin of drug resistance in neoplasms: implications for systemic therapy. *Cancer Res* 1984; 44:3643–3653.
24. Frei E III, Canellos G. Dose: a critical factor in cancer chemotherapy. *Am J Med* 1980; 69:585–594.
25. Pech IV, Peterson K, Cairncross JG. Chemotherapy for brain tumors. *Oncology* 1998; 12(4):537–547.
26. Foth H. Role of the lung in accumulation and metabolism of xenobiotic compounds—implication for chemically induced toxicity. *Crit Rev Toxicol* 1995; 25(2):165–205.
27. Bakhle YS. Pharmacokinetic and metabolic properties of lung. *Br J Anaesth* 1990; 65:79–93.
28. Millay RH, Klein ML, Shults WT, Dahlborg SA, Neuwelt EA. Maculopathy associated with combination chemotherapy and osmotic opening of the blood-brain barrier. *Am J Ophthalmol* 1986; 102:626–632.
29. Neuwelt EA, Hill SA, Frenkel EP. Osmotic blood-brain barrier modification and combination chemotherapy: concurrent tumor regression in areas of barrier opening and progression in brain regions distant to barrier opening. *Neurosurgery* 1984; 15:362–366.
30. Inamura T, Nomura T, Bartus RT, Black KL. Intracarotid infusion of RMP-7, a bradykinin analog: a method for selective drug delivery to brain tumors. *J Neurosurg* 1994; 81:752–758.
31. DeMario MD, Ratain MI. Oral chemotherapy: rationale and future directions. *J Clin Oncol* 1998; 16(7):2557–2567.
32. Shapiro WR, Green SB, Burger PC, et al. A randomized comparison of intra-arterial versus intravenous BCNU, with or without intravenous 5-fluorouracil, for newly diagnosed patients with malignant glioma. *J Neurosurg* 1992; 76:772–781.
33. Wu MB, Liebowitz DN, Mikolajezak, KE, Lin AM, Dolan ME. Sensitivity of mutant 06-alkylguanine-DNA alkyltransferases (AGT) to 06-Benzylguanine (BG) and 06-Benzyl-8-oxoguanine (8-oxoBG). *Proc Am Assoc Ca Res* 1998; 39:517.

2 Regional Administration of Antineoplastic Drugs

Maurie Markman, MD

1. INTRODUCTION

Regional antineoplastic drug delivery is not a new concept. Following the initial recognition that cytotoxic alkylating agents could cause shrinkage of tumor masses and a reduction in the quantity of malignant ascites in patients with advanced ovarian cancer, investigators in the 1950s instilled the drugs directly into the peritoneal cavity in an effort to treat the malignancy *(1)*.

Similarly, intrathecal administration of methotrexate in the treatment and prevention of meningeal leukemia *(2)*, intravesical treatment of superficial bladder cancer *(3)*, and direct administration of drugs into blood vessels feeding a localized cancer *(4)*, have been evaluated for more than a decade as therapeutic strategies in the management of malignant disease.

In this chapter, the basic pharmacokinetic rationale supporting regional antineoplastic drug delivery will be presented, followed by a discussion of theoretical concerns and practical issues associated with this treatment approach. The chapter will conclude with several examples of regional antineoplastic therapy which have been accepted as "standard of care" in the management of certain clinical settings, and other more experimental strategies employing the regional route of drug delivery.

2. PHARMACOKINETIC RATIONALE

The basic aim of regional antineoplastic drug delivery is to deliver a higher concentration of the agent to the tumor present within a particular region of the body, and to

From: *Drug Delivery Systems in Cancer Therapy*
Edited by: D. M. Brown © Humana Press Inc., Totowa, NJ

Table 1
Rationale for Regional Antineoplastic Drug Delivery

1. Higher peak levels of drug in contact with tumor in the region of the body infused/perfused (when compared with systemic compartment).
2. Prolong exposure of tumor present within the region to antineoplastic drugs (particularly relevant for cycle-specific cytotoxic agents).
3. Reduction in systemic toxicity.
4. Improve opportunity to observe clinically relevant concentration-dependent synergy between antineoplastic agents.

expose the tumor to the active drug for longer periods of time than are safely possible with systemic administration (5–9). A favorable pharmacokinetic advantage for exposure of the body compartment (e.g., peritoneal cavity, liver, bladder) compared to that of the systemic compartment can be measured by increases in the peak concentration of drug, a greater AUC (area-under-the-concentration-versus-time curve), or both (Table 1).

The entire pharmacokinetic advantage associated with regional drug delivery occurs during the first pass of the agent through the area perfused or infused. Even if the drug subsequently reaches the tumor through the normal capillary flow into the area, there will be no additional pharmacokinetic benefit associated with this delivery compared to what would have been achieved following systemic administration of the agent.

2.1. Mathematical Model Describing Regional Antineoplastic Drug Delivery

It is possible to define the pharmacokinetic advantage resulting from regional drug delivery by comparing the amount of the agent gaining entry into the region following this method of administration to that achieved with systemic (generally intravenous) treatment (Table 2, Equation 1). A similar calculation can be derived for the relative reduction in systemic exposure associated with regional drug delivery by comparing the concentration of drug found in the systemic compartment after regional and systemic treatments (Table 2, Equation 2).

Combining these two calculations provides an estimate of the overall relative pharmacokinetic advantage resulting from the regional treatment strategy (Table 2, Equation 3).

2.2. Clinical Implications of the Model

Careful examination of Equation 3 (Table 2) leads to several important conclusions relevant to the clinical use of regional antineoplastic drug delivery (Table 3).

The relative pharmacokinetic advantage associated with regional drug administration will be enhanced by measures which either reduce the clearance of the agent from the region and/or increase the clearance from the systemic compartment. Examples of measures which have been employed in the clinical setting to enhance the pharmacokinetic advantage of regional drug delivery are briefly outlined in Table 3.

Analysis of the model leads to several additional implications. First, antineoplastic agents that are not able to be cleared rapidly from the systemic circulation following perfusion/infusion through a region (by first-pass metabolism or artificial removal) will be associated with a relatively less favorable pharmacokinetic advantage, compared to drugs that exhibit this characteristic. However, even in this circumstance there may be

Table 2
Pharmacokinetic Advantage Associated with Regional Antineoplastic Drug Delivery

Equation 1: *Relative increase in exposure to infused/perfused region:*

$$R_{local} = C_{local}(\text{regional})/C_{local}(IV)$$

Equation 2: *Relative decrease in exposure to systemic compartment:*

$$R_{systemic} = C_{systemic}(\text{regional})/C_{systemic}(IV)$$

Equation 3: *Overall pharmacokinetic advantage associated with regional drug delivery:*

$$R = \frac{R_{local}}{R_{systemic}} = \frac{C_{local}(\text{regional})/C_{local}(IV)}{C_{systemic}(\text{regional})/C_{systemic}(IV)}$$

Code: R_{local} = relative increased exposure to infused/perfused region; $R_{systemic}$ = relative decreased exposure to systemic compartment; C_{local}(regional) = local concentration following regional drug delivery; C_{local}(IV) = local concentration following systemic drug delivery; $C_{systemic}$(regional) = systemic concentration following local drug delivery; $C_{systemic}$(IV) = systemic concentration following systemic drug delivery; R = overall pharmacokinetic advantage associated with regional drug delivery.

Table 3
Opportunities to Improve the Pharmacokinetic Advantage Observed
with Regional Antineoplastic Drug Delivery

1. Removal of agent during <u>first pass</u> through perfused organ (e.g., hepatic artery infusion therapy for colon cancer metastatic to the liver).
2. Removal of agent after perfusion through the treated organ, but prior to entry into the systemic circulation (e.g., isolation-perfusion techniques for treating extremity melanomas).
3. Systemic administration of an antagonist for a cytotoxic agent delivered regionally, with the aim to neutralize the drug prior to the production systemic side effects (e.g., intravenous leucovorin following intrathecal methotrexate in the treatment of meningeal leukemia).
4. Use of materials to decrease rate of blood flow through the perfused organ and enhance drug removal (e.g., starch microspheres during hepatic artery infusion).

a valuable contribution associated with regional drug delivery, depending upon other clinical conditions, for example, inherently slow blood flow through a region or highly active cytotoxic drug in the tumor type being treated.

Second, whether the pharmacokinetic advantage associated with regional drug administration of a particular drug is great (e.g., > 100-fold), or relatively minor (e.g., 10-fold), will be only one factor in determining whether a regional treatment strategy is a reasonable therapeutic option in a particular clinical setting.

An important consideration is the actual antineoplastic effectiveness of the agent against the tumor type in question. The regional administration of a drug with a >1000-fold pharmacokinetic advantage (either in peak concentrations or AUC) will not convert a totally inactive drug against a particular tumor type into a useful therapeutic agent.

However, the modest or major increases in tumor–drug interactions possible with regional drug administration have the theoretical potential to result in enhanced cytotoxicity for agents whose activity is known to be *concentration-dependent* or *cycle-specific (10,11)*. In certain clinical circumstances, regional drug delivery can increase both peak levels and duration of exposure far beyond what can be safely accomplished with systemic administration *(8)*. Clinically relevant examples include: the intraperitoneal delivery of cisplatin in patients with ovarian cancer, which achieves a 20-fold increased exposure to the peritoneal cavity when compared with the systemic compartment *(12,13)*, and hepatic artery infusion of floxuridine (FUDR®), which results in 15-fold higher tumor drug levels when compared to those levels resulting from portal vein infusion of the drug *(14)*.

Because significant limitations of preclinical models in predicting activity of antineoplastic drugs in patients are well recognized, data demonstrating the relative importance of concentration and duration of exposure in model systems can be helpful in selecting drug(s) for inclusion in human trials of regional antineoplastic therapy *(15)*. For example, if an in vitro model demonstrates that administering concentrations of drug "A" at levels 100 times higher than are achievable with systemic delivery will *not* produce a significantly greater degree of tumor cell kill, and the regional pharmacokinetic advantage associated with this drug is only 10–50-fold, drug "A" would not be an attractive candidate for this method of delivery.

Conversely, if the cytotoxic potential of drug "B" is demonstrated to be highly concentration-dependent and the levels producing major tumor cell kill can only be achieved (at least in theory) at concentrations attainable following regional delivery (e.g., hepatic arterial infusion for colon cancer metastatic to the liver), drug "B" might be an ideal agent to consider for regional antineoplastic therapy.

3. THEORETICAL CONCERNS WITH REGIONAL ANTINEOPLASTIC DRUG THERAPY

Despite the attraction of regional antineoplastic drug delivery in the management of cancers principally confined to a particular location in the body, there are a number of theoretical objections raised regarding this therapeutic concept.

First, even if one accepts the hypothesis that higher tumor–drug interactions (higher peak levels and AUC) associated with regional therapy will result in enhanced cytotoxicity, there is legitimate concern that the delivery of a drug to cancer cells not directly in contact with the perfused/infused area will not be beneficial. Furthermore, for regional treatments not employing the vascular compartment (e.g., intraperitoneal, intrapleural, intrathecal drug delivery), it might be argued that delivery of drug to tumor by capillary flow will be reduced, resulting in negative impact on therapeutic efficacy. Consideration of this issue leads to the conclusion that it is critically important to measure drug levels in the systemic compartment following regional delivery. If insufficient concentrations of drug are found in the systemic circulation following regional drug administration, it may be necessary to treat patients both regionally and intravenously to achieve optimal therapeutic results.

Second, it is well-recognized that despite the high concentrations achievable at the surface of tumor(s) following regional drug delivery, the actual depth of penetration of these agents directly into tumor tissue is quite limited *(16–21)*.

Thus, the increase in tissue concentrations of drug following regional drug delivery, when compared to standard systemic treatment, is quite modest, despite the often extremely dramatic increases in drug concentration measurable in the plasma or the body cavity containing the tumor. This concern is particularly relevant for regional approaches not employing the vascular compartment, which rely exclusively on direct uptake of drug from the body cavity for any therapeutic advantage associated with regional delivery.

This important issue leads to the logical conclusion that regional therapy will have its greatest theoretical potential for exhibiting an improved clinical outcome in patients with smaller tumor nodules or only microscopic disease in the perfused/infused body compartment. In these patients, the largest possible tumor volume will be exposed to the higher cytotoxic drug concentrations achievable with regional drug administration. Data generated evaluating the role of intraperitoneal therapy in the management of ovarian cancer strongly support this conclusion (22).

A third theoretical concern with regional delivery relates to unique considerations of the specific strategy in question. For example, it has been shown that when a drug is infused into a rapidly flowing blood vessel, the drug does not completely mix in the plasma (the so-called "streaming effect"), resulting in nonuniform drug distribution to the perfused tissue (23,24). The clinical impact of this laboratory observation is uncertain, but the potential exists that portions of the tumor within the organ will be exposed to significantly lower concentrations of drug than are necessary to achieve the desired optimal cytotoxic effect.

A second example is that of the potential for inadequate distribution of an antineoplastic agent instilled into a body cavity (e.g., peritoneum, pleura) (25–27). As blood flow through the region is not employed to deliver drug to the tumor, there is concern that regions of the body compartment will not be exposed to the necessary high concentrations of cytotoxic agent. This may be due to interference with uniform distribution by the presence of normal organs (e.g., bowel), tumor(s), or adhesions.

4. PRACTICAL CONSIDERATIONS ASSOCIATED WITH REGIONAL ANTINEOPLASTIC DRUG THERAPY

A number of practical issues must be considered when designing an experimental regional antineoplastic strategy or when employing a standard regional treatment approach in the clinical management of malignant disease (Table 4).

The establishment of safe, convenient, and cost-effective techniques for the administration of regional antineoplastic therapy is an important issue in the development of these strategies for routine clinical use.

For example, while a peritoneal dialysis catheter can be inserted at the time of each ip treatment, this method of delivery will significantly restrict the application of the regional approach. Only a limited number of physicians will feel comfortable with placing such catheters in patients who have previously undergone one or more laparotomies and who do not have ascites. In addition, time and resources required for this drug delivery technique can be considerable. Finally, even if employed by well-trained physicians, there is a finite risk that catheter insertion performed without direct visualization of the peritoneal cavity will lead to bowel puncture and associated complications (28,29).

The time, effort, and complications associated with achieving access to the arteries can pose greater concerns (30,31). For patients being considered for more than one or two courses of intraarterial therapy, the surgical placement of semipermanent delivery systems would appear to be the optimal method of regional drug delivery (31–33). This situation would also be relevant for patients scheduled to receive weekly or more fre-

Table 4
Practical Considerations in Regional Antineoplastic Drug Delivery

1. Development of a safe, convenient, and cost-effective delivery system (e.g., intraarterial and ip infusion devices).
2. Unique complications associated with regional drug delivery (e.g., peritonitis associated with ip drug administration).
3. Complications associated with drug delivery systems (e.g., infection, bowel perforation, laceration of blood vessel).
4. Requirement to demonstrate improved therapeutic efficacy associated with regional drug delivery (randomized Phase III trials).

quent intrathecal drug administration for the prevention or treatment of meningeal leukemia (34,35).

Considerable caution is advised regarding the potential for unique toxicities associated with regional antineoplastic drug administration. The toxicity profile of an antineoplastic agent may be well-established when the drug is administered systemically at standard dose levels. However, the side effects associated with the extremely high concentrations achievable following regional delivery, or the toxicity to tissues that would normally not come into direct contact with the drug after iv infusion, potentially may be excessive.

For example, the direct hepatic artery administration of FUDR can be associated with the development of sclerosing cholangitis or biliary cirrhosis (36,37); ip delivery of a number of cytotoxic agents, including doxorubicin or mitoxantrone, can lead to severe peritonitis, extensive adhesion formation, and subsequent bowel obstruction (8,38,39).

A number of proposed regional antineoplastic drug delivery methods require extensive surgery (e.g., isolation-perfusion of mesenteric arterial vessels, hyperthermic intraperitoneal chemotherapy), or are associated with considerable risk for the development of serious morbidity or death (40–42). Such strategies will require extensive evaluation and favorable results achieved in well-designed randomized trials before they can leave their current realm of highly experimental treatment programs and be considered reasonable therapeutic regimens in standard clinical practice.

Even regional antineoplastic drug delivery programs which do not require such intensity of treatment or are not associated with excessive toxicity will require the performance of randomized trials to be certain that the theoretical advantages of these novel therapeutic strategies can be translated into clinical benefit for individuals with malignant disease.

5. CLINICAL EXAMPLES OF REGIONAL ANTINEOPLASTIC DRUG DELIVERY

5.1. Intrathecal Therapy for the Prevention and Treatment of Meningeal Leukemia

One of the most established regional antineoplastic drug delivery approaches is that employed to either prevent or treat established leukemia in the central nervous system (2,43–45). In certain specific clinical settings, the risk for the development of meningeal involvement with leukemia has been demonstrated to be substantially reduced with prophylactic intrathecal or intraventricular treatment. Established meningeal leukemia (documented by cerebral spinal fluid cytology) can also be effectively treated in many patients with several established regional antineoplastic drug regimens.

5.2. Intraperitoneal Therapy in the Management of Ovarian Cancer

The ip administration of antineoplastic agents in the management of ovarian cancer has been extensively examined in Phase I toxicity and pharmacology studies and Phase II efficacy trials involving a number of drugs with demonstrated activity in ovarian cancer, for example, cisplatin, carboplatin, paclitaxel, and/or doxorubicin (8,22,46).

More recently, the therapeutic potential of this method of drug delivery has been examined in the randomized Phase III trial setting (47,48). In a study involving newly diagnosed patients with small-volume, residual advanced ovarian cancer following surgical cytoreduction, the ip administration of cisplatin (in combination with iv cyclophosphamide) resulted in an improvement in overall survival, when compared with a control regimen of iv cisplatin administered with iv cyclophosphamide (47).

A recently reported randomized trial comparing iv cisplatin and paclitaxel with a regimen of iv paclitaxel and ip cisplatin has reached similar conclusions (48). This trial, also involving newly diagnosed advanced ovarian cancer patients with small volume residual disease, demonstrated a statistically significant improvement in progression-free survival and borderline improvement in overall survival associated with the regional treatment program. It should be noted that this study employed two courses of moderately dose-intensive iv carboplatin (AUC 9) prior to the administration of the regional program, designed to chemically debulk any residual tumor before the use of the regional drug delivery strategy.

5.3. Intrahepatic Arterial Therapy for Colon Cancer Metastatic to the Liver

Phase III trials have demonstrated a higher objective response rate associated with the direct intrahepatic arterial administration of FUDR, when compared to systemic delivery of the agent in the treatment of colon cancer metastatic to the liver (49–55). Several of these studies have been criticized because a crossover design was employed, whereby the patients randomized to iv drug delivery were permitted to receive intraarterial therapy at the time of disease progression. The impact of such crossover on the ultimate outcome has been debated extensively in the medical literature.

There have also been questions raised regarding the overall benefits of this strategy, in view of the morbidity and costs of the regional treatment approach. However, data available though the conduct of these trials support the clinical utility of this therapeutic strategy in carefully selected individuals with colon cancer metastatic to the liver. These clinical characteristics include adequate patient performance status, absence of serious comorbid medical conditions that might increase potential morbidity of the treatment regimen, and the presence of metastatic disease localized in the liver only.

5.4. Intravesical Therapy of Localized Bladder Cancer

The intravesical administration of both cytotoxic (e.g., mitomycin, thiotepa, doxorubicin) and biological (e.g., bacille Calmette-Guérin [BCG]) agents has been demonstrated to be effective treatment of superficial bladder cancer and carcinoma *in situ* in the bladder (56,57).

The ease of administering high concentrations of antineoplastic drugs directly into the bladder, and the simplicity of measuring the effects of treatment through the performance of urinary cytology and/or bladder wall biopsy, makes the bladder an ideal organ to employ regional therapy.

Intravesical antineoplastic therapy has been shown to prevent the progression from superficial to invasive cancer and to reduce the requirement for more radical surgical interventions, including the performance of a cystectomy.

6. CONCLUSION

Over the past decade, the regional administration of antineoplastic drugs has evolved from a theoretical concept to a rational treatment strategy in a number of clinical settings.

The rather profound pharmacokinetic advantage associated with regional drug delivery is appealing, but a number of theoretical and practical issues limit patient populations where this therapeutic approach is a reasonable option in both clinical trials and standard oncologic practice.

Randomized controlled trials will be required to demonstrate if the potential for enhanced tumor cell kill associated with increased drug concentrations and more prolonged exposure can be translated into improved outcomes for patients with malignant disease.

REFERENCES

1. Weisberger AS, Levine B, Storaasli JP. Use of nitrogen mustard in treatment of serous effusions of neoplastic origin. *JAMA* 1955; 159:1704–1707.
2. Bleyer WA. Current status of intrathecal chemotherapy for human meningeal neoplasms. *Natl Cancer Inst Monogr* 1977; 46:171–178.
3. Jones HC, Swinney J. Thio-TEPA in the treatment of tumours of the bladder. *Lancet* 1961; 2:615–618.
4. Calvo DB, Patt YZ, Wallace S, et al. Phase I–II trial of percutaneous intra-arterial cis-diamminedichloroplatinum (II) for regionally confined malignancy. *Cancer* 1980; 45:1278–1283.
5. Collins JM. Pharmacokinetic rationale for regional drug delivery. *J Clin Oncol* 1984; 2:498–504.
6. Chen H-S, Gross JF. Intra-arterial infusion of anticancer drugs: Theoretic aspects of drug delivery and review of responses. *Cancer Treat Rep* 1980; 64:31–40.
7. Dedrick RL, Myers CE, Bungay PM, DeVita VT Jr. Pharmacokinetic rationale for peritoneal drug administration in the treatment of ovarian cancer. *Cancer Treat Rep* 1978; 62:1–9.
8. Markman M. Intraperitoneal anti-neoplastic agents for tumors principally confined to the peritoneal cavity. *Cancer Treat Rev* 1986; 13:219–242.
9. Sculier JP. Treatment of meningeal carcinomatosis. *Cancer Treat Rev* 1985; 12:95–104.
10. Frei E, Canellos GP. Dose: A critical factor in cancer chemotherapy. *Am J Med* 1980; 69:585–594.
11. Chabner BA, Myers CE, Coleman CN, Johns DG. The clinical pharmacology of antineoplastic agents. *N Engl J Med* 1975; 292:1107–1113.
12. Howell SB, Pfeifle CE, Wung WE, et al. Intraperitoneal cisplatin with systemic thiosulfate protection. *Ann Intern Med* 1982; 97:845–851.
13. Casper ES, Kelsen DP, Alcock NW, Lewis JL. Ip cisplatin in patients with malignant ascites: Pharmacokinetics evaluation and comparison with the iv route. *Cancer Treat Rep* 1983; 67:325–328.
14. Sigurdson ER, Ridge JA, Kemeny N, Daly JM. Tumor and liver drug uptake following hepatic artery and portal vein infusion. *J Clin Oncol* 1987; 5:1836–1840.
15. Alberts DS, Young L, Mason N, Salmon SE. In vitro evaluation of anticancer drugs against ovarian cancer at concentrations achievable by intraperitoneal administration. *Semin Oncol* 1985; 12(3;Suppl. 4):38–42.
16. Blasberg RG, Patlak C, Fenstermacher JD. Intrathecal chemotherapy: Brain tissue profiles after ventriculo-cisternal perfusion. *J Pharmacol Exp Ther* 1975; 195:73–83.

17. Durand RE. Flow cytometry studies of intracellular adriamycin in multicell spheroids in vitro. *Cancer Res* 1981; 41:3495–3498.
18. Los G, Mutsaers PHA, van der Vijgh WJF, Baldew GS, de Graaf PW, McVie JG. Direct diffusion of cis-diamminedichloroplatinum(II) in intraperitoneal rat tumors after intraperitoneal chemotherapy: A comparison with systemic chemotherapy. *Cancer Res* 1989; 49:3380–3384.
19. Nederman T, Carlsson J. Penetration and binding of vinblastine and 5-fluorouracil in cellular spheroids. *Cancer Chemother Pharmacol* 1984; 13:131–135.
20. Ozols RF, Locker GY, Doroshow JH, et al. Pharmacokinetics of adriamycin and tissue penetration in murine ovarian cancer. *Cancer Res* 1979b; 39:3209–3214.
21. West GW, Weichselbau R, Little JB. Limited penetration of methotrexate into human osteosarcoma spheroids as a proposed model for solid tumor resistance to adjuvant chemotherapy. *Cancer Res* 1980; 40:3665–3668.
22. Markman M, Reichman B, Hakes T, et al. Responses to second-line cisplatin-based intraperitoneal therapy in ovarian cancer: influence of a prior response to intravenous cisplatin. *J Clin Oncol* 1991; 9:1801–1805.
23. Dedrick RL. Arterial drug infusion: Pharmacokinetic problems and pitfalls. *JNCI* 1988; 80:83–89.
24. Lutz RJ, Miller DL. Mixing studies during hepatic artery infusion in an in vitro model. *Cancer* 1988; 62:1066–1073.
25. Rosenshein N, Blake D, McIntyre PA, et al. The effect of volume on the distribution of substances instilled into the peritoneal cavity. *Gynecol Oncol* 1978; 6:106–110.
26. Taylor A, Baily NA, Halpern SE, Ashburn WL. Loculation as a contraindication to intracavitary ^{32}P chromic phosphate therapy. *J Nucl Med* 1985; 16:318–319.
27. Vider M, Deland FM, Maruyama Y. Loculation as a contraindication to intracavitary ^{32}P chromic phosphate therapy. *J Nucl Med* 1976; 17:150–151.
28. Runowicz CD, Dottino PR, Shafir MA, Mark MA, Cohen CJ. Catheter complications associated with intraperitoneal chemotherapy. *Gynecol Oncol* 1986; 24:41–50.
29. Kaplan RA, Markman M, Lucas WE, Pfeifle C, Howell SB. Infectious peritonitis in patients receiving intraperitoneal chemotherapy. *Am J Med* 1985; 78:49–53.
30. Sterchi JM. Hepatic artery infusion for metastatic neoplastic disease. *Surg Gynecol Obstet* 1985; 160:477–489.
31. Niederhuber JE, Ensminger WD. Surgical consideration in the management of hepatic neoplasia. *Semin Oncol* 1983; 10:135–147.
32. Williams NN, Daly JM. Infusional versus systemic chemotherapy for liver metastases from colorectal cancer. *Surg Clin North Am* 1989; 69:401–410.
33. Daly JM, Kemeny N, Oderman P, Botet J. Long-term hepatic arterial infusion chemotherapy: Anatomic considerations, operative technique, and treatment morbidity. *Arch Surg* 1984; 119:936–941.
34. Bleyer WA, Pizzo PA, Spence AM, et al. The Ommaya reservoir: Newly recognized complications and recommendations for insertion and use. *Cancer* 1978; 41:2431–2437.
35. Green DM, West CR, Brecher ML, et al. The use of subcutaneous cerebrospinal fluid reservoirs for the prevention and treatment of meningeal relapse of acute lymphoblastic leukemia. *Am J Pediatr Hematol Oncol* 1982; 4:147–154.
36. Kemeny MM, Battifora H, Blayney DW, et al. Sclerosing cholangitis after continuous hepatic artery infusion of FUDR. *Ann Surg* 1985; 202:176–181.
37. Hohn D, Melnick J, Stagg R, et al. Biliary sclerosis in patients receiving hepatic arterial infusions of floxuridine. *J Clin Oncol* 1985; 3:98–102.
38. Litterst CL, Collins JM, Lowe MC, Arnold ST, Powell DM, Guarino AM. Local and systemic toxicity resulting from large-volume Ip administration of doxorubicin in the rat. *Cancer Treat Rep* 1982; 66:157–161.
39. Markman M, Cleary S, Howell SB, Lucas WE. Complications of extensive adhesion formation following intraperitoneal chemotherapy. *Surg Gynecol Oncol* 1986; 112:445–448.
40. Stephens FO. Management of gastric cancer with regional chemotherapy preceding gastrectomy—5-year survival results. *Reg Cancer Treat* 1988; 1:80–82.
41. Aigner KR. Isolated liver perfusion: 5-year results. *Reg Cancer Treat* 1988; 1:11–20.
42. Sugarbaker PH, Zhu B-W, Sese GB, Shmookler B. Peritoneal carcinomatosis from appendiceal cancer: Results in 69 patients treated by cytoreductive surgery and intraperitoneal chemotherapy. *Dis Colon Rectum* 1993; 36:323–329.

43. Aur RJA, Simone J, Hustu HO, et al. Central nervous system therapy and combination chemotherapy of childhood lymphocytic leukemia. *Blood* 1971; 37:272–281.
44. Bleyer WA, Poplack DG. Intraventricular versus intralumbar methotrexate for central-nervous-system leukemia: Prolonged remission with the Ommaya reservoir. *Med Pediatr Oncol* 1979; 6:207–213.
45. Bleyer WA. Intrathecal methotrexate versus central nervous system leukemia. *Cancer Drug Deliv* 1984; 1:157–167.
46. Markman M: Intraperitoneal therapy of ovarian cancer. *Semin Oncol* 1998; 25:356–360.
47. Alberts DS, Liu PY, Hannigan EV, et al. Intraperitoneal cisplatin plus intravenous cyclophosphamide versus intravenous cisplatin plus intravenous cyclophosphamide for stage III ovarian cancer. *N Engl J Med* 1996; 335:1950–1955.
48. Markman M, Bundy B, Benda J, et al. for the Gynecologic Oncology Group. Randomized phase 3 study of intravenous(IV) cisplatin(CIS)/paclitaxel(PAC) versus moderately high dose IV carboplatin(CARB) followed by IV PAC and intraperitoneal(IP) CIS in optimal residual ovarian cancer(OC): An intergroup trial (GOG, SWOG, ECOG). *Proc Am Soc Clin Oncol* 1998; 17:361a (abstract 1392).
49. Chang AE, Schneider PD, Sugarbaker PH, Simpson C, Culnane M, Steinberg SM. A prospective randomized trial of regional versus systemic continuous 5-fluorodeoxyuridine chemotherapy of colorectal liver metastases. *Ann Surg* 1987; 206:685–693.
50. Kemeny N, Daly J, Reichman B, Geller N, Botet J, Oderman P. Intrahepatic or systemic infusion of fluorodeoxyuridine in patients with liver metastases from colorectal carcinoma: A randomized trial. *Ann Intern Med* 1987; 107:459–465.
51. Hohn DS, Stagg RJ, Friedman M, et al. A randomized trial of continuous intravenous versus hepatic intraarterial floxuridine in patients with colorectal cancer metastatic to the liver: The Northern California Oncology Group trial. *J Clin Oncol* 1989; 7:1646–1654.
52. Rougier P, Laplanche A, Huguier M, et al. Hepatic arterial infusion of floxuridine in patients with liver metastases from colorectal carcinoma: Long-term results of a prospective randomized trial. *J Clin Oncol* 1992; 10:1112–1118.
53. Kemeny MM, Goldberg D, Beatty JD, et al. Results of a prospective randomized trial of continuous regional chemotherapy and hepatic resection as treatment of hepatic metastases from colorectal primaries. *Cancer* 1986; 57:492–498.
54. Martin, Jr, JK, O'Connell MJ, Wieand HS, et al. Intra-arterial floxuridine vs systemic fluorouracil for hepatic metastases from colorectal cancer. A randomized trial. *Arch Surg* 1990; 125:1022–1027.
55. Allen-Mersh TG, Earlam S, Fordy C, Abrams K, Houghton J. Quality of life and survival with continuous hepatic-artery floxuridine infusion for colorectal liver metastases. *Lancet* 1994; 344:1255–1260.
56. Soloway MS. Introduction and overview of intravesical therapy for superficial bladder cancer. *Semin Oncol* 1988; 31(3):5–16.
57. Soloway MS. Intravesical therapy for bladder cancer. *Urol Clin North Am* 1988; 15:661–669.

3

Theoretical Analyses and Simulations of Anticancer Drug Delivery

Ardith W. El-Kareh, PhD
and Timothy W. Secomb, PhD

CONTENTS

1. INTRODUCTION

Large amounts of data on tumor cell survival as a function of exposure to anticancer drugs, drug pharmacokinetics, drug distribution in the body, and other aspects of drug delivery and effectiveness are continually being generated. Cancer therapies are becoming increasingly complex, and it is now possible to choose the time schedule of drug delivery, the site of delivery, the size, lipophilicity, release kinetics and other properties of a carrier, and numerous other options. However, it is clearly impossible to perform sufficient animal experiments or clinical trials to determine the optimal choices of all these variables. Even for drugs that have been used for decades, doses and schedules are often based on past experience and medical tradition rather than on rational analysis. These circumstances suggest an increasing need for theoretical models of anticancer drug delivery. Such models can provide a framework for synthesizing and interpreting available experimental data, and a rational basis for optimizing therapies using existing drugs and for guiding development of new drugs.

A synthesis is needed of two main bodies of anticancer drug research: studies on cellular responses to drugs, and studies on how the method of drug administration affects an animal or patient. Improved understanding is needed of the relation between the mode and schedule of therapy and the resulting drug exposure of cancer cells and normal cells that are responsible for limiting toxicities. This requires consideration of

From: *Drug Delivery Systems in Cancer Therapy*
Edited by: D. M. Brown © Humana Press Inc., Totowa, NJ

the steps involved in drug transport from the infusion site to the tumor (1–3). Here, theoretical modeling can play an important role, by predicting cellular exposure and toxicity as a function of treatment mode and schedule, taking into account whole-body pharmacokinetics and transport processes leading to spatial and temporal variations of drug concentrations within the tumor and other tissues.

The focus of this review is on the use of theoretical models to investigate the relationship between delivery of anticancer drugs and their cellular effects, with the goal of optimizing anticancer therapies. First, theoretical models for the dependence of tumor cell kill on cellular drug exposure are considered. The importance of host tissue toxicity is then discussed. Next, studies aimed at optimizing intravenous (iv) delivery are examined, along with studies on alternative delivery methods. Finally, potential directions for future research are considered.

2. ANTITUMOR EFFECTS OF CELLULAR DRUG EXPOSURE

Several theories have been developed to describe the relation between cellular exposure to anticancer drugs and effect, measured as tumor cell kill or surviving fraction of clonogenic cells. In this context, "exposure" refers to the time course of extracellular concentration. Because response to a drug generally increases with increased drug levels and with increased exposure time, the area under the (extracellular) concentration-time curve, generally called AUC, is often used as a predictor of effectiveness. In most in vitro experiments, the extracellular concentration is held constant, so that AUC is $C \times T$, the product of extracellular concentration and exposure time. Data sets with only one exposure time (and several different concentrations) or only one concentration (and varying exposure time) cannot be used to test whether AUC by itself properly predicts drug effect. Data on cell kill for different combinations $C_1 T_1 = C_2 T_2$ where $C_1 \neq C_2$ are needed. Walker et al. (4) and Erlichman et al. (5) obtained such data for two different human bladder cancer cell lines and concluded that AUC alone predicted cell kill. Walker et al. (4) reported this observation for doxorubicin, epodyl, mitomycin C, and thiotepa; Erlichman et al. (5) found it to hold for melphalan, cisplatin, doxorubicin, mitomycin C, and 5-fluorouracil, but not for vincristine. Ozawa et al. (6) concluded that AUC predicts cell kill for Chinese hamster cells exposed to mitomycin C, from their data showing that log(IC_{90}) (where IC_{90} is the concentration required for 90% growth inhibition) plotted vs log(T) is linear with slope –1. Kurihara et al. (7) exposed gastric cancer cell lines to cisplatin for different times, and also concluded that AUC was a predictor of effect.

A cell kill that depends only on AUC, independent of the time course of concentration, is to be expected if the proportional rate of cell kill is linearly related to the concentration. In particular, if cell kill is rapid enough to be considered instantaneous, then cell kill is dependent only on AUC, if and only if the number of cells $n(t)$ satisfies

$$(1/n)\, dn/dt = -kc \qquad \text{[Eq. 1]}$$

where $c(t)$ is the drug concentration and k is a constant. Linear models for cell kill are clearly limited in their applicability. Most pharmacologic responses are nonlinear in concentration, showing saturation at high levels. Furthermore, cooperative behavior is often seen at low-concentration levels, giving a sigmoidal dependence of response on concentration. In such cases, AUC alone cannot predict cell kill. For example, the effects of doubling the concentration and halving the exposure time (while holding AUC constant) do

Table 1
AUC_{50} (in μg-h/mL) for Various Anticancer Drugs, for Different Infusion Times,
Based on Data of Nozue et al., 1995.

A. The GCIY Cell Line

Drug	1 h	6 h	24 h	72 h	Nonmonotonic?
neocarzinostatin	2.0	15.0	33.6	381.6	
mitomycin-C			96.0	237.6	
actinomycin-D	1.18	0.78	1.92	5.76	*
doxorubicin		47.4	105.6	302.4	
pirarubicin	1.40	2.16	7.68	14.4	
epirubicin	>100	28.8	96.0	244.8	*
daunorubicin	5.0	22.2	40.8	111.6	
mitoxantrone	1.80	9.9	13.9	136.8	
vindesine sulfate	5.6	31.2	1.44	0.72	*
SN-38		4.32	18.7	40.3	
cyclophosphamide		4.26	18.7	40.3	
ifosfamide		18.0	67.2	194.4	
cisplatin		24.0	37.2	133.2	
5-fluorouracil			1008.0	2592.0	

B. The JR-St Cell Line

Drug	1 h	6 h	24 h	72 h	Nonmonotonic?
mitomycin-C		50.4	72.0	116.6	
actinomycin-D	0.16	0.36	0.24	0.72	*
doxorubicin	0.9	6.0	4.56	8.64	*
pirarubicin	0.4	2.16	10.56	18.0	
epirubicin	3.3	8.4	14.4	23.0	
daunorubicin	3.3	9.6	38.4	72.0	
mitoxantrone			105.6	316.8	
vincristine	1.45	3.24	20.64	51.8	
vinblastine	0.16	1.02	3.6	0.72	*
vindesine	0.14	0.54	1.44	0.72	*
SN-38	1.6	22.8	81.6	56.16	*
etoposide		420.0	984.0	936.0	*
cisplatin		40.2	79.2	237.6	
5-fluorouracil			432.0	576.0	
methotrexate			24.0	7.92	*

* Denotes a drug for which AUC_{50} does not increase monotonically with exposure time

not cancel each other as they do when the response is linear. Therefore, it is not surprising that AUC has been found to be an inadequate predictor of effect in many studies. For example, Nozue et al. *(8)* determined the (extracellular) drug level needed for 50% growth inhibition (IC_{50}) for a number of anticancer drugs at four different exposure times, for four different cell lines. In Table 1, some of their data are tabulated as AUC_{50} rather than IC_{50}. (Here, AUC_x is defined as the AUC needed to achieve x percent growth inhibition.) If AUC predicted cell kill, AUC_{50} would not vary with exposure time, but Table 1 shows that AUC_{50} does vary. For many drugs, higher AUC_{50} is needed at longer exposure times, while other drugs show nonmonotonic variation of AUC_{50} with exposure time.

Table 2
Studies Showing That Exposure Time is Needed in Addition to AUC to Predict Drug Effect

Drug	Tumor/Cell Type	Source	Replot[e]
Cisplatin	Colon carcinoma	(9), Table 5	yes
Cisplatin	Head and neck cancer	(10), Fig. 4	no
Cisplatin	Chinese hamster cells	(11), Fig. 1	yes
Doxorubicin	Human colorectal carcinoma	(12), Figs. 1 and 2	yes
Doxorubicin	Mouse sarcoma cell line	(13), Table 1	no
Methotrexate	Chinese hamster, HeLa, HAK	(14)	no
Mitomycin-C	Human bladder	(15), Fig. 3	yes
Mitomycin-C	Human ovarian cancer	(16), Fig. 2	yes
Mitomycin-C	Human colon adenocarcinoma	(17), Table 1	yes
Mitomycin-C	Human bladder cancer, human pharynx cancer	(18)	no
3 drugs[a]	Jurkat leukemia	(19)	no
4 drugs[b]	Human ovarian carcinoma	(20)	no
Many drugs[c]	Murine neuroblastoma	(21), Figs. 2 and 3	yes
Many drugs[d]	Human ovarian and ileocecal carcinoma	(22)	no
Many drugs	Human lung adenocarcinoma	(23)	no

[a] Taxol, camptothecin, DACA.
[b] Doxorubicin, cisplatin, vinblastine, and hydroxyurea.
[c] Including doxorubicin, cisplatin, melphalan, methotrexate.
[d] Including cisplatin, doxorubicin, paclitaxel, trimetrexate, raltitrexed, methotrexate, AG2034.
[e] Data are plotted vs extracellular concentration in the cited study.

Many other studies show that drug effect is not predicted by AUC alone, although this may not be readily apparent, because survival fraction is often plotted vs. drug concentration. When the data are plotted as survival fraction vs AUC for different exposure times, failure of the curves to coincide implies that AUC alone is not an adequate predictor of effect. Table 2 lists a number of studies that found such behavior. Some of the drugs appearing in Tables 1 and 2 were also used in studies mentioned earlier that found that AUC alone predicted effect. This suggests that the relation between effect and exposure depends on the cell type. Also, studies reporting a close correlation with AUC might have found the correlation to break down had they sampled more concentrations or exposure times.

Because AUC may not adequately predict effect, the relation $(IC_{50})^n T = k$, or more generally $(IC_x)^n T = k$, where k is a constant and x is percent growth inhibition, has been used by several investigators. If $n = 1$, this reduces to $AUC_{50} = k$, i.e., the effect then depends only on AUC. A larger value of n implies a greater importance of concentration overexposure time; conversely, values of $n < 1$ weight exposure duration as having relatively greater importance. Levasseur et al. (22) gathered a large amount of in vitro dose-response data at different exposure times for a number of drugs, and correlated the data with $IC_{50} T^{(1/n)} = k$, which is equivalent. Their fitted values of n differ significantly from 1 for many drugs. Millenbaugh et al. (18) found n values from 1.04 up to 1.46 for the response of two different cell lines to mitomycin C.

Although it generally allows a better fit to the data, the equation $(IC_{50})^n T = k$ has some limitations. Many drugs have a threshold value below which they will have no effect, no matter how long the exposure time (e.g., methotrexate, Chabner and Longo [24]), but this equation does not allow for such a threshold. Similarly, the equation $(IC_{50})^n T = k$ implies, unrealistically, that if a high enough concentration is used, a response can be achieved in extremely short time. Another limitation of the equation is the fact that it predicts a monotonic increase (if $n > 1$) or decrease (if $n < 1$) of the AUC_{50} with increasing exposure time, i.e., $AUC_{50} = k^{1/n} = T^{1-1/n}$. In Table 1, asterisks indicate drugs that do not exhibit such monotonic behavior. Other data sets exhibiting nonmonotonic behavior include the Schmittgen et al. *(15)* study of mitomycin C acting on human bladder cells (their Fig. 3, although the authors fit this data to the $C^n T$ form) and the Eichholtz-Wirth and Hietel *(11)* data on cisplatin (their Fig. 1).

Apart from the above limitations, a single correlation $(IC_x)^n T = k$ for any particular x (such as 50 or 90) is not sufficient, and a correlation for a range of x values is needed. Recognizing this need, Levasseur et al. *(22)* combined the equation $(IC_{50})^n T = k$ with a Hill model to give mathematical expressions for effect at any concentration and exposure duration. These equations were then fit to a large body of data for seven different anticancer drugs. While this model can describe a wider range of behavior than the correlation $(IC_x)^n T = k$, it does not generalize readily to cases in which concentration varies with time (as generally occurs in vivo). Also, this model cannot be extrapolated to time periods longer than the 24-h range of the fitted data, because the empirical quadratic dependence of one of the parameters on T does not apply for longer periods.

The "exponential kill" model of Gardner *(25)* has the advantage that it is based on a consideration of the kinetics of cell kill. Although results are presented for exposure to constant drug levels, such a model can also be used to predict the response to time-varying concentrations. Other features of this model are that it includes effects of cell cycle time phase on the response of cells to cell-cycle phase-specific drugs, and that it allows for a "plateau" in the response such that cell kill is independent of drug concentration at high concentration levels. However, the applicability of the model is restricted by the assumption that the fractional rate of cell kill at each instant (a quantity having units of inverse time) is given (for cell-cycle phase-nonspecific drugs) by $1-\exp(-aC)$ and a corresponding expression for cell-cycle phase-specific drugs. These expressions are dimensionless, and should therefore be replaced with $k[1-\exp(-aC)]$, where k is an additional parameter with units of inverse time. The need for the parameter k is further shown in the limit of large concentration, where the survival fraction at a fixed exposure time T approaches a plateau at a survival fraction $B(T) = \exp(-T)$. This expression cannot be reconciled with experimental observations because it lacks a parameter to scale the argument of the exponential so that it is dimensionless. With the parameter k, it becomes $B(T) = \exp(-kT)$. Furthermore, the assumed dependence of cell-kill rate on concentration leads to the conclusion (for cell-cycle phase-nonspecific drugs) that the AUC required for a given level of cell kill decreases with increasing exposure time to a constant level of drug, whereas many such drugs show the opposite trend (Table 1).

Different drugs and cell lines show a wide variety of cellular responses to drug dose, and any given model is necessarily restricted in its applicability. Baguley and Finlay *(19)* found that for 1-h exposures to the drug DACA, survival fraction did not always decrease as concentration increased. Rather, there was a maximum cell kill at a finite concentration, indicative of drug self-inhibition. None of the mathematical forms discussed in the foregoing can predict such nonmonotonic behavior of survival fraction with concentration at fixed exposure time. Similarly complex behavior is suggested by data of Slee et al. *(16)*, whose curves for survival fraction of ovarian cancer cells vs mitomycin C concentration at different exposure times intersect. Table 3 of Nozue et al. *(8)*, part of which was retabulated in terms of AUC_{50} (Table 1), also shows a few drugs and cell lines for which IC_{50} does not decrease monotonically in time, including neocarzinostatin, mitoxantrone, SN-38, vincristine, and pirarubicin.

In summary, a number of empirical relationships between cellular exposure and growth inhibition have been proposed. For most anticancer drugs, AUC is not an adequate predictor of effect. The common practice of correlating data on tumor cell kill with the AUC of plasma drug concentration vs time can lead to the incorrect inference that the schedule of drug administration has no bearing on efficacy. Correlations that include exposure time *T* as well as AUC are needed, and may provide a basis for optimizing treatment schedules. A mathematical form that adequately correlates effect with concentration and exposure time for one drug may be inadequate for a different drug or even for the same drug acting on a different cell line. Consideration of the kinetics of cell kill *(25)* may be helpful in developing improved models.

Many anticancer drugs must enter tumor cells before they can take effect and this takes finite time. For example, equilibration of extracellular and intracellular concentrations of doxorubicin takes hours *(26)*. A deficiency of the models described so far is that they do not take into account the kinetics of this transport process. Experimental studies are needed in which intracellular concentration is measured along with growth inhibition. Such data can provide a basis for more realistic models to predict antitumor effect. Other factors may have to be included in some cases, such as self-inhibition of toxicity, cell-cycle specificity, and different mechanisms of cell kill at different concentrations *(27)*.

3. DRUG EXPOSURE AND HOST TOXICITY

Information on the relation between host toxicity and exposure is essential for optimization of drug delivery. All anticancer therapies are subject to limits on allowable host toxicity. A crude measure of host toxicity is maximum tolerated dose (MTD), determined as an average over some patient population. Use of MTD has serious limitations. Some patients have medical conditions besides cancer that give them lower tolerance, such as renal and liver failure, or heart disease. For example, Sadoff *(28)* found severe enhancement of 5-fluorouracil toxicity in patients with diabetes. Clearance of drug shows considerable individual variation. Patients with more rapid than average drug clearance might receive suboptimal treatment if given an average MTD. These considerations have led to the use of pharmacokinetic monitoring to individualize the dose so that patients have equivalent plasma levels rather than equivalent injected dose *(29)*. However, as with drug effectiveness, toxicity may depend not only on the total amount of drug, but also on the schedule of administration. For example, total lifetime limits of doxorubicin are around 500 mg/m^2 for bolus injection, but have been pushed to 700 mg/m^2 with continuous infusion *(30)*.

Many researchers have correlated host toxicity with AUC. However, just as AUC has limitations as a predictor of antitumor drug effect, AUC is not necessarily a good pre-

Table 3A
Reported Correlations of Host Hematological Toxicity with Drug AUC

Drug	Toxicity	Source
Carboplatin	Thrombocytopenia	31
Cisplatin	Thrombocytopenia	32
Pyrazine diazohydroxide	Leukopenia	33
Topotecan	Myelosuppression	34
Many drugs	Hematological	35

Table 3B
Reported Correlations of Host Toxicity with Measures of Drug Exposure Other Than AUC

Drug	Toxicity	Correlating factor	Source
Cisplatin	Nephrotoxicity	Duration above threshold level (plasma)	36,37
Doxorubicin	Cardiotoxicity	Peak plasma levels	38
Etoposide	Myelosuppression	Peak plasma levels	39
Methotrexate	Neurotoxicity	Duration above threshold level (plasma)	24
Paclitaxel	Myelosuppression	Duration above threshold level (plasma)	40

dictor of host toxicity. Table 3A lists some studies, including a review (35), that found correlations of hematological toxicity with AUC. Table 3B lists studies that found other measures of exposure to be more relevant.

Lokich and Anderson (41) surveyed anticancer drugs to determine whether the maximum tolerated dose and dose intensity were different for bolus injection and for infusion. Dose intensity is a measure of plasma exposure rather than amount injected, and reflects the individual variation in clearance of drug or other factors such as binding of drug to plasma proteins, and so on. Unfortunately, they defined bolus administration as any taking less than 24 h, and continuous infusion as any taking longer than 24 h. Significant variation of response with infusion times may be overlooked when schedules of administration are lumped in these two categories. Even so, that review (41) shows that the schedule of administration influences the maximum tolerated dose, and therefore must influence toxicity.

Although the studies in Table 3A reported a correlation of toxicity with AUC, they did not establish that these correlations would apply to schedules or modes of administration that differ significantly from the type used in obtaining the correlation. For example, Dhodapkar et al. (33) give correlations for the hematological toxicity of pyrazine dizohydroxide that involve AUC. They note that "Since AUC and C_{peak} were highly correlated, either parameter may be used to predict hematologic toxicity." For bolus iv infusion, AUC and C_{peak} may indeed be correlated. However, with another schedule such as long-time continuous infusion, a high AUC may be achieved with a low C_{peak}. For such schedules, it is important to determine whether AUC or C_{peak} determines the hematological toxicity, or whether neither quantity provides a reliable indicator of toxicity.

Several of the studies in Table 3B correlated toxicity with the period that plasma drug concentrations exceeded a threshold level. Although such correlations may be adequate to fit a data set wherein the threshold was exceeded in all cases, their form is not suitable for determining optimum exposure. Mathematically, they suggest that the optimum schedule is a plasma concentration just below the threshold for infinite time. This is clearly unrealistic. Mathematical forms that do not include artificial discontinuities (e.g., toxicity dropping abruptly to zero) are more likely to lead to plausible results when used to optimize exposure.

In conclusion, quantitative relations between the limiting toxicities of anticancer drugs and exposure, including schedule dependence, are needed. Studies correlating hematological toxicities with AUC or steady-state plasma values should be reexamined to determine whether the findings apply only for a particular schedule of administration, or whether they are schedule-independent. More in vitro studies relating host cell toxicity to extracellular drug level would also be valuable.

4. OPTIMIZATION OF INTRAVENOUS DELIVERY

To address the question of what therapy offers the best probability of success, results of studies at the cellular level should ideally be incorporated into models for cost and benefit for the whole body. Optimization should obviously involve maximization of benefit with minimization of cost, but this involves the difficult problem of choosing measures of cost and benefit. At the cellular level, survival fraction or percent growth inhibition are obvious measures of effect. At the whole-body level, the most indisputable measure of benefit is statistically significant prolonged survival of a human patient population (perhaps with quality-of-life considerations added). However, controlled clinical trials are scarce, take many years to yield long-term survival data, seldom analyze more than one variable relating to treatment, and often have several confounding variables. Therefore, it is extremely difficult to relate long-term survival to the numerous factors that could be varied to optimize treatment. For this reason, most theoretical studies use survival fraction or percent growth inhibition for tumor cells as measures of benefit at the whole-body level. This admittedly has a serious drawback, in that treatments leading to greater short-term response (e.g., greater immediate tumor cell kill) do not necessarily lead to improved long-term survival. For example, intraarterial delivery of 5-fluorouracil for liver metastases of colon cancer gives better short-term response than iv therapy, but does not result in increased survival *(42)*. Similarly, long-time infusion of 5-fluorouracil produces a higher response rate than bolus injection for colorectal cancer, but with no statistically significant increase in survival *(43)*.

Minimization of "cost" is also complicated for cancer therapy. Given that many cancers are life-threatening diseases, significant permanent damage to the host may be acceptable if it is accompanied by sufficient tumor cell kill. Thus, for many life-threatening cancers, cost should logically be fixed at the highest level short of killing or too severely disabling the patient (a subjective choice in some cases). Rather than setting toxicity at the maximum tolerable level, some investigators have used the steepness of the dose-response curve as a criterion *(12,35)*. For therapy that has a chance of cure, the rationale for stopping at the point of diminishing returns is not clear, however, since an increase in toxicity to achieve a small additional cell kill can be worthwhile if it results in prolonged survival. On the other hand, for palliative therapy (i.e., therapy that is known *a priori* to have no chance of being curative), the acceptable level of toxicity should perhaps be lower. Whereas not all toxicities are easily quantified, certain common dose-limiting toxicities such as thrombocytopenia and leukopenia have objective measures. These measures can be correlated with probability of surviving treatment, so that the remaining subjective element is choosing an acceptable level of risk. It may be best to optimize therapy as a function of this risk level, leaving it as a parameter to be chosen for each patient.

4.1. Optimization of Plasma Exposure

Several researchers have used data on the dependence of tumor cell toxicity on exposure schedule to determine optimal delivery schedules. Some of these studies assume implicitly that tumor extracellular exposure is identical with plasma exposure, even though other researchers have emphasized that this is not necessarily the case *(1–3)*. Such studies are reviewed here, with particular attention to the criteria chosen to optimize treatment.

Millenbaugh et al. *(18)* fitted the relation $C^nT = h$, where h is a measure of drug effect, to cell kill data for mitomycin C, and stated that "when the n value deviates from 1.0, even to a relatively minor extent, different treatment schedules can result in large differences in the C^nT product" and that this is "important for deciding on the treatment schedules that produce the highest effect." Many years earlier, Skipper *(44)* made the key observation that the basis of successful therapy is the *difference* between the n values for tumor and host tissue. If $C^nT = h$ holds with different n values for the tumor cells and the normal cells that give rise to dose-limiting toxicity, then therapy can be optimized by changing the schedule of administration.

In an in vitro study screening 24 drugs for effect on gastric cancer, Nozue et al. *(8)* maximized the quantity $AUC/\Delta IC_{50}$, where ΔIC_{50} is a composite measure of IC_{50} for four different gastric cancer cell lines and AUC is the clinically achievable exposure, as a criterion for effectiveness. The rationale was that a large achievable AUC is favorable since it means that more drug can be administered, whereas a low IC_{50} means that less drug is needed to achieve 50% growth inhibition. One drawback was noted: the achievable AUC is actually schedule-dependent, and use of a single value neglects substantial variation that might be achieved by changing the schedule of administration. A further drawback is that the schedule dependence of the tumor cell kill was neglected. Moreover, IC_x can show complicated dependence on x. Since therapy aims for a much higher fractional cell kill than 50%, it is not clear that behavior at 50% cell kill (i.e., IC_{50}) should be used in optimization. Nozue et al. *(8)* noted that their predictions for 5-fluorouracil and mitomycin C did not agree well with clinical observations.

Link et al. *(12)* determined optimal exposure times by another criterion. They determined survival vs. concentration curves for various exposure times. Then for each exposure time, the concentration IC_{50} and the slope of the curve at that point (α) were determined. The time T for which $IC_{50} T/\alpha$ was minimum was taken as optimum. The rationale for this choice was not stated, but appears to be as follows. $IC_{50} T$ is AUC, assumed to measure toxicity to normal tissue. Where $1/\alpha$ is smallest, the benefit from increasing the concentration is largest. However, as mentioned previously, the logic of using the steepness of the dose-response curve as a criterion is questionable. Furthermore, the dose-response curves are nonlinear, and the behavior at 50% cell kill may

differ from that at higher cell kill. The scatter in the data makes accurate estimation of
α difficult. A simpler and more robust approach, retaining the assumption that AUC
measures toxicity, would be to plot survival as a function of AUC and choose the exposure time that maximizes the cell kill when AUC is set at the maximum tolerable level.

In summary, some studies attempted to optimize treatment schedules under the
assumption that tumor cell extracellular exposure can be approximated by plasma
exposure. Some of the optimization criteria, e.g., use of single parameters such as IC_{50}
or the slope of the dose-response curve at one point to create a measure of drug effectiveness, have questionable rationales. Taking into account the entire three-dimensional
concentration-time-effect surface might give significantly different predictions, given
the nonlinearity of drug exposure-effect relations (22). In particular, the relative performance of various drugs at 50% growth inhibition will not necessarily be the same as at,
say, 95% growth inhibition. Despite studies showing schedule-dependence of toxicity
to normal tissues for many drugs, AUC is generally used as a measure of toxicity.
Future work in this area should aim to develop consistent criteria for optimization of
therapy, with attention given to the dependence of host toxicity on treatment schedule.

4.2. Mathematical Models

Mathematical models for pharmacokinetics, pharmacodynamics, and tissue transport of intravenously injected drugs have existed for some time. However, the synthesis
of these separate components into a single model predicting effect and toxicity for typical tumors in the human body has been addressed by few researchers. Early whole-
body models for anticancer drugs (e.g., 45–47) neglected the time lags associated with
transport of drug from plasma to tumor, and also spatial gradients within the tumor,
which can be important (1–3).

Some recent studies have addressed the question of optimal schedule and dose of
chemotherapeutic agents, with models that include tumor growth kinetics (48–50).
Such studies raise the question of whether tumor growth over the time interval of treatment is significant. The mean volume doubling time for human tumors is in the range
17–632 d (51). For optimizing treatments with durations up to 24 h, tumor growth during treatment seems unlikely to be a major factor, although growth may be relevant in
optimization of fractionated therapy of faster-growing tumors, with treatment cycles
separated by 1 wk or more.

The predictions of such models are sensitive to the assumed dependence of cell proliferation and death on cell population (n) and on drug concentration (c). The simplest
assumption is linear dependence on both quantities:

$$dn/dt = k_1\, n - k_2\, c\, n \qquad \text{[Eq. 2]}$$

a generalization of Eq. 1. This equation may be solved explicitly, giving a survival
fraction

$$n_{final}/n_{initial} = exp[k_1\, T - k_2\, (AUC)] \qquad \text{[Eq. 3]}$$

independent of the time course of c(t), where T is the duration of drug administration
and k_1 and k_2 are constants. In this case, for a given AUC, the survival fraction is independent of the treatment schedule. Optimization of the treatment schedule, if toxicity
is assumed measured by AUC, is possible only if nonlinear dependence on n and/or c
is included.

In the model of Jackson and Byrne *(49)*, nonlinear (saturable) dependence of cell growth rate on population is assumed, but the rate of cell kill is assumed to be directly proportional to drug concentration. The conclusion is that bolus injection gives a slight advantage over continuous infusion, for a given AUC. However, most anticancer drugs have a saturable response to increasing dose *(22)*. Inclusion of this effect in the model would likely lead to the opposite conclusion, because a saturable response reduces the effectiveness of short, high-level doses relative to slower infusions.

Apart from this saturation effect, other factors influence the choice between bolus injection and continuous infusion. For cell cycle-specific drugs, if the drug is administered over too short a time, it is possible that some cells not in the sensitive part of the cell cycle will escape therapy *(48)*. Iliadis and Barbolosi *(50)* point out that the AUC is not necessarily a good predictor of dose-limiting hematological toxicity. Instead, they model white cell population kinetics, and impose the constraint that the number of white cells must not fall below a certain level. Their model includes nonlinear (Gompertzian) growth kinetics, and linear dependence of cell kill on concentration above a threshold level. The optimal therapy is then an initial high-dose infusion, until the white cells reach their nadir, followed by a "maintenance" continuous infusion at a lower level. This approach has the potential problem that while most patients can recover from a certain level of leukopenia, the outcome may be less favorable if this level is maintained over an extended period.

Consideration of transport processes between plasma and tumor cells may also affect the optimization of iv drug delivery. To a first approximation, transport between plasma and tumor space may be represented by a compartmental model, as assumed in *(50)*. Spatial gradients within tumors may be significant as a result of boundary effects or variations in vascular density or flow. The model of Jackson and Byrne *(49)* is formulated for a spherical tumor and includes terms representing diffusive and convective transport of cells and drug resulting from spatial gradients. The convective velocity for drugs is assumed equal to the cell velocity associated with tumor growth, but this neglects convective fluid motion through the extracellular spaces driven by filtration from blood vessels *(52)*. Also, the extracellular fraction may vary depending on whether the tumor is growing or regressing. These factors, which may significantly influence spatial gradients of drugs in tumors, are not included in the model.

Many drugs must enter cells to kill them, and kinetics of cellular uptake of the drug may therefore be significant. This aspect of drug transport is considered in a model *(53)* comparing bolus injection of doxorubicin with continuous infusion of varying duration. Because the doxorubicin molecule is small, spatial variations in concentration within the extracellular space of the tumor are neglected, assuming that the tumor is adequately vascularized. The time scales for drug clearing from plasma, crossing the vessel wall, and crossing the cell membrane are accounted for. Published data *(54)* show that fractional survival depends on peak cellular levels rather than cellular AUC and that transport of doxorubicin from the extracellular space to the cell interior is saturable with slow equilibration *(26)*. Based on these data, the model predicts dose-dependent optimal durations of continuous infusion in the range of 1–3 h. Bolus injection or shorter infusion times are less favorable because the resulting high drug concentrations lead to saturation of cellular uptake, whereas the low plasma levels corresponding to longer infusion times limit the peak cellular level that can be achieved. This study shows that the kinetics of drug uptake by cells can be a key factor in determining optimal treatment schedules. In the model, the hematological toxicities limiting the dose that can be administered on a single cycle are assumed to be predicted by AUC *(55)*. As discussed in Subheading 3, more detailed studies might show that the toxicity is schedule-dependent, and the model would then require modification.

Once a drug has entered the cell, it may be retained there and remain active even when drug is not present outside the cell. In the models *(49,50)* and also in *(25)* discussed earlier, the rate of cell kill is assumed to be a function of the instantaneous extracellular concentration. In a study of effects of paclitaxel on six human cancer cell lines in vitro, Au et al. *(56)* found the delayed response (survival fraction measured at 96 h) to be substantially different from the immediate response (survival fraction measured at cessation of extracellular exposure) for exposure durations of 3–72 h. This suggests that intracellular drug continues to contribute to cell kill after extracellular levels are reduced to zero. The concept of noninstantaneous response is suggested in Panetta's model *(48)* which has an "active time" for the drug that may exceed the exposure time, due to the finite time for drug clearance from the body.

The models discussed so far have explicitly computed tumor cell kill. Some other models have focused on predicting extracellular concentration profiles of drug, without attempting to relate these to cell kill *(52,57,58)*. Baxter and Jain *(52)* included convective currents due to the absence of tumor lymphatics, and predicted highly nonuniform concentration profiles for large drugs that are transported primarily by convection. Although these models provide insight into effects of spatial gradients, they have yet to be integrated into models that predict antitumor response.

In summary, development of theoretical models to predict optimal schedules of iv drug delivery is at a relatively early stage. Several models have been developed, but most have significant deficiencies. In particular, nonlinear dependence of cell kill or growth inhibition on concentration has been neglected in some models, but can strongly influence the results. Other factors that may need more attention include drug transport in tissue and spatial gradients in concentration, the kinetics of drug uptake and retention by cells, cell-cycle specificity of some drugs, and measures of host toxicity.

5. CARRIERS FOR INTRAVENOUS ADMINISTRATION

Carriers have been developed for anticancer drugs, with the goal of reducing either toxicity or altering pharmacokinetics (e.g., keeping a drug in circulation longer). Liposomes have received the most attention *(59)*. For drugs encapsulated in liposomes, several additional parameters can potentially be optimized, including liposome size, rate of drug release, charge, and other surface properties. Of these, only the rate of drug release appears to have been examined with mathematical modeling *(53,60,61)*.

For doxorubicin, Harashima et al. *(61)* considered the dependence of tumor extracellular AUC on clearance rates of drug and liposomes and on liposome release kinetics. Comparing three values of the first-order kinetic rate constant for release by liposomes, i.e., 0.6, 0.06, and 0.006 h^{-1}, they concluded that 0.06 h^{-1} was the optimal value. As discussed earlier, AUC is not a good predictor of cell kill for doxorubicin. Use of a more realistic predictor might lead to a different conclusion regarding the optimal release rate.

As aforementioned, data for doxorubicin *(54)* indicate that peak intracellular concentration is a good predictor of cell survival fraction. This information and data on the kinetics of doxorubicin uptake by cells formed the basis for the model *(53)* described in

Subheading 4.2, which was also used to determine optimal release rates of doxorubicin from liposomes. The resulting optimal time constants were relatively short (1–2 h) and dose-dependent. With more rapid release than this, drug enters the extracellular space faster than cells can incorporate it, because of the saturable uptake kinetics, and drug clears back into the plasma and is wasted. On the other hand, slower release of drug leads to extracellular and intracellular levels that are always low.

In contrast, the results of Harashima et al. *(61)* imply a much longer release time constant of about 17 h. This discrepancy illustrates that different assumptions for the dependence of cell kill on exposure can result in very different conclusions regarding optimal treatment methods. As shown in Subheading 2, the dependence of antitumor effect on exposure may vary considerably even for the same drug acting on different cell lines. Clearly, more data on the relationship between effect and exposure for different drugs and different cell types is needed as a basis for optimizing rates of drug release by carriers.

6. REGIONAL DELIVERY MODALITIES

A number of alternatives to iv injection have been developed, with the goal of providing regional delivery, that is, selective delivery to the tumor region. Examples of such "regional" therapies are polymeric implants, ip infusion, intrapleural infusion, intra-arterial delivery, chemoembolization, and inhalation of aerosols. An important question is whether these therapies actually achieve selective delivery to tumors. When such therapies are found clinically to give improved outcome, this may be caused by altered pharmacokinetics. Theoretical considerations can be used to address this issue, and to examine whether such treatments are likely to be superior to intravenous delivery.

6.1. Intraperitoneal Delivery

Intraperitoneal (ip) administration of chemotherapy has been studied extensively for ovarian carcinoma and other abdominal tumors. Despite clinical trials *(62,63)*, it is still not clear how this modality compares to intravenous administration. Few controlled comparisons of ip and iv delivery using equivalent patient populations and the same doses of the same drugs are available. The recent study of Polyzos et al. *(64)* did not confirm the survival benefit for ip vs iv found by Alberts et al. *(63)*, but found reduced toxicity, suggesting the possibility of using higher doses with ip delivery. Polyzos et al. *(64)* suggested differences in tumor size as a possible reason for the different findings.

Using a rat model to study the penetration of cisplatin into intraperitoneal tumors, Los et al. *(65)* found that ip delivery gave a higher concentration in the periphery of tumors than iv delivery, with the advantage extending up to 1.5 mm inward. This suggests a limit on size of nodules for which drug can diffuse from the cavity into the tumor during the time that ip levels remain elevated. A molecule the size of cisplatin has a diffusivity in tissue about 2×10^{-6} cm^2/s, and would therefore take about 3 h to diffuse the distance of 1.5 mm. By comparison, the half-life of cisplatin in the peritoneal cavity is about 1.8 h *(66)*, and plasma drug concentration reaches significant levels within less than 1 h (because of capillary uptake; *65*).

An unresolved question is whether convection could have a significant role in transporting small-molecular-weight drugs (such as cisplatin) from the cavity to adjacent peritoneal metastases. If k represents a rate constant for drug uptake by capillaries and cells, the penetration distance resulting from diffusive transport scales as $(D/k)^{1/2}$ *(67)*.

Similarly it can be shown that the penetration distance from convection scales as u/k, where u is the fluid velocity. A fluid loss rate of 5 mL/h can be obtained in dialysis of 200–300 g rats *(68)*. Such rats have peritoneal surface area 450 cm^2 *(69)*, giving an approximate fluid velocity near the peritoneal surface of 3×10^{-6} cm/s. For a drug the size of cisplatin, diffusion results in much further penetration for this rate of fluid loss. However, higher convective flow rates could in principle be achieved by either increasing hydrostatic pressure inside the cavity, or infusing with hypotonic solution, which causes convective flow out of the cavity *(70)*. Tsujitani et al. *(71)* and Kondo et al. *(72)* found that cisplatin administered ip in hypotonic solutions enhanced therapeutic effect in a mouse model, but this was attributed to increased cellular uptake rather than tissue convection.

For larger drugs, convective transport outpaces diffusive transport in normal tissue *(73)*. However, the model of Baxter and Jain *(52)* predicts a convective current directed from the interior of a tumor nodule outward (because of the absence of lymphatics in the tumor to absorb fluid that has transported out of microvessels into tissue). The convective flow out of the cavity would have to be strong enough to overcome this current, which rises rapidly for tumors up to about 2 mm, and levels off around 7×10^{-6} cm/s for larger tumors (based on parameter values from [*52*]).

Intraperitoneal administration is referred to as a "regional" means of delivery, implying that drug reaches peritoneal metastases primarily through direct diffusion or convection from the peritoneal cavity rather than from the circulation. However, the outcome of ip delivery may also differ from that of iv delivery because it results in altered plasma pharmacokinetics. In the study of Los et al. *(65)*, the plasma AUC was approx the same for iv and ip administration, but the exposure was more prolonged for ip administration. As discussed in Subheading 2, the time-course of exposure may significantly alter cell kill, even for a fixed AUC.

6.2. Intraarterial Delivery

Intraarterial therapy is used extensively in Japan, especially for primary liver tumors, but appears to be less popular in the United States. Several early theoretical studies predicted benefits of intraarterial delivery *(74–77)*, but clinical trials did not match these expectations, as discussed by Dedrick *(78)*. A possible explanation, not mentioned by Dedrick *(78)*, is offered here. Theoretical studies to date have assumed that tumor cell kill is directly correlated either with plasma concentrations in the tumor microvascular bed, or with total tumor or tumor extracellular uptake. However, most chemotherapeutic drugs must enter tumor cells to be effective, and equilibration of intracellular with extracellular or plasma concentrations is not instantaneous. Intraarterial delivery is based on the premise of significant drug extraction on the first pass through the tumor microcirculatory bed, but the processes of cellular uptake—and for some drugs, extravasation and diffusion to the tumor cells—may take longer than the residence time of blood in the tumor microvasculature.

A consideration of time scales illustrates this. The time for circulation of plasma through the body is approx 1 min, and transit times through the microcirculation are approx 5–10 s. Small molecular weight chemotherapeutic drugs will be considered here since their case is the most favorable. Sufficient quantities of drug to supply the tissue surrounding each microvessel can transport across the vessel wall in 1–10 min (depending on whether vascular density is high or low), and can diffuse through the extracellular space to tumor cells most distant from microvessels in 1–26 min (depending again on vascular density) *(3)*. Equilibration of intracellular with extracellular drug concentrations takes hours for doxorubicin *(26)*, and over 20 min for melphalan and methotrexate *(79,80)*. Maximal accumulation of free intracellular 5-fluorouracil occurs within 200 s, but the drug continues to transport inside the cell subsequent to this, because of binding within the cell *(24)*. Based on these time scales, the intracellular concentration achieved on the first pass is probably small or negligible for the drugs mentioned above. Short-term high extracellular concentrations do not result in significant cell kill if the drug clears out of the extracellular space before it can be taken up by the cells *(53)*. These factors should be considered in studies *(12)* aiming to determine optimal infusion times for intraarterial delivery of various drugs. Future studies of intraarterial delivery should emphasize drugs that enter cells quickly.

6.3. Chemoembolization

Chemoembolization has been developed mainly for primary liver tumors *(81)* but also for liver metastases of other cancers. The premise is that simultaneous intraarterial delivery of the drug and an agent that occludes the supplying vessels results in regional delivery to the tumor. Occlusion has been accomplished with iodized oils or gelfoams, and also with microparticles of varying sizes. One clinical trial (Kato et al. [*81*]) used 225 µm particles, but smaller ones (10–30 µm [*82*]) have been developed in preclinical studies. Theoretical considerations of diffusion times indicate that such therapy is feasible only if the drug penetrates the entire microvasculature of the tumor bed, because even small molecular weight drugs cannot diffuse from arterioles to all the surrounding tissue in reasonable time. Particles of 225 µm size cannot enter capillaries, which generally have diameters of 8–30 microns. Even 10–30 µm particles cannot readily enter liver sinusoids, with a typical diameter of 7 µm. Further understanding of the effects of chemoembolization on microvascular flow is needed to predict the effect of such therapies, since even a small residual microvascular flow could strongly enhance drug distribution.

7. FUTURE DIRECTIONS AND CONCLUSIONS

Use of theoretical analyses for investigating and optimizing anticancer therapies is at an early stage. In addition to the topics discussed previously, many other effects will eventually have to be considered. The earlier discussion has focused on commonly used chemotherapeutic drugs, but other agents such as antibody immunoconjugates and prodrugs should be considered. A number of strategies have been developed, aimed at improving the effectiveness or delivery of anticancer drugs, including hyperthermia, agents that alter tumor blood flow, and agents that alter tumor oxygenation. The effect of these interventions on drug transport and on toxicity to both tumor and normal cells must be better understood in order to optimize their use with anticancer drugs. Tumors have special properties compared to most normal tissues, such as irregular vessel architecture, which can lead to heterogeneous drug delivery, poor oxygenation, low pH, and so on (Table 3 in ref. [*3*]). These properties can affect drug response and transport. In some cases, incorporation of these factors into theoretical models must await the availability of more complete experimental data.

Predictions of the optimal schedule and mode of administration of an anticancer drug require knowledge in three main areas: how cellular exposure affects response; what cellular exposure results from a certain therapy; and what host toxicity results from the therapy. This article has reviewed work on quantifying these three issues, as well as on the synthesis of these types of information into whole-body theoretical models that can be used to optimize therapies. Even the fundamental issue of how cellular exposure is related to growth inhibition is not well understood. Simplistic and sometimes misleading assumptions, such as that plasma AUC predicts antitumor response, continue to be made despite studies refuting them. More work remains to be done in many areas. Computational complexity associated with the models is not the main limiting factor. A major obstacle is lack of experimental data to quantify the various input functions and parameters needed for theoretical models. Relations between exposure, antitumor effect, and toxicity should be quantified in forms that are valid over the entire range of possible therapies. Where possible, experimental data should not be presented in forms that presuppose particular types of correlations, as this can severely limit the usefulness of the data. For example, data on cell kill should not be presented only in terms of its dependence on a single measure of drug exposure, such as AUC, peak concentration, or period above a given threshold. Data showing the dependence on both duration and intensity of exposure are much more useful.

Some researchers take the viewpoint that each individual cancer patient or tumor is so different from others, and that the parameters needed for optimizing drug therapy vary so widely, that a theoretical approach is useless. Nonetheless, the studies reviewed here suggest considerable scope for more rational choice of therapies if improved understanding of basic principles of drug delivery can be achieved. Progress is slowed by lack of communication between theoretical modelers and clinicians, even though such communication is increasingly needed. On the clinical side, therapies are becoming too complex to be understood solely by a trial-and-error approach. On the theoretical side, the utility of models is limited if they are based on poor assumptions, do not address relevant problems, or do not present their results in forms that clinicians can use. It is hoped that this article will help to facilitate the interaction of theoretical modelers and clinicians in this area, with the ultimate goal of developing improved anticancer drug therapies.

ACKNOWLEDGMENTS

This work was supported by NSF Grant 0074985 and NIH Grant CA40355.

REFERENCES

1. Jain RK. Barriers to drug delivery in solid tumors. *Sci Am* 1994; 271(1):58–65.
2. Jain RK. Delivery of molecular and cellular medicine to solid tumors. *Science* 1997; 271(5252): 1079–1080.
3. El-Kareh AW, Secomb TW. Theoretical models for drug delivery to solid tumors. *Crit Rev Biomed Engin* 1997; 25(6):503–571.
4. Walker MC. Intravesical chemotherapy: in vitro studies on the relationship between dose and cytotoxicity. *Urol Res* 1986; 14:137–140.
5. Erlichman C, Vidgen D, Wu A. Antineoplastic drug cytotoxicity in a human bladder cancer cell line: implications for intravesical chemotherapy. *Urol Res* 1987; 15:13–16.
6. Ozawa S, Sugiyama Y, Mitsuhashi Y, Kobayashi T, Inaba M. Cell killing action of cell cycle phase-non-specific antitumor agents is dependent on concentration-time product. *Cancer Chemother Pharmacol* 1988; 21(3):185–190.
7. Kurihara N, Kubota T, Hoshiya Y, Otani Y, Kumai K, Kitajima M. Antitumor activity of cis-diamminedichloroplatinum (II) depends on its time x concentration product against human gastric cancer cell lines in vitro. *J Surg Oncol* 1995; 60(4):238–241.

8. Nozue M, Nishida M, Todoroki T, Fukao K, Tanaka M. Selection of three out of 24 anti-cancer agents in poorly-differentiated gastric cancer cell lines, evaluated by the AUC/ΔIC_{50} ratio. *Anticancer Drugs* 1995; 6:291–302.
9. Los G, Verdegaal E, Hub PJM, et al. Cellular pharmacokinetics of carboplatin and cisplatin in relation to their cytotoxic action. *Biochem Pharmacol* 1991; 42(2):357–363.
10. Troger V, Fischel JL, Formento P, Gioanni J, Milano G. Effects of prolonged exposure to cisplatin on cytotoxicity and intracellular drug concentration. *Eur J Cancer* 1992; 28(1):82–86.
11. Eichholtz-Wirth H, Hietel B. The relationship between cisplatin sensitivity and drug uptake into mammalian cells in vitro. *Br J Cancer* 1986; 54:239–243.
12. Link KH, Leder G, Pillasch J, et al. In vitro concentration response studies and in vitro Phase II tests as the experimental basis for regional chemotherapeutic protocols. *Sem Surg Oncol* 1998; 14:189–201.
13. Nguyen-Ngoc T, Vrignaud P, Robert J. Cellular pharmacokinetics of doxorubicin in cultured mouse sarcoma cells originating from autochthonous tumors. *Oncology* 1984; 41:55–60.
14. Eichholtz H, Trott KR. Effect of methotrexate concentration and exposure time on mammalian cell survival in vitro. *Br J Cancer* 1980; 41(2):277–284.
15. Schmittgen TD, Wientjes MG, Badalament RA, Au JLS. Pharmacodynamics of mitomycin C in cultured human bladder tumors. *Cancer Res* 1991; 51:3849–3856.
16. Slee PHThJ, de Bruijn EA, Leeflang P, Kuppen PJK, van den Berg L, van Oosterom AT. Variations in exposure to mitomycin C in an in vitro colony-forming assay. *Br J Cancer* 1986; 54:951–955.
17. Barlogie B, Drewinko B. Lethal and cytokinetic effects of mitomycin C on cultured human colon cancer cells. *Cancer Res* 1980; 40:1973–1980.
18. Millenbaugh NJ, Wientjes MG, Au JSL. A pharmacodynamic analysis method to determine the relative importance of drug concentration and treatment time on effect. *Cancer Chemother Pharmacol* 2000; 45:265–272.
19. Baguley BC, Finlay GJ. Pharmacokinetic/cytokinetic principles in the chemotherapy of solid tumours. *Clin Exp Pharmacol Physiol* 1995; 22(11):825–828.
20. Rupniak HT, Whelan RDH, Hill BT. Concentration and time-dependent inter-relationships for antitumour drug cytotoxicities against tumour cells in vitro. *Int J Cancer* 1983; 32:7–12.
21. Hill BT, Whelan RDH, Rupniak HT, Dennis LY, Rosholt MA. A comparative assessment of the in vitro effects of drugs on cells by means of colony assays of flow microfluorimetry. *Cancer Chemother Pharmacol* 1981; 7:21–26.
22. Levasseur LM, Slocum HK, Rustum YM, Greco WR. Modeling of the time-dependency of in vitro drug cytotoxicity and resistance. *Cancer Res* 1998; 58:5749–5761.
23. Matsushima Y, Kanzawa F, Hoshi A, et al. Time-schedule dependence of the inhibiting activity of various anticancer drugs in the clonogenic assay. *Cancer Chemother Pharmacol* 1985; 14:104–107.
24. Chabner BA, Longo DL. *Cancer Chemotherapy and Biotherapy.* 2nd ed. Lippincott-Raven, New York, 1996.
25. Gardner SN. A mechanistic, predictive model of dose-response curves for cell cycle phase-specific and -nonspecific drugs. *Cancer Res* 2000; 60:1417–1425.
26. Kerr DJ, Kerr AM, Freshney RI, Kaye SB. Comparative intracellular uptake of adriamycin and 4'-deoxydoxorubicin by non-small cell lung tumor cells in culture and its relationship to cell survival. *Biochem Pharmacol* 1986; 35:2817–2823.
27. Gerwitz DA. A critical evaluation of the mechanisms of action proposed for the antitumor effects of the anthracycline antibiotics adriamycin and daunorubicin. *Biochem Pharmacol* 1999; 57:727–741.
28. Sadoff L. Overwhelming 5-fluorouracil toxicity in patients whose diabetes is poorly controlled. *Am J Clin Oncol* 1998; 21(6):605–607.
29. Balis FM, Holcenberg JS, Bleyer WA. Clinical pharmacokinetics of commonly used anticancer drugs. *Clin Pharmacokinet* 1983; 8:202–232.
30. Legha SS, Benjamin RS, Mackay B, et al. Reduction of doxorubicin cardiotoxicity by prolonged continuous intravenous infusion. *Ann Intern Med* 1982; 96:133–139.
31. Duffull SB, Robinson BA. Clinical pharmacokinetics and dose optimisation of carboplatin. *Clin Pharmacokinet* 1997; 33(3):161–183.
32. Groen HJM, van der Leest AHD, de Vries, EGE, Uges DRA, Szabo BG, Mulder NH. Continuous carboplatin infusion during 6 weeks' radiotherapy in locally inoperable non-small-cell lung cancer: a phase I and pharmacokinetic study. *Br J Cancer* 1995; 72:992–997.
33. Dhodapkar MV, Richardson RL, Reid JM, Ames MM. Pyrazine diazohydroxide (NSC-361456). Phase I clinical and pharmacokinetic studies. *Invest New Drugs* 1994; 12(3):207–216.

34. Stewart CF, Baker SD, Heideman RL, Jones D, Crom WR, Pratt CB. Clinical pharmacodynamics of continuous infusion topotecan in children: systematic exposure predicts hematological toxicity. *J Clin Oncol* 1994; 12(9):1946–1954.
35. Kobayashi K, Jodrell DI, Ratain MJ. Pharmacodynamic-pharmacokinetic relationships and therapeutic drug monitoring. *Cancer Surv* 1993; 17:51–78.
36. Nagai N, Kinoshita M, Ogata H, et al. Relationship between pharmacokinetics of unchanged cisplatin and nephrotoxicity after intravenous infusions of cisplatin to cancer patients. *Cancer Chemother Pharmacol* 1996; 39:131–137.
37. Kelsen DP, Alcock N, Young CW. Cisplatin nephrotoxicity. Correlation with plasma platinum concentrations. *Am J Clin Oncol* 1985; 8:77–80.
38. Vora J, Boroujerdi M. Pharmacokinetic-toxicodynamic relationships of adriamycin in rat: prediction of butylated hydroxyanisole-mediated reduction in anthracycline cardiotoxicity. *J Pharm Pharmacol* 1996; 48:1264–1269.
39. Greco FA. Etoposide: seeking the best dose and schedule. *Sem Oncol* 1992; 19:59–63.
40. Danesi R, Conte PF, Del Tacca M. Pharmacokinetic optimisation of treatment schedules for anthracycline and paclitaxel in patients with cancer. *Clin Pharmacokin* 1999; 37(3):195–211.
41. Lokich J, Anderson N. Dose intensity for bolus versus infusion chemotherapy administration: review of the literature for 27 anti-neoplastic agents. *Ann Oncol* 1997; 8:15–25.
42. Lorenz M, Heinrich S, Staib-Sebler E, et al. Relevance of locoregional chemotherapy in patients with liver metastases from colorectal primaries. *Swiss Surg* 2000; 6(1):11–22.
43. Hansen RM, Ryan L, Anderson T, et al. Phase III study of bolus versus infusion fluorouracil with or without cisplatin in advanced colorectal cancer. *J Natl Cancer Inst* 1996; 88(10):668–674.
44. Skipper HE. The effects of chemotherapy on the kinetics of leukemic cell behavior. *Cancer Res* 1965; 25:1544–1550.
45. Bischoff KB, Dedrick R, Zaharko DS, Longstreth JA. Methotrexate pharmacokinetics. *J Pharm Sci* 1971; 60(8):1128–1133.
46. Collins JM, Dedrick RL, King FG, Speyer JL, Myers CE. Nonlinear pharmacokinetic models for 5-fluorouracil in man: intravenous and intraperitoneal routes. *Clin Pharmacol Ther* 1980; 28(2):235–246.
47. Farris FF, Dedrick RL, King FG. Cisplatin pharmacokinetics: applications of a physiological model. *Toxicol Lett* 1998; 43:117–137.
48. Panetta JC. A mathematical model of breast and ovarian cancer treated with paclitaxel. *Math Biosci* 1997; 146:89–113.
49. Jackson TL, Byrne HM. A mathematical model to study the effects of drug resistance and vasculature on the response of solid tumors to chemotherapy. *Math Biosci* 2000; 164:17–38.
50. Iliadis A, Barbolosi D. Optimizing drug regimens in cancer chemotherapy by an efficacy-toxicity mathematical model. *Comput Biomed Res* 2000; 33:211–226.
51. Steel GG. *Growth Kinetics of Tumors: Cell Population Kinetics in Relation to the Growth and Treatment of Cancer.* Clarendon, Oxford, 1977.
52. Baxter LT, Jain RK. Transport of fluid and macromolecules in tumors. I. Role of interstitial pressure and convection. *Microvasc Res* 1989; 37:77–104.
53. El-Kareh AW, Secomb TW. A mathematical model for comparison of bolus injection, continuous infusion, and liposomal delivery of doxorubicin to tumor cells. *Neoplasia* 2000; 2(4):325–338.
54. Durand RE, Olive PL. Flow cytometry studies of intracellular adriamycin in single cells in vitro. *Cancer Res* 1981; 41:3489–3494.
55. Walkman P. Infusional anthracyclines: is slower better? If so, why? *Ann Oncol* 1992; 3(8):591–594.
56. Au JL-S, Li D, Gan Y, et al. Pharmacodynamics of immediate and delayed effects of paclitaxel: role of slow apoptosis and intracellular drug retention. *Cancer Res* 1998; 58:2141–2148.
57. Lankelma J, Fernandez Luque R, Dekker H, Schinkel W, Pinedo HM. A mathematical model of drug transport in human breast cancer. *Microvasc Res* 2000; 59:149–161.
58. Subramanian B, Claudius JS. Effect of intravenous drug administration mode on drug distribution in a tumor slab: a finite Fourier transform analysis. *J Theor Biol* 1990; 143:55–76.
59. Allen TM. Liposomes: opportunities in drug delivery. *Drugs* 1997; 54Suppl 4:8–14.
60. Tsuchihashi M, Harashima H, Kiwada H. Development of a pharmacokinetic/pharmacodynamic (PK/PD)-simulation system for doxorubicin in long circulating liposomes in mice using peritoneal P388. *J Controlled Release* 1999; 61:9–19.
61. Harashima H, Iida S, Urakami Y, Tsuchihashi M, Kiwada H. Optimization of antitumor effect of liposomally encapsulated doxorubicin based on simulations by pharmacokinetic/pharmacodynamic modeling. *J Controlled Release* 1999; 61:93–106.

62. Kirmani S, Braly PS, McClay EF, et al. A comparison of intravenous versus intraperitoneal chemotherapy for the initial treatment of ovarian cancer. *Gynecol Oncol* 1994; 54(3):338–344.
63. Alberts DS, Liu PY, Hannigan EV, et al. Intraperitoneal cisplatin plus intravenous cyclophosphamide versus intravenous cisplatin plus intravenous cyclophosphamide for Stage III ovarian cancer. *N Engl J Med* 1996; 335:1950–1955.
64. Polyzos A, Tsavaris N, Kosmas C, et al. A comparative study of intraperitoneal carboplatin versus intravenous carboplatin with intravenous cyclophosphamide in both arms as initial chemotherapy for Stage III ovarian cancer. *Oncology* 1999; 56:291–296.
65. Los G, Mutsaers PHA, van der Vijgh WJF, Baldew GS, de Graaf PW, McVie JG. Direct diffusion of cis-diamminedichloroplatinum(II) in intraperitoneal rat tumors after intraperitoneal chemotherapy: a comparison with systemic chemotherapy. *Cancer Res* 1989; 49:3380–3384.
66. O'Dwyer PJ, LaCreta FP, Daugherty JP, et al. Phase I pharmacokinetic study of intraperitoneal etoposide. *Cancer Res* 1991; 51(8):2041–2046.
67. Dedrick RL, Flessner MF. Pharmacokinetic problems in peritoneal drug administration: tissue penetration and surface exposure. *J Natl Cancer Inst* 1997; 89:480–487.
68. Flessner MF, Schwab A. Pressure threshold for fluid loss from the peritoneal cavity. *Am J Physiol* 1996; 270:F377–F390.
69. Kuzlan M, Pawlaczyk K, Wieczorowska-Tobis K, Korybalska K, Breborowicz A, Oreopoulos DG. Peritoneal surface area and its permeability in rats. *Perit Dial Int* 1997; 17:295–300.
70. Stephen RL, Novak JM, Jensen EM, Kablitz C, Buys SS. Effect of osmotic pressure on uptake of chemotherapeutic agents by carcinoma cells. *Cancer Res* 1990; 50:4704–4708.
71. Tsujitani S, Oka A, Kondo A, et al. Administration in a hypotonic solution is preferable to dose escalation in intraperitoneal cisplatin chemotherapy for peritoneal carcinomatosis in rats. *Oncology* 1999; 57:77–82.
72. Kondo A, Maeta M, Oka A, Tsujitani S, Ikeguchi M, Kaibara N. Hypotonic intraperitoneal cisplatin chemotherapy for peritoneal carcinomatosis in mice. *Br J Cancer* 1996; 73(10):1166–1170.
73. Flessner MF, Dedrick RL. Monoclonal antibody delivery to intraperitoneal tumors in rats: effects of route of administration and intraperitoneal solution osmolality. *Cancer Res* 1994; 54:4376–4384.
74. Collins JM. Pharmacologic rationale for regional drug delivery. *J Clin Oncol* 1984; 2(5):498–504.
75. Eckman WW, Patlak CS, Fenstermacher JD. A critical evaluation of the principles governing the advantages of intra-arterial infusions. *J Pharmacokin Biopharm* 1974; 2(3):257–285.
76. Fenstermacher JD, Cowles AL. Theoretic limitations of intracarotid infusions in brain tumor chemotherapy. *Cancer Treatment Rep* 1977; 61(4):519–526.
77. Chen HSG, Gross JF. Intra-arterial infusion of anti-cancer drugs: theoretic aspects of drug delivery and review of responses. *Cancer Treatment Rep* 1980; 64(1):31–40.
78. Dedrick RL. Arterial drug infusion: pharmacokinetic problems and pitfalls. *J Natl Cancer Inst* 1988; 80(2):84–89.
79. Begleiter A, Froese EK, Goldenberg GJ. A comparison of melphalan transport in human breast cancer cells and lymphocytes in vitro. *Cancer Lett* 1980; 10:243–251.
80. Sirotnak FM, Donsbach RC. Kinetic correlates of methotrexate transport and therapeutic responsiveness in murine tumors. *Cancer Res* 1976; 36:1151–1158.
81. Kato T, Sato K, Sasaki R, Kakinuma H, Moriyama M. Targeted cancer chemotherapy with arterial microcapsule chemoembolization: review of 1013 patients. *Cancer Chemother Pharmacol* 1996; 37:289–296.
82. Willmott N, Chen Y, Goldberg J, Mcardle C, Florence AT. Biodegradation rate of embolized protein microspheres in lung, liver and kidney of rats. *J Pharm Pharmacol* 1989; 41(7):433–438.

II TECHNOLOGIES AVAILABLE FOR USE IN CANCER DRUG DELIVERY SYSTEMS

Biopolymers for Parenteral Drug Delivery in Cancer Treatment

Wolfgang Friess, PhD

CONTENTS

1. INTRODUCTION

Traditional chemotherapy treats tumors by systemic treatment via parenteral or oral application, by intratumoral injection, or by interstitial placement of drugs. New drug delivery systems can be used for local delivery to reduce side effects, to improve the bioavailability, or to target specific sites. Most of these specifically designed dosage forms in cancer treatment are based on polymeric materials to control the release of the active agent via dissolution, matrix erosion and degradation, diffusion, or cleavage of prodrugs. The focus of this chapter is on parenteral biodegradable carrier systems, which present a main form of drug delivery or targeting in local or systemic chemotherapy. Enhanced local drug retention at the tumor site can be achieved by administration of drug-loaded monolithic polymer implants of different shapes, microparticles, or a polymeric gel vehicle. In addition, chemoembolization provides higher local therapeutic concentrations. The expression chemoembolization connotes a bipartite anticancer effect through occlusion of the tumor vascular bed via metal coils, ethanol, glues, or particulate systems *(1)* coupled with cytotoxic drug administration either via embolization followed by chemotherapy or embolization with microparticulate drug delivery systems *(2,3)*. In systemic chemotherapy, biomaterials can also be used for sustained-release formulations that yield steady drug levels and avoid side effects caused by toxic peaks or for dosage forms that allow drugs to selectively lodge

From: *Drug Delivery Systems in Cancer Therapy*
Edited by: D. M. Brown © Humana Press Inc., Totowa, NJ

in tumors. Furthermore, prodrugs based on a drug attached to a polymer are utilized, which liberate the active drug in vivo through an enzymatic or chemical cleavage process. This bioreversible polymeric modification can result in enhanced permeability retention in tumor tissue *(4)*, a change in the in vivo drug distribution *(5)*, and alteration of the drug pharmacokinetics *(6)*, as well as selective activation in target cells *(7)*.

The development of new biomaterials represents a key to successful drug delivery, and many researchers are engaged in devising polymeric materials based on new chemical entities, tailoring degradation properties, improving compatibility, evaluating new composites or organic/inorganic hybrid materials, and optimizing drug release profiles. A broad spectrum of synthetic polymers has been designed for cancer treatment, ranging from polyvinyl alcohol, polyanhydrides, poly-α-hydroxyacids, and cyanoacrylates, to polyorthoesters. In contrast to this, synthetic approach scientists also look to nature as a source for macromolecules. The natural materials used for drug delivery can generally be classified based on their chemical character into proteinous materials such as collagen, gelatin, or albumin and carbohydrates such as chitosan, hyaluronic acid, or starch. These materials of biological origin frequently claim to be relatively safer and more biocompatible, readily available, relatively inexpensive, and capable of a multitude of chemical modifications. However, the pros and cons of each natural material have to be weighed individually. This chapter will evaluate the properties and applications of biopolymers in cancer treatment.

2. COLLAGEN

A variety of proteinous biomaterials have been described for local drug delivery in cancer treatment (Table 1) with collagen, gelatin, albumin, and fibrin being the most thoroughly investigated materials. Most synthetic polymers represent mixtures of chains with variable length composed of repeating units. They show physical and chemical properties that are, to a considerable extent, determined by polymerization steps. In contrast, proteins have a specific amino acid sequence, molecular weight, and structure, all of which define their basic qualities as a biomaterial suitable for medical products.

2.1. Chemical and Biological Properties

Collagen comprises a family of more than 20 genetically distinct molecules that are constructed from three polypeptide chains, each consisting of more than 1000 amino acids. Here, the discussion will be limited to collagen type I, which is the chief structural protein of tendon, bone, and skin with only minor differences in its amino acid sequences between vertebrate species *(8)*. Most collagenous biomaterials are based on this type. Its primary sequence is characterized by glycine as every third amino acid allowing for close package into a helix (Fig. 1A). Approximately one-fourth of the sequence is occupied by proline and hydroxyproline, which stiffen the triple helix because of their alicyclic nature, forming hydrogen bonds that limit rotation *(9)*. As a secondary arrangement, the chains represent left-handed helices (Fig. 1B) and on the third level three polypeptide chains intertwine to form a right-handed triple helix with an average molecular weight of approx 300 kD, a length of 300 nm, and a diameter of 1.5 nm (Fig. 1C). In addition, short telopeptide regions at both ends of the molecule are not incorporated into the helical structure. On the fourth level of order, the triple helical molecules are staggered into fibrils of 10 to 500 nm in diameter depending on the type

Table 1
Amino Acid Composition of Type I Collagen from Calfskin[a]

Amino Acid	α(I)-Chain	α2(I)-Chain
alanine	124 (2)	111 (3)
arginine	53 (2)	56 (1)
asparagine	13	23
aspartic acid	33 (3)	24 (2)
glutamic acid	52 (2)	46 (2)
glutamine	27 (3)	24 (1)
glycine	345 (6)	346 (6)
histidine	3 (1)	8
hydroxylysine	4	9
hydroxyproline	114	99
isoleucine	9 (1)	18
leucine	22 (3)	33
lysine	34 (2)	21 (1)
methionine	7	4
phenylalanine	13 (1)	15 (3)
proline	127 (4)	108 (1)
serine	37 (5)	35 (1)
threonine	17 (1)	20
tyrosine	5 (5)	4 (3)
valine	17 (1)	34
TOTAL	1056 (42)	1038 (24)

[a] The values in parentheses are the residues contributed by the non-helical telopeptide regions (data from Piez, 1985).

of tissue and developmental stage (Fig. 1D) *(10)*. This packaging of the triple helices provides tensile strength and resilience to collagen fibers. Further mechanical and chemical stability derives from intra- and intermolecular crosslinks.

Probably as a result of its function as the primary structural protein in the body, collagen is peculiarly resistant to attacks by neutral proteases. At neutral pH, only specific collagenases assisted by elastase and cathepsins cleave the native helix *(11)*. Once the triple helix is split, the collagen molecule is further degraded by gelatinases and nonspecific proteinases. Activation of macrophages has been shown to cause a pH decrease *(12)* and together with the excretion of cathepsin *(13)* this creates an acidic path for collagen breakdown. In vitro the degradation is usually simulated by incubation with bacterial collagenase, cathepsin, pepsin, or trypsin.

Cattle are the main source for collagen. In addition to porcine, equine, ovine, and marine collagen varieties, recombinant human collagen expressed in *Escherichia coli* or derived from transgenic animals have been described *(10)*. An alternative offers autologous collagen material *(14)*. Collagen is known for excellent biocompatibility caused by low toxicity and mild antigenicity *(15,16)*. Bovine collagen poses the risk of bovine spongiform encephalopathy (BSE) or transmissible spongiform encephalopathy (TSE) contamination, which has to be evaluated based on the country of origin and animal environment, the starting material, risk-reducing procedures during manufacturing such as alkali treatment, the amount of animal raw material required to produce the daily dose, the number of daily doses, and the route of administration *(17,18)*. The

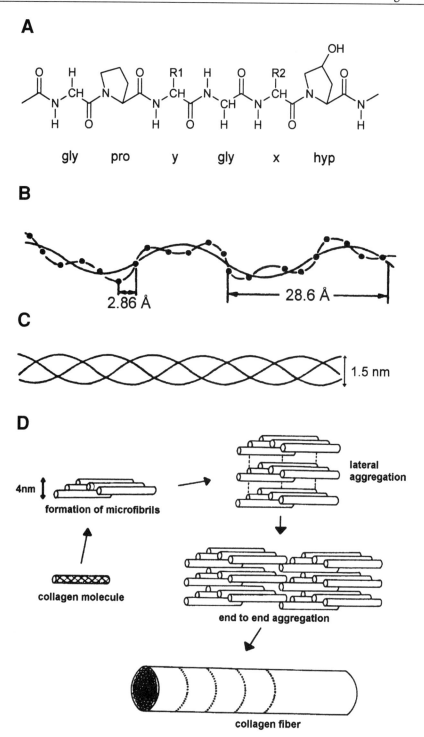

Fig. 1. Chemical structure of collagen type I: (**A**) *primary* amino acid sequence. (**B**) *secondary* left-handed helix. (**C**) triplehelical *tertiary* arrangement. (**D**) staggered *quaternary* structure (with permission from Friess, 2000).

most commonly used extraction media are neutral salt solution or dilute acid *(19)*, which dissolve freshly synthesized and negligibly crosslinked collagen molecules. Dilute acidic solvents are more efficient because labile intermolecular crosslinks are dissociated *(20)*. These solubilized collagen molecules can be reconstituted into large fibrils by adjusting pH or temperature of the solution. The remaining insoluble collagen can be further disintegrated by alkali *(21)* or enzyme treatment *(9)* to cleave additional crosslinks and truncate the nonhelical telopeptide regions. Instead of disintegration and transfer into soluble material, extensively crosslinked collagen can be dispersed as fibrillar suspensions after chemical and mechanical fragmentation, usually at acidic pH. In additional steps, collagen can be subjected to chemical modifications such as succinylation, acetylation, methylation, mineralization, grafting of polymers, or attachment of molecules via biotinylation *(10)*.

Owing to dissociation of natural crosslinks in the course of the aforementioned isolation processes, reconstituted forms of collagen can lack sufficient strength and resistance to biodegradation. This can be compensated by the introduction of exogenous crosslinking. Chromium or aluminum tanning results in formation of ionic bonds *(22)*. Covalent crosslinks in collagen can be created by various organic reagents such as formaldehyde, glutaraldehyde, hexamethylenediisocyanate or polyepoxy reagents, preferably with the ε-amino groups of lysine and hydroxylysine residues *(23)*. Albeit approved for medical devices, general concerns arise from cytotoxicity due to primary release of extractables and secondary degradation and monomer release *(24–27)*. Crosslinking with water soluble carbodiimides or via acyl azide intermediate formation offers the advantage that this only facilitates the formation of amide bonds without becoming part of the actual linkage, and the material is well tolerated *(28,29)*. Dehydrothermal treatment (e.g., at 110°C and 50 mtorr for a few days) and UV irradiation results in both additional crosslinking and partial denaturation *(30,31)*. Sterility of the material can be achieved by aseptic processing or sterile filtration of soluble collagen. Ethylene oxide gas treatment leads to little denaturation, but it reacts with amino groups, causes decrease in helix stability, and changes enzymatic degradation rate *(32)*. In contrast, both γ-irradiation and dry heat induce chain scission and crosslinks simultaneously *(33,34)*.

Collagen has found broad use in medical practice as aqueous injectable solutions or dispersion or dried into a variety of forms such as sheets, tubes, sponges, and powders *(35)*. Attempts have been made to apply these systems for drug delivery in ophthalmology or tissue engineering. Successful uses in cancer treatment are injectable gels for intratumoral injection, injectable collagen rods, and chemoembolization using collagen materials.

2.2. Anticancer Application of Collagen

2.2.1. AQUEOUS INJECTABLES FOR INTRATUMORAL DELIVERY

Collagen gels are primarily used for subcutaneous (sc) injection for the repair of dermatological defects. For this application, crosslinking with GTA can be used to reduce the rate of biodegradation. The biological response is characterized by fibroblast invasion, neovascularization and little, if any, evidence of inflammation *(36)*. Calcification was found and certain areas were undergoing ossification which identified a potential complication in various treatment modalities. Hyaluronic acid, polymers such as dextran, and small molecules such as maltose can be used as lubricants to improve the ease of intrusion into soft tissue *(37,38)*. The delivery of small molecules via injectable collagen preparations is pursued emphatically under the aspect of intratumoral cytostatica injection. Typically, not more than 12% of a systemically applied dose reaches the tumor, with the remainder distributed to healthy tissues all over the body, resulting in side effects. Injection of drug solution directly into solid tumors has not been successful because the drug levels in the tumor drop off rapidly and are typically cleared within 20–30 min after injection. Matrix Pharmaceutical, Inc. (technology now owned by Chiron Corporation), investigated two gels based on approx 2% bovine collagen and 0.1% epinephrine loaded with either CDDP or 5-FU. The CDDP/epinephrine system was studied in Phase III clinical trials for treatment of head-and-neck cancer and other solid tumors such as metastatic breast cancer, esophageal cancer, or malignant melanoma, and in Phase II studies in treatment of liver tumors both primary and metastatic *(39)*. Prior to application, the formulation is prepared by combination of a CDDP/epinephrine preparation and a bovine collagen dispersion via syringe-to-syringe mixing *(40)*.

The system resulted in 8.4-fold increase in intratumoral concentration of 5-FU 30 min postinjection and a 7–9-fold increase in the local AUC when compared with a local injection of drug solution tested in a human pancreatic cancer xenograft model in mice (Fig. 2) *(40,41)*. It is important to note that the effect can be attributed to both the collagen network and the effect of the vasoconstrictor epinephrine, which temporarily reduces the local body fluid supply (Fig. 3) *(42)*. In vitro, 50% was released after 4 h and 80% after 24 h from 5-FU gel *(43)*. In patients with malignant tumors of various types repeated intratumoral injection was performed for 4 wk with an initial dose of 1 mg CDDP per cm^3 tumor volume, with escalation to 6 mg CDDP per cm^3 allowed. The overall tumor response rate was 50%, with 40% of these complete responses *(44)*. The CDDP/epinephrine gel treatments were generally well tolerated in the clinical trials and no nephro-, neuro-, or ototoxic effects were reported *(44,45)*.

The collagen gel loaded with 5-FU has been tested in Phase I/II studies for treatment of tumors in the chest wall from advanced or recurrent breast cancer. It was applied shortly prior to radiation treatment and the combination resulted in more severe damage to tumor cells than radiation alone or 5-FU in solution administered intravenously with or without radiation treatment. Thus, the formulation is considered a radiopotentiator. The matrix with 5-FU has also proved to be highly effective in studies against superficial squamous cell carcinoma with 96% complete tumor clearing *(45)*, basal cell carcinoma with 91% complete tumor resolution *(46)*, and condylomata acuminata with 77% complete response *(47,42)*. Intratumoral administration of 4 mg/mL CDDP using the collagen/epinephrine-gel into a murine SCCVII squamous cell carcinoma model resulted in an average tumor growth delay time of 1.5 ± 2.8 d, approximately six times longer than CDDP suspension applied intratumorally or intraperitoneally. When combined with a single dose radiation of 10 gy, CDDP in the collagen matrix was 2.0–3.6-fold more effective than when administered as intratumoral suspension or intraperitoneal (ip) solution *(48)*.

The collagen gel conveying CDDP provides advantage after perinephric VX-2 tumor resection bed injection in rabbits. The matrix prevented tumor recurrence in all animals and led to a significant increase in local CDDP levels at days 1, 4, 20, and 7 *(49)*. The system may also allow for improvement in the therapeutic index of radioimmunotherapy. As a study with ^{111}In or ^{90}Y attached to monoclonal antibodies demonstrated, the use of the collagen system markedly enriched the radioisotopes in tumors,

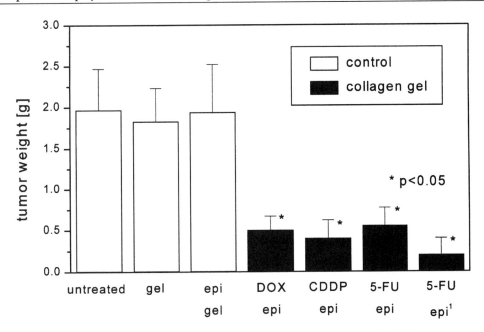

Fig. 2. Effects of intratumorally administered collagen/epinephrin gels on BxPC-3 human pancreatic tumor weight in athymic mice (8 mg/kg doxorubicin, 8 mg/kg cisplatin or 60 mg/kg 5-fluorouracil) at day 28 after the first treatment (injection on Days 1 and 4; [1] injection on days 1, 4, 8, and 12) (modified from Smith et al., 1995)—a second study demonstrated no effect of 5-FU solution injected intratumorally.

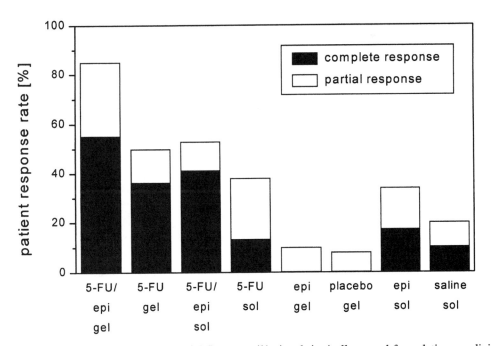

Fig. 3. Contribution of components of 5-fluorouracil/epinephrine/collagen gel formulation on clinical efficacy after intralesional injection in condylomata acuminata in human (modified from Swinehart et al., 1997b).

enhanced the antitumor efficacy, and reduced systemic toxicity when compared with systemic administration *(50)*. Application of the CDDP collagen/epinephrine gel also improved the treatment of advanced head-and-neck cancer by intratumoral injection followed by interstitial laser hyperthermia *(51)*. Combination chemotherapy using both 5-FU and CDDP gels has also been tested and proved to be more effective than both drugs given intraperitoneally or application of either drug alone. Treatment sequences starting with 5-FU were superior in delaying tumor growth when compared with courses initiated with CDDP gel *(43)*.

In order to diffusionally control the release rate of a drug that is soluble in the aqueous collagen matrix it is necessary that the mesh size of the protein fiber network approach the size of the drug molecule *(52)*. Fibrillar collagen matrices were capable of moderating the release rates of fibrinogen (mol wt, 340 kD) only and a significant non-fibrillar content was necessary to modulate the diffusivity of smaller proteins such as chymotrypsinogen (mol wt, 23 kD). Drug release from collagen gels can also be affected by interactions with collagen and the release of positively charged lysozyme (mol wt, 14 kD; isoelectrical point, approx 11.0) could be further reduced by an increase in negative net charge of the native collagen molecules by succinylation *(53)*. Low apparent diffusivities of lysozyme from collagen matrices were not only because of electrostatic interactions, but also hydrophobic interactions *(54)*. It is important to note that the source of collagen material plays a crucial role for the binding capacity of collagen as a result of differences in amino acid composition and isoelectrical point. The viability of adsorption/desorption and subsequent diffusion as a release mechanism was also evaluated for gentamicin *(53)*. Owing to small size and, hence, large diffusion coefficients of the antibiotic, as well as its high water solubility, a prolonged release cannot be obtained by simple Fickian diffusion or interactions with collagen. Consequently, cytostatica retention in the collagen matrices presents more of a mechanical effect of the intact gel formulation forming a three-dimensional depot as compared to a liquid that spreads rapidly. Rapid diffusion of water-soluble compounds or slower dissolution for drugs which are insoluble in the gel matrix should be decisive.

Thus, the collagen gel system is designed to be used with a variety of cancer treatment modalities. It focuses high drug concentrations for hours to days in solid tumors, increases the exposure of the cancer cells to the chemotherapeutic agent to allow more cancer cells to be attacked during their vulnerable stage of growth and replication, and limits total body confrontation with the cytotoxic agent.

2.2.2. Dense Collagen Matrices

For local treatment of soft tissue and bony tumors, the use of a collagen sponge was suggested by Stemberger *(55)*. Collagen sponges were originally developed as wound dressings and hemostats. They are used in combination with growth factors for tissue repair *(56,57)* and with antibiotics in the treatment and prophylaxis of soft tissue infections *(58)*. Drug release occurs rapidly because of minimal hindrance of diffusion but the liberation of mitoxantrone in vitro could be sustained for several days with different poly(α)-hydroxyester coatings *(55)*. Dense collagen films can be formed by air-drying casted collagen preparation. Their main biomaterial application is as barrier membranes. These systems exhibit substantial swelling and rapid release of low and high molecular weight drug compounds within several hours in vitro *(59)*. Introduction of exogenous crosslinks yields reduction in swelling and enclosure of macromolecular

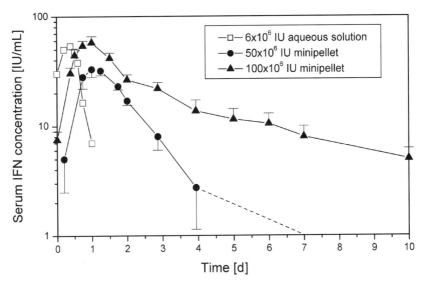

Fig. 4. Interferon-α serum concentration in healthy volunteers after subcutaneous administration of interferon-α minipellet and aqueous solution (modified from Fujioka et al., 1998).

compounds in the fibrous matrix network. Concomitantly, crosslinking reduces the rate of degradation and the dense crosslinked collagen systems are characterized by diffusional release of a fraction of the loaded drug as systems swell, followed by liberation of the proportion mechanically entrapped in the devices as cleavage of the matrix proceeds. In mice, significant activity of an immunostimulating extract from Mycobacterium bovis (bacille Calmette-Guérin; BCG vaccine) against S180 murine sarcoma cells was sustained for at least 32 h after sc insertion *(60)*. The systems activated a pronounced cellular response and an almost complete resorption of the carrier system after 14 d. In order to tailor the release profile, several collagen layers can be laminated *(61)*.

Besides films, injectable drug-loaded collagen rods approx 1 mm in diameter and 10–15 mm length, called minipellets, have been tested intensively. The systems are prepared by extrusion of a highly concentrated (up to 30%) gel of atelocollagen without further crosslinking or modification *(15)*. The starting material is obtained by solubilization through pepsin treatment, resulting in removal of telopeptide moieties and reduced immunogenicity. Initial investigations demonstrated only rather short-release periods for low-molecular weight drugs such as 5-FU after sc injection *(62)*. However, the results achieved with interferon-α (IFN) and interleukin 2 (IL-2) are very promising. Most currently available IFN preparations must be administered intramuscularly several times per week because of the rapid elimination of IFN from the body. After sc injection of the minipellet system, an initial-burst phenomenon was suppressed and adequate plasma levels of IFN were sustained for more than 1 wk (Fig. 4) *(15,63)*. In contrast, the plasma level peaked 30 min after injection of the aqueous solution and after 48 h the detection limit was reached. The in vitro and in vivo release profile depends on various processing parameters such as gel concentration prior to drying and the drying process itself *(64)*. After a short lag phase, the release can be explained by the infiltration of water and swelling of the system over 24 h, with the protein dissolv-

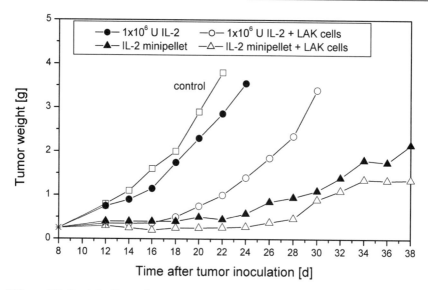

Fig. 5. Effect of IL-2 minipellet and aqueous solution (administered twice on days 8 and 10) in conjunction with lymphokine-activated killer cells (LAK) on murine fibrosarcoma (modified from Fujioka et al., 1998).

ing simultaneously. The protein is retained within the collagen matrix in a dissolved state and after a short lag phase is gradually released by diffusion *(15)*. In vivo, the IFN-loaded minipellet still maintained its original shape after 1 wk, indicating that erosion of the matrix is of minor impact on drug release. However, a clear relationship between the protein molecular weight and its diffusion rate was not found *(65)*. Moreover, the release profile might be influenced by binding of the protein to the collagen fibers. Two sc administrations at an interval of 10 d significantly inhibited the growth of nude mouse-implantable human renal tumor cells and the effect was more prominent than with an aqueous solution *(15)*. In humans, both time of peak drug concentration and half-life of IFN were increased with fewer side effects due to a reduction in the peak drug concentration *(66)*. Local treatment with the IFN minipellet was evaluated after sc injection vs peritumor injection in mice carrying human renal cell carcinoma. Substantial IFN levels remained detectable in both tumor tissue and serum up to 10 d after peritumor injection of the minipellet, and tumor growth was inhibited significantly with the effect being superior to sc application *(67)*.

The second protein drug tested with the minipellet system is IL-2. High-dose intravenous (iv) injection of IL-2 and adoptive immunotherapy consisting of IL-2 injection and lymphokine activated killer (LAK) cells have been introduced for cancer treatment *(68)*. Following sc injection of the IL-2 minipellet in mice, the serum IL-2 concentration reached its peak after 6 h and IL-2 was detectable in the serum for up to 72 h after injection with an increase in half-life from 15 to 360 min *(69)*. The IL-2 minipellet system induced natural killer and lymphokine-activated killer cells in mice, and was studied against murine tumors testing LAK cells administered concomitantly with IL-2 as an aqueous solution or with the IL-2 minipellet *(70)*. The collagen matrix formulation was most powerful and its effect was further augmented by simultaneous use of adoptive immunotherapy (Fig. 5). Histological studies revealed significant infiltration of lymphocytes into the tumor region and the parenchyma, as well as necrosis of tumor cells in the IL-2 minipellet-treated groups. Furthermore, therapy with the IL-2 minipellet in a colorectal adenocarcinoma liver metastases model resulted in elevated killer cell activities as well as a reduced number of metastatic nodules (71). Thus, the collagen minipellet appears to be a promising candidate for sustained-release formulation of protein drugs used in anticancer therapy.

2.2.3. CHEMOEMBOLIZATION

For chemoembolization in hepatic and renal cancer, microfibrillar collagen material has been developed (Angiostat®, Regional Therapeutic Inc., Pacific Palisades, CA; Avitene®, Alcon Laboratories Inc., Fort Worth, TX). A study in 1998 with 30 patients undergoing one to three hepatic artery chemoembolizations by injection of bovine collagen material with CDDP, doxorubicin, and mitomycin C demonstrated a decrease in lesion density or size and a decrease in the baseline carcinoembryonic antigen levels, with transient mild-to-moderate toxicity (72). However, the responses are measured in months and all patients had eventual progression of disease. Another study in patients with liver metastasis from colorectal cancer treated with two or three cycles of chemoembolization using a collagen suspension with doxorubicin, mitomycin C, and CDDP combined with systemic chemotherapy did not yield an improvement in complete response rate or time to progression when compared with standard systemic chemotherapy (73). The tissue platinum deposition 2.5 h following left renal injection in rabbits with CDDP increased dose-dependently, being 220 times that in the contralateral kidney at 10 mg/mL collagen. At 10 mg/mL of Angiostat, chemoembolized porcine liver had two times the hepatic platinum concentration when compared with iv and intraarterial infusion of CDDP (74). In mongrel dogs, hepatic ischemic injury was shown to be transient and to reverse within 48–72 h by recanalization. Over 2–3 mo, the collagen was removed and normal vascular anatomy was restored (75). The prophylactic use of antibiotics decreased the prevalence of infectious complications (76). Thus, chemoembolization using other biopolymers like starch or gelatin, as well as using polyvinyl alcohol, may be superior and has been studied more thoroughly. In conclusion, collagen gels and dense collagen matrices may play a more important role in intratumoral and systemic drug delivery in the future as commercial products arrive on the market.

3. GELATIN

3.1. Chemical and Biological Properties

Gelatin is obtained by extraction and purification following either acid or alkaline treatment of collagenous parts of the body, especially white connective tissue, bone, and hide from swine and cattle. Partial hydrolysis of collagen yields gelatin and renders the tough fibrous precursor structures into water-soluble material by cleavage of natural crosslinks, dissolution of the helical arrangement, and cleavage of the polypeptide chain. Based on the method of disintegration gelatin is differentiated into an acid type (pH 6–9) and an alkaline type (pH ~5.0). The amino acid composition is similar to that of collagen, but a difference in the isoelectrical point is caused by conversion of asparagin and glutamin into the corresponding acid in the presence of alkali (Table 1). Gelatin contains fractions termed α, β, and γ, which represent single chains, dimeric species, and triple helical forms similar to the higher order structures present in collagen (Subheading 2.1.). In addition, higher molecular weight oligomeric species and a microgel fraction of approx 1.5×10^7 Da are found in size exclusion chromatography *(77)* as well as lower molecular weight fractions starting at approx 10,000. For process engineering reasons, gelatin is technically characterized by its gel strength, given in Bloom, and not by its molecular weight. The gel strength reflects the weight necessary to give a 4-mm depression in a gel containing 6.67% gelatin in water using a defined plunger *(78)*. For gelatin material of 250 Bloom and 50–60 Bloom, mean molecular weights of approx 120 and 60–80 kD, respectively, were found *(79)*. These properties can be manipulated by treatment time (several weeks) and temperature. Gelatin is practically insoluble in common organic solvents, but can easily be dissolved in water forming a colloidal solution by warming after swelling in chilled water. The aqueous solution reversibly changes from the sol to the gel state upon cooling. In order to stabilize gelatin formulations which otherwise rapidly dissolve in water, the systems are stabilized via crosslinking, preferably by means of glutaraldehyde or heat treatment (Subheadings 2.1. and 4.2.1.).

Gelatin is described as biocompatible with low toxicity and antigenicity *(80)*. One of its major medical applications is as porous gelatin sponges for hemostasis. In surgical wounds, gelatin sponges are resorbed within 4–6 wk *(81)*, whereas the sponges liquidify on mucosa within 2–5 d. In addition, plasma expanders have been developed based on modified gelatin, e.g., succinylated gelatin. After iv administration, the gelatin half-life ranges from 7.8 min for 2700 da to 315 min for 99,000 da material; it is barely accumulated in heart, lung, and spleen, mostly accumulated in carcass, and is finally excreted via kidneys with the rate increasing with molecular weight *(80)*.

3.2. Anticancer Application of Gelatin

Gelatin has been extensively studied as a natural polymer from microencapsulation to sustained drug release. In addition, gelatin binds to fibronectin, and gelatin microspheres have a similar avidity as, for example, BCG cells, which are used in treatment of bladder cancer. Thus, gelatin particles may enhance interaction with fibronectin-bearing surfaces of tumors *(77,82)*. Fujita tested viscous gelatin solutions for ip application of mitomycin C in mice. This formulation led to a significantly higher mean residence time and time of peak drug concentration, whereas the peak drug concentration was decreased (Fig. 6) *(83)*. Consequently, the lifespan of S-180 sarcoma ascites tumor-bearing mice was increased. For treatment of resected non-small cell lung cancer with positive surgical margin, radioactive ^{125}I or [103]Pd seeds embedded in gelatin plaque have been successfully utilized. Patients received an intraoperative lung implant with gelatin pellets in combination with external beam radiation, and the technique is described as safe, reproducible, and effective *(84)*. However, the most important application is gelatin microspheres.

3.2.1. GELATIN MICROSPHERES AND NANOSPHERES FOR SUSTAINED RELEASE

Microspheres of 15–40 μm can be obtained from an emulsion of an aqueous drug containing gelatin solution in, for example, paraffin oil at 80°C, which is cooled; the particles are hardened with glutaraldehyde, separated, and washed *(85)*. The degree of crosslinking is a decisive factor for drug release *(86)*, and emulsification and surfactant concentration are important for particle size *(87)*. Incorporated TAPP-Br (2-bromo derivative of p-amidino phenoxy *neo*-pentane) was still active in vitro against human leukemia cells *(85)*, but release was incomplete (approx 60% maximum reached after 40 h). Oxidized sugars or dextran offer alternatives as crosslinking agents *(88–90)*.

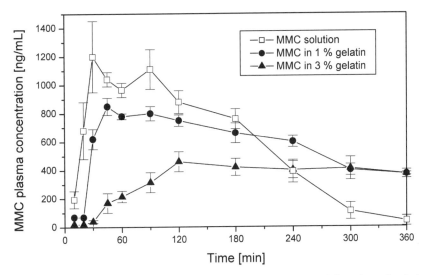

Fig. 6. Plasma concentration of mitomycin C after intraperitoneal administration of gelatin viscous solution (7.5 mg/kg MMC) in rats (modified from Fujita et al., 1997).

Studies with MTX incorporated in gelatin microspheres of 5–25 μm indicated that the lung-targeting efficiency in mice was increased 3 to 35 times, and the kinetic of the drug in the lung could be described by an open one-compartment model, with the residual time increased by 10 h *(91)*.

Small gelatin microparticles crosslinked with glutaraldehyde of approx 2 μm can also be loaded by swelling in drug solution, for example, thiotepa. Upon iv injection, the AUC was strongly increased and the clearance rate reduced *(92)*. Similarly, PS1, a polysaccharide complex derived from Mycobacterium bovis (BCG) with immunostimulating antitumor activity *(93)*, was loaded onto gelatin microspheres. In vitro dissolution experiments demonstrated sustained-release behavior, with a half-life of approx 8 h. Injected into mice bearing S180 sarcoma cells, PS1 in solution and the suspension of PS1-loaded gelatin microparticles resulted in almost identical dose-related suppression of the tumor cell growth, but only PS1 formulated in gelatin microspheres presented an enhanced activity over 24–48 h *(94)*. The effect may be related to activation of macrophages (*see* Subheading 3.2.2.).

3.2.2. GELATIN MICROSPHERES FOR ACTIVATION OF MACROPHAGES

Gelatin microspheres may also be used to deliver drugs to macrophages. Macrophage activation by biological response modifiers is potentially of great importance for stimulation of the host defense against primary and metastatic tumors. However, macrophage-activating agents are rapidly catabolized and cleared, which make high doses necessary with the risk of serious side effects *(95)*. One way to overcome this hurdle is to target the stimulants to the macrophages via particulate carriers. This approach takes advantage of the inherent avidity of macrophages to ingest foreign material, and gelatin in particular works as a strong opsonin which enhances phagocytosis *(96)*. The incorporated microspheres will be degraded and the conveyed drug will slowly be released in the macrophages and can more effectively activate the antitumor activity.

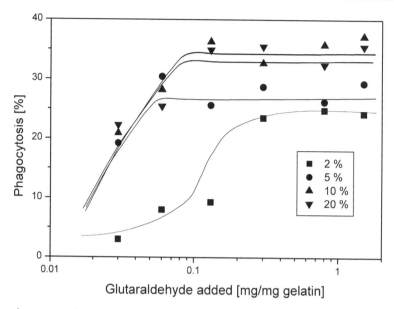

Fig. 7. In vitro macrophage phagocytosis of gelatin microspheres with different glutaraldehyde amounts and gelatin concentrations used in microsphere preparation (modified from Tabata & Ikada, 1996).

In another study, gelatin microparticles were prepared using glutaraldehyde crosslinking of alkaline-type gelatin emulsion droplets containing recombinant human interferon alpha A/D (IFN) which were dispersed in a mixture of toluene, chloroform, and Span 80®. The size was adjusted to 1.5 μm by sonication to allow for macrophage phagocytosis *(97)*. In vitro degradation and IFN release can be controlled via the crosslinking degree. The numbers of microspheres taken up by macrophages were proportional to the numbers of microspheres added until saturation of phagocytosis process was observed (Fig. 7). The extent of phagocytosis was reduced with decreasing concentration of gelatin and glutaraldehyde used in the manufacturing process which was related to changes in swelling and surface properties *(7)*. The phagocytosed microspheres were gradually degraded and IFN was released based on enzymatic hydrolysis. Whereas macrophages in cell culture pretreated with free IFN scarcely inhibited the growth of murine fibrosarcoma cells, the inhibitory activity was drastically augmented by addition of gelatin microspheres containing IFN, and the amount of IFN required for activity induction was strongly reduced *(7)*. Intratumoral injection of gelatin microspheres containing IFN and free IFN into mouse footpads bearing solid tumors indicated that the microspheres were more effective in suppressing tumor growth. Moreover, a distinct preventive effect of the iv injection of gelatin microspheres containing IFN on the incidence of pulmonary metastasis was observed. However, in an experiment with ascitic tumors in mice, the intraperitoneally applied gelatin microspheres containing IFN were not consistent in the suppression of tumor growth, which was caused by the absence of systemic antitumor effects of IFN *(98)*. As an alternative, muramyl-dipeptide *(99)*, interferon *(100)*, IL-1 *(101)*, and tumor necrosis factor *(102)* were conjugated to gelatin via carbodiimide. The conjugates were effectively taken up by macrophages via pinocytosis and this augmented macrophage recruitment and activity in treatment of ascitic tumor growth in the peritoneal cavity in contrast to gelatin microspheres loaded with IFN.

The same macrophage targeting approach via gelatin microspheres can be used to enhance antibody production. In mice, IgG antibody levels after immunization with gelatin microspheres containing the model proteinaceous antigen human γ-globulin were higher than those after application of antigen incorporated in Freund's incomplete adjuvant. The IgG antibody production was dependent on the size of the microspheres, and the balance between the extent of macrophage phagocytosis and the rate of antigen release *(7)*.

An alternative approach used gelatin nanoparticles for liver targeting *(103)*. After iv injection, selective uptake by the liver occurs, depending on particle diameter, like other colloidal preparations of similar size, and could allow delivery of drugs to the liver. The nanoparticles can be made by adding a desolvating agent to a gelatin solution and then the particles have to be stabilized by chemical crosslinking *(77,104)*. Gelatin micro- and nanoparticles have also been tested as carriers for recombinant adenoviruses. Administration of the adenovirus-containing microspheres to human tumor nodules engrafted in mice showed that the viral transgene was transferred to the tumor cells *(105)*.

3.2.3. GELATIN MICROPARTICLES FOR EMBOLIZATION

Besides PVA and starch, gelatin is one of the major sources for biodegradable embolic particles to infarct tumors and to locally enhance therapeutic drug levels caused by shifts in the local blood supply. The normal liver has a double circulation but is primarily supplied from portal circulation. In contrast, in malignant primary and secondary tumors, the blood supply is provided more than 90% by the hepatic artery *(106)*. Thus, closure of the hepatic artery is a valuable target to trigger the effect of chemotherapeutic agents. Physicians are most familiar with the absorbable gelatin powder, Gelfoam® (Pharmacia & Upjohn, Kalamazoo, MI). The crosslinked pork skin gelatin has its primary use in hemostasis. In soft tissue, the material is absorbed completely within 4–6 wk. During intravascular catheterization, the gelatin particles produce vessel occlusion, hasten clot formation, and become liquefied within 1 wk or less.

Transcatheter arterial chemoembolization using gelatin microparticles has become a standard procedure in the treatment of hepatocellular carcinoma *(107–111)*. Chemoembolization with gelatin particles causes massive shrinkage as a result of ischemia and increases local drug exposure. Some of the major complications are acute hepatic failure, liver infarction or abscess, intrahepatic biloma, multiple intrahepatic aneurysms, cholecystitis, and gastrointestinal bleeding *(112,113)*. Gelatin particles have also been used in treatment of bone metastasis and spinal column neoplasms *(114,115)*, adrenal tumors *(116)*, and embolization of various arteries for treatment of soft tissue carcinomas *(117)*. Testing of different particle sizes in transcatheter arterial embolization in patients and mongrel dogs suggest that the optimal size of gelatin sponge particles is between 500 and 1000 μm *(118,119)*.

There are many different protocols for treatment of inoperable tumors or for metastatic liver tumors, for example, regimens prior to surgery or transplantation *(120)*. The chemoembolization with gelatin particles may be performed in combination with many different drugs such as mitomycin C, CDDP, 5-FU, or epirubicin, or in an emulsion of iodized poppy-seed oil (Lipiodol®) *(121,122)*, as well as in combination with irradiation or systemic chemotherapy protocols. Therefore, the results are difficult to compare *(110,123–125)*.

A few studies describe the use of drug-loaded gelatin microspheres for emboliza-tion. Particles of 50 μm loaded with mitomycin C were developed for transcatheter arterial embolization, but mitomycin C was rapidly released from the microspheres *(6)*. In order to overcome this problem, mitomycin C was conjugated with dextran, which liberated mitomycin C by a base-catalyzed hydrolysis with a half-life of approx 24 h. Thus, hydrolysis became the rate-limiting step in the release of mitomycin C from gelatin microparticles loaded with dextran-conjugated mitomycin C *(6)*. Remainders of gelatin microspheres of 70 μm loaded with mitomycin C and ^{131}I were found 1 mo after hepatic embolization and still exhibited radioactivity *(126)*. These particles allowed local internal radiation to be concentrated in the tumor along with local chemotherapeutic treatment *(127)*. In addition to biodegradable gelatin microspheres, nonresorbable particles have been developed as particulate embolization material based on a trisacryl gelatin polymer core and hydrophilic surface characteristics *(128,129)*. In summary, the application of gelatin microspheres proceeded in human studies only for chemoembolization. Both chemoembolization using drug-loaded spheres, macrophage targeting, and sustained-release formulations have been evaluated to different degrees, but have not been pursued further up to the end of the 1990s.

4. ALBUMIN

4.1. Chemical and Biological Properties

Albumin is one of the most frequently investigated proteins for medical use. Its main source include human (HSA) and bovine (BSA) material. Albumin (mol wt, approx 65,000) represents the major plasma protein (approx 55%). It consists of 585 amino acids, has an ellipsoid form with diameters of 14.0 and 4.0 nm, respectively, and does not show glycosilation sites. Because of its isoelectrical point of 4.8, it is negatively charged under physiological conditions. Albumin has a high water-binding capacity and is involved in maintaining the colloid osmotic pressure in the blood. In addition, it binds to a number of endogenous and exogenous substances including bilirubin, steroid hor-mones, and many mainly acidic drugs *(130)*. Albumin is separated by ion-exchange chromatography or Cohn fractionation using ethanol at low temperature, with albumin being one of the last plasma proteins to precipitate (Cohn fraction V) *(131)*. Albumin can be stabilized in solution by the addition of sodium acetyltryptophanate and sodium caprylate, which allows for pasteurization at 60 °C for at least 10 h *(132)*.

Albumin solutions of 4–5% are used for plasma volume replacements, and to restore colloid osmotic pressure in case of acute hypovolemic shock, burns, and severe acute albumin loss; these also serve as an exchange fluid in therapeutic plasmapheresis or in cases of neonatal hyperbilirubinemia *(133,134)*. Concentrated albumin solutions of 15–25% have been suggested for short-term management of edema, hypoproteinemia in hepatic diseases, and in diuretic-resistant patients with nephrotic syndrome. Adverse effects to albumin infusion occur rarely, and include nausea, vomiting, increased sali-vation, febrile reactions, and allergic reactions *(130)*. Upon infusion, albumin is distrib-uted throughout the intravascular space, partially passes into the interstitium, but is recirculated via the lymphatic system, showing a half-life of approx 19 d *(131)*. Besides infusion, the second medical application for albumin is diagnostic, with a number of official pharmacopeia monographs about ^{125}I, ^{131}I, and ^{99m}Tc-labeled solutions and aggregated albumin injections. Technetium labeled albumin solutions are used in diagnostics of hemodynamics, as the radioactivity remains in the vascular system for an adequate time to allow arterio- or phleboscintigraphy. Labeled albumin particles, crosslinked by heat treatment (see Subheading 4.2.1.) with a diameter just slightly above the lumina of the terminal blood vessels, are retained in the capillaries and allow imaging of the local blood flow in the terminal artery region. Because the microspheres are degradable, the vessels are not permanently blocked. Biodegradability is strongly dependent on the manufacturing process, especially temperature, but usually degradation occurs within 12–24 h (ranging from 2.4 h to 144 h with temperature treatment increasing from 118 to 165°C) (135). Particles injected intravenously enable imaging of the perfusion conditions of the lung, whereas intraarterial injection allows for imaging of the situation in the supplied region, for example, a tumor, or to control the position of a selectively placed arterial catheter. The aggregated albumin may also be used for embolization (136). The European Pharmaceopeia (137) describes ^{99m}Tc macrosalb albumin particles, which can also contain nondenatured albumin, with the particle size limited between 10 and 150 µm. The macrosalb particles are introduced into the blood capillaries of the lung for imaging and then degrade with a half-life of 4–8 h (138). Smaller nanoparticles pass through the capillaries, are ingested by the reticuloendothelial system, and enable its imaging. Whereas the surface charge of the nanoparticles influences the phagocytic uptake in vitro, differences in the in vivo distribution of albumin carriers in rats could not be observed (139). The effect is probably due to adsorption of plasma components on the surface which leads to a similar surface charge for all spheres.

In addition, air-filled albumin microspheres of 3–5 µm (maximum, 32 µm) produced by sonification are used as an aid for ultrasound contrast enhancement of ventricular chambers, and with transvaginal ultrasound to assess fallopian tube patency. The gas microspheres are stabilized by a thin shell of heat-modified human albumin. Applied iv via catheter, the microspheres are cleared via phagocytosis in the liver with a plasma half-life of less than 1 min; after 24 h, 75% of radioactively labeled material is excreted in the urine as free iodide (140). In order to visualize myocardial perfusion, a gas of low blood solubility, octafluoropropane, is used to fill particles that remain echogenic in the blood for more than 5 min (141).

4.2. Anticancer Application of Albumin Microspheres

These particulate albumin systems for diagnostic use form the basis for application as micro- or nanoparticles loaded with or without drug for chemoembolization in cancer treatment. The manufacturing process has been transferred to drug-loaded microparticles (142–144). For drug-loaded microparticle preparation, usually a 10–30% albumin solution is dispersed in an immiscible oil with or without stabilizer (e.g., Span 80, Span 85, hydroxypropylcellulose) and albumin covalently crosslinked by heating (100–180°C) or by adding a crosslinking agent (e.g., glutaraldehyde, formaldehyde, 2,3-butanedione). Upon thermal treatment, crosslinking through formation of lysinoalanine occurs (145). As the number of crosslinks increase, the protein becomes water-insoluble and swells less in an aqueous environment, resulting in retardation of drug release and biodegradation. Compounds with reasonably high solubility in oil, for example, 5-FU, are not totally incorporated *(146)*. In general, the encapsulation process has to be adjusted for drugs that are susceptible to heat decomposition, e.g., adriamycin and mitomycin C, or for drugs that interact with crosslinking agents, e.g., methotrexate. Because a crosslinking process cannot be omitted, application to peptide or protein drugs must take into account the risk of denaturation, aggregation, and conjugation of the drug with the carrier material, which could result in inactivation or increased toxicity, specifically immunogenicity *(146)*.

Drug release is generally biphasic: an initial fast-release phase followed by slower first-order release by diffusion through the hydrated swollen matrix and aqueous channels *(147)*. Release of water-soluble drugs occurs rapidly whereas release of hydrophobic drugs such as 5-FU is retarded by dissolution as the rate-limiting step rather than diffusion through the matrix or erosion of the carrier. In addition, drug release can be influenced by particle size, drug loading, pH and concentration of the albumin solution, degree and nature of crosslinking, interaction between drug and matrix, as well as the presence of additives *(146)*.

Detailed toxicity studies carried out with albumin microspheres have demonstrated LD_{50} values of 200 mg/kg or 30,000 particles per gram of body weight in mice. Over 30 d, 50 mg per animal did not lead to distressful side effects without indications of inflammation or necrosis after multiple im and sc injections *(144)*. In vivo degradation of the crosslinked albumin spheres by proteases is hard to predict from the in vitro results.

4.2.1. Intravenous Application of Albumin Spheres

Albumin spheres have been investigated for targeted delivery of anticancer agents by nanospheres for passive targeting and by microspheres for active targeting via intraarterial delivery of magnetic delivery. In general, particle size plays a major role, not only for the release properties but also for distribution in the body. It can be reduced by increasing the oil viscosity, stirring speed, and oil amount, or by decreasing the amount of protein or aqueous phase *(146)*. After iv application of 1 µm, microspheres localize mainly in the liver. Microspheres of 15 µm or larger are entrapped in the first capillary bed they encounter, for example, in the tumor region after intraarterial injection (second-order targeting) and predominantly in the lungs (first-order targeting) owing to mechanical filtration after iv application *(144)*.

Adriamycin-loaded albumin microspheres of 7–80 µm, crosslinked with glutaraldehyde, have been evaluated for drug targeting to lungs in rats. Whereas free adriamycin was detectable in serum for only 6 h, administration through microspheres led to six times lower initial concentrations of 40 ng/mL in the serum, approx 5 ng/mL after 48 h, and the detection limit was reached after 4 d. The adriamycin microspheres were entrapped in the lung with 50% left after 24 h, and became completely degraded after 4 d *(148)*. Following administration of 5-FU entrapped in submicron microspheres, almost 45% of the dose was maintained in the liver for 24 h when compared with only 3% found after 2 h after injection as free drug *(149)*. Whereas drug release was hardly influenced by the crosslinking process, swelling and thus particle size in vivo was reduced at higher stabilization temperatures, resulting in decreased lung deposition.

Albumin nanoparticles can be prepared via desolvation of an aqueous solution, resulting in a coacervation phase. Standard methods include crosslinking with glutaraldehyde, removal of excess crosslinking agent by addition of sodium metabisulfite, and purification via gel permeation chromatography, yielding nonporous particles *(150)*. As an alternative procedure, a nanoemulsion in the inner-phase size range below 200 nm can be prepared using ultrasound, and the particles are subsequently crosslinked *(151)*. The drug-payload ranges from 0.2% to 15%. Beside the standard crosslinking agents for microspheres (Subheading 4.2.), methyl polyethylene glycol-modified oxidized dextran has been tested as a possible crosslinker, which results in a polyethylene oxide surface layer *(152)* and other surface modifications that change plasma protein adsorption *(153)*. The nanoparticles appear to be endocytosed by tumor cells. In vitro sensitivity of B16 and MMTV cells was reduced when 5-FU or doxorubicin was incorporated in albumin nanoparticles. These results correlated with studies of the two cell types injected in mice; the increase in animal survival time required higher doses of the nanoparticulate form intravenously vs free drug, whereas toxicity seemed to be reduced, and the therapeutic index was increased from approx 1.5 for 5-FU and doxorubicin to approx 2.5 *(150)*. Nanoparticles are taken up by the spleen *(154)* and could also be capable of targeting macrophages for activation of the immune system *(155)*. In addition, nanoparticles with a monoclonal antibody coupled to albumin and containing adriamycin have been tested in vitro and exhibited strong activity against bladder cancer cells *(156)* as antibody-linked particles might be capable of enhancing binding to tumor cells *(157)*.

Another approach to target albumin particles to the tumor site is the incorporation of magnetic material into the particles to apply an extracorporal magnetic field. After intraarterial injection, the magnetically responsive particles containing adriamycin or doxorubicin and magnetite could be selectively localized with an efficiency of 50–80% in the capillaries of Yoshida sarcoma tumors in rat tails exposed to a 5.5 kGauss external field for 30 min *(158)*. The particles led to sustained release of the drug with substantially reduced delivery to nontarget tissues and marked tumor regression. Similar results could be demonstrated with albumin particles injected intravenously and directed magnetically to lung metastases from AH 7974 tumor cells *(159)*. The presence of magnetite increased the level of drug entrapment and the initial burst, but significantly reduced the release rate of entrapped adriamycin from albumin microspheres *(147)*.

4.2.2. Intraperitoneal Application of Albumin Microspheres

Beside the targeting aspect of the iv administration of albumin microspheres, research groups focused their interest on local drug retention by injecting the particles intraperitoneally, intratumorally, or intraarterially for chemoembolization. Albumin microspheres loaded with adriamycin and 5-FU have been tested for potential application in the treatment of ovarian cancer. Truter found that, whereas activity of 5-FU against tumor cells was maintained in vitro, toxic effects in rats were only mild to moderate *(160)*. In a study in S-180 sarcoma ascites-bearing mice, it was demonstrated that 30% of the animals survived for more than 6 mo after ip treatment with daunomycin incorporated into human albumin microspheres, whereas all the animals in the control groups treated with daunomycin solution or no treatment died within 21 and 14 d, respectively *(161)*. Considering the fact that a single microsphere dose may not deliver effective amounts of drug for an adequate duration due to fast release, a multiple-dosing regimen of adriamycin microspheres was tested against Ehrlich ascites. Administration on days 1, 5, and 9 was superior in increasing the lifespan of mice when compared with multiple doses of free drug *(162)*.

The adriamycin payload can be increased, the release prolonged, and local adverse effects reduced by incorporation or conjugation of albumin with anionic polymers such as heparin *(163)* or polyglutamic acid *(164)*. The ip injection of adriamycin-loaded albumin-heparin-conjugate microspheres led to enhanced survival times of L1210 tumor-bearing mice and improved tumor growth delay in CC531 tumor-bearing rats *(163)*. Such albumin-heparin microspheres can be obtained via double crosslinking technique by stabilization of an aqueous mixture of albumin and heparin with 1-ethyl-3-(3-dimethylaminopropyl)carbodiimide followed by glutaraldehyde. The process allows control of particle size, swelling, and enzymatic degradation rate *(165)*. After intrahepatic administration the microspheres were degraded within 2 wk with a half-life of approx 1 d without adverse effects *(166)*.

Souza and Pourfarzib examined a combination therapy of iv methotrexate and intraperitoneal recombinant human macrophage colony-stimulating factor ip against melanoma induced by sc injection of B-16 tumor cells in mice *(167)*. The group that received both methotrexate solution and rhM-CSF in albumin microparticles demonstrated significant increase in survival time (30.4 ± 3.3 d) vs the no treatment group (11.8 ± 1.9 d), the methotrexate treatment only group (19.4 ± 5.0 d), and the methotrexate treatment + rhM-CSF solution intraperitoneal group (21.0 ± 2.2 d). The increases in TNF-α and IL-1β levels upon treatment with encapsulated rhM-CSF indicated macrophage activation as could be demonstrated by the same group in other studies using albumin microspheres *(168,169)*.

4.2.3. INTRATUMORAL APPLICATION OF ALBUMIN SPHERES

The antitumor activity of drugs in tumor tissue can be potentiated using albumin microspheres for local injection. Cummings et al. investigated pharmacokinetics and metabolism of mitomycin C after intratumoral injection in mice bearing MAC 16 colon adenocarcinoma. The microspheres produced steady drug levels when compared with injection of free mitomycin C, avoiding an early peak (20.5 vs 98.9 μg per tumor) and reducing the systemic levels (1.8 vs 6.8 μg/mL·h) *(170)*. In contrast, the key intermediate in mitomycin C quinone bioreduction, 2,7-diaminomitosene, reached peak levels that were 10-fold higher with an AUC that was fivefold higher than those with the particulate formulation. Intratumoral injection of albumin microspheres containing epirubicin resulted in a steady release in vitro over 3 d; the growth of solid MDA-MB-231 breast cancer was reduced (Fig. 8) with marked intracellular calcification and necrosis in the group treated with the microsphere-entrapped epirubicin *(171)*.

4.2.4. ALBUMIN MICROSPHERES FOR EMBOLIZATION

Embolization with albumin microparticles has been tested in different clinical settings using drug-free and drug-loaded microspheres, primarily for liver cancer *(172)*. Drug-free albumin microspheres were studied in a Phase II trial in a combined intrahepatic treatment administering angiotensin II to redistribute the arterial blood flow toward the tumor, intraarterially injecting albumin microspheres every 4–6 wk, and giving 5-FU bolus in the intervening weeks. Toxicity was minimal, response was seen in seven of 21 patients *(173)*, and survival was prolonged. However, benefits were modest. Studies with radiolabeled microspheres in patients demonstrated a median biological half-life of 2.4 d (1.5–11.7 d) *(174)*.

In patients with liver tumors, Fujimoto et al. have reported superior tumor response to intraarterial chemoembolization with BSA microspheres (approx 45 μm) incorporat-

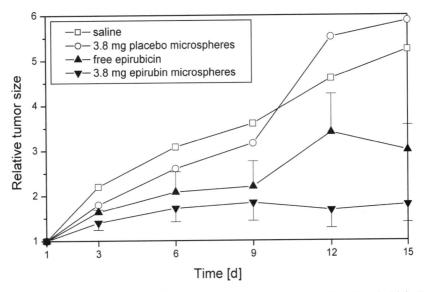

Fig. 8. Size of breast cancer implanted into mice treated on day 1, 5, and 9 with epirubicin (5 mg/kg) containing albumin microspheres (modified from Novotny & Zinek, 1994).

ing 5% mitomycin when compared with conventional infusion *(175)*. This trial was preceded by animal studies employing rabbits bearing VX-2 tumors on the hind leg. After application through the femoral artery, the microspheres were detected in the arterioles of the tumor tissue *(176)*. The microspheres led to sustained high drug levels in the tumor tissue of approx 1 µg/mL for up to 8 h, whereas injection of mitomycin C solution resulted in less than 0.003 µg/mL up to 4 h. During manufacturing of the particles, it should be noted that mitomycin C is susceptible to heat decomposition, and glutaraldehyde crosslinking results in a covalent adduct and an isomeric form of intact mitomycin C as the two major decomposition products, totaling approx 10% *(177)*.

In another clinical study, second-order drug targeting with CDDP-loaded albumin microspheres in patients with hypervascular liver tumors was performed. Following administration of 15–35 µm spheres through the artery, particles were predominantly retained in the tumor vasculature *(178)*. The retention of CDDP in albumin microspheres could be enhanced by admixing chitin or chitosan. CDDP albumin microspheres were prepared with various chitin concentrations, and CDDP release in vitro and antitumor effect in a VX-2 hepatocellular tumor model in rabbits following injection into the hepatic artery were determined. As the concentration of chitin increased, CDDP entrapment in the microspheres increased, enhancing the antitumor effect *(179,180)*. The results also indicated that the size of the microspheres and the CDDP dose were strongly correlated with the augmentation of the antitumor effect by the composite microspheres *(181)*.

Furthermore, Doughty et al. treated a breast cancer patient with adriamycin-loaded albumin microspheres. A complete response was observed and prolonged local control was achieved until the patient's death from disseminated disease *(182)*. No systemic toxicity was observed.

The interest in albumin as a biomaterial for drug delivery peaked in the 1980s and early 1990s and has markedly receded. The most encouraging activities were directed toward embolization, and both intratumoral and ip applications may have higher potential. However, no major clinical trials evaluating these approaches are underway despite the vast experience with albumin spheres in diagnostics.

5. FIBRIN/FIBRINOGEN

Fibrin sealant is used for local cancer treatment with the idea that in combination with surgical resection the intraoperative application may reduce the tumor recurrence rate (183) or to treat local cancerous lesions, for example, superficial gastric cancer (184).

5.1. Chemical and Biological Properties

Fibrin glue consists of two components: fibrinogen (factor I, mol wt, $3.6 \cdot 10^5$ D) concentrate, also containing factor XIII, and thrombin, containing factor IIa (Fig. 9). When combined, thrombin activates the removal of two fibrinopeptides from the fibrinogen molecules in the presence of calcium and incites polymerization of the resulting fibrin monomers (185). In addition, thrombin cleaves an activation peptide from factor XIII, creating an active transglutaminase (factor XIIIa) which immediately (within 3–5 min) induces the formation of covalent bonds between the fibrin molecules. Thus, fibrin glue reflects the last step of the blood clotting cascade. In order to avoid early fibrinolysis and removal of the clot by plasmin, a suitable protease inhibitor such as aprotinin is added. Consequently, an insoluble, mechanically stable clot is formed. Fibrin glue is generally created in situ from the two components using, for example, a double syringe. It is used clinically as a temporary tissue replacement, a surgical sealant to improve wound healing, or a spray to bleeding surfaces to control hemorrhage (186). The fibrin clot degrades by enzymatic fibrinolysis, complemented by cellular metabolism and phagocytosis by granulocytes and macrophages, with only mild foreign-body reaction (187). The resorption rate depends on the local fibrinolytic activity, the thickness of the sealant layer, and the amount of aprotinin present.

5.2. Anticancer Application of Fibrin/Fibrinogen

The fibrin meshwork formed within the clot will provide a matrix that slows the liberation of drug. In local chemotherapy mitomycin C/fibrin glue exhibits stronger effects in vitro and in animals when compared with mitomycin C solution on gastric and esophageal cancer cell lines (188) and a glioma cell line (189). In vitro release from the coagulate testing of 0.3, 0.6, and 1 mg mitomycin C/100 µL fibrin glue demonstrated that 54, 18, and 15%, respectively, were released after 30 min, and the 1 mg dose was the most suitable with a steady release for at least 24 h (190,191). Inoculation of tumor tissue with mitomycin C/fibrin glue resulted in replacement of the tumor tissue by plasma cells and lymphocytes. Injection of the combination in Balb/c mice into the tumor or the direct local application of the gel to the tumor surface significantly decreased the tumor growth rate and increased the survival time when compared with injection of mitomycin C solution or drug-free fibrin glue (Fig. 10). In addition, the abdominal aorta, vena cava, and intestine were not damaged by the local application at the high dose (190).

Fibrin glue was also tested in animals in combination with CDDP for treatment of osteosarcoma (192) and with 5-FU for head and neck cancer (193). Almost all of the MTX was released from fibrin glue within 1–3 d, and murine 9L-gliosarcoma decreased soon after administration and disappeared in four out of five animals after 10 d (194). In

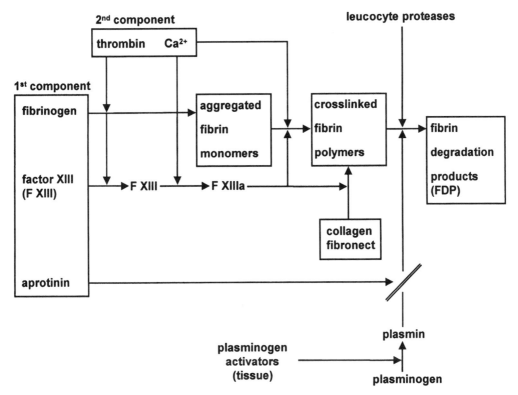

Fig. 9. Reaction scheme of fibrin sealent (modified from Redl et al., 1985).

patients with a malignant brain tumor, sustained-release drug was detected for more than 1 wk, and tumor decrease occurred. Kabuto et al. found that the local concentration after covering C6 gliomas in rat brains with fibrin glue containing nitrosourea was more than sufficient for 50% inhibition of cell growth in vitro for 12 h; after 5 d tumor cell damage could be shown to a depth of 2–3 mm *(183)*.

Fibrin glue has not only been successfully used for local retention of low molecular weight cytostatica but, as no chemical crosslinking agent or temperature is applied, can be used to embed more sensitive agents. OK-432, an attenuated strain of *Streptococcus pyogenes,* induces the production of various cytokines by monocytes and lymphocytes, and has been recognized as an effective biological response modifier *(195)*. The effect of OK-432 on colorectal cancer is markedly augmented when it is injected intratumorally together with fibrinogen. Extensive fibrin meshwork formation is induced in cancer tissues with high urokinase-type plasminogen activator levels such as colorectal cancer. Subsequently, macrophages infiltrate along the fibrin meshwork leading to granuloma development with giant cells followed by extensive tumor necrosis *(196,197)*. The inflammatory cells that migrate into the fibrin matrix phagocytose OK-432 produce chemotactic factors and cytokines that promote antitumor immunity, and numerous cytotoxic CD4+ lymphocytes surround the residual cancer cells *(198)*. The concept has been applied for treatment of patients with pancreatic cancer *(199)* but it was less effective for breast cancer. When fibrinogen is injected into breast cancer, which has low urokinase-type plasminogen activator levels, a dense fibrin clot is formed instead of a loose fibrin meshwork suitable for macrophage migration *(200)*.

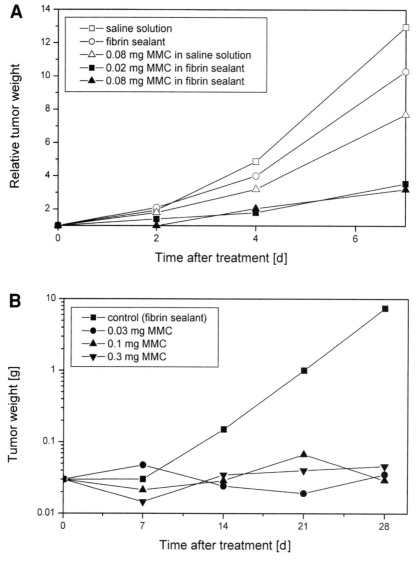

Fig. 10. Growth inhibition effects of mitomycin C in 100 1 fibrin sealant against (**A**) Meth A tumor in mice (intratumoral injection) and (**B**) SCC-131 tumor in rats (spread superficially onto tumors) (modified from Matsuoka et al., 1996).

Addition of activated macrophages that produce urokinase-type plasminogen activators assists in the formation of a loose fibrin meshwork and results in tumor regression.

In order to enhance local drug retention, polymers can be added to the fibrin glue to obtain a denser network or charge interactions. Sugitachi showed that a fibrin clot containing gelatin and loaded with adriamycin or CDDP, when placed intra-abdominally in ascites hepatoma AH130-bearing rats, exhibited sustained-release drug levels for approx 14 d and substantially increased the antitumor effect when compared with intraperitoneally injected adriamycin or CDDP *(201)*. Whereas almost all rats treated with the conventional formulation died within 20 d with massive ascites and metastasis, 68% of the fibrin glue/gelatin/adriamycin-treated animals survived for more than 200 d and evidence of malignancy disappeared. A similar system has been used in patients for therapy of serious malignant pleural effusion *(202)*. Enhanced drug retention was demonstrated for a combination fibrin glue/sodium alginate/doxorubicin in vitro and in vivo using microdialysis to assess the concentration in the extracellular fluid of an AH60C tumor in the back of rats *(203)*. The tumor volume was inversely correlated with tumor extracellular-fluid AUC to plasma AUC ratios.

In a pilot study, spraying of fibrin glue in combination with CDDP offered an alternative in the treatment of lung cancer, especially as an adjuvant for postoperative purification *(204)*, but further studies have not been reported. Furthermore, bovine fibrinogen microspheres containing 5-FU, adriamycin or mitomycin C, prepared by an emulsion heat-hardening method, have been described *(147)*.

Thus, fibrin glue appears to a promising candidate to sustain local drug retention after surgical tumor resection with encouraging results. In addition, the simple mode of application by admixing drug to commercially available fibrin glues and the avoidance of additional chemical or heat crosslinking offer major advantages.

6. CHITOSAN

6.1. Chemical and Biological Properties

Chitosan is a polysaccharide obtained by deacetylation of chitin, which is the major constituent of the exoskeleton of crustaceous water animals and insects and is found in the cell wall of bacteria and fungi. At present, most chitosan is obtained by a concentrated alkali treatment of chitin using the shells of crab, shrimp, lobster, and krill, being the most available sources, but production in fungus cell culture has also been evaluated *(205)*. Chitin represents a mucopolysaccharide family consisting predominantly of water-insoluble, unbranched $\beta1\rightarrow4$-*N*-acetyl-D-glucosamine chains having a molecular weight $> 1 \cdot 10^6$ (Fig. 11A). Purity, polymorphous structure, the degree of deacetylation (usually 70–95%), and the molecular weight of chitosan ($1 \cdot 10^5$ D–$1.2 \cdot 10^6$ D) can vary widely because many factors in the manufacturing process influence the characteristics of the final product. Chitosan is insoluble in water, alkali, and organic solvents but is soluble and forms viscous preparations in aqueous media at pH < 6.0. Different methods have been described to obtain low-molecular weight and water-soluble chitosan *(205)*. Chemical modification, e.g., succinylation, can also render water-soluble material.

Different types of chitin and chitosan materials have been described as biocompatible and biodegradable *(206,207)*. Tissue response to implanted chitin and chitosan is mild, except for highly deacetylated, rapidly degrading material, in which case significantly larger quantities of low molecular weight compounds are rapidly formed that elicit an acute inflammation reaction *(208)*. Some recent reports indicate problems of chitosan with respect to blood compatibility and cell viability after parenteral application; the drawbacks seem to depend on chemical and physical characteristics such as deacetylation degree, molecular weight, and counter ion species *(209,210)*. Upon ip injection, chitosan (50% hydrolyzed) moves rapidly into kidney and urine and is scarcely distributed into liver, spleen, abdominal edema, and plasma. It is hydrolyzed to small molecular weight products and excreted into urine typically within 2 wk *(209)*. Chitosan is mainly depolymerized enzymatically by lysozyme *(211)*, which binds to specific chitosan sequences *(212)*. The degradation rate decreases with an increase in

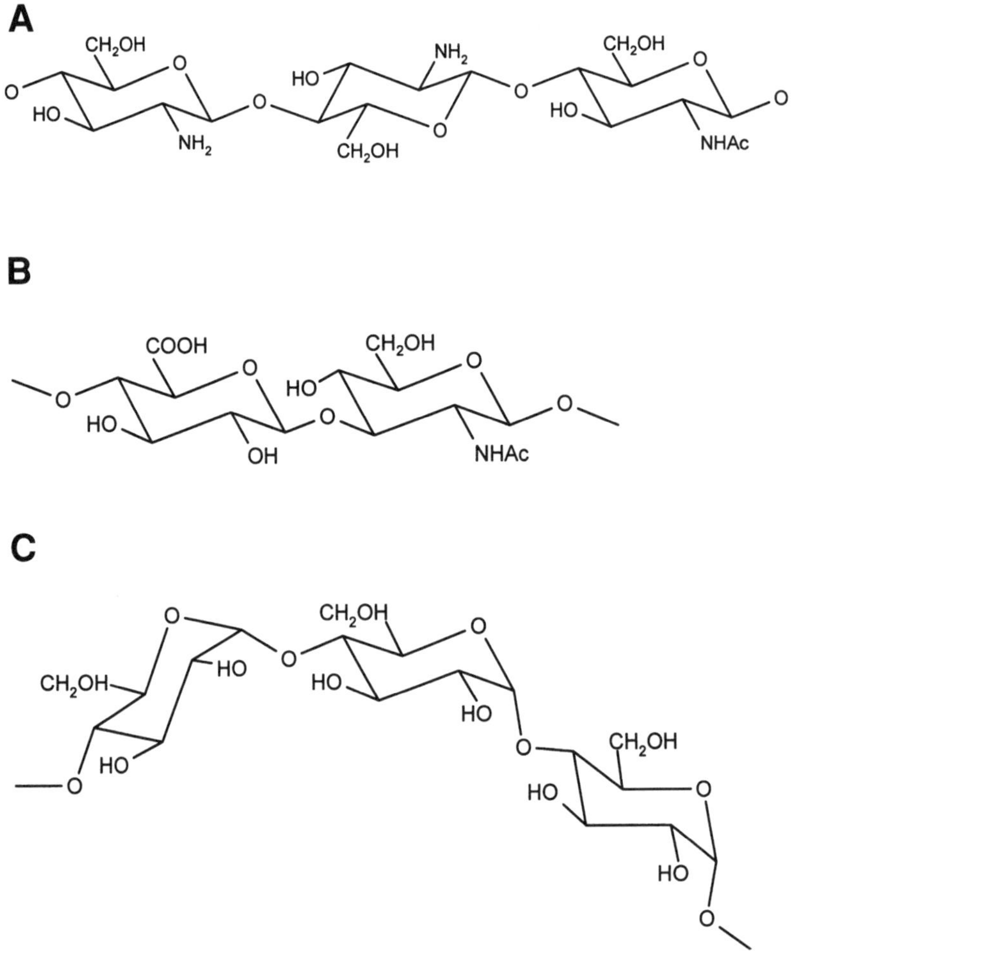

A

B

C

Fig. 11. Repeating units of chitosan (**A**), hyaluronan (**B**), starch—amylose (**C**), starch—amylopectin (**D**), and dextran (**E**).

the degree of deacetylation *(208,211)*. Therefore, lysozyme is used for in vitro assays testing chitosan degradation. Intravenous administration of succinylated chitosan and glycolchitosan as water-soluble materials demonstrated half-lives in the blood circulation of more than 2 d. For succinylated material only marginal distribution into other tissues occurred, whereas the glycol derivative was found to a high extent in the kidney. Furthermore, succinylated material was less partitioned to the tumor tissue but accumulated there more easily than glycol-chitosan. This suggests an enhanced permeability and retention (EPR) effect for succinylated chitosan and may explain the increase in antitumor activity by conjugation of cytostatica to water-soluble succinylated chitosan (Subheading 6.2.2.) *(213)*.

A variety of biological effects have been attributed to chitosan ranging from marked affinity for proteins, for example, laminin which is considered to be involved in tumor invasion *(214)* to the inhibition of tumor cells *(215)*, antimicrobial activity, acceleration of wound healing, and stimulation of the immune system *(216–219)*. Oral administra-

D

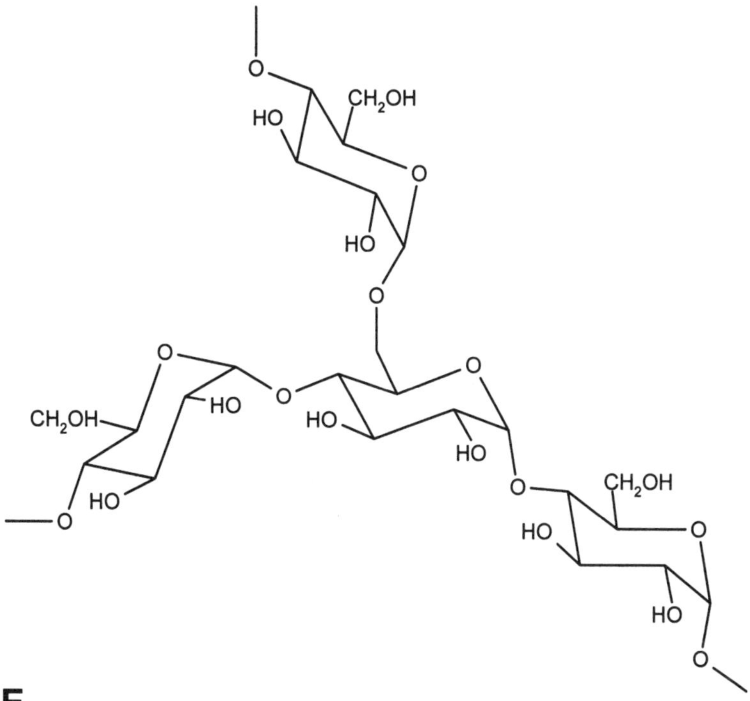

E

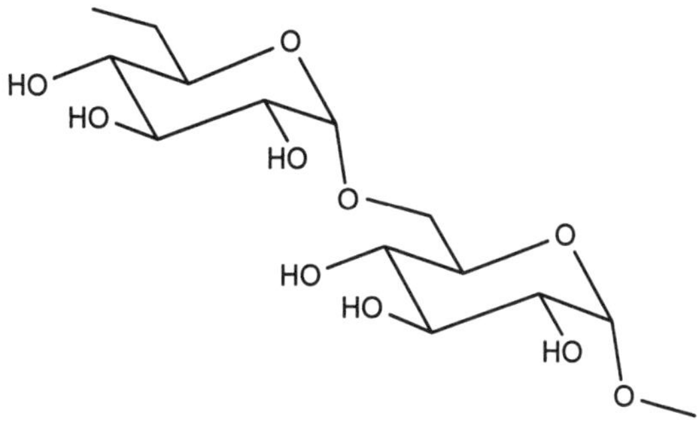

Fig. 11. *(Continued)*

tion of chitosan stimulated an increase in IgA, IgG, and IgM concentrations in serum and mesenteric lymph nodes lymphocytes *(219)*. In contrast, intravenous application of phagocytosable chitin particles primed alveolar macrophages due to, at least in part, direct activation by IFN-γ which is produced by NK1.1+CD4-cells. In addition, chitosan stimulates the migration of cells and accelerates reformation of connective tissue and angiogenesis *(205)*, probably because of induction of IL-8 *(220)*. Additionally, it has been shown that chitosan is mucoadhesive *(221)* and increases the permeability of epithelial tight junctions which may enhance, e.g., nasal or intestinal drug absorption and may affect gating properties of the blood–brain barrier *(222)*. The biomedical applications of chitosan include bandages and sponges as wound dressings (taking advantage of its hemostatic properties), artificial blood vessels, and matrices for cell encapsulation *(223)*. It has been tested for numerous other applications, for example, oral controlled-release formulations *(224)* and cosmetic products, especially hair conditioner or fixative *(225)*. The properties can be adapted by formation of macromolecular complexes between the polycationic chitosan and other polymers *(226)*. Compared to other biopolymers such as collagen or hyaluronic acid, chitosan is relatively heat stable and less sensitive to electrolytes.

6.2. Anticancer Application of Chitosan

The application of chitosan in cancer treatment has two major aspects: microparticles and conjugates with drugs attached via the amino groups or complexes with holmium or platinum. In addition, chitosan can be used to prepare gels for photosensitizer-enhanced laser treatment *(227,228)*. This study combined the photosensitizer with glycated chitosan as an immunoadjuvant which also functioned as the gel-former and prolonged retention of the dye at the injection site. After the immediate photothermal destruction of neoplastic cells, the treatment stimulated the immunological defense system against residual and metastatic tumor cells in rats. It was hypothesized that chitosan elicits an immune reaction against the remaining tumor cell population by combining with cellular antigens released from the disrupted tumor cells to form an *in situ* autovaccine *(227)*. The treatment resulted in an increase in survival rate, the eradication of tumor burden, both primary and metastatic, as well as an augmentation of resistance to rechallenge. Because of its highly positive charges, chitosan can be used for DNA delivery and offers possibilities in gene delivery *(229,230)*.

6.2.1. CHITOSAN MICROSPHERES

Chitosan microspheres can be prepared by emulsifying a drug-containing acidic aqueous chitosan solution in an oil phase (e.g., rape-seed oil or paraffin) followed by crosslinking with glutaraldehyde, or via heat *(231,232)* and final particle separation. Drug release from microparticles occurs relatively fast in vitro for both hydrophobic and hydrophilic drugs *(233)* and is mostly controlled by dissolution and diffusion rather than matrix degradation *(233)*. Drug liberation is affected to some extent by size, drug loading, and additional coats of chitosan or derivatives that delay the release from the particles *(234)*. In vivo degradation occurs within 1–2 mo after sc injection *(235)*.

The ability of chitosan to chelate metal ions *(236)* has been used to form a chemical complex between CDDP and chitosan named plachitin, which is transferred into microparticles. Chemoembolization with CDDP-chitosan microspheres (approx 75 μm; 20% CDDP) in dogs resulted in a reduction of the AUC and hepatic tissue concentrations three times higher after infusion into the hepatic artery when compared with a CDDP solution *(91,237)*. Angiograms revealed a decrease in the number of arterioles in liver, necrosis, and hepatic cell degeneration in the embolized region, with particles still present after 4 wk. The addition of chitin to CDDP-chitosan-microspheres reduced the CDDP release rate and enhanced the efficacy for embolization through the hepatic artery *(91)*. Successful use in liver cancer patients was reported with transient and few adverse effects *(91,238)*. The material can also be used for intraperitoneal chemotherapy of gastrointestinal cancer *(239)* and as a local agent for treatment of solid tumors *(240,241)*. The potential of mitoxantrone-loaded chitosan microspheres for sustained drug delivery has been shown in vitro and in vivo *(242)*. The mean survival time of

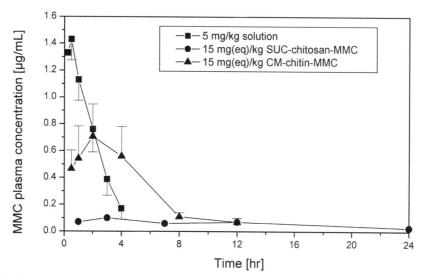

Fig. 12. Plasma concentration of MMC after intraperitoneal injection of 5 mg/kg MMC and 15 mg(eq)/kg MMC conjugated with *N*-succinyl-chitosan or with 6-*O*-carboxymethyl-chitin (modified from Onishi et al., 1997).

Ehrlich ascites carcinoma bearing mice upon intraperitoneal injection was increased from 4.6 d for 2 mg of free mitoxantrone to 50 d with an equivalent amount of microspheres. Chitosan itself has been shown to diminish glycolysis in Ehrlich ascites tumor cells and to decrease glucose uptake and ATP levels. This is caused by inhibition of a tumor-specific variant of pyruvate kinase from fraction B *(215)* and may enhance the effect of cytostatica. Magnetic chitosan microspheres of approx 0.5 µm loaded with oxantrozole were shown to enhance delivery to the brain after injection with the head under a magnetic field. Oxantrozole concentrations were at least 100-fold increased after application of the magnetic microsphere system *(243,244)*.

6.2.2. DRUG CONJUGATES WITH CHITOSAN

Drug conjugates with chitosan can profit from the continuous drug release by prodrug cleavage. In addition, the enhanced permeability and retention effect of chitosan materials in tumor tissue, and their immunostimulating and anti-tumor effects, can improve cancer therapy. Cytarabine, which is rapidly inactivated and excreted from the body, can be conjugated using N^4-(4-carboxybutyryl)-cytarabine in the presence of carbodiimide. Cytarabine generation from the conjugate was shown to be pH-dependent with approx 56% at pH 7.4 within 7 d *(235)*. The conjugate significantly enhanced the survival time of leukemia-bearing mice whereas neither chitosan nor cytarabine exhibited a positive effect. In addition, toxicity studies after ip injection showed that the maximum tolerable dose was more than 3 g/kg.

For local delivery of mitomycin C, conjugates have been presented. In vitro, drug release from the conjugates followed a mono-exponential liberation profile with an apparent half-life of 180 h and 6.2 h for mitomycin C conjugated with N-succinyl-chitosan and 6-O-carboxymethyl-chitin, respectively (Fig. 12). Such water-soluble conjugates show long systemic retention and tumor accumulation *(213)*. Upon intraperitoneal injection of 15 mg mitomycin C/kg, the mitomycin C plasma level reached its maximum at 30 min after injection of mitomycin C solution. Injecting 6-*O*-carboxymethyl-chitin conjugated mitomycin C, the time of peak plasma concentration was at 2 h and *N*-succinyl-chitosan conjugates resulted in low consistent levels over the 24-h test period. The water-soluble conjugates did not show a substantial improvement in the survival time of tumor-bearing mice. But whereas survival time was inversely related to the dose of free mitomycin C injected indicating toxic effects, the lifespan was extended with increasing conjugated mitomycin C dose *(235,245)*.

Chitin may also be coupled to polypeptide sequences which interfere with cell adhesion and may be used to control cancer metastasis *(246,247)*. Synthetic peptides derived from adhesion molecules have been shown to be involved in regulation of the metastatic process. RGDS (Arg-Gly-Asp-Ser), a sequence that is based on fibronectin, has been shown to interfere with tumor metastasis in murine tumor models. Studies employing spontaneous metastasis models indicated that 6-*O*-sulfated- and 6-*O*-carboxymethyl-chitin inhibit metastasis and lung tumor colonization of murine melanoma *(248)*. In addition, chitin suppressed tumor cell invasion of the reconstituted basement membrane and tumor—induced angiogenesis by its specific binding to laminin and fibronectin and/or by inhibiting enzymatic activities of cell-derived heparanase and type IV collagenase. Therefore, conjugates of cell adhesive RGDS peptide with 6-*O*-sulfated- and 6-*O*-carboxymethyl-chitin, which are structurally related to heparin, were developed. These macromolecular compounds are more effective for inhibition of liver and lung metastasis than chitin, RGDS, or their mixture after intravenous injection *(246,248,249)*. The ip injection of RGDS conjugates increased the survival time of mice carrying extensive peritoneal-seeding tumor cells and may present a treatment option against the dissemination of scirrhous gastric cancer *(247)*.

Similar to platinum, holmium may interact with chitosan, and this phenomenon can be used to enhance the retention of [166]Ho for internal radionuclide therapy. Analysis after intrahepatic injection in rats and mice revealed that most of the radioactivity is localized at the administration site; only low levels are detected in liver, spleen, lung, and bone. Application of free [166]Ho results in high radioactive concentrations in the blood and many organs and tissues *(250)*. After intratumoral administration of the complex in B16 melanoma, the radioactivity is localized at the site of administration without distribution to other organs and tissues *(250)*. Toxicity of the complex results in a slight decrease in erythrocyte number and an increase in liver and lung weight at an early stage after administration, but this is reversible within 14 d *(251)*.

In summary, chitosan and its derivatives have recently demonstrated great potential in cancer treatment. Leading candidates will be conjugates with platinum, holmium, or RGDS, all of which still require thorough investigation and clinical evaluation.

7. HYALURONAN

7.1. Chemical and Biological Properties

Hyaluronic acid is a naturally occurring polyanionic linear polysaccharide composed of disaccharide units with the structure D-glucuronic acid-β (1,3)-*N*-acetyl-D-glucosamine-β(1,4) (Fig. 11B). Its molecular weight ranges from several hundred to $> 10^6$ D, with an average of $1–2 \cdot 10^6$ D *(252)*. Hyaluronic acid and sodium hyaluronate, which represent the predominant entity under physiological conditions, together form hyaluronan (HA). HA acts as a lubricant and shock absorbant throughout the body, stabilizing the cartilage matrix and controlling the water homeostasis of tissues *(253,254)*. It binds to proteins in the extracellular matrix and on cell surfaces, and influences the migration, adhesion, proliferation of cells, and the leukocyte functions *(252)*. Hyaluronan was previously isolated from disparate sources such as bovine vitreous humor, rooster comb, or umbilical cord. The resulting material varies in molecular weight, its three-dimensional organization of chains, as well as the degree of contamination with other tissue constituents *(254)*. Development of HA production from *Streptococcus zooepidemicus* cell culture gave access to material of higher purity at a more reasonable price, and the procedure is now applied on industrial scale *(255)*. The unique physicochemical properties of HA, such as the rheological behavior of aqueous solutions, its polyelectrolytic properties, and molecular weight characteristics have been described in detail by Berriaud *(256)*.

In vivo, HA is degraded by a slow, specific enzymatic pathway via hyaluronidase and/or in a fast process by hydroxyl radicals. Hyaluronidase is present in various mammalian tissues with the highest activity in hepatic and lymphatic lysosomes. It randomly cleaves the 1,4-linkages between the *N*-acetyl-β-D-glucosamine and the D-glucuronate units. Hyaluronidase typically displays its maximum activity at an acidic pH *(257)*. HA has a half-life of 0.5–2.5 d in tissues; it is rapidly cleared from plasma by HA receptor-mediated uptake in the liver with a half-life of several minutes and an upper limit for renal excretion of approx 25,000 D *(258)*. A variety of chemically modified HA-based materials have been developed by crosslinking with glutaraldehyde or EDC, as well as by esterification of the carboxylic groups with reduced susceptibility to enzymatic degradation *(252)*. Generally, good biocompatibility of HA materials has been reported *(259–262)*, and HA does not induce antibody-formation following injection into animals or humans *(254)*.

The major clinical applications of HA are for injectable treatment of osteoarthritis in the knee, and in the field of viscosurgery or viscosupplementation in ophthalmology to maintain eye shape and protect delicate tissues during cataract removal, corneal transplantation, or glaucoma surgery *(252)*. Furthermore, the cosmetic industry takes advantage of the moisturizing properties *(225)*. HA has been tested as a base material for barrier membranes *(263)*, as an injectable formulation in combination with basic fibroblast growth factor to accelerate bone fracture healing *(264)*, and as an adjuvant in ophthalmic drug delivery to enhance drug absorption through mucus tissue *(252)*. A project to commercialize an injectable HA formulation with enhanced local retention of diclofenac was discontinued *(265)*.

7.2. Anticancer Application of Drug Conjugates with Hyaluronan

Considerable progress has been made in understanding the physiological and pathophysiological importance of HA-receptors located on cell surfaces. The two selective receptors, CD44 and RHAMM, are involved in cell adhesion *(266)*, proliferation, migration *(267)*, and metastasis of tumors *(268)*. The synthesis and accumulation of HA is associated with the migration of cells not only as part of developmental and wound healing events, but also in tumorigenesis and metastasis *(254)*. It could be shown that the receptors are overexpressed in metastatic cells, and a high proportion of HA-positive cancer cells appears to be predictive for poor survival rate of patients *(269,270)*. HA specifically binds to colon cancer cells in a saturable mechanism, is specifically taken up by the cells through endocytosis *(271)*, and upon iv injection, HA targets liver metastases of a colon adenocarcinoma in rats *(272)*. Thus, using HA-bioconjugates could allow cell-selective targeting of anticancer drugs and localizing of a slow release formulation at a specific site in the body.

Akima coupled mitomycin C to HA and epirubicin to acetylated HA. The antitumor activity was evaluated by the inhibition of lymph node metastasis, growth suppression of implanted MH-134 ascites tumor, and reduction of Lewis lung carcinoma metastasis. After sc injection, the HA-epirubicin conjugate concentration in the regional lymph nodes was significantly higher than that in the liver *(5)*. The HA-mitomycin C conjugate exhibited higher antitumor activity against MH-134 tumors than did free mitomycin C and proved to be a potent antimetastatic agent at a dose of only 0.01 mg/kg. In addition, toxicity was strongly reduced by coupling mitomycin C to HA. The Lewis lung carcinoma cells also internalize HA but the HA-epirubicin complex did not show a clear advantage over free epirubicin. Coradini et al. evaluated a conjugate of sodium butyrate to HA in order to increase the half-life of sodium butyrate and found an improvement in the antiproliferative activity against mamma adenocarcinoma cells in mice *(273)*. Thus, the idea of HA-conjugates is intriguing but major effort is necessary to follow-up on the initial studies.

7.3. Anticancer Application of Hyaluronidase

Cancer cells not only overexpress HA receptors, but also produce high levels of hyaluronan, forming a halo that protects them against lymphocytes or macrophages, shields them from cytostatics, and additionally promotes migration and metastasis. This raises the question about the biological role of hyaluronidase and its potential application to tumor treatment which is discussed briefly here in the context of HA. On the one hand, increased hyaluronidase activity in the extracellular space can facilitate invasiveness and, on the other hand, enhanced levels of hyaluronidase activity in the serum can provide better protection against the development of tumors *(257)*. In addition, hyaluronidase increases TNF sensitivity of cancer cells and counteracts with TGF-β mediated TNF-resistance, and suppresses TGF-β1 gene expression in L929 cells in a serum-dependent manner *(274)*. Moreover, hyaluronidase antagonized TGF-β-mediated inhibition of epithelial cell growth. Hyaluronidase has also been shown to reduce the interstitial fluid pressure in solid tumors *(275)*. Several working groups have focused on the addition of hyaluronidase to chemotherapy in order to attack the HA coating surrounding the tumor cells, loosening the cell-to-cell contact and the interstitial connective tissue, making them more easily accessible to both the anticancer drug and cytotoxic lymphocytes *(257)*.

Hyaluronidase was shown to enhance the efficacy of cytostatic agents in a number of preclinical and clinical trials *(257,276–278)*. Muckenschnabel and colleagues could show that the intratumoral concentration after sc administration of vinblastine in murine melanoma was significantly increased by simultaneous local injection of hyaluronidase *(279)*. Hyaluronidase could also lead to selective melphalan enrichment in malignant melanoma *(280)*. Kohno could show that the addition of hyaluronidase enhanced the penetration and cell-killing effect of doxorubicin *(281)*. The approach was also successfully used in the treatment of bladder cancer with mitomycin C *(282)* and of head-and-neck carcinoma with polychemotherapy, radiation, and hyaluronidase *(277)*. Ex vivo experiments with vital brain tumor samples demonstrated that hyaluronidase promoted the penetration of CDDP into tumor tissue with a matrix rich in hyaluronic acid. In a corresponding pilot study with 19 children suffering from malignant brain tumors, supportive hyaluronidase resulted in significantly fewer relapses and better survival *(283)*. Furthermore, hyaluronidase offers potential to reverse forms of both intrinsic and acquired drug resistance in solid tumors that are sensitive to its antiadhesive effects as shown for multidrug resistant EMT-6 tumors in mice *(284,285)*. Disa reported an additional protection by local hyaluronidase injection against the ulcer formation upon sc injection with doxorubicin in an animal model. This phenomenon was referred to the ability of hyaluronidase to temporarily decrease the viscosity of the extracellular matrix, increasing the transport of doxorubicin into surrounding tissue *(286)*. A similar effect has been shown for paclitaxel *(287)*. Although proven to be effective as additive to local chemotherapy, a randomized study failed to show synergy to chemotherapy after systemic application in high-grade astrocytomas *(288)*. In addition, a supportive effect of hyaluronidase in treatment of adenocarcinoma in the liver of rats with mitomycin C could not be demonstrated *(289)*. Further clinical studies have to be awaited.

8. OTHER BIOPOLYMERS FOR PARENTERAL DRUG DELIVERY IN CANCER TREATMENT

8.1. Starch

Next to cellulose, starch is one of the most abundant polysaccharides available for industrial exploitation. It is isolated commercially from a variety of crop plants as starch granules. The isolated granules represent clusters of tightly bound starch molecules, composed of two basic polysaccharides: amylopectin and amylose (Fig. 11C,D). Both are based on repeating α-D-(1,4)-glucose chains, with amylose presenting a linear chain forming tight helices (approx $1 \cdot 10^6$ D) and amylopectin with additional randomly attached α-D-(1,4)-glucose chains (approx $5 \cdot 10^8$ D). Dissolution in water is difficult due to strong hydrogen bonds, especially in amylose and frequently starch is supplied in a prehydrolyzed version obtained by temperature, acid, or oxidation treatment. Degradable starch microspheres (DSM) of approx 45 μm in diameter have been specifically developed for chemoembolization (Spherex®, Pharmacia & Upjohn, Kalamazoo, MI). The particles are produced from partially hydrolyzed potato starch in a common emulsion process and crosslinked with epichlorohydrin, also called amilomer *(290)*. After intraarterial administration of DSM, the particles settle in precapillary vessels, slowing the blood flow through the arteriolar-capillary bed. The particles are disintegrated into oligomeric fragments (mol wt, approx 1 kD) by serum α-amylase and subsequently further digested *(290)*. The in vitro half-life in serum is approx 25 min and is proportional to the diameter and the degree of crosslinking *(291,292)*. Thus, DSMs induce a transient ischemia for 15–80 min permitting repetitive cycles as compared to collagen, gelatin, albumin, or polyvinyl alcohol, which occlude the blood flow for 1.5 d up to several weeks *(293)*. DSMs are well tolerated, nonimmunogenic, and no adverse effects associated with DSM injection were observed *(290)*.

DSMs have been shown to enhance the antitumor efficacy of several cytotoxic drugs in animal experimental models, and in a number of noncomparative and randomized clinical trials in more than 1000 patients suffering from unresectable, advanced, malignant liver tumors, and in patients with pancreatic or breast cancer *(291,294–296)*. In addition, DSMs reduce energy dissipation in heated tumors and have been found to aid localized hyperthermia treatment *(297)*. DSMs are administered via the artery prior to regional cytotoxic delivery. The transient circulatory arrest and redistribution provide time for local drug deposition in the organ, reduce systemic cytotoxic exposure and toxicity, and enhance tumor response when compared with drug alone. In different studies, the ratios of doxorubin and fluoxuridine concentrations in tumor/liver were increased by factors between 2.5 and 5 by intrahepatic coadministration of DSM *(291)*. Peak plasma concentrations and plasma AUCs of a variety of drugs have been found to be significantly reduced following intraarterial coadministration with DSM *(290,291,293)*. In order to take advantage of the pharmacokinetic modulation and the redistribution of blood flow to hypovascular tumor areas, a near-complete occlusion without causing unacceptable toxicity should be achieved by individual adjustment of the DSM dose *(293)*. Deurloo and coworkers describe the intratumoral administration of CDDP in starch rods, but release was completed within 2 h *(298,299)*. Swelling and rapid degradation are the main obstacles for application of starch as a carrier material for drug delivery systems. Thus, starch is currently limited to DSMs, which are coadministered with drugs for chemoembolization.

8.2. Dextran

Dextran is based on poly α-(1→6)-D-glucose chains with a high number of α-(1→4)-branches (Fig. 11E). The base material of approx $4 \cdot 10^7$ Da is produced in *Leuconoster mesenteroides* cultures *(300)* and subsequently becomes hydrolyzed to any desired molecular weight, typically $4–8 \cdot 10^5$ D. Dextran is enzymatically cleaved in vivo and lacks intrinsic toxicity *(301)*. Primarily it is used as a plasma expander and as an iron complex for treatment of anemia. However, it represents a potent antigen, but antibody production in vivo does not occur when infused, probably because of an "immunological paralysis" *(302)*.

Dextran has been conjugated with different anticancer drugs, such as mitomycin C, to form long-acting prodrugs (Subheading 3.2.3.). Recently, iv injections of platinum complexes with oxidized dextran and dicarboxymethyldextran have been demonstrated to be effective in mice against colon 26 tumors (Fig. 13) *(303,304)*. The results of further studies have to be awaited. Dextran magnetite has been reported to be an agent for selective heating by electromagnetic induction *(305,306)* and can be used as a nanoparticulate superparamagnetic contrast agent *(307,308)*. Such magnetic dextran nanospheres (10–20 nm) have been described to surpass the blood–brain barrier. Brain tumor targeting was demonstrated by a 2–21-fold increase in magnetite concentrations in brain tumors when compared with normal brain in rats bearing RG-2 tumors. Animals were sacrificed after 30 min and 6 h, respectively, and levels of 41–48% of the dose were found in the presence of a magnetic field *(309)*. The concentrations were significantly higher than those achieved with microspheres (approx 1 μm) of cationic aminodextran which, again, were superior to neutral dextran *(310)*. Neutral magnetic microspheres loaded with mitomycin C conjugated to dextran were significantly enriched in the brain tumor; however, within 45 min following application, all animals treated with particles died, possibly because of redistribution of particles to the lung *(311,312)*. Additionally, sulfated dextran, which is used for gel permeation chromatography, has also been proposed as microparticulate carrier *(313)*. Thus, dextran conjugates, especially magnetic and nanoparticulate forms, have demonstrated their positive effects in cancer treatment but still lack sufficient clinical data.

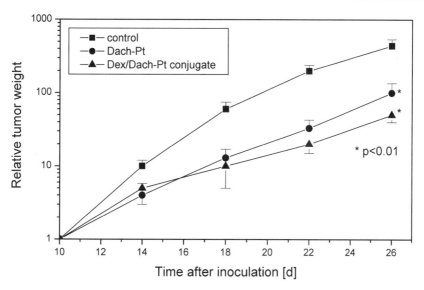

Fig. 13. Growth inhibition effects of Dach-Pt platinum complex (8 mg/kg) as conjugate with oxidized dextran or as free drug in colon 26 tumor bearing mice intravenously injected on days 10, 14, and 18 (modified from Ohya et al., 1998).

8.3. Cellulose and Derivates

Cellulose is the major structural polysaccharide; it is composed of β-D-(1,4)-glucose chains (approx $1–2 \cdot 10^6$ Da). As it slowly degraded in vivo, cellulose was evaluated in a preliminary clinical trial for permanent vascular occlusion *(314)*. Two cellulose derivates, hydroxypropylcellulose and ethylcellulose, have been used as drug carriers in cancer treatment. Kato et al. reviewed their experience with intraarterial infusion of mitomycin C, CDDP, or peplomycin encapsulated in ethylcellulose microcapsules in 1013 patients *(315)*. The particles were prepared by coating mitomycin C crystals in an organic solution of ethylcellulose *(316)*. The target sites in the 1996 trial were mostly liver, kidney, intrapelvic organs, lung, and head-and-neck tumors. A tumor reduction of more than 50% was seen in 28% of the tumors. The response rate depended on both tumor size and treatment number, with the highest response rate obtained for mitomycin C. Local mitomycin C activity could still be found 6 h after injection, whereas mitomycin C as free drug was not detectable after injection and mitomycin C serum levels were decreased in the microencapsulated form. Hydroxypropylcellulose-doxorubin conjugates were of interest owing to the mucoadhesive properties that enhanced retention after installation within the urinary bladder in a trial to treat superficial bladder carcinoma *(317)*. The doxorubicin concentration in tumors were increased and the antitumor effect in patients could be further improved by combination with local hyperthermia treatment *(318)*. An alternative offers the application of the cytotoxic drug, peplomycin, in a 1% hydroxypropylcellulose formulation *(319)*. A single application when compared with 10 repetitive doses of peplomycin in saline resulted in significantly higher response rates in the peplomycin-hydroxypropylcellulose group.

9. SUMMARY

Biopolymers have been shown to be useful in drug delivery for cancer therapy, especially in local treatment, with chemoembolization as the most frequent application. Many clinical trials of different dosage forms and carriers failed to produce evidence of an advantage in survival when compared with systemic therapy. Clinical data are often limited to Phase II studies. However, a few applications, such as collagen gels, were carried toward approval. Most natural polymers are hydrophilic and require dissolution or suspension in aqueous media, as well as chemical crosslinking to stabilize forms such as microspheres. This hydrophilicity leads to rapid water uptake, swelling, and diffusional drug release. Thus, synthetic polymers such as poly-α-hydroxyacids may be superior to achieve systemic controlled release from microspheres. Therefore, interactions between polymer and drug (e.g., between chitosan and platinum) and specific biological activities of the biopolymers (e.g., enhancement of tissue regeneration by collagen, infiltration of macrophages along a fibrin meshwork, or inhibition of tumor cells by chitosan) have to be the tools that researchers use in cancer treatment.

REFERENCES

1. Coldwell DM, Stokes KR, Yakes WF. Embolotherapy: agents, clinical applications, and techniques. *Radiographics* 1994; 14:623–643.
2. Kerr DJ, Kaye SB. Chemoembolism in cancer chemotherapy. *Crit Rev Ther Drug Carrier Syst* 1991; 8:19–37.
3. McCullogh P. Nonsurgical treatment of liver metastases. *Curr Opin Gen Surg* 1994; 151–155.
4. Maeda H. Polymer conjugated macromolecular drugs for tumor-specific targeting, in *Polymeric Site-Specific Pharmacotherapy* (Domb AJ, ed). Wiley, New York, 1994, pp. 96–117.
5. Akima K, Ito H, Iwata Y, et al. Evaluation of antitumor activities of hyaluronate binding antitumor drugs: synthesis, characterization and antitumor activity. *J Drug Target* 1996; 4:1–8.
6. Hashida M, Sezaki H. Specific delivery of mitomycin C: combined use of prodrugs and spherical delivery systems, in *Microspheres and drug therapy. Pharmaceutical, immunological and medical aspects* (Davis SS, Illum L, McVie JG, Tomlinson E, eds). Elsevier Science, New York, 1984, pp. 281–293.
7. Tabata Y, Ikada Y. Biodegradable gelatin microspheres for drug delivery to macrophages, in *Microparticulate systems for the delivery of proteins and vaccines* (Cohen S, Bernstein H, eds). Marcel Dekker, New York, 1996, pp. 407–423.
8. Timpl R. Immunology of the collagens, in *Extracellular matrix biochemistry* (Piez KA, Reddi AH, eds). Elsevier, New York, 1984, pp. 159–190.
9. Piez KA. Molecular and aggregate structures of the collagens, in *Extracellular matrix biochemistry* (Piez KA, Reddi AH, eds). Elsevier, New York, 1984, pp. 1–39.
10. Friess W. Collagen - biomaterial for drug delivery. *Europ J Pharm Biopharm* 1998; 45:113–136.
11. Cawston TE, Murphy G. Mammalian collagenases, in *Methods in Enzymology* (Lorand L, ed). Vol. 80, *Proteolytic Enzymes.* Academic, London, UK, 1981, pp. 711–722.
12. Etherington DJ, Pugh D, Silver IA. Collagen degradation in an experimental inflammatory lesion: studies on the role of the macrophage. *Acta Biol Med Germ* 1981; 40:1625–1636.
13. Hunt JA, van der Laan JS, Schakenraad J, Williams DF. Quantitative in vivo assessment of the tissue response to dermal sheep collagen in abdominal wall defects. *Biomaterials* 1993; 15:378–382.
14. DeVore DP, Kelman CD, Fagien S, Casson P. Autologen: autologous, injectable, dermal collagen. In: Principles and practice of ophthalmic plastic and reconstructive surgery. Chapter 65. W.B. Saunders, Philadelphia, PA, 1996, pp. 670–675.
15. Fujioka K, Maeda M, Hojo T, Sano A. Protein release from collagen matrices. *Adv Drug Del Rev* 1998; 31:247–266.
16. Ellingsworth LR, DeLustro F, Brennan JE, Sawamura S, McPherson J. The human response to reconstituted bovine collagen. *J Immunol* 1986; 136:877–882.
17. Bader F, Davis G, Dinowitz M, et al. Assessment of risk of bovine spongiform encephalopathy in pharmaceutical products, Part I. *BioPharm* 1998a; 11(1):20–31.

18. Bader F, Davis G, Dinowitz M, et al. Assessment of risk of bovine spongiform encephalopathy in pharmaceutical products, Part II. *BioPharm* 1998b; 11(3):18–30.
19. Fielding AM. Preparation of neutral salt soluble collagen, in *The Methodology of Connective Tissue Research* (Hall DA, ed). Joynson-Bruvvers Ltd. Oxford, UK, 1976, pp. 9–12.
20. Trelstad RL. Immunology of collagens, in *Immunochemistry of the extracellular matrix* (Furthmayer H, ed). Vol.I Methods. CRC, Boca Raton, FL, 1982, pp. 32–39.
21. Collagen preparation for the controlled release of active substances. Roreger M. (LTS Lohmann Therapie-systeme GmbH und Co. KG, Germany). PCT Int. Appl. (1995). 37 pp. CODEN: PIXXD2 WO 9528964 A1 19951102 Designated States W: AU, CA, CZ, FL, HU, JP, KR, NO, NZ, PL, SI, SK, US. Designated States RW: AT, BE, CH, DE, DK, ES, FR, GB, GR, IE, IT, LU, MC, NL, PT, SE. Patent written in German. Application: WO 95-EP1428 19950415. Priority: DE 94-4414755. CAN 124:66603 AN 1995:998164 CAPLUS.
22. Heidemann E. The chemistry of tanning, in Nimni E (ed), Collagen Vol. III–Biotechnology. CRC, Boca Raton, FL, 1988, pp. 39–61.
23. Khor E. Methods for the treatment of collagenous tissues for bioprostheses. *Biomaterials* 1997; 18:95–105.
24. van Luyn MJA, van Wachem PB, Olde Damink L, et al. Relations between in vitro cytotoxicity and crosslinked dermal sheep collagens. *J Biomed Mater Res* 1992a; 26:1091–1110.
25. van Luyn MJA, van Wachem PB, Olde Damink L, et al. Secondary cytotoxicity of cross-linked dermal sheep collagens during repeated exposure to human fibroblasts. *Biomaterials* 1992b; 13:1017–1024.
26. Naimark WA, Pereira CA, Tsang K, Lee JM. HMDC crosslinking of bovine pericardial tissue: a potential role of the solvent environment in the design of bioprosthetic materials. *J Mater Sci Mater Med* 1995; 6:235–241.
27. Nishi C, Nakajima N, Ikada Y. In vitro evaluation of cytotoxicity of diepoxy compounds used for biomaterial modification. *J Biomed Mater Res* 1995; 29:829–834.
28. Olde Damink LHH, Dijkstra PJ, van Luyn MJA, et al. In vitro degradation of dermal sheep collagen cross-linked using a water-soluble carbodiimide. *Biomaterials* 1996; 17:679–684.
29. Petite H, Duval JL, Frei V, et al. Cytocompatibilty of calf pericardium treated by glutaraldehyde and by the acyl azide methods in an organotypic culture model. *Biomaterials* 1995; 16:1003–1008.
30. Wang M-C, Pins GD, Silver FH. Collagen fibres with improved strength for the repair of soft tissue injuries. *Biomaterials* 1994; 15:507–512.
31. Weadock KS, Miller EJ, Bellincampi LD, Zawadsky JP, Dunn MG. Physical crosslinking of collagen fibers: comparison of ultraviolet iradiation and dehydrothermal treatment. *J Biomed Mater Res* 1995; 29:1373–1379.
32. Friess W, Uludag H, Foskett S, Biron R. Bone regeneration with recombinant human bone morphogenetic protein-2 (rhBMP-2) using absorbable collagen sponges (ACS): influence of processing on ACS characteristics and formulation. *Pharm Dev Technol* 1999; 4:387–396.
33. Cheung DT, Perelman N, Tong D, Nimni ME. The effect of γ-irradiation on collagen molecules, isolated α-chains, and crosslinked native f Wallace, D. G., Rhee, W., Reihanian, H., Ksander, G., Lee, R., Braun, W. B., Weiss, B. A., Pharriss, B. B., Injectable cross-linked collagen with improved flow properties. *J Biomed Mater Res* 1989; 23:931–945.ibers. *J Biomed Mater Res* 1990; 24:581–589.
34. Olde Damink LHH, Dijkstra PJ, van Luyn MJA, van Wachem PB, Nieuwenhuis P, Feijen J. Changes in the mechanical properties of dermal sheep collagen during in vitro degradation. *J Biomed Mater Res* 1995; 29:139–147.
35. Gorham SD. Collagen, in *Biomaterials* (Byrom D, ed). Stockton, New York, 1991, pp. 55–122.
36. Wallace DG, Pherson JM, Ellingsworth L, et al. Injectable collagen for tissue augmentation. In: Nimni ME ed). Collagen Vol. III-Biotechnology. CRC, Boca Raton, FL, 1988a, pp. 117–144.
37. Wallace DG, Reihanian H, Pharriss BB, Braun WG. Injectable implant composition having improved intrudability. *Europ Patent* 87305651.9 (1988b).
38. Wallace DG, Rhee W, Reihanian H, et al. Injectable cross-linked collagen with improved flow properties. *J Biomed Mater Res* 1989; 23:931–945.
39. Malhotra H, Plosker GL. Cisplatin/epinephrine injectable gel. *Drugs Aging* 2001;18:787–793.
40. Smith JP, Stock E, Orenberg EK, et al. Intratumoral chemotherapy with a sustained-release drug delivery system inhibits growth of human pancreatic cancer. *Anti-Cancer Drugs* 1995; 6:717–726.
41. Smith JP, Kanekal S, Patawaran MB, et al. Drug retention and distribution after intratumoral chemotherapy with fluorouracil/epinephrine injectable gel in human pancreatic cancer xenografts. *Cancer Chemother Pharmacol* 1999; 44:267–274.

42. Swinehart JM, Sperling M, Phillips S, et al. Intralesional fluorouracil/epinephrine injectable gel for treatment of condylomata acuminata. A phase 3 clinical study. *Arch Dermatol* 1997b; 133:67–73.
43. Yu NY, Patawaran MB, Chen JY, et al. Influence of treatment sequence on efficacy of fluorouracil and cisplatin intratumoral drug delivery in vivo. *Cancer J Sci Am* 1995; 1:215–221.
44. Burris HA 3rd, Vogel CL, Castro D, et al. Intratumoral cisplatin/epinephrine-injectable gel as a palliative treatment for accessible solid tumors: a multicenter pilot study. *Otolaryngol Head Neck Surg* 1998; 118:496–503.
45. Kraus S, Miller BH, Swinehart JM, et al. Intratumoral chemotherapy with fluorouracil/epinephrine injectable gel: a nonsurgical treatment of cutaneous squamous cell carcinoma. *J Am Acad Dermatol* 1998; 38:438–442.
46. Miller BH, Shavin JS, Cognetta A, et al. Nonsurgical treatment of basal cell carcinomas with intralesional 5-fluorouracil/epinephrine injectable gel. *J Am Acad Dermatol* 1997; 36:72–77.
47. Swinehart JM, Skinner RB, McCarty JM, et al. Development of intralesional therapy with fluorouracil/adrenaline gel for management of condylomata acuminata: two phase II clinical studies. *Genitourin Med* 1997a; 73:481–487.
48. Ning S, Yu N, Brown DM, Kanekal S, Knox SJ. Radiosensitization by intratumoral administration of cisplatin in a sustained-release drug delivery system. *Radiother Oncol* 1999; 50:215–223.
49. Davidson BS, Izzo F, Cromeens DM, et al. Collagen matrix cisplatin prevents local tumor growth after margin-positive resection. *J Surg Res* 1995; 58:618–624.
50. Ning S, Trisler K, Brown DM, et al. Intratumoral radioimmunotherapy of a human colon cancer xenograft using a sustained-release gel. *Radiother Oncol* 1996; 39:179–189.
51. Graeber IP, Eshraghi AA, Paiva MB, et al. Combined intratumor cisplatinum injection and Nd:YAG laser therapy. *Larongoscope* 1999; 109:447–454.
52. Rosenblatt J, Rhee W, Wallace D. The effect of collagen fiber size distribution on the release rate of proteins from collagen matrices by diffusion. *J Contr Rel* 1989; 9:195–203.
53. Singh MP, Stefko J, Lumpkin JA, Rosenblatt J. The effect of electrostatic charge interactions on release rates of gentamicin from collagen matrices. *Pharm Res* 1995; 12:1205–1210.
54. Singh MA. Fundamental study of electrostatic effects on release of polypeptides from collagen hydrogels. PhD thesis, University of Maryland, 1994.
55. Stemberger A, Unkauf M, Arnold DE, Blümel G. Drug carrier systems based on resorbable polyester collagen and/or biomaterial combinations. In *Cosm Pharm Appl Polym* (Gebelein CG, Cheng TC, Yang CCM, eds). Plenum Press, New York, 1990, pp. 263–268.
56. Fujisato T, Sajiki T, Liu Q, Ikada Y. Effect of basic fibroblast growth factor on cartilage regeneration in chondrocyte-seeded collagen sponge scaffold. *Biomaterials* 1996; 17:155–162.
57. Winn SR, Uludag H, Hollinger JO. Sustained release emphasizing recombinant human bone morphogenetic protein-2. *Adv Drug Del Rev* 1998; 31:303–318.
58. Stemberger A, Grimm H, Bader F, Rahn HD, Ascherl R. Local treatment of bone and soft tissue infections with the collagen-gentamicin sponge. *Eur J Surg* 1997; 163 Suppl. 578:17–26.
59. Friess W, Lee G, Groves MJ. Insoluble collagen matrices for prolonged delivery of proteins. *Pharm Dev Technol* 1996a; 1:185–193.
60. Friess W, Zhou W, Groves MJ. In vivo activity of collagen matrices containing PS1, an antineoplastic glycan, against murine sarcoma cells. *Pharm Sci* 1996b; 2:1–4.
61. Song S-Z, Morawiecki A, Pierce GF, Pitt CG. Collagen film for sustained delivery of proteins. *Europ Patent* 92305467.3 (1992).
62. Pharmaceutical carriers from collagens. (Koken Co., Ltd., Japan). Jpn. Kokai Tokkyo Koho (1981), 6 pp. CODEN: JKXXAF JP 56122317 19810925 Showa. Patent written in Japanese. Application: JP 80-25806 19800229. CAN 95:225688 AN 1981:625688 CAPLUS.
63. Takenaka H, Fujioka K, Takada Y.: New formulations of bioactive materials. *Pharm Tech Japan* 1986; 2:1083–91.
64. Fujioka K, Takada Y, Sato S, Mitata T.: Novel delivery system for proteins using collagen as a carrier material: the minipellet. *J Contr Rel* 1995; 33:307–315.
65. Aisaka A, Hojo T, Maeda M, et al. Novel sustained release formulation using collagen as a carrier material (2) – in vivo characterization of interferon-minipellet. *Drug Deliv Syst* 1996; 11:337–343.
66. Nakajima S, Kuroki T, Nishiguchi S, et al. Phase I trial of long-acting preparation (SM-10500) of a natural interferon-α (HLBI), Kiso to Risho (Clinical Report), 1994; 28:4219–4232.
67. Marumo K, Oya M, Murai M. Application of the interferon minipellet to human renal cell carcinoma in nude mice. *Int J Urol* 1997; 4:55–61.

68. Rosenberg SA, Lotze MT, Muul LM, et al. A progress report on the treatment of 157 patients with advanced cancer using lymphokine-activated killer cells and interleukin-2 or high-dose interleukin-2 alone. *New Engl J Med* 1987; 316:889–897.

69. Matsuoka J, Sakagami K, Shiozaki S, et al. Development of an interleukin-2 slow delivery system. *Trans Am Soc Artif Intern Organs* 1988; 34:729–731.

70. Fujiwara T, Sakagami K, Orita K. Antitumor effects of a new interleukin-2 slow delivery system on methylcholanthrene-induced fibrosarcoma in mice. *J Cancer Res Clin Oncol* 1990a; 116:141–148.

71. Fujiwara T, Sakagami K, Matsuoka J, et al. Application of an interleukin-2 slow delivery system to the immunotherapy of established murine colon 26 adenocarcinoma liver metastases. *Cancer Res* 1990b; 50:7003–7007.

72. Tellez C, Benson AB 3rd, Lyster MT, et al. Phase II trial of chemoembolization for the treatment of metastatic colorectal carcinoma to the liver and review of the literature. *Cancer* 1998; 82:1250–1259.

73. Leichman CG, Jacobson JR, Modiano M, et al. Hepatic chemoembolization combined with systemic infusion of 5-fluorouracil and bolus leucovorin for patients with metastatic colorectal carcinoma: a southwest oncology group pilot trial. *Cancer* 1999; 8:775–781.

74. Daniels JR, Sternlicht M, Daniels AM. Collagen chemoembolization: pharmacokinetics and tissue tolerance of cis-diamminedichloroplatinum(II) in porcine liver and rabbit kidney. *Cancer Res* 1988; 48:2446–2450.

75. Daniels JR, Kerlan RK Jr, Dodds L, et al. Peripheral hepatic arterial embolization with crosslinked collagen fibers. *Invest Radiol* 1987; 22:126–131.

76. Reed RA, Teitelbaum GP, Daniels JR, Pentecost MJ, Katz MD. Prevalence of infection following hepatic chemoembolization with cross-linked collagen with administration of prophylactic antibiotics. *J Vasc Interv Radiol* 1994; 5:367–371.

77. Farrugia CA. The formulation of gelatin nanoparticles and their effect on melanoma growth in vivo. Ph.D. Thesis, University of Illinois at Chicago, IL, 1998.

78. European Pharmacopoeia, Monograph 330: Gelatin. European Department for the Quality of Medicines within the Council of Europe, Strasbourg, France, 2002 4th ed., Supp. 4.5, p. 3699.

79. Moßhammer P, Spongoide Systeme – Darstellung und galenisch relevante Eigenschaften von Gelatine-Xerogelen zur vaginalen Anwendung. PhD Thesis, University of Erlangen, Germany, 1992.

80. Yamaoka T, Tabata Y, Ikada Y. Body distribution of intravenously administered gelatin with different molecular weights. *J Contr Rel* 1994; 31:1–8.

81. Pharmacia & Upjohn, Gelfoam – absorbable gelatin sterile powder. Package insert, 1997.

82. Gao X, Groves MJ. Fibronectin-binding peptides. Isolation and characterization of two unique fibronectin-binding peptides from gelatin. *Eur J Pharm Biopharm* 1998; 45:275–284.

83. Fujita T, Tamura T, Yamada H, Yamamoto A, Muranishi S. Pharmacokinetics of mitomycin C (MMC) after intraperitoneal administration of MMC-gelatin gel and its anti-tumor effects against sarcoma-180 bearing mice. *J Drug Target* 1997; 4:289–296.

84. Nori D, Li X, Pugkhem T. Intraoperative brachytherapy using gelfoam radioactive plaque implants for resected stage III non-small cell lung cancer with positive margin: a pilot study. *J Surg Oncol* 1995; 60:257–261.

85. Nastruzzi C, Pastesini C, Cortesi R, et al. Production and in vitro evaluation of gelatin microspheres containing an anti-tumour tetra-amidine. *J Microencapsul* 1994; 11:249–260.

86. Vandelli MA, Forni F, Coppi G, Cameroni R. The effect of the cross-linking time period upon the drug release and the dynamic swelling of gelatin microspheres. *Pharmazie* 1991; 46:866–869.

87. Ugwoke MI, Kinget R. Influence of processing variables on the properties of gelatin microspheres prepared by the emulsification solvent extraction technique. *J Microencapsul* 1998; 15:273–281.

88. Cortesi R, Nastruzzi C, Davis SS. Sugar cross-linked gelatin for controlled release: microspheres and disks. *Biomaterials* 1998; 19:1641–1649.

89. Cortesi R, Esposito E, Osti M, et al. Dextran cross-linked gelatin microspheres as a drug delivery system. *Eur J Pharm Biopharm* 1999; 47:153–160.

90. Draye J-P, Delaey B, van de Voorde A, et al. In vitro and in vivo biocompatibility of dextran dialdehyde cross- linked gelatin hydrogel films. *Biomaterials* 1998; 19:1677–1687.

91. Wang JH, Lu B, Xu PL, Bao DY, Zhang ZR. Studies on lung targeting gelatin microspheres of mitoxantrone. *Yao Hsueh Hsueh Pao* 1995; 30:549–555.

92. Lou Y, Groves MJ. In-vitro and in-vivo evaluation of an intravenous formulation of the antineoplastic agent thiotepa. *Pharm Sci* 1995; 1:355–358.

93. Lou Y, Klegerman ME, Muhammad A, Dai X, Groves MJ. Initial characterization of an antineoplastic polysaccharide-rich extract of mycobacterium bovis BCG, Tice substrain. *Anticancer Res* 1994b; 14:1469–1476.

94. Lou Y, Groves MJ, Klegerman ME. In-vivo and in-vitro targeting of a murine sarcoma by gelatin microparticles loaded with a glycan (PS1). *J Pharm Pharmacol* 1994a; 46:863–866.

95. Tabata Y, Ikada Y. Drug delivery systems for antitumor activation of macrophages. *Crit Rev Ther Drug Carrier Syst* 1990a; 7:121–148.

96. Tabata Y, Ikada Y. Phagocytosis of polymer microspheres by macrophages. *Adv Polym Sci* 1990c; 94:107–114.

97. Tabata Y, Ikada Y. Synthesis of gelatin microspheres containing interferon. *Pharm Res* 1989; 6:422–427.

98. Tabata Y, Uno K, Muramatsu S, Ikada Y. In vivo effects of recombinant interferon alpha A/D incorporated in gelatin microspheres on murine tumor cell growth. *Jpn J Cancer Res* 1989; 80:387–393.

99. Tabata Y, Ikada Y. Macrophage activation for antitumour function by muramyl dipeptide-protein conjugates. *J Pharm Pharmacol* 1990b; 42:13–19.

100. Tabata Y, Uno K, Yamaoka T, Ikada Y, Muramatsu S. Effects of recombinant alpha-interferon-gelatin conjugate on in vivo murine tumor cell growth. *Cancer Res* 1991; 51:5532–5538.

101. Tabata Y, Uno K, Ikada Y, Kishida T, Muramatsu S. Potentiation of in vivo antitumor effects of recombinant interleukin-1 alpha by gelatin conjugation. *Jpn J Cancer Res* 1993a; 84:681–688.

102. Tabata Y, Uno K, Ikada Y, Muramatsu S. Suppressive effect of recombinant TNF-gelatin conjugate on murine tumour growth in-vivo. *J Pharm Pharmacol* 1993b; 45:303–308.

103. Oppenheim RC, Marty JJ, Stewart NF. The labelling of gelatin nanoparticles with 99mTechnetium and their in vivo distribution after intravenous injection. *Austral J Pharm Sci* 1978; 7:113–117.

104. Marty JJ, Oppenheim RC, Speiser P. Nanoparticles – a new colloidal drug delivery system. *Pharm Acta Helv* 1978; 53:17–23.

105. Kalyanasundaram S, Feinstein S, Nicholson JP, Leong KW, Garver RI Jr. Coacervate microspheres as carriers of recombinant adenoviruses. *Cancer Gene Ther* 1999; 6:107–112.

106. Venook AP, Warren RS. Regional chemotherapy approaches for primary and metastatic liver tumors. *Surg Oncol Clin N Amer* 1996; 5:411–427.

107. Lu CD, Peng SY, Jiang XC, Chiba Y, Tanigawa N. Preoperative transcatheter arterial chemoembolization and prognosis of patients with hepatocellular carcinomas: retrospective analysis of 120 cases. *World J Surg* 1999; 23:293–300.

108. Seong J, Keum KC, Han KH, et al. Combined transcatheter arterial chemoembolization and local radiotherapy of unresectable hepatocellular carcinoma. *Int J Radiat Oncol Biol Phys* 1999; 43:393–397.

109. Chung JW, Park JH, Han JK, Choi BI, Kim TK, Han MC. Transcatheter oily chemoembolization of the inferior phrenic artery in hepatocellular carcinoma: the safety and potential therapeutic role. *J Vasc Interv Radiol* 1998; 9:495–500.

110. Bartolozzi C, Lencioni R, Armillotta N. Combined treatment of hepatocarcinoma with chemoembolization and alcohol administration. Long-term results. *Radiol Med Torino* 1997; 94:19–23.

111. Hatanaka Y, Yamashita Y, Takahashi M, et al. Unresectable hepatocellular carcinoma: analysis of prognostic factors in transcatheter management. *Radiology* 1995; 195:747–752.

112. Sakamoto I, Aso N, Nagaoki K, et al. Complications associated with transcatheter arterial embolization for hepatic tumors. *Radiographics* 1998; 8:605–619.

113. Chung JW, Park JH, Han JK, et al. Hepatic tumors: predisposing factors for complications of transcatheter oily chemoembolization. *Radiology* 1996; 198:33–40.

114. Layalle I, Flandroy P, Trotteur G, Dondelinger RF. Arterial embolization of bone metastases: is it worthwhile? *J Belge Radiol* 1998; 81:223–225.

115. Smith TP, Gray L, Weinstein JN, Richardson WJ, Payne CS. Preoperative transarterial embolization of spinal column neoplasms. *J Vasc Interv Radiol* 1995; 6:863–869.

116. O'Keeffe FN, Carrasco CH, Charnsangavej C, Richli WR, Wallace S. Arterial embolization of adrenal tumors. *Am J Roentgenol* 1988; 151:819–822.

117. Nagata Y, Mitsumori M, Okajima K, et al. *Cardiovasc Intervent Radiol* 1998; 21:208–213.

118. Sonomura T, Yamada R, Kishi K, et al. Dependency of tissue necrosis on gelatin sponge particle size after canine hepatic artery embolization. *Cardiovasc Intervent Radiol* 1997; 20:50–53.

119. Sonomura T. Optimal size of embolic material in transcatheter arterial embolization of the liver. *Nippon Igaku Hoshasen Gakkai Zasshi* 1994; 54:489–499.

120. Cherqui D, Piedbois P, Pierga J-Y, et al. Multimodal adjuvant treatment and liver transplantation for advanced hepatocellular carcinoma. *Cancer* 1994; 73:2721–2726.

121. Higashi S, Shimizu M, Nakashima T, et al. Arterial-injection chemotherapy for hepatocellular carcinoma using monodispersed poppy-seed oil microdroplets containing fine aqueous vesicles of epirubicin. Initial medical application of a membrane-emulsification technique. *Cancer* 1995; 75:1245–1254.

122. Sanz-Altamira PM, Spence LD, Huberman MS, et al. Selective chemoembolization in the management of hepatic metastases in refractory colorectal carcinoma: a phase II trial. *Dis Colon Rectum* 1997; 40:770–775.

123. Fiorentini G, Campanini A, Dazzi C, et al. Chemoembolization in liver malignant involvement. *Minerva Chir* 1994; 49:281–285.

124. Ruszniewski P, Rougier P, Roche A, et al. Hepatic arterial chemoembolization in patients with liver metastases of endocrine tumors. *Cancer* 1993; 71:2624–2630.

125. Shimizu T, Endou H. SMANCS/TAE for hepatocellular carcinoma: comparison with SMANCS/TAI. *Gan To Kagaku Ryoho* 1998; 25:80–83.

126. Yan C, Li X, Chen X, et al. Anticancer gelatin microspheres with multiple functions. *Biomaterials* 1991; 12:640–644.

127. Chen QH, Lu WG, Ge QH, et al. Study on targeting drug delivery system – the characteristics of methotrexate microsphere and experimental treatment of hepatic tumor in rats by arterial embolization. *Yao Hsueh Hsueh Pao* 1991; 26:293–298.

128. Laurent A, Beaujeux R, Wassef M, et al. Trisacryl gelatin microspheres for therapeutic embolization I: development and in vitro evaluation. *Am J Neuroradiol* 1996; 17:533–540.

129. Beaujeux R, Laurent A, Wassef M, et al. Trisacryl gelatin microspheres for therapeutic embolization. II: preliminary clinical evaluation in tumors and arteriovenous malformations. *Am J Neuroradiol* 1996; 17:541–548.

130. Martindale. The Extra Pharmacopoeia Monograph: Albumin. Reynolds JEF (Ed). The Pharmaceutical Press, London, UK, 1996a, pp. 754.

131. Moser U, Albuminlösung vom Menschen – Kommentar A 18 zum Deutschen Arzneibuch 1996, Wiss. Verlagsg., Stuttgart, 1997.

132. Shrake A, Finlayson JS, Ross PD. Thermal stability of human albumin measured by differential scanning calorimetry. *Vox Sang* 1984; 47:7–18.

133. Tullis JL. Albumin. 1. Background and use. *JAMA* 1977a; 237:355–360.

134. Tullis JL, Albumin. 2. Guidelines for clinical use. *JAMA* 1977b; 237:460–463.

135. Pechtold F, Steinsträßer A, [99mTc] Technetium-Mikrosphären-Injektionslösung. Kommentar T 14 zum Deutschen Arzneibuch, 10. Aufl Wiss Verlagsg., Stuttgart 1995b.

136. Order SE, Siegel JA, Lustig RA, et al. A new method for delivering radioactive cytotoxic agents in solid cancers. *Int J Radiat Oncol Biol Phys* 1994; 30:715–720.

137. European Pharmacopoeia, Monograph 570: European Pharmacopoeia, Monograph 570: Technetium (99mTc) macrosalb injection, 2002. European Department for the Quality of Medicines within the Council of Europe, Strasbourg, France, 2002.

138. Pechtold F, Steinsträßer A, [99mTc] Technetium-Macrosalb-Injektionslösung. Kommentar T 12 zum Deutschen Arzneibuch, 10. Aufl, Wiss. Verlagsg., Stuttgart, 1995a.

139. Roser M, Fischer D, Kissel T. Surface-modified biodegradable albumin nano- and microspheres. II: effect of surface charges on in vitro phagocytosis and biodistribution in rats. *Eur J Pharm Biopharm* 1998; 46:255–263.

140. Walday P, Tolleshaug H, Gjoen T, et al. Biodistributions of air-filled albumin microspheres in rats and pigs. *Biochem J* 1994; 299:437–443.

141. Cohen JL, Cheirif J, Segar DS, et al. Improved left ventricular endocardial border delineation and opacification with optison (FS069), a new echocardiographic contrast agent. Results of a phase III multicenter trial. *J Am Coll Cardiol* 1998; 32:746–752.

142. Arshady R. Albumin microspheres and microcapsules: methodology of manufacturing techniques. *J Contr Rel* 1990; 14:111–131.

143. Gupta PK, Hung C-T. Albumin microspheres I: physico-chemical characteristics. *J Microencapsul* 1989a; 6:463–472.

144. Gupta PK, Hung C-T. Albumin microspheres II: applications in drug delivery. *J Microencapsul* 1989b; 6:473–484.

145. Sokoloski TD, Royer GP. Drug entrapment within native albumin beads, in *Microspheres and drug therapy. Pharmaceutical, immunological and medical aspects* (Davis SS, Illum L, McVie JG, Tomlinson E, eds). Elsevier Science, New York, 1984, pp. 295–307.

146. Tomlinson E, Burger JJ, Schoonderwoerd EMA, McVie JG. Human serum albumin microspheres for intraarterial drug targeting of cytostatic compounds. Pharmaceutical aspects and release characteris-

tics, in *Microspheres and drug therapy. Pharmaceutical, immunological and medical aspects* (Davis SS, Illum L, McVie JG, Tomlinson E, eds). Elsevier Science, New York, 1984, pp. 75–89.

147. Okada H, Togouchi H. Biodegradable microspheres in drug delivery. *Crit Rev Ther Drug Carrier Syst* 1995; 12:1–99.

148. Willmott N, Kamel HMH, Cummings J, Stuart JFB, Florence AT. Adriamycin-loaded albumin microspheres: Lung entrapment and fate in the rat, in *Microspheres and drug therapy. Pharmaceutical, immunological and medical aspects* (Davis SS, Illum L, McVie JG, Tomlinson E, eds). Elsevier Science, New York, 1984, pp. 205–215.

149. Sugibayashi K, Morimoto Y, Nadai T, Kato Y. Drug carrier property of albumin microspheres in chemotherapy. 1. Tissue distribution of microsphere entrapped 5-fluorouracil in mice. *Chem Pharm Bull* 1977; 25:3433–3434.

150. Oppenheim RC, Gipps EM, Forbes JF, Whitehead RH. Development and testing of proteinaceous nanoparticles containing cytotoxics, in *Microspheres and drug therapy. Pharmaceutical, immunological and medical aspects* (Davis SS, Illum L, McVie JG, Tomlinson E, eds). Elsevier Science, New York, 1984, pp. 117–128.

151. Müller BG, Leuenberger H, Kissel T. Albumin nanospheres as carriers for passive drug targeting: an optimized manufacturing technique. *Pharm Res* 1996; 13:32–37.

152. Lin W, Coombes AGA, Garnett MC, et al. Preparation of sterically stabilized human serum albumin nanospheres using a novel dextranox-MPEG crosslinking agent. *Pharm Res* 1994; 11:1588–1592.

153. Lin W, Garnett MC, Davies MC, et al. Preparation of surface-modified albumin nanospheres. *Biomaterials* 1997; 18:559–565.

154. Demoy M, Andreux JP, Weingarten C, et al. In vitro evaluation of nanoparticles spleen capture. *Life Sci* 1999; 64:1329–1337.

155. Schafer V, von Briesen H, Rubsamen-Waigmann H, et al. Phagocytosis and degradation of human serum albumin microspheres and nanoparticles in human macrophages. *J Microencapsul* 1994; 11:261–269.

156. Sheng J, Samten BK, Xie SS, Wei SL. Study on the specific killing activity of albumin nanoparticles containing adriamycin targeted by monoclonal antibody BDI-1 to human bladder cancer cells. *Yao Hsueh Hsueh Pao* 1995; 30:706–710.

157. Akasaka Y, Ueda H, Takayama K, Machida Y, Nagai T. Preparation and evaluation of bovine serum albumin nanospheres coated with monoclonal antibodies. *Drug Des Deliv* 1988; 3:85–97.

158. Widder KJ, Morris RM, Poore GA, Howard DP, Senyei AE. Selective targeting of magnetic albumin microspheres containing low-dose doxorubicin: total remission in Yoshida sarcoma-bearing rats. *Eur J Cancer Clin Oncol* 1983; 19:135–139.

159. Gupta PK, Hung C-T. Targeted delivery of low dose doxorubicin hydrochloride administered via magnetic albumin microspheres in rats. *J Microencapsul* 1990; 7:85–94.

160. Truter EJ. Heat-stabilized albumin microspheres as a sustained drug delivery system for the antimetabolite, 5-fluorouracil. *Art Cells Blood Subs Immob Biotech* 1995; 23:579–586.

161. Wang RZ, Zhong WQ, Guan SR. Daunomycin-human albumin microspheres (dau-ha-ms) – preparation, characterization and use in experimental cancer therapy. *Chung Hua Chung Liu Tsa Chih* 1994; 16:98–101.

162. Morimoto Y, Akimoto M, Sugibayashi K, Nadai T, Kato Y. Drug carrier property of albumin microspheres in chemotherapy. IV. Antitumour effect of single shot or multiple shot administration of microspheres entrapped 5-fluorouracil on Ehrlich ascites or solid tumour in mice. *Chem Pharm Bull* 1980; 28:3087–3092.

163. Cremers HFM, Seymour LW, Lam K, et al. Adriamycin-loaded albumin-heparin conjugate microspheres for intraperitoneal chemotherapy. *Int J Pharmaceut* 1994b; 110:117–124.

164. Goldberg EP, Iwata H, Longo W. Hydrophilic albumin and dextran ion-exchange microspheres for localized chemotherapy, in *Microspheres and drug therapy. Pharmaceutical, immunological and medical aspects* (Davis SS, Illum L, McVie JG, Tomlinson E, eds). Elsevier Science, New York, 1984, pp. 309–325.

165. Cremers HFM, Kwon G, Bae YH, et al. Preparation and characterization of albumin-heparin microspheres. *Biomaterials* 1994a; 15:38–48.

166. Cremers HFM, Wolf RFE, Blaauw EH, et al. Degradation and intrahepatic compatibility of albumin-heparin conjugate microspheres. *Biomaterials* 1994c; 15:577–585.

167. D'Souza MJ, Pourfarzib R. Improved efficacy of a microencapsulated macrophage colony stimulating factor and methotrexate in melanoma. *Drug Dev Ind Pharm* 1999; 25:583–590.

168. D'Souza MJ, Oettinger CW, Milton GV. Evaluation of microspheres containing cytokine neutralizing antibodies in endotoxemia. *Drug Dev Ind Pharm* 1999; 25:727–734.

169. Oettinger CW, D'Souza M, Milton GV. Targeting macrophages with microspheres containing cytokine-neutralizing antibodies prevents lethality in gram-negative peritonitis. *J Interferon Cytokine Res* 1999; 19:33–40.

170. Cummings J, Allan L, Smyth JF. Encapsulation of mitomycin C in albumin microspheres markedly alters pharmacokinetics, drug quinone reduction in tumour tissue and antitumour activity. Implications for the drugs' in vivo mechanism of action. *Biochem Pharmacol* 1994; 47:1345–1356.

171. Novotny J, Zinek K. Application of epirubicin containing albumin microspheres in the experimental therapy of breast cancer. *Neoplasma* 1994; 41:201–204.

172. Morimoto Y, Fujimoto S. Albumin microspheres as drug carriers. *Crit Rev Ther Drug Carrier Syst* 1985; 2:16–63.

173. Goldberg JA, Kerr DJ, Wilmott N, McKillop JH, McArdle CS. Regional chemotherapy for colorectal metastases: a phase II evaluation of targeted hepatic arterial 5-fluorouracil for colorectal liver metastases. *Br J Surg* 1990; 77:1238–1240.

174. Goldberg JA, Willmott NS, Anderson JH, et al. The biodegradation of albumin microspheres used for regional chemotherapy in patient with colorectal liver metastases. *Nucl Med Commun* 1991; 12:57–63.

175. Fujimoto S, Miyazaki M, Endoh F, et al. Biodegradable mitomycin C microspheres given intra-arterially for inoperable hepatic cancer. With particular reference to a comparison with continuous infusion of mitomycin C and 5-fluorouracil. *Cancer* 1985; 56:2404–2410.

176. Fujimoto S, Endoh F, Kitsukawa Y, et al. Continued in vitro and in vivo release of an antitumor drug from albumin microspheres. *Experientia* 1983; 39:913–916.

177. Allan L, Cummings J, Willmott N, Whateley TL, Smyth JF. Incorporation and release of chemically intact mitomycin C from albumin microspheres: a high performance liquid chromatography evaluation. *J Drug Target* 1993; 1:317–323.

178. Tomlinson E, Burger JJ. Incorporation of water-soluble drugs in albumin microspheres. *Methods Enzymol* 1985; 112:27–43.

179. Nishioka Y, Kyotani S, Okamura M, et al. A study of embolizing materials for chemo-embolization therapy of hepatocellular carcinoma: effects of chitin concentration on cis-diamminedichloroplatinum(II) albumin microsphere properties and antitumor effect in VX2 hepatocellular carcinoma model rabbits. *Biol Pharm Bull* 1993; 16:1136–1139.

180. Kyotani S, Nishioka Y, Okamura M, et al. A study of embolizing materials for chemo-embolization therapy of hepatocellular carcinoma antitumor effect of cis-diamminedichloroplatinum(II) albumin microspheres, containing chitin and treated with chitosan on rabbits with VX2 hepatic tumors. *Chem Pharm Bull* 1992; 40:2814–2816.

181. Nishioka Y, Kyotani S, Okamura M, et al. A study of embolizing materials for chemo-embolization therapy of hepatocellular carcinoma: effects of particle size and dose on chitin-containing cis-diamminedichloroplatinum(II) albumin microsphere antitumor activity in VX2 hepatic tumor model rabbits. *Biol Pharm Bull* 1994; 17:1251–1255.

182. Doughty JC, Anderson JH, Willmott N, McArdle CS. Intra-arterial administration of adriamycin-loaded albumin microspheres for locally advanced breast cancer. *Postgrad Med J* 1995; 71:47–49.

183. Kabuto M, Kubota T, Kobayashi H, et al. Experimental study of intraoperative local chemotherapy with fibrin glue containing nitrosourea for malignant gliomas. *Surg Neurol* 1995; 44:151–156.

184. Takahashi Y, Minami S, Ohta T, et al. Experimental study on local attachment of Beriplast P membrane including MMC. *Gan To Kagaku Ryoho* 1991; 18:1944–1946.

185. European Pharmacopoeia, Monograph 903: Fibrin Sealant Kit. European Department for the Quality of Medicines within the Council of Europe, Strasbourg, France, 2002 4th ed., Supp. 4.6, p. 4003.

186. Martindale, The Extra Pharmacopoeia, Monograph: Fibrin. Reynolds, JEF (Ed). The Pharmaceutical Press, London, UK, 1996b, pp. 766.

187. Redl H, Schlag G, Dinges HP. The use and biomcompatibility of a human fibrin sealant for heamostasis and tissue sealing, in *Biocompatibility of tissue analogs* (Williams D, ed). Vol. I. CRC, Boca Raton, FL, 1985, pp. 136–157.

188. Tanaka T, Yamana H, Fujita H, et al. An experimental study on antitumor effect of MMC-fibrin glue mixture. *Gan To Kagaku Ryoho* 1996; 23:1400–1402.

189. Kawasaki H, Shimizu T, Takakura K, Umezawa Y. Pharmacodynamic study of mitomycin C mixed with fibrin glue for treatment of malignant brain tumors. *No Shinkei Geka* 1994; 22:819–825.

190. Matsuoka H, Yano K, Katsuta Y, et al. Advantages and safety of local treatment with MMC/Beriplast P for cancer tumors. *Cancer Chemotherap Pharmacol* 1996; 38:508–512.

191. Yano K, Matsuoka H, Baba H, et al. Antitumor effect of MMC mixed in Beriplast P. *Gan To Kagaku Ryoho* 1995; 22:1629–1631.

192. Miura S, Mii Y, Miyauchi Y, et al. Efficacy of slow-releasing anticancer drug delivery systems on transplantable osteosarcomas in rats. *Jpn J Clin Oncol* 1995; 25:61–71.
193. Kubota T, Matsui K, Ohtani M, Takasaki S. Local chemotherapy by a sustained-release preparation with fibrin seal against the operative wound in head and neck cancer. *Gan To Kagaku Ryoho* 1995; 22:877–882.
194. Hirakawa W, Kadota K, Asakura T, et al. Local chemotherapy for malignant brain tumors using methotrexate-containing fibrin glue. *Gan To Kagaku Ryoho* 1995; 22:805–809.
195. Ishiko T, Sakamoto K, Mita S, Kamohara H, Ogawa M. Evidence that eosinophil infiltration in the OK-432/fibrinogen-injected Meth-A tumor in mice is mediated by locally produced IL-5. *Int J Immunopharmacol* 1997; 19:405–412.
196. Monden T, Morimoto H, Shimano T, et al. Use of fibrinogen to enhance the anti-tumor effect of OK-432. A new approach to immunotherapy for colorectal cancer. *Cancer* 1992; 69:636–642.
197. Yoshida T, Osato H, Sakon M, et al. Locoregional injection of OK-432/fibrinogen/thrombin for unresectable metastatic liver tumors. *Gan To Kagaku Ryoho* 1996; 23:1575–1577.
198. Takeda T, Ito Y, Wakasugi E, Kobayashi T, Monden M. Role of urokinase-type plasminogen activator in local immunotherapy. *Oncol Rep* 1998; 5:329–333.
199. Takekuni K, Sakon M, Kishimoto S, et al. A patient with unresectable cancer of pancreas head, effectively treated by a local injection of the mixture of OK-432, fibrinogen and thrombin. *Gan To Kagaku Ryoho* 1996; 23:1621–1623.
200. Takeda T, Kobayashi T, Monden T, et al. The effect of local immunotherapy for breast cancer using a mixture of OK-432 and fibrinogen supplemented with activated macrophages. *Biotherapy* 1994; 7:47–54.
201. Sugitachi A, Shindo T, Matsuda Y, Sakamoto I. A newly designed anticancer tumor immunity drug delivery system. *ASAIO Trans* 1991; 37:M177–178.
202. Sugitachi A, Kawahara T, Kido T, Shindoh T, Sakamoto I. Loco-regional cancer chemotherapy in patients with malignant pleural effusion – improving the QOL of patients. *Gan To Kagaku Ryoho* 1990; 17:1583–1587.
203. Kitazawa H, Sato H, Adachi I, Masuko Y, Horikoshi I. Microdialysis assessment of fibrin glue containing sodium alginate for local delivery of doxorubicin in tumor-bearing rats. *Biol Pharm Bull* 1997; 20:278–281.
204. Ishihama H, Nagai S, Umezu H, et al. The usefulness of fibrin glue spraying combined with CDDP for lung cancer. *Gan To Kagaku Ryoho* 1997; 24:981–985.
205. Muzzarelli R, Baldassarre V, Conti F, et al. Biological activity of chitosan: ultrastructural study. *Biomaterials* 1998; 9:247–252.
206. Rao SB, Sharma CP. Use of chitosan as a biomaterial: study on its safety and hemostatic potential. *J Biomed Mater Res* 1997; 34:21–28.
207. Lee KY, Ha WS, Park WH. Blood compatibility and biodegradability of partially N-acetylated chitosan derivatives. *Biomaterials* 1995; 16:1211–1216.
208. Tomihata K, Ikada Y. In vitro and in vivo degradation of films of chitin and its deacetylated derivatives. *Biomaterials* 1997; 18:567–575.
209. Ohnishi H, Machida Y. Biodegradation and distribution of water-soluble chitosan in mice. *Biomaterials* 1999; 20:175–182.
210. Carreno-Gomez B, Duncan R. Evaluation of the biological properties of soluble chitosan and chitosan microspheres. *Int J Pharm* 1997; 148:231–240.
211. Varum KM, Myhr MM, Hjerde RJ, Smidsrod O. In vitro degradation rates of partially N-acetylated chitosans in human serum. *Carbohydr Res* 1997; 299:99–101.
212. Kristiansen A, Varum KM, Grasdalen H. Quantitative studies of the non-productive binding of lysozyme to partially N-acetylated chitosans. Binding of large ligands to a one-dimensional binary lattice studied by a modified McGhee and von Hippel model. *Biochim Biophys Acta* 1998; 1425:137–150.
213. Kamiyama K, Ohnishi H, Machida Y. Biodisposition characteristics of N-succinyl-chitosan and glycol-chitosan in normal and tumor-bearing mice. *Biol Pharm Bull* 1999; 22:170–186.
214. Saiki I, Murata J, Nakajima M, Tokura S, Azuma I. Inhibition by sulfated chitin derivatives of invasion through extracellular matrix and enzymatic degradation by metastatic melanoma cells. *Cancer Res* 1990; 50:3631–3637.
215. Guminska M, Ignacak J, Wojcik E. In vitro inhibitory effect of chitosan and its degradation product on energy metabolism in Ehrlich ascites tumour cells (EAT). *Pol J Pharmacol* 1996; 48:495–501.
216. Azuma I. Synthetic immunoadjuvants: application to non-specific host stimulation and potentiation of vaccine immunogenicity. *Vaccine* 1992; 10:1000–1006.

217. Shibata Y, Foster LA, Metzger WJ, Myrvik QN. Alveolar macrophage priming by intravenous administration of chitin particles, polymers of N-acetyl-D-glucosamine, in mice. *Infect Immun* 1997a; 65:1734–1741.

218. Shibata Y, Metzger WJ, Myrvik QN. Chitin particle-induced cell-mediated immunity is inhibited by soluble mannan: mannose receptor-mediated phagocytosis initiates IL-12 production. *J Immunol* 1997b; 159:2462–2467.

219. Lim BO, Yamada K, Nonaka M, et al. Dietary fibers modulate indices of intestinal immune function in rats. *J Nutr* 1997; 127:663–667.

220. Mori T, Okumura M, Matsuura M, et al. Effects of chitin and its derivatives on the proliferation and cytokine production of fibroblasts in vitro. *Biomaterials* 1997; 18:947–951.

221. Lehr CM, Bouwstra JA, Schacht EH, Junginger HE. In vitro evaluation of mucoadhesive properties of chitosan and some other natural polymers. *Int J Pharm* 1992; 78:43–48.

222. Artursson P, Lindmark T, Davis SS, Illum L. Effect of chitosan on the permeability of monolayers of intestinal epithelial cells (caco-2). *Pharm Res* 1994; 11:1358–1361.

223. Li Q, Dunn ET, Grandmaison EW, Goosen MFA. Applications and properties of chitosan, in *Applications of chitin and chitosan* (Goosen MFA, ed). Technomic Publ. Comp., Lancaster, PA, 1997, pp. 3–30.

224. Bodmeier R, Chen H, Paeratakul O. A novel approach to the oral delivery of micro- or nanoparticles. *Pharm Res* 1989; 6:413–417.

225. Gruber JV. Polysaccharide-based polymers in cosmetics, in *Principles of polymer science and technology in cosmetics and personal care* (Goddard ED, Gruber JV, eds). Marcel Dekker Inc., New York, 1999, pp. 325–389.

226. Kubota N, Kikuchi Y. Macromolecular complexes of chitosan, in *Polysaccharides: structural diversity and functional versatility* (Dumitriu S, ed). Marcel Dekker, New York, 1998, pp. 595–628.

227. Chen WR, Adams RL, Carubelli R, Nordquist RE. Laser-photosensitizer assisted immunotherapy: a novel modality for cancer treatment. *Cancer Lett* 1997; 115:25–30.

228. Xu F, Liu H, Wu X, et al. Measurement of x-ray attenuation coefficients of aqueous solutions of indocyanine green and glycated chitosan. *Med Phys* 1999; 26:1371–1374.

229. Richardson SCW, Kolbe HVJ, Duncan R. Potential of low molecular mass chitosan as a DNA delivery system: biocompatibility, body distribution and ability to complex and protect DNA. *Int J Pharm* 1999; 178:231–243.

230. Leong KW, Mao H-Q, Truong-Le VL, et al. DNA-polycation nanospheres as non-viral gene delivery vehicles. *J Contr Rel* 1998; 53:183–193.

231. Berthold A, Cremer K, Kreuter J. Influence of crosslinking on the acid stability and physicochemical properties of chitosan microspheres. *STP Pharma Sci* 1996; 6:358–364.

232. Lim LY, Wan LSC. Heat treatment of chitosan films. *Drug Dev Ind Pharm* 1995; 21:839–846.

233. Patashnik S, Rabinovich L, Golomb G. Preparation and evaluation of chitosan microspheres containing bisphosphonates. *J Drug Target* 1997; 4:371–380.

234. Giunchedi P, Genta I, Conti B, Muzzarelli RAA, Conte U. Preparation and characterization of ampicillin loaded methylpyrrolidinone chitosan and chitosan microspheres. *Biomaterials* 1998; 19:157–161.

235. Ohnishi H, Nagai T, Machida Y. Applications of chitin, chitosan, and their derivatives to drug carriers for microparticulated or conjugated drug delivery sytems, in *Applications of chitin and chitosan* (Goosen MFA, ed). Technomic Publ. Comp., Lancaster, PA, 1997, pp. 3–30.

236. Muzzarelli RAA, Muzzarelli B. Structural and functional versatility of chitins, in *Polysaccharides: structural diversity and functional versatility* (Dumitriu S, ed). Marcel Dekker, New York, 1998, pp. 569–594.

237. Wang YM, Shi TS, Pu YL, Zhu JG, Zhao YL. Studies on preparation and characteristics of cisplatin chitosan microspheres. *Yao Hsueh Hsueh Pao* 1996; 31:300–305.

238. Tabara H, Matsuura H, Kohno H, et al. Intraarterial chemoembolization therapy for unresectable liver cancer using plachitin particles. *Gan To Gakaku Ryoho* 1994; 21:2225–2228.

239. Tabara H, Kinusaga S, Tachibana M, et al. Pharmacokinetic study of intraperitoneally administered plachitin for non-curative gastrointestinal. *Gan To Gakaku Ryoho* 1995; 22:1473–1476.

240. Suzuki K, Nakamura T, Matsuura H, Kifune K, Tsurutani R. A new drug delivery system for local cancer chemotherapy using cisplatin and chitin. *Anticancer Res* 1995; 15:423–426.

241. Suzuki K, Matsuura H, Yoshimura H, et al. Slow releasing anticancer drug containing CDDP for intraoperative use in residual cancer cells. *Gan To Gakaku Ryoho* 1992; 19:1728–1730.

242. Jameela SR, Jayakrishnan A. Glutaraldehyde cross-linked chitosan microspheres as a long-acting biodegradable drug delivery vehicle: studies on the in vitro release of mitoxantrone and in vivo degradation of microspheres in rat muscle. *Biomaterials* 1995; 16:769–775.

243. Hassan EE, Parish RC, Gallo JM. Optimized formulation of magnetic chitosan microspheres containing the anticancer agent oxantrazole. *Pharm Res* 1992; 9:390–397.

244. Hassan EE, Gallo JM. Targeting anticancer drugs to the brain. I. Enhanced brain delivery of oxantrazole following administration in magnetic cationic microspheres. *J Drug Target* 1993; 1:7–14.

245. Sato M, Onishi H, Takahara J, Machida Y, Nagai T. In vivo drug release and antitumor characteristics of water-soluble conjugates of mitomycin C with glycol-chitosan and N-succinyl-chitosan. *Biol Pharm Bull* 1996; 19:1170–1177.

246. Azuma I, Saiki I. Prevention of cancer metastasis in mice with fibronectin-related substances. *Princess Takamatsu Symp* 1994; 24:125–141.

247. Matsuoka T, Hirakawa K, Chung YS, et al. Adhesion polypeptides are useful for the prevention of peritoneal dissemination of gastric cancer. *Clin Exp Metastasis* 1998; 16:381–388.

248. Komazawa H, Saiki I, Nishikawa N, et al. Inhibition of tumor metastasis by arg-gly-asp-ser (RGDS) peptide conjugated with sulfated chitin derivative, SCM-chitin-RGDS. *Clin Exp Metastasis* 1993; 11:482–491.

249. Murata J, Saiki I. Inhibition of tumor metastasis by synthetic peptide analogues of cell-adhesive RGD sequence of fibronectin. *Nippon Rinsho* 1995; 53:1653–1659.

250. Suzuki YS, Momose Y, Higashi N, et al. Biodistribution and kinetics of holmium-166-chitosan complex (DW-166HC) in rats and mice. *J Nucl Med* 1998; 39:2161–2166.

251. Lee WY, Moon EY, Lee J, et al. Toxicities of 166holmium-chitosan in mice. *Arzneimittelforschung* 1998; 48:300–304.

252. Vercruysse KP, Prestwich GD. Hyaluronate derivatives in drug delivery. *Crit Rev Ther Drug Carrier Syst* 1998; 15:513–555.

253. Stedman's Medical Dictionary, Hyaluroanic acid. Williams & Wilkins, Baltimore, MD, 26th ed., 1995, p. 813.

254. Swann DA, Kuo J. Hyaluronic acid, in *Biomaterials* (Byrom D, ed.) Stockton Press, New York, 1991, pp. 287–305.

255. Jann K, Jann B. Bacterial polysaccharides related to mammalian structures, in *Polysaccharides: structural diversity and functional versatility* (Dumitriu S, ed). Marcel Dekker, New York, 1998, pp. 211–236.

256. Berriaud N, Milas M, Rinaudo M. Characterization and properties of hyaluronic acid (hyaluronan), in *Polysaccharides: structural diversity and functional versatility* (Dumitriu S, ed). Marcel Dekker, New York, 1998, pp. 313–334.

257. Demeester J, Vercruysse KP. Hyaluronidase, in *Pharmaceutical enzymes* (Lauwers A, ed). Marcel Dekker, New York, 1997, pp. 155–186.

258. Fraser JRE, Laurent TC, Laurent UBG. Hyaluronan: its nature, distribution, functions, and turnover, *J Intern Med* 1997; 242:27–33.

259. Sourdille P, Santiago PY, Villain F, et al. Reticulated hyaluronic acid implant in perforating trabecular surgery. *J Cataract Refract Surg* 1999; 25:332–329.

260. Abatangelo G, Barbucci R, Brun P, Lamponi S. Biocompatibility and enzymatic degradation studies on sulphated hyaluronic acid derivatives. *Biomaterials* 1997; 18:1411–1415.

261. Benedetti L, Cortivo R, Berti T, et al. Biocompatibility and biodegradation of different hyaluronan derivatives (Hyaff) implanted in rats. *Biomaterials* 1993; 14:1154–1160.

262. Larsen NE, Pollak CT, Reiner K, Leshchiner E, Balazs EA. Hylan gel biomaterial: dermal and immunologic compatibility. *J Biomed Mater Res* 1993; 27:1129–1134.

263. Haney AF, Doty E. A barrier composed of chemically cross-linked hyaluronic acid (Incert) reduces postoperative adhesion formation. *Fertil Steril* 1998; 70:145–151.

264. Radomsky ML, Aufdemorte TB, Swain LD, et al. Novel formulation of fibroblast growth factor-2 in a hyaluronan gel accelerates fracture healing in nonhuman primates. *J Orthop Res* 1999; 17:607–614.

265. Hyal Pharmaceutical, Press Release, Hyal announces revised agreement with debenture holders, 1/12/1998.

266. Nomura M, Sugira Y, Tatsumi Y, Miyamoto K. Adhesive interaction of highly malignant hepatoma AH66F cells with mesothelial cells. *Biol Pharm Bull* 1999; 22:738–740.

267. Hayen W, Goebeler M, Kumar S, Riessen R, Nehls V. Hyaluronan stimulates tumor cell migration by modulating the fibrin fiber architecture. *J Cell Sci* 1999; 112:2241–2251.

268. Kaystha S, Freedman AN, Piver MS, et al. Expression of hyaluronan receptor, CD44S, in epithelial ovarian cancer is an independent predictor of survival. *Clin Cancer Res* 1999; 5:1073–1076.

269. Ropponen K, Tammi M, Parkkinen J, et al. Tumor cell-associated hyaluronan as an unfavorable prognostic factor in colorectal cancer. *Cancer Res* 1998; 58:342–347.

270. Itano N, Sawai T, Miyaishi O, Kimata K. Relationship between hyaluronan production and metastatic potential of mouse mammary carcinoma cells. *Cancer Res* 1999; 59:2499–2504.

271. Samuelsson C, Gustafson S. Studies on the interaction between hyaluronan and a rat colon cancer cell line. *Glycoconj J* 1998; 15:169–175.
272. Mahmete H, Graf W, Larsson BS, Gustafson S. Uptake of hyaluronan in hepatic metastases after blocking of liver endothelial cell receptors. *Glycoconj J* 1998; 15:935–939.
273. Coradini D, Pellizzaro C, Miglierini G, Daidone MG, Perbillini A. Hyaluronic acid as drug delivery sodium butyrate: improvement of the anti-proliferative activity on a breast-cancer cell line. *Int J Cancer* 1999; 81:411–416.
274. Chang NS. Transforming growth factor-beta protection of cancer cells against tumor necrosis factor cytotoxicity is counteracted by hyaluronidase. *Int J Mol Med* 1998; 2:653–659.
275. Brekken C, de Lange-Davies C. Hyaluronidase reduces the interstitial fluid pressure in solid tumours in a non-linear concentration-dependent manner. *Cancer Lett* 1998; 131:65–70.
276. Baumgartner G. The impact of extracellular matrix on chemoresistance of solid tumors – experimental and clinical results of hyaluronidase as additive to cytostatic chemotherapy. *Cancer Lett* 1998; 131:1–2.
277. Klocker J, Sabitzer H, Raunik W, Wieser S, Schumer J. Hyaluronidase as additive to induction chemotherapy in advanced squamous cell carcinoma of the head and neck. *Cancer Lett* 1998; 131:113–115.
278. Haselsberger K, Radner H, Pendl G. Boron neutron capture therapy for glioblastoma: improvement of boron biodistribution by hyaluronidase. *Cancer Lett* 1998; 131:109–111.
279. Muckenschnabel I, Bernhardt G, Spruss T, Dietl B, Buschauer A. Quantitation of hyaluronidases by the Morgan-Elson reaction: comparison of the enzyme activities in the plasma of tumor patients and healthy volunteers. *Cancer Lett* 1998; 131:13–20.
280. Muckenschnabel I, Bernhardt G, Spruss T, Buschauer A. Hyaluronidase pretreatment produces selective melphalan enrichment in malignant melanoma implanted in nude mice. *Cancer Chemother Pharmacol* 1996; 38:88–94.
281. Kohno N, Ichikawa G, Kawasaki K, Kawaida M, Ohnuma T. Combination chemotherapy of solid tumor: effects of hyaluronidase on doxorubicin (DXR) penetration into multicellular tumor spheroids (MTS). *Gan To Kagaku Ryoho* 1992; 19:981–986.
282. Höbarth K, Maier U, Marberger M. Topical chemoprophylaxis of superficial bladder cancer with mitomycin C and adjuvant hyaluronidase. *Eur Urol* 1992; 21:206–210.
283. Pillwein K, Fuiko R, Slavc I, et al. Hyaluronidase additional standard chemotherapy improves outcome for children with malignant brain tumors. *Cancer Lett* 1998; 131:101–108.
284. St.-Croix B, Man S, Kerbel RS. Reversal of intrinsic and acquired forms of drug resistance by hyaluronidase treatment of solid tumors. *Cancer Lett* 1998; 131:35–44.
285. Kerbel RS, St.-Croix B, Florenes VA, Rak J. Induction and reversal of cell adhesion-dependent multicellular drug resistance in solid breast tumors. *Hum Cell* 1996; 8:247–264.
286. Disa JJ, Chang RR, Mucci SJ, Goldberg NH. Prevention of adriamycin-induced full-thickness skin loss using hyaluronidase infiltration. *Plast Reconstr Surg* 1998; 101:370–374.
287. Dorr RT, Snead K, Liddil JD. Skin ulceration potential of paclitaxel in a mouse skin model in vivo. *Cancer* 1996; 78:152–156.
288. Baumgartner G, Gomar-Hoss C, Sakr L, Ulsperger E, Wogritsch C. The impact of extracellular matrix on the chemoresistance of solid tumors – experimental and clinical results of hyaluronidase as additive to cytostatic chemotherapy. *Cancer Lett* 1998; 131:85–99.
289. Harnek J, Cwikiel W, Zoucas E, Seiving B, Stenram U. Treatment of adenocarcinoma of the liver with mitomycin, hyaluronidase, and ethanol: an experimental study in the rat. *Cardiovasc Intervent Radiol* 1998; 21:57–62.
290. Lindberg B, Lote K, Teder H. Biodegradable starch microspheres – a new medical tool, in *Microspheres and drug therapy. Pharmaceutical, immunological and medical aspects* (Davis SS, Illum L, McVie JG, Tomlinson E, eds). Elsevier Science, New York, 1984, pp. 153–188.
291. Hakansson L, Hakansson A, Morales O, Thorelius L, Warfving T. Spherex (degradable starch microspheres) chemo-occlusion – enhancement of tumor drug concentration and therapeutic efficacy: an overview. *Semin Oncol* 1997; 24:S6-100–S6-109.
292. Hamdi G, Ponchel G. Enzymatic degradation of epichlorohydrin crosslinked starch microspheres by α-amylase. *Pharm Res* 1999; 16:867–875.
293. Taguchi T. Chemo-occlusion for the treatment of liver cancer – a new technique using degradable starch microspheres. *Clin Pharmacokinet* 1994; 26:275–291.
294. Wollner IS, Walker-Andrews SC, Smith JE, Ensminger WD. Phase II study of hepatic arterial degradable starch microspheres and mitomycin. *Cancer Drug Deliv* 1986; 3:279–284.

295. Carr BI, Zajko A, Bron K, Orons P, Sammon J, Baron R. Phase II study of spherex (degradable starch microspheres) injected into the hepatic artery in conjunction with doxorubicin and cisplatin in the treatment of advanced-stage hepatocellular carcinoma: interim analysis. *Semin Oncol* 1997; 23:S6-97–S6-99.

296. Civalleri D, Pector J-C, Hakansson L, et al. Treatment of patients with irresectable liver metastases from colorectal cancer by chemo-occlusion with degradable starch microspheres. *Brit J Surg* 1994; 81:1338–1341.

297. Murata T, Akagi K, Imamura M, et al. Studies on hyperthermia combined with arterial therapeutic blockade for treatment of tumors (part III): effectiveness of hyperthermia combined with arterial chemoembolization using degradable starch microspheres on advanced liver cancer. *Oncol Rep* 1998; 5:709–712.

298. Deurloo MJM, Bohlken S, Kop W, et al. Intratumoral administration of cisplatin in slow-release devices: I. tumour response and toxicity. *Cancer Chemother Pharmacol* 1990a; 27:135–140.

299. Deurloo MJM, Kop W, van Tellingen O, Bartelink H, Begg AC. Intratumoral administration of cisplatin in slow-release devices: II. pharmacokinetics and intratumoural distribution. *Cancer Chemother Pharmacol* 1990b; 27:347–353.

300. Popa VI, Spiridon I. Hemicelluloses: structure and properties, in *Polysaccharides: structural diversity and functional versatility* (Dumitriu S, ed). Marcel Dekker, New York, 1998, pp. 297–312.

301. Martindale. The Extra Pharmacopoeia, Monograph: Dextran. Reynolds, JEF, (Ed.), The Pharmaceutical Press, London, UK, 1996c, pp. 760–762.

302. Mudge GH, Weiner IM. Agents affecting volume and composition of body fluids, in *Goodman and Gilman's – The Pharmacological Basis of Therapeutics* (Goodman Gilman A, Rall TW, Nies AS, Taylor P, eds). Pergamon, New York, 1990, pp. 682–707.

303. Ohyo Y, Masunaga T, Ouchi T, et al. Antitumor drug delivery by dextran derivatives immobilizing platinum complex (II) through coordination bond, in *Tailored polymeric materials for controlled delivery systems* (McCulloch I, Shalaby WS). ACS Symposium Series, American Chemical Society, Washington, USA, 1997, pp. 266–278.

304. Nakashima M, Ichinose K, Kanematsu T, et al. In vitro characteristics and in vivo plasma disposition of cisplatin conjugated with oxidized and dicarboxymethylated dextrans. *Biol Pharm Bull* 1999; 22:756–761.

305. Mitsumori M, Hiraoka M, Shibata T, et al. Targeted hyperthermia using dextran magnetite complex: a new treatment modality for liver tumors. *Hepatogastroenterology* 1996; 43:1431–1437.

306. Viroonchatapan E, Ueno M, Sato H, et al. Preparation and characterization of dextran magnetite-incorporated thermosensitive liposomes: an on-line flow system for quantifying magnetic responsiveness. *Pharm Res* 1995; 12:1176–1183.

307. Rousseau V, Pouliquen D, Darcel F, Jallet P, Le-Jeune JJ. NMR investigation of experimental chemical induced brain tumors in rats, potential of a superparamagnetic contrast agent (MD3) to improve diagnosis. *MAGMA* 1998; 6:13–21.

308. Caramella D, Jin XN, Mascalchi M, et al. Liver and spleen enhancement after intravenous injection of carboxydextran magnetite: effect of dose, delay of imaging, and field strength in an ex vivo model. *MAGMA* 1996; 4:225–230.

309. Pulfer SK, Ciccotto SL, Gallo JM. Distribution of small magnetic particles in brain tumor-bearing rats. *J Neurooncol* 1999; 41:99–105.

310. Pulfer SK, Gallo JM. Enhanced brain tumor selectivity of cationic magnetic polysaccharide microspheres. *J Drug Target* 1998; 6:215–227.

311. Devineni D, Blanton CD, Gallo JM. Preparation and in vitro evaluation of magnetic microsphere-methotrexate conjugate drug delivery systems. *Bioconjug Chem* 1995a; 6:203–210.

312. Devineni D, Klein-Szanto A, Gallo JM. Tissue distribution of methotrexate following administration as a solution and as a magnetic microsphere conjugate in rats bearing brain tumors. *J Neurooncol* 1995b; 34:143–152.

313. Liu Z, Wu XY, Bendayan R. In vitro investigation of ionic polysaccharide microspheres for simultaneous delivery of chemosensitizer and antineoplastic agent to multidrug-resistant cells. *J Pharm Sci* 1999; 88:412–418.

314. Hamada J, Kai Y, Nagahiro S, et al. Embolization with cellulose porous beads, II: clinical trial. *Am J Neuroradiol* 1996; 17:1901–1906.

315. Kato T, Sato K, Sasaki R, Kakinuma H, Moriyama M. Targeted cancer chemotherapy with arterial microcapsule chemoembolization: review of 1013 patients. *Cancer Chemother Pharmacol* 1996; 37:289–296.

316. Nemoto R, Kato T. Microencapsulation of anticancer drug for intraarterial infusion, and its clinical application, in *Microspheres and drug therapy. Pharmaceutical, immunological and medical aspects* (Davis SS, Illum L, McVie JG, Tomlinson E, eds). Elsevier Science, New York, 1984, pp. 153–188.

317. Ueda K, Sakagami H, Okamura T, Masui Y. Studies on the retention of the mucous-membrane-adhesive anticancer agent hydroxypropylcellulose doxorubicin. *Eur Urol* 1992; 21:250–252.

318. Ueda K, Sakagami H, Masui Y, Okamura T. Single instillation of hydroxypropylcellulose-doxorubicin as treatment for superficial bladder carcinoma. *Cancer Chemother Pharmacol* 1994; 35 Suppl:S81–83.

319. Horii A, Kyo M, Yasumoto R, et al. Clinical effect on tumor regression and tissue concentration of peplomycin treated with peplomycin emulsion in hydroxypropylcellulosum. *Hinyokika Kiyo* 1991; 37:21–24.

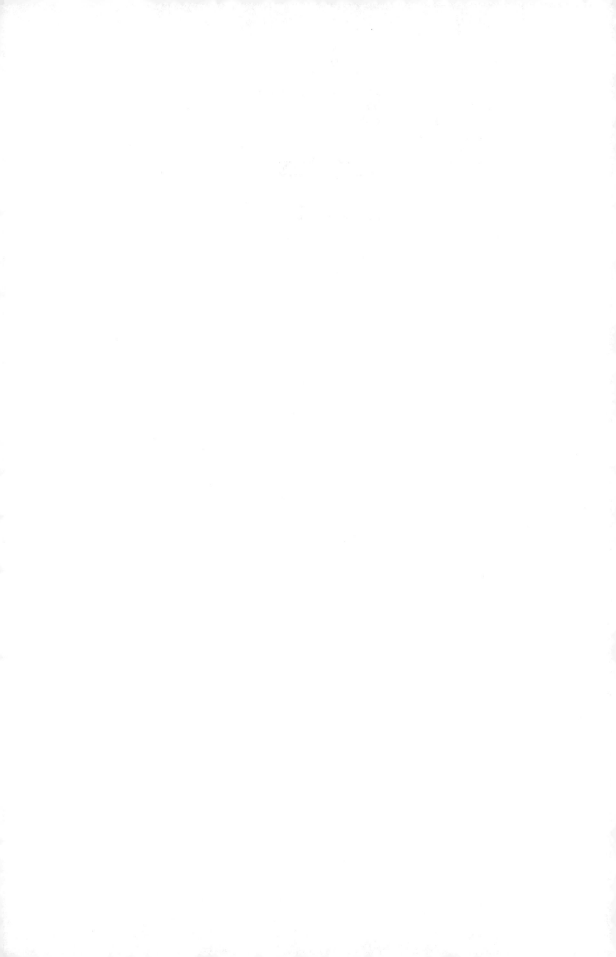

5

Hydrogels in Cancer Drug Delivery Systems

Sung-Joo Hwang, PhD, Namjin Baek, PhD, Haesun Park, PhD, and Kinam Park, PhD

CONTENTS

1. INTRODUCTION TO HYDROGELS

Hydrogels have played a vital role in the development of controlled-release drug delivery systems. A hydrogel (also called an aquagel) is a three-dimensional (3-D) network of hydrophilic polymers swollen in water *(1)*. The 3-D polymer network of a hydrogel is maintained in the form of elastic solid in the sense that there exists a remembered reference configuration to which the system returns even after being deformed for a very long time. By definition, hydrogels usually contain water at least 10% of the total weight. The term hydrogel implies that the material is already swollen in water. Dried hydrogels (or xerogels) absorb water to swell, and the size of the swollen gel depends on how much water is absorbed. A hydrogel swells for the same reason that an analogous linear polymer dissolves in water to form an ordinary polymer solution. The extent of swelling is usually measured by the swelling ratio, which is the volume (or weight) of the swollen gel divided by the volume (or weight) of the xerogel. If the weight of absorbed water exceeds 95% of the total weight, a hydrogel is often called a superabsorbent. Thus, 20 g of fully swollen superabsorbent will have 1 g or less of polymer network and 19 g or more of water (i.e., the swelling ratio is more than 20). The swelling ratio of many hydrogels can easily reach greater than 100. Despite such a large quantity of water, highly swollen hydrogels still maintain solid forms.

1.1. Preparation of Hydrogels

Hydrogels can be divided into chemical and physical gels depending on the nature of the crosslinking. Figure 1 shows chemical and physical gels. Chemical gels are those that have covalently crosslinked networks. Thus, chemical gels will not dissolve in water or other

From: *Drug Delivery Systems in Cancer Therapy*
Edited by: D. M. Brown © Humana Press Inc., Totowa, NJ

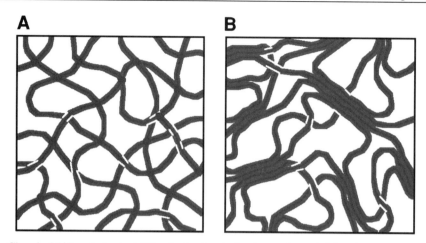

Fig. 1. Chemical (**A**) and physical (**B**) gels. In physical gels, a substantial fraction of a polymer chain is involved in the formation of stable contacts between polymer chains. Association of certain linear segments of long polymer molecules form extended "junction zones," which is distinguished from well-defined point crosslinks of chemical gels.

organic solvent unless covalent crosslinks are cleaved. Chemical gels can be prepared by two different approaches. First, chemical gels can be made by polymerizing water-soluble monomers in the presence of bi- or multifunctional crosslinking agents (i.e., by crosslinking polymerization). Second, chemical gels can be prepared by crosslinking water-soluble polymer molecules using typical organic chemical reactions that involve functional groups of the polymers. Physical gels (also called physical networks, association networks, or pseudogels) are the continuous, disordered 3-D networks formed by associative forces capable of forming noncovalent crosslinks. The point covalent crosslinks found in chemical gels are replaced by weaker and potentially more reversible forms of chain–chain interactions. These interactions include hydrogen bonding, ionic association, hydrophobic interaction, stereocomplex formation, and solvent complexation.

A weak and noncovalent molecular association is sometimes more than sufficient to result in a supramolecular assembly. For example, pullulan, which was partly substituted by cholesterol moieties (i.e., cholesterol-bearing pullulan, or CHP), formed monodispersive nanoparticles (20–30 nm) as shown in Fig. 2 *(2)*. The CHP self-aggregate can be regarded as a hydrogel, in which microdomains provided noncovalent crosslinking points arising from the association of hydrophobic cholesterol moieties. One of the advantages of this type of physical gel nanoparticles is that complexes can be formed with various hydrophobic substances such as adriamycin, and even various soluble proteins and enzymes. Physical and biochemical stability of insulin, for example, is known to be drastically increased upon complexation *(2,3)*. When a 3-D structure of a chemical gel is formed, the network extends from one end to the other and occupies the entire reaction vessel. For this reason, the hydrogel formed is essentially one molecule, no matter how large the hydrogel is. Thus, there is no concept of molecular weight for hydrogels. Hydrogels can be prepared in various sizes and shapes, depending on the application.

1.1.1. MONOMERS USED FOR MAKING HYDROGELS

Any monomers that become hydrophilic polymers can be used to make hydrogels. Table 1 lists some of the monomers and crosslinkers commonly used to prepare hydro-

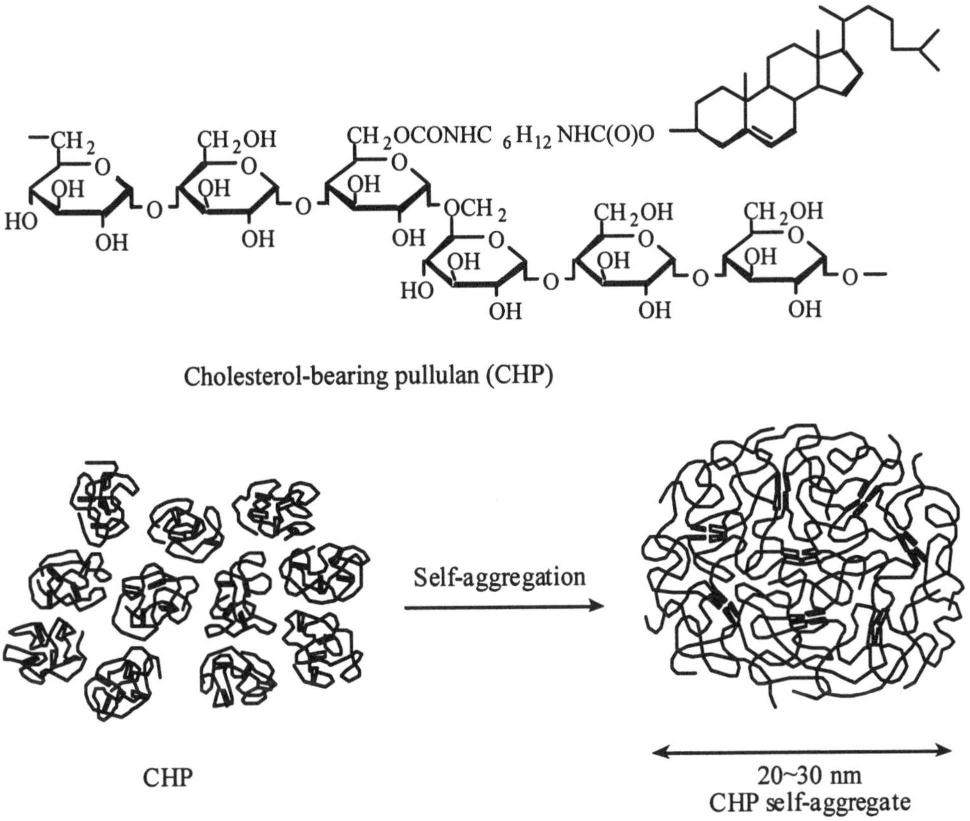

Cholesterol-bearing pullulan (CHP)

Self-aggregation

CHP

20~30 nm
CHP self-aggregate

Fig. 2. Chemical structure of cholesterol-bearing pullulan (CHP) and schematic representation of self-aggregation of CHP into a hydrogel nanoparticle. From *ref. (2)* with permission.

gels. The monomers shown in Table 1 are all vinyl monomers, since they are most widely used in preparation of hydrogels. Most monomers in Table 1 are hydrophilic and highly water-soluble. Some monomers are not freely water-soluble. For example, hydroxyethyl methacrylate (HEMA) is not hydrophilic enough to be soluble in water, but a poly(hydroxyethyl methacrylate) (polyHEMA) matrix, whether crosslinked or not, takes up sufficient amount of water to be called a hydrogel. PolyHEMA does not dissolve in water even in the absence of crosslinking. To form a crosslinked network, a crosslinking agent is added to a monomer solution, and the mixture is polymerized using an initiator. Any combination of monomer and crosslinker in Table 1 can be used to form hydrogels. More than one type of monomer can be used to form hydrogels. It is quite common to use two different types of monomers, and in this case, the obtained polymer is known as a copolymer instead of a homopolymer. For example, if acrylic acid and HEMA are used as monomers, the obtained hydrogel is known as crosslinked poly(acrylic acid-co-HEMA). Vinyl monomers are polymerized by free radical polymerization using an initiator. Commonly used initiators are azo initiators (e.g., azobisisobutyronitrile), peroxide (e.g., benzoyl peroxide), persulfate (ammonium persulfate), and redox initiators (e.g., ammonium persulfate and tetramethylethylenediamine). The monomer concentration is adjusted by diluting with suitable solvents, usually water. The monomer mixture containing a crosslinking agent and an initiator can be dispersed in organic solvent to form hydrogels in droplets. Hydrogels can also be prepared by

Table 1
Examples of Monomers, Crosslinkers, and Initiators Frequently
Used for Preparation of Hydrogels by Free Radical Polymerization

1. Monomers

Acrylamide	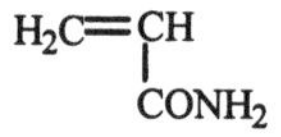 $H_2C=CH$ $\quad\quad\vert$ $\quad\quad CONH_2$	Methacrylic acid
Acrylic acid	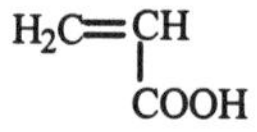 $H_2C=CH$ $\quad\quad\vert$ $\quad\quad COOH$	Methyl methacrylate
Hydroxyethyl methacrylate (HEMA)	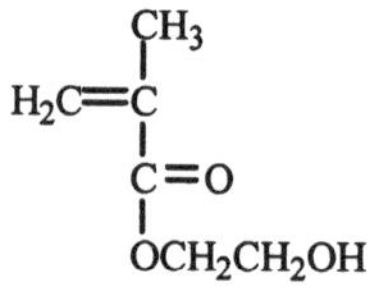 $\quad\quad CH_3$ $\quad\quad\vert$ $H_2C=C$ $\quad\quad\vert$ $\quad\quad C=O$ $\quad\quad\vert$ $\quad\quad OCH_2CH_2OH$	Monomethyl itaconate
Hydroxypropyl methacrylate (HPMA)	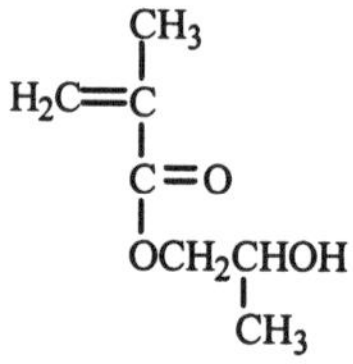 $\quad\quad CH_3$ $\quad\quad\vert$ $H_2C=C$ $\quad\quad\vert$ $\quad\quad C=O$ $\quad\quad\vert$ $\quad\quad OCH_2CHOH$ $\quad\quad\quad\quad\vert$ $\quad\quad\quad\quad CH_3$	Vinylpyrrolidone
N-isopropylacrylamide (NIPAM)	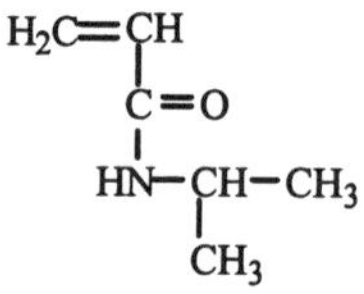 $H_2C=CH$ $\quad\quad\vert$ $\quad\quad C=O$ $\quad\quad\vert$ $\quad HN-CH-CH_3$ $\quad\quad\quad\vert$ $\quad\quad\quad CH_3$	

(continues)

mixing different types of polymers. The concentrations of monomer and crosslinking agent affect the mesh size of the polymer network and thus, the release property of the loaded drugs from a hydrogel matrix. The drug release rate from collagen-poly(HEMA) hydrogels is known to be controlled by adjusting the crosslinking density of the hydrogels. Crosslinked hydrogels released methotrexate (MTX) at a slower rate than an uncrosslinked hydrogel *(4)*.

1.1.2. POLYMERS USED FOR MAKING HYDROGELS

Hydrophilic polymers can be crosslinked, either by chemical reaction or by physical associations, to form hydrogels. Hydrophilic polymers include not only synthetic polymers, but also natural polymers such as proteins and polysaccharides. Commonly used proteins are collagen, gelatin, fibrin, and mucin. Widely used polysaccharides are agarose, alginate, carrageenan, cellulose derivatives, chitosan, chondroitin sulfate, dextran, guar gum, heparin, hyaluronic acid, pectin, and starch. To make a

Table 1
(Continued)

2. Crosslinkers

Dimethacryloyl hydroxylamine

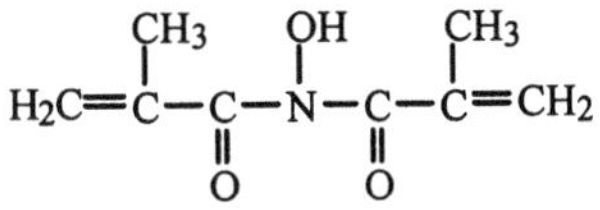

$$H_2C=\overset{CH_3}{\underset{\underset{O}{\|}}{C}}-\overset{}{\underset{\underset{O}{\|}}{C}}-\overset{OH}{\underset{}{N}}-\overset{}{\underset{\underset{O}{\|}}{C}}-\overset{CH_3}{\underset{}{C}}=CH_2$$

Divinyl glycol (1,5-hexadiene-3,4-diol)

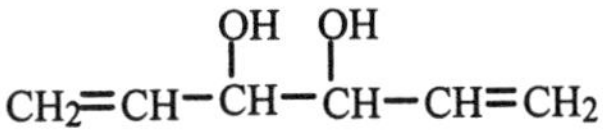

$$CH_2=CH-\overset{OH}{\underset{}{CH}}-\overset{OH}{\underset{}{CH}}-CH=CH_2$$

Ethylene diacrylate

$$H_2C=CH-\overset{\overset{O}{\|}}{C}-O-CH_2-CH_2-O-\overset{\overset{O}{\|}}{C}-CH=CH_2$$

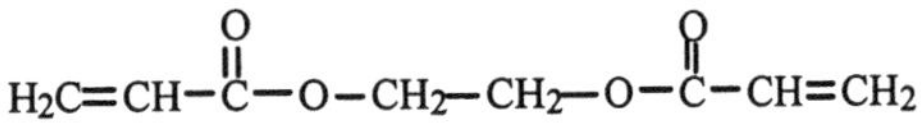

Ethylene glycol dimethacrylate (EGDMA) or ethylene dimethacrylate (EDMA)

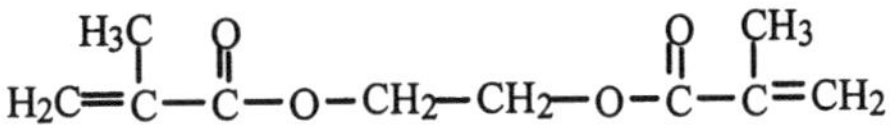

$$H_2C=\overset{H_3C}{\underset{}{C}}-\overset{\overset{O}{\|}}{C}-O-CH_2-CH_2-O-\overset{\overset{O}{\|}}{C}-\overset{CH_3}{\underset{}{C}}=CH_2$$

Glutaraldehyde

$$OHC-CH_2-CH_2-CH_2-CHO$$

N,N'-methylene-bisacrylamide (BIS)

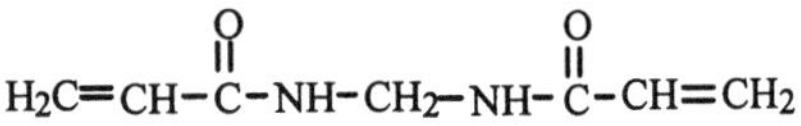

$$H_2C=CH-\overset{\overset{O}{\|}}{C}-NH-CH_2-NH-\overset{\overset{O}{\|}}{C}-CH=CH_2$$

PEG diacrylate

$$CH_2=CH-\overset{\overset{O}{\|}}{C}-O-\left(CH_2-CH_2-O\right)_n-\overset{\overset{O}{\|}}{C}-CH=CH_2$$

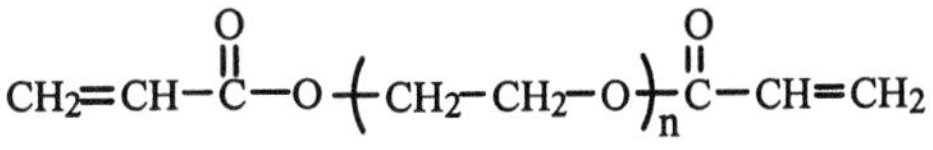

Trimethylolpropane trimethacrylate (TMPTMA)

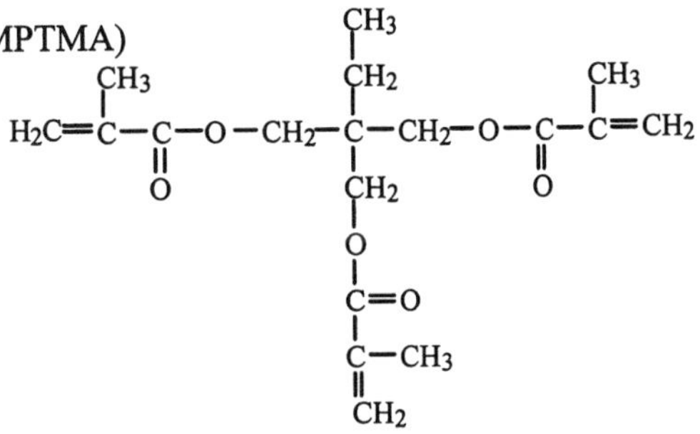

$$H_2C=\overset{CH_3}{\underset{\underset{O}{\|}}{C}}-C-O-CH_2-\overset{\overset{CH_3}{|}\overset{CH_2}{|}}{\underset{\underset{\underset{\underset{CH_2}{\|}}{C-CH_3}}{C=O}}{\underset{O}{|}}{C}}-CH_2-O-\overset{CH_3}{\underset{\underset{O}{\|}}{C}}-C=CH_2$$

crosslinked network from polymer molecules, the polymers have to possess chemically active functional groups for crosslinking. Thus, polymers with carboxyl groups, such as acrylic acid, or with amine groups, such as chitosan, can be easily crosslinked to form hydrogels. Polymers with hydroxyl groups can also be easily crosslinked.

1.2. Drug Loading into Hydrogels and Release
from Hydrogels

Anticancer drugs and imaging agents, such as X-ray contrast or radiopaque materials, can be loaded into hydrogels by a number of methods. Drugs can be added to the monomer solution before crosslinking polymerization or to the polymer solution before crosslinking reaction. In this case, relatively large concentrations of drugs can be added, but the prepared hydrogels may have to be purified to remove residual initiators, monomers, and crosslinkers, although their concentrations may be small. However, the washing step may remove the loaded drugs as well. Ara-C was added to the mixture of monomers (HEMA and vinylpyrrolidone) and a crosslinking agent (EGDMA) at the concentration of 34% (v/v). The solution was then polymerized to obtain an optically transparent hydrogel, indicating complete solubility of ara-C in the matrix *(5)*. The same approach was used to load ara-C into poly(HEMA) hydrogel crosslinked with EGDMA *(6,7)*. Prepared hydrogels can be dried for storage. The prepared hydrogel was cut into disks which contain ara-C from 5 to 25 mg/disk. Release of ara-C from disks was varied from 1 d to 16 d by adjusting the concentration of the crosslinking agent used *(5)*.

The drug can be loaded into hydrogels after they are purified. In this case, the concentration of the loaded drug will be rather limited because the drug loading is limited by the concentration of the drug in the loading solution. 5-Fluorouracil (5-FU), MTX, and ara-C were loaded into poly(HEMA) hydrogels by immersing the hydrogels into aqueous solutions saturated with drug molecules *(8,9)*. Since purified hydrogels are used in this approach, the prepared drug-loaded hydrogels are ready to use. 5-FU was also loaded into hydrogels of poly(acrylamide-co-monomethyl itaconate) and poly(acrylamide-co-monopropyl itaconate). Sodium salt of 5-FU has a solubility of 65 mg/mL, which is five times higher than that of 5-FU (13 mg/mL). Thus, in order to trap the maximum amount of 5-FU in the xerogel (dried hydrogel) disk, aqueous solutions of 5-FU neutralized with NaOH were used instead of water in the feed mixture of polymerization *(10,11)*. Adriamycin (ADR) was loaded into CHP aggregates by simply mixing ADR with CHP suspensions. ADR formed complexes with hydrophobic cholesterol moieties of CHP. ADR was spontaneously dissociated from the complex as a function of time. Less than 30% of complexed ADR was released even after 7 d in phosphate buffered saline (PBS, pH 7.4) at 25°C. The dissociation significantly increased as the medium temperature increased to 37°C and/or the medium pH decreased to 5.9 or 3.7. Approximately 20% of the loaded ADR was released at pH 7.4, whereas more than 50% was released at lower pH readings in 24 h (Fig. 3). The enhanced dissociation of ADR from the complex at lower pH is expected to be caused by the increase in its water solubility in an acidic medium. The chemical stability of ADR was largely improved by the complexation. The in vitro cytotoxicity of ADR was also diminished by the complexation. The diminished cytotoxicity of the CHP-ADR complex would be ascribed to either retarded release of ADR from the complex or decreased cell internalization of the complex *(2,3)*.

If both polymer chains and drug molecules have chemically active groups, drug molecules can be covalently attached to the polymer chains. The immobilized drug molecules are released by chemical or enzymatic dissociation from polymer chains.

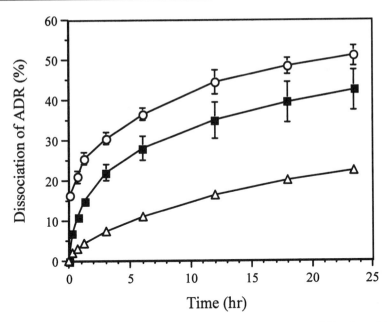

Fig. 3. Dissociation of adriamycin (ADR) from CHP-ADR complex at 37°C and at pH 3.7 (○), 5.9 (■), and 7.4 (△). The concentrations of ADR and CHP were $3.6 \times 10^{-6}M$ and $4.1 \times 10^{-8}M$, respectively. From *ref. (2)* with permission.

One of the advantages of this approach is that the drug-polymer conjugates can be purified without losing the grafted drug molecules.

1.3. Swelling Kinetics

As it is preferred to prepare final hydrogel dosage forms in the dried state (i.e., xerogels) for long-term storage before in vivo applications, the swelling kinetics of the xerogels also contribute significantly to controlling the drug release kinetics. During the drying process of hydrogels, water evaporates from a gel and the surface tension of water causes collapse of polymer chains and thus shrinking of the hydrogel body to only a small fraction of its swollen size. The physical state of xerogels is known to be glassy. Water absorption into the glassy polymer occurs by diffusion, which is a very slow process, leading to very slow swelling. This slow swelling property is used to slowly release loaded drug molecules.

If water is removed without collapsing the polymer network either by lyophilization (i.e., freeze drying) or by extraction with organic solvents, then a xerogel is porous. The pore size is typically less than 10 μm. When bubbles of air (or nitrogen or carbon dioxide) are introduced during hydrogel formation, the formed hydrogel contains very large pores of approx 100 μm even in the dried state. These hydrogels are called superporous hydrogels *(12)*. Superporous hydrogels absorb water through the interconnected pores forming open channels (i.e., by capillary action); the water absorption is very fast and swelling can be completed in a matter of minutes instead of hours for the glassy xerogels. Swelling ratios can be as high as a few hundred. The rapid and large swelling properties can be highly useful in certain applications, such as endovascular chemoembolization.

2. HYDROGELS IN ANTICANCER THERAPY

2.1. Endovascular Chemoembolization

Blocking the blood vessel feeding a tumor and thus starving the tumor of blood and oxygen is an effective way of treating cancer. In addition to antiangiogenesis therapy, endovascular chemoembolization is another means of blocking the blood supply to a tumor. Endovascular chemoembolization is the method of simultaneously administering into the blood vessel of the tumor tissue the vascular occlusion materials and antitumor agents that block the supply of nutrients to the tumor tissue as well as contribute cytotoxic action of the anticancer agents. Blocking of the artery decreases the blood flow rate, thereby increasing the dwell time and the concentration of anticancer agents in the tumor tissue. Arterial chemoembolization with microencapsulated drugs has been used clinically since 1978 *(13)*. This mode of treatment can be applied to a variety of tumor lesions with remarkable therapeutic effect and minimal systemic cytotoxicity. Vascular occlusion in chemoembolization has been accomplished by using different embolizing agents as listed in Table 2. All materials in Table 2, except Lipiodol®, are hydrogels in a microparticulate form. Degradable starch microspheres (Spherex®, Pharmacia, Sweden) without anticancer drug have been frequently used for embolization *(14)*. Starch microspheres, which were first used for scintigraphic imaging in the diagnosis of lung emboli, are currently used for transient occlusion of blood flow *(14)*. The most important feature of degradable starch microspheres is that the degradation time can be regulated by means of the degree of crosslinking to suit various organs and applications. Degradable starch microspheres have been delivered to the liver, kidney, and mesenterium without harm. Poly(HEMA) microparticles grafted with MTX were also used for chemoembolization *(15)*. Unlike starch microspheres, poly(HEMA) microparticles are not degradable. Although many materials were used for the purpose of embolization and drug reservoir, there was no effort to control the drug release. Adverse effects of anticancer agents are frequent, involving more than 60% of patients, although they are often transitory. The adverse effects were caused by rapid release of drug from embolization materials. Thus, it is necessary to use embolizing materials with the ability to control the drug release rate.

When injected intraarterially into the target organ, microparticles of a suitable size (e.g., 500 μm) become trapped in arteriolae. The hydrogel microparticles can release anticancer drugs locally for extended periods of time. The locally released drug from microspheres can cross the capillary walls and enter the cells of the target organ within the time of circulatory arrest. This targeted delivery of anticancer drugs would reduce the systemic concentration significantly *(22,23)*. This regional cancer chemotherapy can strongly increase the efficiency of the drug, while limiting the toxic effects. One of the advantages of this approach is that chemotherapy can be combined with embolization. Hydrogel microparticles can swell to block blood vessels and thus the supply of blood to tumors. For this particular application, fast-swelling superporous hydrogels are more useful than conventional hydrogels. For biodegradable hydrogels, the occlusion of the blood vessels can be transient until all drug is released. Permanent occlusion for tumor necrosis can be achieved using nondegradable hydrogel microparticles. Endovascular embolization before surgery (i.e., preoperative embolization) is thought to reduce the risk of hemorrhage and to decrease the release of tumor cells into the blood stream during surgical removal of solid tumors *(24)*. Successful emboli materials

Table 2
Examples of Materials Used in Chemoembolization

Name	Component	Size	References
Gelfoam®	Gelatin	90 μm in diameter	16,17
Ivalon®	Poly(vinyl alcohol)	150–250 μm in diameter	18
Spherex®	Starch	45 μm in diameter	19
Angiostat®	Microfibrillar collagen (Crosslinked)	5 μm × 75 μm (diameter × length)	20
Albumin microspheres	Albumin + chitosan (glutaraldehyde crosslinked)		21
Lipiodol®	Iodised poppyseed oil	25 μm in diameter	18

are expected to be nontoxic, nonantigenic, hydrophilic, nonthrombogenic, chemically stable, and radiopaque. At present, there is no standard emboli material that meets all the required properties. Rapid advances in polymer chemistry, however, are expected to produce ideal emboli materials in the near future. In addition to endovascular embolization, microparticles can also be employed for intratumoral, subcutaneous, extravascular, and intravascular administration.

Chemoembolization using different microparticles has been used for metastatic colorectal carcinoma of the liver and hepatocellular carcinoma *(18,20)*. Although there was an increase in the mean survival time in many cases, there was no statistical significance for most of materials used. This is mainly due to the use of inadequate embolization materials. For this approach to work effectively, hydrogel microparticles should swell rapidly to a size large enough to block the blood vessel. Currently, there are no hydrogels that can swell rapidly in blood, especially when they are dried. Recent development of superporous hydrogels that swell extremely fast in aqueous solution *(12)* provides an approach to develop effective chemoembolization or embolization materials.

2.2. Intratumoral Administration

Higher anticancer concentrations in tumors during the course of a fractionated irradiation treatment are known to increase therapeutic efficacy *(25)*. One way of achieving localized high concentrations is to implant a rod-shaped hydrogel in the center of subcutaneous tumors. The drug enhancement ratio for the group of mice treated with intratumoral hydrogel rods was higher than those for other groups where drug in solution was administered intraperitoneally or intratumorally. In this approach, the release kinetics of cisplatin from the implanted hydrogel rods was important. If the drug release was too slow, the drug distribution within tumors became inhomogeneous, resulting in low therapeutic effect *(26)*. The highest response, which showed a delay of tumor growth for 55 d, was obtained with a hydrogel formulation that released 56% of cisplatin in 4 d with 14% of water uptake. Figure 4 shows in vitro release profiles of platinum [i.e., *cis*-diamminedichloroplatinum(II) or cisplatin] from polyether hydrogels. The water uptakes of three different polyether hydrogel rods (1.5 mm diameter × 5 mm length) containing 10% (w/w) cisplatin were 4%, 14%, and 40% (w/w). The polyether hydrogel rods, which absorbed only 4% of water, are by definition not hydrogels. Polyether hydrogel rods released only 10% of cisplatin in 4 d and 17% in 11 d.

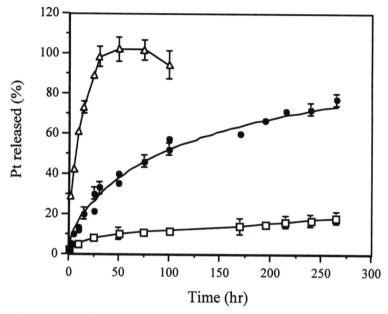

Fig. 4. In vitro release of Pt(or cisplatin) from polyether hydrogel rods with water uptake of 4% (□), 14% (●), and 40% (△). The hydrogel rods contained 10% (w/w) cisplatin. From *ref. (27)* with permission.

The 14%-hydrogel released 56% and 75% of the incorporated cisplatin in 4 d and 11 d, respectively. The 40%-hydrogel released almost 90% on day 1 and the remaining drug was released on day 2. The absolute amount of the drug released from hydrogels increased with increasing the payload (i.e., loading amount), but the cumulative fractional release decreased with increasing the payload *(27)*. The intratumoral implants have a therapeutic advantage over systemic therapy. Implantation of hydrogel rods, which release cisplatin during the period of a fractionated radiotherapy, was shown to be an effective method of administering the drug. Such treatment may be useful in patients with inoperable pelvic or head-and-neck tumors in which hydrogel rods could be implanted under ultrasound guidance *(25)*.

Complexes of hydrogels with radiotherapeutic agents were also used to maintain high concentrations of therapeutic agents *(28)*. Chitosan is soluble under acidic conditions, but becomes gel under basic conditions. The Holmium-166-chitosan complex solution becomes a gel upon administration into the body. Higher radioactivity at the administration site was obtained with the administration of the complex than that of Holmium-166 alone *(29)*.

Hydrogels can also be used to deliver α-interferon. Ocular inserts were made of hybrid polymers of maleic anhydride-alkyl vinyl ether copolymers and human serum albumin *(30)*. α-Interferon was loaded into transparent, flexible, and coherent hydrogel films by a low temperature casting procedure. The ocular inserts exhibited a gel-like behavior with a strong morphological stability even at a fairly high level of water uptake. The water uptake into the inserts showed that about 90% of the equilibrium swelling was observed after 10–12 h. The swelling ratio was more than 30 and the insert diameter was increased from 3 mm to 10–12 mm, while maintaining the shape and integrity of disk-like inserts *(30)*. The most hydrophilic matrix, based on the

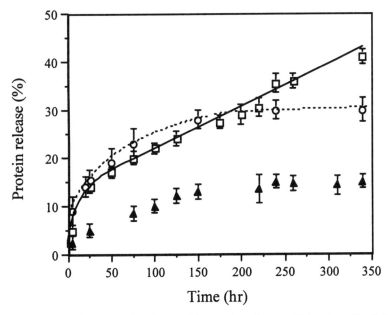

Fig. 5. Kinetic profiles of the protein release of inserts based on partial esters of poly(maleic anhydride-alt-alkyl vinyl ether)s in PBS at 37°C. Samples MP1m (○), MP1b (□), and MP3m (▲). From *ref. (30)* with permission.

methyl ester of poly(MAn-alt-Peg3VE), showed the lowest hydration, probably owing to the stronger interactions occurring between the hydrophilic portions of the polymer and the protein. The percent released protein was proportional to polymer hydrophobicity (*see* Fig. 5). Initial-burst release was observed during the first 18 h, and it was more pronounced for the esters of copolymer based on maleic anhydride and mono-*O*-methyloligoethyleneglycol vinyl ether. The initial-burst release was followed by an almost constant release for the next 10–15 d. During this period, the percent releases of the protein virtual load were 40%, 30%, and 15%, respectively, for the inserts based on butyl ester of poly(MAn-alt-Peg1VE) (MP1b in Fig. 5), methyl ester of poly(MAn-alt-Peg1VE) (MP1m in Fig. 5), and methyl ester of poly(MAn-alt-Peg3VE) (MP3m in Fig. 5) *(30)*. The more hydrophobic hydrogels released more proteins. Again, this may be because of the interaction of hydrophilic polymer chains with proteins, resulting in an increase of effective crosslinking density. The study indicated that erosion of hydrogel matrices also contributed to the initial-burst releases. This was supported by kinetic measurements of weight losses of hydrogel inserts, which showed rapid weight loss in the first several hours *(30)*.

2.3. Implantation of Hydrogels

One of the most effective ways for treating cancer could be delivering high concentrations of anticancer drugs to the cancerous lesions for periods long enough to kill all of the cancer cells. Anticancer drugs can be infused directly into the artery supplying blood to the neoplastic tissue. While this approach achieves targeted introduction of anticancer drugs into tumor tissues, its effect is only short-term unless the catheter is left in the vessel for a long time *(15)*. A pronounced therapeutic effect usually requires

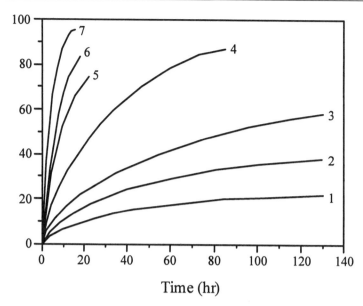

Fig. 6. Release profiles of narciclasin from polyHEMA matrices containing different concentration (v/v) of TMPTMA or MPEG. 1, HEMA:TMPTMA (80:20); 2, HEMA:TMPTMA (85:15); 3, HEMA:TMPTMA (90:10); 4, HEMA; 5, HEMA:MPEG (90:10); 6, HEMA:MPEG (75:25); and 7, HEMA:MPEG (50:50). From *ref. (32)* with permission.

that the procedures must be repeated many times. In addition, such treatment may still be accompanied by the same toxic side effects as conventional treatments. An alternative approach may be local delivery of anticancer agents from controlled-release devices, such as drug-loaded hydrogels. Various hydrogels have been used for subcutaneous delivery of anticancer agents. Examples are narciclasine-containing poly(HEMA) *(31,32)*, cytarabine (ara-C)-containing α, β-polyasparthydrazide hydrogel *(33)*, and 5-fluorouracil-containing poly(acrylamide-co-monomethyl itaconate) or poly(acrylamide-co-monopropyl itaconate) *(10,11)*.

The drug release rate from hydrogel implants can be controlled by adjusting crosslinking density and/or by adding water-soluble components. Figure 6 shows examples of narciclasin release from polyHEMA implants. PolyHEMA forms hydrogels even in the absence of a crosslinking agent, but addition of a crosslinking agent delays the drug release. The addition of TMPTMA, a crosslinking agent shown in Table 1, to the narciclasin-HEMA mixture significantly delayed the drug release. In the absence of a crosslinking agent (Fig. 6, line 4), more than 80% of the drug was released in 3 d. On the other hand, when the TMPTMA concentration was 20% (v/v) (Fig. 6, line 1), only about 20% of the drug was released even after several days. The addition of poly(ethylene glycol) methyl ether (MPEG), a water-soluble component, resulted in release of most of the drug within a day (Fig. 6, lines 5–7).

Hydrogels swell to a large extent in aqueous solution and this effect tends to result in mechanically weak structures that may limit their pharmaceutical and medical applications *(34)*. The mechanical strength of hydrogels can be improved by making an interpenetrating network with collagen. Collagen-poly(HEMA) hydrogel pellets were loaded with drugs, such as 5-fluorouracil, mitomycin C, bleomycin A2 *(35,36)*, and

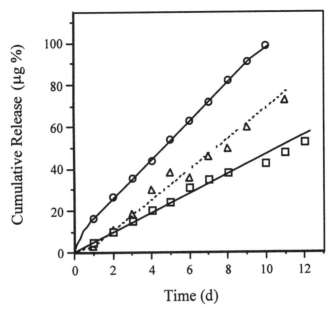

Fig. 7. In vitro cumulative release of 5-fluorouracil (○), mitomycin C (□), and bleomycin A2 (△) from collagen-poly(HEMA) hydrogel matrices. From *ref. (35)* with permission.

camptothecin derivatives *(37)*. The drug-loaded collagen-poly(HEMA) hydrogel pellets were subcutaneously implanted into rats with solid tumor fibrosarcoma *(37,38)* or into mice *(37)*. In both cases, the drug was released at zero-order rate for more than several days. The main advantage of using implantable hydrogels is that the long-term delivery of anticancer agents can eliminate daily administration of the drugs and reduce the potential side effects *(33)*. Figure 7 shows the in vitro cumulative drug release profiles of 5-fluorouracil, mitomycin C, bleomycin A2 from the hydrated collagen-poly(HEMA) hydrogel pellets (10 mm diameter × 3 mm thick) in phosphate buffer at 37°C and pH 7.4 *(35)*. As shown in Fig. 7, the release profiles were different. The release of 5-fluorouracil indicated burst release followed by the zero-order release, whereas that of bleomycin showed the lag-time effect before reaching the steady state. No burst release or lag time was observed with mitomycin C. The burst release of 5-fluorouracil is most likely owing to migration of the drug to the surface during drying. The molecular weights of 5-fluorouracil, mitomycin C, and bleomycin A2 are 130, 334, and 1400, respectively *(35)*. The highest molecular weight of bleomycin A2 may be responsible for the observed lag time. The hydrogel may have to swell before allowing diffusion of large molecules such as bleomycin A2. Because all three drugs showed the zero-order release at steady state, the release rate decreased in the order of 5-fluorouracil > bleomycin A2 > mitomycin C. The slow release of mitomycin C may be owing to interaction with collagen in the hydrogel pellets *(35)*.

Copolymers of *N*-(2-hydroxypropyl)methacrylamide and *N,O*-dimethacryloyl hydroxylamine were used to prepare hydrolytically degradable hydrogels for the release of doxorubicin and polymer-doxorubicin conjugates *(39,40)*. D-galactosamine was attached to the polymer-doxorubicin conjugate as a targeting moiety to hepatocytes. When the hydrogel was implanted intraperitoneally into DBA2 mice, 35% of the targeted conjugates accumulated in the liver, whereas only 2% of the control conjugates were found in the liver 48 h after implantation.

Albumin microparticular (100–500 μm) hydrogels were prepared by crosslinking albumin with polyethylene glycol disuccinate (41,42). Anticancer agents and diagnostic agents were covalently attached in stoichiometric quantities. The hydrogel microparticles effectively reduced the risk of local tumor recurrence in a rat model when implanted locally after surgical tumor removal. The albumin microparticles were degraded by proteases released from macrophages. Typically, 1-mL samples that were implanted into paraspinal muscles of rats were completely absorbed within 4 wk and its constituents were metabolized.

2.4. Peroral and Oral Administration of Hydrogels

α, β-Polyasparthydrazide microparticles have been used for peroral administration of anticancer agents (43). α, β-Polyasparthydrazide is a linear polymer and a promising plasma expander and drug carrier with interesting properties such as water-solubility, and absence of toxicity and antigenicity (44). A different crosslinking degree was obtained by varying the ratio of crosslinking agent/polymer that influenced the swelling behavior of the gel. 5-Fluorouracil was incorporated into the matrices during the crosslinking reaction, and in vitro release studies were performed in simulated gastric juice (pH 1.1) and in pH 7.4 buffer solution. The dried hydrogel samples were ground, and the particles obtained were analyzed by sieving on a mechanical shaker to obtain sizes ranging 20–90 μm. The prepared hydrogels were chemically stable in the dissolution media. The observed data demonstrated the potential application of these new matrices for peroral administration of anticancer agents (43).

One of the salient features of the gastrointestinal (GI) tract is the large pH change from stomach to intestine. Quite often, such a pH change is exploited for targeted delivery of drugs either to the stomach or to the intestine. A semi-interpenetrating polymer network of poly(vinylpyrrolidone-co-acrylic acid) and poly(ethylene glycol) containing 5-fluorouracil was prepared (45). Poly(vinylpyrrolidone-co-poly[ethylene glycol]) containing 5-fluorouracil was also synthesized using poly(ethylene glycol diacrylate) (46). Because these dosage forms were able to release the entrapped drug for periods of days/weeks, their clinical applicability is highly limited as the GI transit time is only several hours or less. The hydrogel formulation for the delivery of anticancer agent in the GI tract requires an effective platform that maintains the delivery module at the area of tumors.

2.5. Topical Applications

Gel-forming hydrophilic polymers are commonly used to prepare semisolid dosage forms, such as dermatological, ophthalmic, dental, rectal, vaginal, and nasal hydrogels. These are especially useful for application of therapeutic agents to mucous membranes and ulcerated tissues because their high water content reduces irritation (47). Carbopol® hydrogels, which are loosely crosslinked poly(acrylic acid), were used to formulate topical delivery systems for treatment of multiple actinic keratoses and superficial basal cell carcinoma with 5-fluorouracil (47,48). Mycosis fungoides, the most common type of cutaneous T-cell lymphoma, progresses in three clinical phases: the premycotic, mycotic, and tumor stages. Treatment with chemotherapy and radiotherapy in the earlier stages can result in cure of mycosis fungoides. Topically treated hydrogels in sheet form (Nu-Gel® Wound Dressing, Johnson & Johnson Medical, Inc., Arlington, TX) can absorb exudate, contain odor, and reduce pain upon dressing removal from patients in the tumor stage of mycosis fungoides *(49)*. Hydrogel sheets have also been used to deliver recombinant interferon α2c and interferon β for treatment of condylomata acuminata *(50,51)*.

2.6. Rectal Applications

Eudispert® hydrogels were used for rectal delivery of hydrophilic 5-fluorouracil in rats *(52)*. The addition of capric acid or linolenic acid to the hydrogel increased the permeability of 5-fluorouracil through the rectal membranes. Eudispert hydrogels with capric acid may be a useful preparation for increasing the maximum plasma level and improving the absolute bioavailability of 5-fluorouracil after rectal administration.

3. APPLICATIONS OF HYDROGELS IN THE CANCER-RELATED AREA

3.1. Assessment of Tumor Cell-Induced Angiogenesis

Hydrogels were used to develop a quantitative assay system for in vivo evaluation of angiogenesis induced by human tumor cells in mice *(53,54)*. The human epidermoid carcinoma A431 cells cultured on microcarriers were microencapsulated with agarose hydrogel to isolate them from the immune system of the C57BL/6 mice after subcutaneous dorsal midline implantation. When A431 cell-containing microcapsules (diameter, 300 μm) were subcutaneously injected into mice, notable angiogenesis was observed at the site of implantation. The extent of angiogenesis was quantitated by measuring the hemoglobin content in the implanted site using a mouse hemoglobin (mHb) enzyme-linked immunosorbent assay system. This type of simple system allows quantitative evaluation of angiogenesis in mice induced by xenogeneic cells such as human tumor cells. This may be useful in testing antiangiogenic properties of various agents using human tumor cells. There are many hydrogel systems that can be used to microencapsulate cells. Alginate has been commonly used to encapsulate cells and proteins in various sizes and shapes.

3.2. Removal of Adriamycin from Blood

Anthracyclines, such as adriamycin, generally possess a long plasma half-life that might produce serious toxicity to myeloproliferative and cardiac cells. In patients with impaired liver function or biliary obstruction, cytotoxic blood levels tend to be maintained for excessive periods with resultant severe, and potentially lethal, acute toxicity. Acrylic hydrogel-coated activated charcoal was used for hemoperfusion of beagle dogs 4 h after an intravenous bolus of adriamycin (2.5 mg/kg) *(55–57)*. Throughout the 3-h hemoperfusion period, the extraction of adriamycin averaged 43%, which was a 20-fold increase in total body elimination of adriamycin. The extended hemoperfusion would have resulted in reduction of tissue concentrations of adriamycin. The role of the hydrogel coating was to increase blood compatibility. Hemoperfusion using hydrogel-coated activated charcoal may be useful in reducing blood levels of adriamycin in cases of accidental overdose or in patients with hepatic disease.

3.3. Solid-Phase Radioimmunoassay

A sensitive, rapid method for the measurement of MTX in biologic fluids has been developed using hydrogel-based, solid-phase radioimmunoassay. Rabbit antimethotrexate antisera were added to hydroxyethylmethacrylate monomer before polymerization. The resultant hydrogel was lyophilized, ground to fine powder, and aliquoted into 3-mL syringes fitted with a fritted filter disk *(58)*. A dose-response curve expressing percent bound MTX versus antiserum concentration allowed measurement of drug concentrations less than 1 ng/mL. The controlled entrapment of antiserum into a hydrogel matrix was shown to be simple, inexpensive, and stable. The porosity of the hydrogels, which is related to the utility of the hydrogel as a solid phase, can be easily controlled by the concentration of crosslinking agent.

3.4. Hydrogels as a Culture Medium

Agar has been commonly used as the supporting gel for testing of antimicrobial susceptibility. The results of such testing are known to be influenced by both the nutrient milieu and the supporting gel *(59)*. Agar, obtained from red seaweed, is a complex mixture of neutral and acidic polysaccharides with variable quantities of lipids, metallic cations, and other unknown substances. Some of the components in agar may antagonize or boost certain antimicrobial or anticancer agents. Synthetic hydrogels with well-defined amino acid medium may yield reproducible solid medium without potential antagonistic or booster effects of some components of agar. Such a medium could be used as a reference medium for testing anticancer effects of various drugs.

4. FUTURE HYDROGEL TECHNOLOGIES

Hydrogels possess many properties useful for controlled drug delivery. Because of very high water content, hydrogels are known to be biocompatible, however, most polymers used in hydrogel synthesis are not degradable in the body. Thus, to avoid manual removal of hydrogel matrices after all drug is released, the use of biodegradable hydrogels is preferred. One way of preparing biodegradable hydrogels is to use proteins and polysaccharides. Currently available biodegradable polymers, such as poly(lactic acid) or poly(glycolic acid), are not water-soluble and cannot be used for making hydrogels. Synthesis of new biodegradable, hydrophilic polymers is needed. Another property that will make hydrogels even more useful is improved mechanical strength. Because of the absorption of large amounts of water, hydrogels are usually weak and may not be able to withstand pressures occurring in the body. Currently, hydrogels can be made to swell rapidly with large swelling ratios by making interconnected pores inside the hydrogels *(12)*. Such superporous hydrogels can be effectively used for chemoembolization, and the high mechanical strength of such hydrogels would make them more useful. Certain types of anticancer drugs have high molecular weights. For example, many angiogenesis inhibitors *(60,61)* are peptides or proteins. Delivery of peptide and protein drugs can be easily achieved using macro (or super) porous hydrogels and/or biodegradable hydrogels.

It is only 40 yr since the first synthetic hydrogels were proposed for bioapplications *(62)*. During this relatively short time period, remarkable advances have been made in the development of hydrogels with numerous properties. Hydrogels that respond (i.e., either expand, shrink, or degrade) to changes in environmental factors, such as temperature, pH, or salt concentration, are known as smart hydrogels *(63)*. Poly(acrylic acid) hydrogels respond to changes in environmental pH or salt concentration, while poly(*N*-isopropylacrylamide) hydrogels respond to temperature changes. These smart hydrogels can be used to target delivery of anticancer agents by exploiting small changes in pH naturally occurring in the body as well as artificial changes in local temperatures. Further advances in hydrogel research will undoubtedly result in hydrogels with new properties ideal for anticancer therapy.

REFERENCES

1. Park K, Shalaby SWS, Park H. *Biodegradable Hydrogels for Drug Delivery* Technomic, Lancaster, PA. 1993, Ch. 1.
2. Akiyoshi K, Taniguchi I, Fukui H, Sunamoto J. Hydrogel nanoparticle formed by self-assembly of hydrophobized polysaccharide: stabilization of adriamycin by complexation. *Eur J Pharm Biopharm* 1996; 42:286–290.
3. Akiyoshi K, Deguchi S, Tajima H, Nishikawa T, Sunamoto J. Microscopic structure and thermoresponsiveness of a hydrogel nanoparticle by self-assembly of a hydrophobized polysaccharide, *Macromolecules* 1997; 30:857–861.
4. Narayani R, Panduranga Rao K. Collagen-poly (HEMA) hydrogels for the controlled delivery of methotrexate and cisplatin, *Int J Pharm* 1996; 138:121–124.
5. Blanco MD, Trigo RM, Garcia O, Teijon JM. Controlled release of cytarabine from poly(2-hydroxyethyl methacrylate-co-n-vinyl-2-pyrrolidone) hydrogels, *J Biomater Sci Polymer Edn* 1997; 8:709–719.
6. Teijon JM, Trigo RM, Garcia O, Blanco MD. Cytarabine trapping in poly(2-hydroxyethyl methacrylate) hydrogels—drug delivery studies, *Biomaterials* 1997; 18:383–388.
7. Beyssac E, Bregni C, Aiache JM, Gerula S, Smolko E. Hydrogel implants for methotrexate obtained by ionizing radiation, *Drug Devel Ind Pharm* 1996; 22:439–444.
8. Garcia O, Trigo RM, Blanco MD, Teijon JM. Influence of degree of crosslinking on 5-fluorouracil release from poly(2-hydroxyethyl methacrylate) hydrogels, *Biomaterials* 1994; 15:689–694.
9. Trigo RM, Blanco MD, Teijon JM, Sastre R. Anticancer drug, ara-C, release from pHEMA hydrogels, *Biomaterials* 1994; 15:1181–1186.
10. Blanco MD, Garcia O, Trigo RM, Teijon JM, Katime I. 5-Fluorouracil release from copolymeric hydrogels of itaconic acid monoester, *Biomaterials* 1996; 17:1061–1067.
11. Blanco MD, Garcia O, Olmo R, Teijon JM, Katime I. Release of 5-fluorouracil from poly(acrylamide-co-monopropyl itaconate) hydrogels, *J Chromatogr B: Biomed Appl* 1996; 680:243–253.
12. Chen J, Park H, Park K. Synthesis of superporous hydrogels: hydrogels with fast swelling and superabsorbent properties, *J Biomed Mater Res* 1999; 44:53–62.
13. Kato T. Encapsulated drugs in targeted cancer therapy, in *Controlled Drug Delivery. Vol. II. Clinical Applications* (Bruck SD, ed). CRC, Boca Raton, FL, 1983, pp 189–240.
14. Lindberg B, Lote K, Teder H. Dioderadable starch microspheres—A new medical tool, in *Microspheres and Drug Therapy—Pharmaceutical, Immunological and Medical Aspects* (Davis SS, Illum L, McVie JG, Tomlinson E, eds). Elsevier, New York, 1983, pp 153–188.
15. Horak D, Svec F, Adamyan A, et al. Hydrogels in endovascular embolization. V. Antitumour agent methotrexate-containing p(HEMA), *Biomaterials* 1992; 13:361–366.
16. Fiorentini G, Campanini A, Dazzi C, et al. Chemoembolization in liver malignant involvement. Experiences on 17 cases, *Minerva Chirurgica* 1994; 49:281–285.
17. Päuser S, Wagner S, Lippman M, et al. Evaluation of efficient chemoembolization mixtures by magnetic resonance imaging therapy monitoring: An experimental study on the VX2 tumor in the rabbit liver, *Cancer Res* 1996; 56:1863–1867.
18. Colleoni M, Audisio RA, De Braud F, Fazio N, Martinelli G, Goldhirsch, A. Practical considerations in the treatment of hepatocellular carcinoma, *Drugs* 1998; 55:367–382.
19. Taguchi T. Liver tumor targeting of drugs: Spherex, a vascular occlusive agent, *Jap J Cancer & Chemotherapy* 1995; 22:969–976.
20. Tellez C, Benson AB, Lyster MT, et al. Phase II trial of chemoembolization for the treatment of metastatic colorectal carcinoma to the Liver and review of the literature, *Cancer* 1998; 82:1250–1259.
21. Kyotani S, Nishioka Y, Okamura M, et al. A study of embolizing materials for chemo-embolization therapy of hepatocellular carcinoma: antitumor effect of cis-diamminedichloroplatinum(II) albumin microspheres, containing chitin and treated with chitosan on rabbits with VX2 hepatic tumors, *Chem Pharmaceut Bull* 1992; 40:2814–2816.

22. Teder H, Johansson CJ. The effect of different dosages of degradable starch microspheres (Spherex) on the distribution of doxorubicin regionally administered to the rat, *Anticancer Res* 1993; 13:2161–2164.

23. Chang D, Jenkins SA, Grime SJ, Nott DM, Cooke T. Increasing hepatic arterial flow to hypovascular hepatic tumours using degradable starch microspheres, *Br J Cancer* 1996; 73:961–965.

24. Horak D, Svec F, Isakov Y, et al. Use of poly(2-hydroxyethyl methacrylate) for endovascular occlusion in pediatric surgery, *Clin Mater* 1992; 9:43–48.

25. Begg AC, Deurloo MJ, Kop W, Bartelink H. Improvement of combined modality therapy with cisplatin and radiation using intratumoral drug administration in murine tumors, *Radiother Oncol* 1994; 31:129–137.

26. Deurloo MJ, Kop W, van Tellingen O, Bartelink H, Begg AC. Intratumoural administration of cisplatin in slow-release devices: II. Pharmacokinetics and intratumoural distribution, *Cancer Chemother Pharmacol* 1991; 27:347–353.

27. Deurloo MJ, Bohlken S, Kop W, et al. Intratumoural administration of cisplatin in slow-release devices. I. Tumour response and toxicity, *Cancer Chemotherapy & Pharmacology* 1990; 27:135–140.

28. Park KB, Kim YM, Kim JR. Radioactive chitosan complex for radiation therapy. U.S. Patent 1998; 5:762,903.

29. Suzuki Y, Momose Y, Higashi N, et al. Biodistribution and kinetics of Holmium-166-chitosan complex (DW-166HC) in rats and mice, *J Nucl Med* 1998; 39:2161–2166.

30. Chiellini E, Solaro R, Leonardi G, Giannasi D, Mazzanti G. New polymeric hydrogel formulations for the controlled release of alpha-interferon, *J Controlled Rel* 1992; 22:273–282.

31. Veronese FM, Ceriotti G, Keller G, Lora S, Carenza M. Controlled release of narciclasine from poly(hema) matrices polymerized by a chemical initiator and by gamma irradiation, *Radiation Physics & Chemistry* 1990; 1990:88–92.

32. Veronese FM, Ceriotti G, Caliceti P, Lora S, Carenza M. Slow release of narciclasine from matrices obtained by radiation-induced polymerization, *J Controlled Rel* 1991; 16:291–298.

33. Giammona G, Pitarresi G, Tomarchio V, Cavallaro G, Mineo M. Crosslinked alpha, beta-polyasparthydrazide hydrogels: effect of crosslinking degree and loading method on cytarabine release rate, *J Controlled Rel* 1996; 41:195–203.

34. Jeyanthi R, Panduranga Rao K. In vivo biocompatibility of collagen-poly(hydroxyethyl methacrylate) hydrogels, *Biomaterials* 1990; 11:238–243.

35. Jeyanthi R, Panduranga Rao K. Controlled release of anticancer drugs from collagen-poly(HEMA) hydrogel matrices, *J Controlled Rel* 1990; 13:91–98.

36. Jeyanthi R, Panduranga Rao K. Equilibrium swelling behavior of collagen-poly (HEMA) copolymeric hydrogels, *J App Polymer Sci* 1991; 43:2332–2336.

37. Uemura K, Kurono Y, Ikeda K. Application of implantable collagen-poly (hydroxyethyl methacrylate) hydrogels containing camptothecin derivative to solid tumor chemotherapy, *Jpn J Hosp Pharm Byoin Yakugaku* 1994; 20:33–40.

38. Jeyanthi R, Nagarajan B, Panduranga Rao, K. Solid tumor chemotherapy using implantable collagen-poly(HEMA) hydrogel containing 5-fluorouracil, *J Pharm Pharmacol* 1991; 43:60–62.

39. Ulbrich K, Subr V, Seymour LW, Duncan R. Novel biodegradable hydrogels prepared using the divinylic crosslinking agent N,O-dimethacryloylhydroxylamine. Part 1. Synthesis and characterization of rates of gel degradation, and rate of release of model drugs, in vitro and in vivo, *J Controlled Rel* 1993; 24:181–190.

40. Ulbrich K, Subr V, Podperova P, Buresova M. Synthesis of novel hydrolytically degradable hydrogels for controlled drug release, *J Controlled Rel* 1995; 34:155–165.

41. Weissleder R, Bogdanov A, Frank H, et al. AUR Memorial Award 1993. A drug system (PDH) for interventional radiology. Synthesis, properties, and efficacy, *Investigative Radiology* 1993; 28:1083–1089.

42. Weissleder R, Poss K, Wilkinson R, Zhou C, Bogdanov A, Jr. Quantitation of slow drug release from an implantable and degradable gentamicin conjugate by in vivo magnetic resonance imaging, *Antimicrobial Agents & Chemoth* 1995; 39:839–845.

43. Giammona G, Pitarresi G, Carlisi B, Cavallaro G. Crosslinked alpha, beta-polyasparthydrazide micromatrices for controlled release of anticancer drugs, *J Bioact Compat Polymers* 1995; 10:28–40.

44. Giammona G, Carlisi B, Cavallaro G, Pitarresi G, Spampinato S. A new water-soluble synthetic polymer, alpha, beta -polyasparthydrazide, as poential plasm expander and drug carrier, *J Controlled Rel* 1994; 29:63–72.

45. Ravichandran P, Shantha KL, Rao KP. Preparation, swelling characteristics and evaluation of hydrogels for stomach specific drug delivery, *Int J Pharm* 1997; 154:89–94.

46. Yamini C, Shantha KL, Rao KP. Synthesis and characterization of poly[n-vinyl-2-pyrrolidone-polyethylene glycol diacrylate] copolymeric hydrogels for drug delivery, *J Macromol Sci Pure Appl Chem A34* 1997; 12:2461–2470.

47. Dolz M, Gonzalez F, Herraez M, Diez O. Influence of polymer concentration on the 5-fluorouracil release rate from Carbopol hydrogels, *J Pharmacie de Belgique* 1994; 49:509–513.

48. Dolz M, Rodriguez FG, Dominguez MH. The influence of neutralizer concentration on the rheological behavior of a 0.1% Carbopol hydrogel, *Pharmazie* 1992; 47:351–355.

49. Gelliarth KA, DeSantis P. A brief review of the pathophysiology and treatment of cutaneous T-cell lymphoma "mycosis fungoides", *Ostomy Wound Manag* 1995; 41:44–48.

50. Gross G, Roussaki A, Pfister H. Postoperative interferon hydrogel treatment. A method for the successful therapy of chronic persistent giant condylomas in an immunologically deficient patient with Hodgkin's disease, *Hautarzt* 1988; 39:684–687.

51. Fierlbeck G, Rassner G, Pfister H. Condylomata acuminata in children—detection of HPV 6/11 and 2. Local therapy with interferon-beta hydrogel, *Hautarzt* 1992; 43:148–151.

52. Umejima H, Kikuchi A, Kim NS, Uchida T, Goto S. Preparation and evaluation of Eudragit gels. VIII. Rectal absorption of 5-fluorouracil from Eudispert hv gels in rats, *J Pharm Sci* 1995; 84:199–202.

53. Okada N, Fushimi M, Nagata Y, et al. A quantative in vivo method of analyzing human tumor-induced angiogenesis in mice using agarose microencapsulation and hemoglobin enzyme-linked immunosorbent assay, *Jap J Cancer Res* 1995; 86:1182–1188.

54. Okada N, Kaneda Y, Miyamoto H, et al. Selective enhancement by tumor necrosis factor-alpha of vascular permeability of new blood vessels induced with agarose hydrogel-entrapped Meth-A fibrosarcoma cells, *Jap J Cancer Res* 1996; 87:831–836.

55. Winchester JF, Rahman A, Tilstone WJ, Kessler A, Mortensen L, Schreiner GE, Schein PS. Sorbent removal of adriamycin in vitro and in vivo, *Cancer Treatment Rep* 1979; 63:1787–1793.

56. Plate NA, Valuev LI, Valueva TA, Chupov VV. Biospecific haemosorbents based on proteinase inhibitor. I. Synthesis and properties, *Biomaterials* 1993; 14:51–56.

57. Plate NA, Valuev LI. Affinity chemotherapy and diagnostics using some novel polymeric hydrogels, *Polymers Adv Technol* 1994; 5:634–644.

58. Tracey KJ, Mutkoski R, Lopez JA, Franzblau W, Franzblau C. Radioimmunoassay for methotrexate using hydroxyethylmethacrylate hydrogel, *Cancer Chemother Pharmacol* 1983; 10:96–99.

59. Lawrence RM, Hoeprich PD. Totally synthetic medium for susceptibility testing, *Antimicrobial Agents Chemother* 1978; 13:394–398.

60. Teicher, BA. *Antiangiogenic Agents in Cancer Therapy* Humana Press, Totowa, NJ, 1999.

61. Arap W, Pasqualini R, Ruoslahti E. Cancer treatment by targeted drug delivery to tumor vasvularture in a mouse model, *Science* 1998; 279:377–380.

62. Wichterle O, Lim D. Hydrophilic gels for biological use, *Nature* 1960; 185:117–118.

63. Park K, Park H. Smart hydrogels, in *Concise Polymeric Materials Encyclopedia* (Salamone JC, ed). CRC, Boca Raton, FL, 1999, pp 1476–1478.

6 Microparticle Drug Delivery Systems

Duane T. Birnbaum, PhD
 and Lisa Brannon-Peppas, PhD

CONTENTS

1. INTRODUCTION

Tremendous opportunities exist for utilizing advanced drug delivery systems for cancer treatments. One such formulation type that has already begun to fulfill its promise is injectable microencapsulated delivery systems. Biodegradable microspheres containing leutinizing hormone-releasing hormone (LHRH) are already used for treatment of hormone dependent cancers and precocious puberty. This product is the Lupron® Depot and its in vivo results will be discussed later in this chapter. In addition, other in vitro and in vivo results from microparticulate delivery systems for traditional cancer-fighting agents will be described. The more recent developments in gene delivery and utilization of targeted delivery and angiogenic factors will be discussed briefly with an emphasis on the possibilities that have yet to be realized. A more complete analysis of some of these future directions of cancer therapy may be found in Part IV of this volume.

2. MICROENCAPSULATION TERMINOLOGY

First, some of the more basic information on the methods of preparing microparticulate formulations must be discussed, with an emphasis on biodegradable microparticles. The terminology used to describe microparticulate formulations can sometimes be inconsistent and confusing to readers unfamiliar with the field. Essentially, the term "microparticle" refers to a particle with a diameter of 1–1000 μm, irrespective of the precise interior

From: *Drug Delivery Systems in Cancer Therapy*
Edited by: D. M. Brown © Humana Press Inc., Totowa, NJ

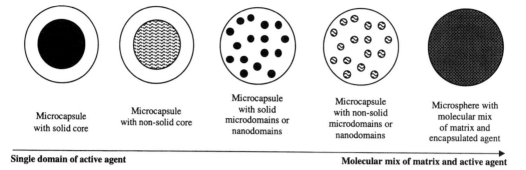

Microcapsule with solid core | Microcapsule with non-solid core | Microcapsule with solid microdomains or nanodomains | Microcapsule with non-solid microdomains or nanodomains | Microsphere with molecular mix of matrix and encapsulated agent

Single domain of active agent   **Molecular mix of matrix and active agent**

Fig. 1. Variations of microparticle formulations.

or exterior structure. Within the broad category of microparticles, "microspheres" specifically refers to spherical microparticles and the subcategory of "microcapsules" applies to microparticles which have a core surrounded by a material which is distinctly different from that of the core. The core may be solid, liquid, or even gas.

Despite the specific and logical subcategories, many researchers use the terms interchangeably, often to the confusion of the reader. It is usually assumed that a formulation described as a microparticle is comprised of a fairly homogeneous mixture of polymer and active agent, whereas microcapsules have at least one discrete domain of active agent and sometimes more. Some variations on microparticle structures are given in Fig. 1. As the domains and subdomains of active agent within microcapsules become progressively smaller, the microcapsules become microparticles.

3. PREPARATION OF MICROPARTICLES

There are innumerable methods for preparing microparticles for use in applications as diverse as carbonless paper to ion exchange resins to cosmetics to drug delivery. Here, we will concentrate on the materials, biodegradable and nonbiodegradable, which have been studied for drug delivery specifically for cancer treatment.

An overwhelming majority of methods used for encapsulating drugs in a submillimeter spherical polymer matrix involve the use of liquid emulsions. A simple definition of an emulsion as applied to liquids is the dispersion and stabilization of one liquid within another to which it is immiscible. The most common emulsion type is oil-in-water, however, oil-in-oil and multiple emulsions (water-oil-water, oil-oil-water, solid-oil-water, and so on) are used frequently *(1–14)*. There are numerous materials available for creating these emulsions and we discuss a few specific examples here. The main criterion for creating an emulsion is that the dispersed phase (solution containing polymer and drug) must be immiscible (or nearly so) in the continuous phase (external phase containing dissolved surfactant).

4. PREPARATION OF BIODEGRADABLE MICROPARTICLES

4.1. Poly(lactic-co-glycolic Acid)

Most systems that use oil–water emulsions to prepare microparticles consist of an organic phase comprised of a volatile solvent with dissolved polymer and the drug to be encapsulated, emulsified in an aqueous phase containing dissolved surfactant (*see* Fig. 2).

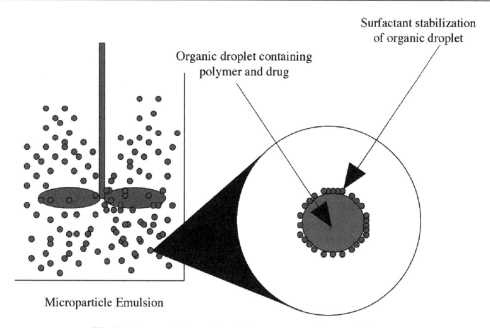

Organic droplet containing
polymer and drug

Surfactant stabilization
of organic droplet

Microparticle Emulsion

Fig. 2. Encapsulation using oil-in-water emulsion technique.

Two common examples of volatile organic solvents used for the organic-phase solvent are dichloromethane and ethyl acetate. There are numerous examples of biodegradable polymers that can be used for the microparticle matrix, however, polylactic acid (PLA) and the copolymer of lactic and glycolic acid (PLAGA) are the most frequently used due to their high biocompatibility and government approval *(15)*. The PLAGA polymer degrades hydrolytically over time to its monomeric components, which are easily removed from the body through natural life processes. A surfactant is also included in the aqueous phase to prevent the organic droplets from coalescing once they are formed. Once the droplets are formed via physical means, the organic solvent leaches out of the droplet into the external aqueous phase before evaporating at the water–air interface. Emulsions are simply created by using a propeller or magnetic bar for mixing the organic and aqueous phases. The organic-phase solvent should be able to dissolve the polymer up to reasonably high concentrations, preferably in the hundreds of mg/mL, but does not necessarily need to be a good solvent for the drug. The solvent should be completely or almost completely immiscible in water such that a two-phase system can be easily obtained. If the solvent is slightly soluble in water, then steps to control the extraction rate of the solvent into the external aqueous phase need to be considered. A high extraction rate will result in the formation of microparticles with a high porosity that could lead to the untimely and immediate release of drug *(16,17)*. Scanning electron microscopy (SEM) images of microparticles prepared using poly(lactic acid-co-glycolic acid) (PLAGA) and ethyl acetate dispersed in an aqueous PVA solution are shown in Fig. 3. Since ethyl acetate is slightly soluble in water (10% v/v) it partitions upon mixing to the external phase at an increased rate, relative to an immiscible solvent such as dichloromethane, such that the resultant microparticles are highly porous and/or hollow. Saturating the external aqueous phase with ethyl acetate and minimizing its volume will significantly reduce the extraction rate of the ethyl acetate leading to the formation of microparticles with reduced porosity.

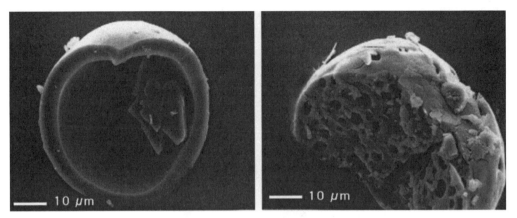

Fig. 3. Hollow and porous microparticles of PLAGA prepared using ethyl acetate and poly(vinyl alcohol) at a magnification of ×1250.

When the drug is not soluble in the organic solvent, it may be encapsulated as a solid provided its form is of small size. Nominally, the size of the drug crystals should be at least an order of magnitude smaller than the desired microparticle diameter in order to avoid large bursts associated with dissolution of larger crystals. Smaller crystals will be more homogeneously distributed throughout the organic droplets created in the emulsion. This results in a solid-in-oil-in-water emulsion (S/O/W) and may be used with any hydrophilic drug (e.g., cisplatin, 5-fluorouracil, and doxorubicin).

The most serious challenge with encapsulating hydrophilic materials is loss of drug to the external aqueous phase during the formation of the microparticles. Along with the loss of drug to the external phase, the remaining material may migrate to the surface of the droplet before hardening. To minimize these problems, the organic droplets should be hardened into microparticles as quickly as possible following their formation. An in-liquid drying process is often used to harden the organic droplets into solid microparticles (*see* Fig. 4) *(18)*. The method typically involves the use of a viscous organic solution of polymer and drug and a large secondary volume of water that essentially extracts the organic solvent into the external aqueous phase immediately, thus leaving only the microparticle with encapsulated drug. Again, care has to be taken to ensure that high-quality microparticles are produced. Parameters that control the porosity of the resultant microparticles formed from an in-liquid drying/extraction process include the viscosity of the organic solution, volume of organic solvent used, time interval at which the large volume of water is added, and the volume of water used to extract the organic solvent from the particles. The highly viscous dispersed phase serves two purposes. First, the volume of volatile organic solvent is at a minimum, facilitating its quick removal from the droplet. Second, highly viscous material will make the migration of the solid drug particles/crystals to the surface of the droplet more difficult, resulting in a more homogenous distribution of drug within the microparticle.

As an alternative to S/O/W emulsions, hydrophilic drugs may be encapsulated in a polymer matrix using a multiple water-in-oil-in-water (W/O/W) or oil-in-oil (O/O) emulsions. If a W/O/W emulsion is used, the drug is first dissolved in water and emulsified in an organic phase containing the polymer and a surfactant (*see* Fig. 5). This emulsion is then dispersed in another aqueous phase containing more surfactant. A complication with this

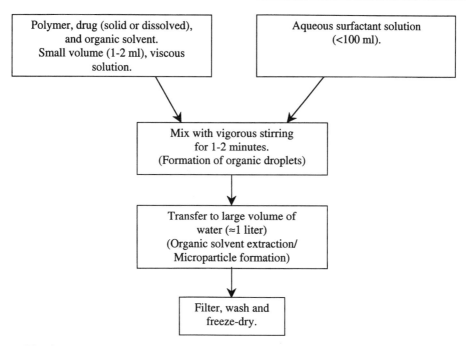

Fig. 4. Schematic diagram of in-liquid drying process for microparticle preparation.

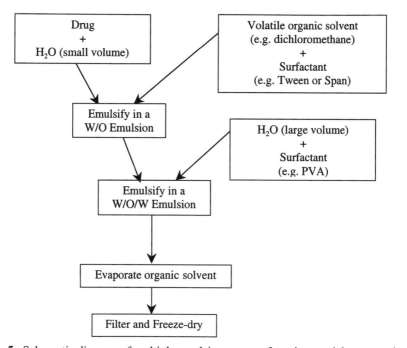

Fig. 5. Schematic diagram of multiple emulsion process for microparticle preparation.

type of emulsion occurs when the inner emulsion is not sufficiently stabilized such that aqueous droplets containing dissolved drug are lost to the external aqueous phase. The choice of surfactants that can be used to stabilize the inner emulsion is limited to materials that will dissolve in the organic solvent. Typically, the fatty acid esters of polyoxyethylene sorbitan or sorbitan are used due to their high solubility in organic solvents and good bio-compatibility. With the O/O method, the drug may be suspended or dissolved in the oil phase before being dispersed in another oil phase. One example might use dichloromethane as the solvent for the polymer and dispersant for the drug, and cottonseed oil with the appropriate surfactant added as the external phase in the emulsion. The greatest concern with using highly viscous oil such as cottonseed oil for the external phase is the difficulty in collection and washing of the particles. Filtration of viscous material is signifi-cantly more difficult than filtering aqueous suspensions, and washing the microparticles requires the use of yet another organic solvent (typically hexane or heptane).

Encapsulation of hydrophilic drugs may also be achieved by chemically conjugating the drug to the polymer *(19–28)*. The synthesis of such materials will not be discussed here, but typically involves the activation of hydroxyl groups on the polymer, which then react with amino groups located on the drug *(24,29)*. Polyethylene glycol and dextran are often used as the drug carriers; however, it is also possible to conjugate drugs to PLAGA and other biodegradable polymers *(30–33)*. These polymeric "prodrugs" are often administered as intravenous (iv) solutions (if they are soluble in water, dextrans, PEGs, and so on), however, they also may be fashioned into microparticles using the same methods discussed above. The overall drug encapsulation efficiency may not be better than other methods but, assuming all of the drug that ends up attached to the polymer is encapsulated in the microparticles, it allows for easier and more reproducible control over the quantity of drug in the microparticles. Furthermore, because drug will not be released from the microparticles until the hydrolytic degradation of the bond between drug and polymer, there is usually little burst of drug from such particles.

Hydrophobic drugs are typically much easier to encapsulate because they are often highly soluble in the volatile organic solvents used in the formulations and thus lack the thermodynamic drive to partition to the external aqueous phase. Encapsulation efficien-cies greater than 90% are typical, with little manipulation of formulation parameters. Challenges arise only when the solubility of the drug is low in the desired dispersed-phase solvent. In these cases, drug loadings may have to be limited to the maximum concentra-tion obtained in the dispersed phase. Alternatively, it may be possible to use a cosolvent system (e.g., dichloromethane and methanol) where the second component is used to increase the concentration of drug in the dispersed phase. If a cosolvent is used for the dis-persed phase, it is best if both components are immiscible in water, however, this may not be possible depending on the solubility of the active agent in the various components available. The problems associated with using acetone or methanol as the second compo-nent in the dispersed phase is that these are both soluble in water in all proportions. Thus, if acetone or methanol is used to increase the solubility of active agent in the dispersed phase, they may also serve to carry the active agent to the surface of the droplet before partitioning to the aqueous phase. This leaves microparticles with an inordinate amount of active agent at or near the surface, resulting in undesirable release kinetics.

The last method for preparing biodegradable PLAGA microparticles that we will mention here is spray-drying as it is a widely used method in the pharmaceutical indus-try and has been investigated by several researchers as a method for formulating biodegradable microparticles *(34–40)*. Although no such studies attempting to encapsulate anticancer agents in biodegradable microparticles using this technique are found in the literature, there is no reason this method could not be used for this purpose. This method for formulating microparticles typically uses drug dissolved or suspended in a polymer solution (either organic or aqueous solvent, depending on the polymer used). This solution/suspension is then fed into the spray-drying apparatus, of which the most important component is the nozzle. Nebulization of the polymer/drug solution may be carried out at the nozzle using different mechanisms *(40)*. Basically, the polymer/drug solution is mixed rapidly with air and forced through a small diameter orifice. Nebulization of the polymer/drug solution occurs at the nozzle and the resultant droplets are very quickly dried by evaporation (under high-pressure air) before collection. Significant advantages of using this technique include high encapsulation efficiencies and no residual surfactant on the surface of the microparticles. There is no external aqueous phase that can act as a sink for the drug, and of course there is no surfactant present anywhere in the formulation. Parameters that can affect microparticle size and morphology are temperature, pressure (air used for drying), nozzle diameter, air/solution volume mixture, and of course, polymer/drug concentrations as is the case for emulsions.

4.2. Albumin-Containing Microparticles

Microparticles of bovine serum albumin (BSA) may be prepared using an emulsion of aqueous BSA in cottonseed oil *(41)*. Sufficient elevation of the temperature of the emulsion will set the BSA microparticles. Any drug may be included, either in solution along with the BSA or in suspension, for water-insoluble drugs. The microparticles are cooled and then washed with ether (or another appropriate solvent) and collected usually by filtration or centrifugation.

To add greater functionality to albumin microspheres, some research groups have included other biodegradable polymers in the microparticles. Specifically, dextran sulfate has been added to these microparticles to add ion-exchange characteristics *(42)*. For this microparticle synthesis, a bovine serum albumin solution was made which also contained sodium dodecyl sulfate and dextran sulfate sodium salt. This phase was emulsified in olive oil, and an aqueous solution of glutaraldehyde was then added to chemically crosslink the albumin. These particular particles were washed with light petroleum, followed by isopropanol followed by distilled water.

4.3. Fibrinogen Microparticles

Microparticles may be prepared from fibrinogen using procedures very similar to those used to make albumin microparticles. One specific method combines fibrinogen and drug in an aqueous solution and then emulsifies this solution in cottonseed oil containing 10% Span 85® *(43)*. This emulsion is added to more cottonseed oil and heated to 100 or 140°C to set the fibrinogen. After 30 min of stirring, the solution is cooled, the particles are washed with ether and dried. Clearly, all of these methods for preparing microparticles of albumin and fibrinogen should be effective for encapsulating water-soluble drugs, which are not proteins, for cancer treatment. Drugs that are more soluble in the oil phase can easily partition out of the microparticles during the stirring step, as the microparticles are in a swollen state during preparation. Also, it is impossible to encapsulate active proteins within these microspheres as the drug will be denatured during the setting or crosslinking step when the microparticles are formed.

5. PREPARATION OF NONBIODEGRADABLE MICROPARTICLES

For nonbiodegradable microparticles to be useful in drug delivery, the active agents must be adsorbed onto the surface of the particles. Such solid particles have been used in specific treatments of embolization to block the blood flow to cancer tissue. Very few permanent microparticle systems have been studied, with the exception of magnetic microparticles that are currently being used by FeRx Incorporated. FeRx uses magnetic targeted carriers as delivery vehicles for the site-specific targeting, retention, and sustained release of cancer-fighting active agents. These carriers approx 0.5 to 5 µm in diameter and are composed of elemental iron and activated carbon. The drugs to be delivered are bound to the surface of the particles, which are then localized using a small externally positioned magnetic field that directs the particles, and the drug adsorbed on them, specifically to the cancerous tissue.

6. RELEASE BEHAVIOR OF ANTICANCER COMPOUNDS FROM MICROPARTICLES

This and following sections present predominately a review of the work published in the last five years, categorized according to the active agent being delivered. This direct comparison should help to point out the diverse approaches using microencapsulation techniques that are being investigated and used to control the delivery of cancer-treating drugs. Of course, with the approval already in place for PLAGA for in vivo applications, many different research groups have focused their work on that polymer family. This chapter will not be addressing formulations that are either liposomes, micelles, or polymer conjugates as those topics are covered elsewhere in this volume.

7. ENCAPSULATION AND IN VITRO RELEASE

7.1. Hydrophilic Drugs

The encapsulation of hydrophilic compounds such as doxorubicin and 5-fluorouracil within hydrophobic biodegradable polymers presents a serious challenge because of the thermodynamic drive of these drugs to partition to the aqueous external phase in an O/W emulsion. Some methods used to alleviate these challenges include using O/O emulsions to avoid the use of water, in-liquid drying processes to harden the microparticles quickly, and covalently attaching the drug to the polymer used for the biodegradable matrix before preparing the microparticles.

7.1.1. DOXORUBICIN

Doxorubicin is widely used for the treatment of many types of cancer and is moderately hydrophilic, with a solubility of the hydrochloride salt in water of approx 10 mg/mL. Doxorubicin has been encapsulated in a wide range of microparticles prepared from albumin, albumin-dextran sulfate, fibrinogen, and poly(lactic acid) *(41–44)*. Methods involved W/O emulsion for fibrinogen or albumin microparticles, O/W emulsion for PLA, and an ion-exchange W/O method for albumin-dextran sulfate. It should also be possible to encapsulate doxorubicin using W/O/W or S/O/W methods.

Albumin particles with an average diameter of approx 1 µm encapsulating doxorubicin were prepared using a W/O emulsion *(41)*. Encapsulation efficiencies were low (23%) and the resulting drug loading was slightly over 2% by mass. Because cottonseed oil was used as the external phase, very high encapsulation efficiencies would have been expected. The authors did not discuss the unusually low encapsulation efficiency of the doxorubicin in their formulation. The in vitro release of doxorubicin from these particles in tris buffer was biphasic with approx 1/3 of the drug released in the first 6 h, followed by the release of the remaining drug over the next 90 h. The initial burst of drug is typically due to surface-bound drug. The relatively short release time (approx 4 d) is a function of the microparticle size (1 μm) and the nature of the material used for the microparticle matrix, in this case, water-soluble bovine serum albumin (BSA).

Another microparticle formulation containing doxorubicin and prepared from bovine serum albumin using a W/O emulsion resulted in particles with a size range of 20–60 μm *(42)*. Dextran sulfate was also encapsulated into the albumin microparticles. In this case, doxorubicin was loaded after the preparation of the microparticles. The particles were first swollen with ethanol, and water was then added to a doxorubicin solution. After 1 h, essentially all the drug was taken up by the particles via an ion-exchange mechanism with the sulfate groups of the derivatized dextran already encapsulated in the albumin microparticles. Drug loadings were as high as 50% by mass as a result of the very efficient ion exchange process. Release of doxorubicin in phosphate buffered saline (PBS) was nearly constant and lasted for approx 10 h. The release time was doubled by including iron in the formulation, which is known to complex with doxorubicin.

Although these microparticles containing albumin and dextran are considerably larger than those previously mentioned containing only albumin, the total time required to release the doxorubicin is considerably less (90 h vs 10 h). This is owing to the method used to encapsulate the drug. The ion-exchange method encapsulates the doxorubicin after the microparticles are formed. Therefore, the drug diffuses into the microparticles and is held there only by the strength of the ionic interaction with the sulfate groups of the derivatized dextran. Consequently, the release of doxorubicin under sink conditions will be governed primarily by this ionic interaction because diffusion is quite rapid. The release of doxorubicin from the smaller diameter microparticles mentioned earlier will be governed by degradation and diffusion as the drug was encapsulated at the time of microparticle formation.

Fibrinogen particles containing doxorubicin have also been prepared from a W/O emulsion *(43)*. Again, the external oil phase used was cottonseed oil. Drug loadings were approx 10% with encapsulation efficiencies of 40–45%. Particle diameters averaged 2–3 μm with all particles under 10 μm in diameter. Sustained release of the drug had occurred for at least 7 d when the studies were stopped after 10–20% of the drug had been released. There was no initial burst from the fibrinogen microspheres, indicating that the fibrinogen was a very effective encapsulant for the doxorubicin. The fibrinogen microparticles appear to swell much less than albumin microparticles, even when preparation conditions are similar. The degradation, both in vitro and in vivo, may also be slower for the fibrinogen.

Doxorubicin has also been encapsulated in varying molecular weight oligomers of polylactic acid with particle diameters of approx 100 μm using an O/W emulsion *(44)*. Drug loadings ranged from 0.5 to 2.5% by mass with encapsulation efficiencies of 30–90%. The relatively high encapsulation efficiencies were attributed to the doxorubicin being slightly soluble in the dichloromethane (2–3 μg/mL) that was used as the organic solvent for the dispersed phase. Thus, the drug will partition to the external aqueous phase at a decreased rate relative to a formulation in which doxorubicin is insoluble in the organic solvent. There was also a strong correlation between doxorubicin encapsulation efficiency and molecular weight of PLA used for the matrix. The lower molecular weight PLA used resulted in higher doxorubicin encapsulation efficiencies. Sustained release of drug was observed in tris buffer for a period of several days with an initial burst that increased with increased drug loadings.

7.1.2. CISPLATIN

Significant efforts have also focused on the encapsulation of cisplatin in biodegradable microspheres. Cisplatin is slightly soluble in water (1 mg/mL), making it a candidate for S/O/W and W/O/W emulsions. Because it is less soluble in water than doxorubicin, encapsulation efficiencies are typically higher when using an aqueous external phase in the emulsion. Cisplatin has been encapsulated in PLAGA/PLA microparticles by a number of research groups *(44–51)*. Particle size ranges have varied between 1 and 300 µm with high encapsulation efficiencies (> 90%). However, depending on the type of emulsion used, a large burst was often observed in the in vitro release profiles. Release times, in vitro, vary between a few days to months depending on the diameter of the microparticles and the molecular weight of the polymer used.

Cisplatin encapsulated in PLA microspheres and prepared using an O/O method produced particles with a diameter of 100 µm *(48)*. Dimethyl formamide and castor oil were used for the dispersed and external-phase solvents, respectively. The microparticles contained 4% drug by mass and released their contents in vitro within 3 d. This is an unexpectedly fast release considering the diameter of the spheres involved. The quick release of cisplatin from these microparticles was attributed to the burst effect from surface-bound drug, suggesting that all encapsulated cisplatin was at or near the surface of the microparticles. Similar results have been obtained by other researchers when encapsulating cisplatin in PLAGA microparticles using an O/O emulsion *(44,47–49)*. High encapsulation efficiencies and drug loadings are achieved, but the in vitro release displays large bursts within the first few hours that increase with the drug loading. These initial bursts of drug may be as high as 80% of the total amount of drug encapsulated in the microparticles. As the amount of the drug in the particles increased so did the burst, and the subsequent duration of the controlled release decreased significantly.

More satisfactory results were obtained by using a more traditional S/O/W method with dichloromethane as the dispersed-phase solvent and a PVA solution for the external phase *(45)*. Microparticles of a diameter between 100–200 µm exhibited a slow sustained release of drug in vitro for a period of 60 d before the remaining drug was released over a period of approx 1 wk. The release of drug in this manner is consistent with a diffusion mechanism that is followed by the degradation of the polymer to a point where the microparticles release the remaining drug. Similar results have been obtained with 5-fluorouracil encapsulated in PLAGA microspheres, as discussed in the following section. Other studies have also used the S/O/W emulsions to encapsulate cisplatin in PLAGA microparticles with excellent results showing high encapsulation efficiencies and little or no burst *(46,50,51)*.

7.1.3. 5-FLUOROURACIL

Another slightly hydrophilic drug widely used in cancer treatments, with a solubility in water of approx 1 mg/mL, is 5-fluorouracil (5-FU). Microparticles (3–6 µm) prepared from PLA using a S/O/W emulsion contained 5–15% 5-FU by mass and released

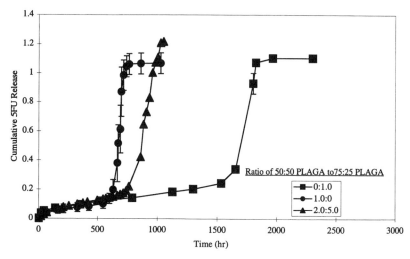

Fig. 6. In vitro drug delivery in buffered saline at 37°C for 5-fluorouracil from microparticles prepared from various ratios of 50:50 PLAGA (mol wt: 13,000) and 75:25 PLAGA (mol wt: 65,000).

drug in vitro over a period of about 5 d *(52)*. There was a substantial burst (20–40% of encapsulated drug) from these particles that increased with the initial drug loading. Microparticles using cross-linked chitosan and containing 5-FU have been prepared using a W/O emulsion *(53)*. Drug loadings were as high as 20% by mass. However, these particles released the drug in saline in just a few hours despite their relatively large diameters (490–760 μm), indicating that any crosslinking was not effective in controlling the release of the 5-FU.

As with cisplatin, it is possible to encapsulate the hydrophilic drug 5-FU with high efficiency and drug loadings and still obtain a desirable release profile with little to no burst and relatively constant release. In our research group, we have prepared 5-FU microparticles from high and low molecular weight PLAGAs as well as a mixture of molecular weights. A S/O/W emulsion was used in conjunction with a highly viscous organic phase and an in-liquid drying process. The resulting microparticles were 50–60 μm in diameter with encapsulation efficiencies as high as 75% and drug loadings as high as 25%. Release profiles in buffered saline from PLAGA microparticles are shown in Fig. 6. The initial release is slow and sustained with no burst and lasts three or more weeks, depending on the molecular weight of the PLAGA samples used, with higher molecular weight polymers yielding formulations with longer controlled-release duration. After the polymer degradation reaches a critical phase, the remaining drug is quickly released over a period of about 1 wk. Thus the release is controlled by both diffusion and polymer hydrolysis rates, resulting in a biphasic release profile. The time lag between the slower release phase and the faster release phase can be controlled by using different molecular weight PLAGA or a blend of PLAGA polymers with differing molecular weights. Because higher molecular weight PLAGA will hydrolyze at a slower rate, the initial slow-release phase will last longer when using higher molecular weight PLAGA, either alone or in a blend. The release profile can be made monophasic by including low molecular weight PLAGA and hydrophilic polyethylene glycol (PEG) in the formulation, as shown in Fig. 7. At

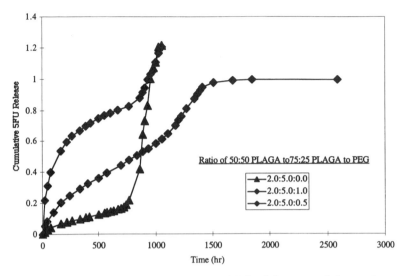

Fig. 7. In vitro drug delivery in buffered saline at 37°C for 5-fluorouracil from microparticles prepared from various ratios of 50:50 PLAGA (mol wt: 13,000), 75:25 PLAGA (mol wt: 65,000), and PEG (mol wt: 6,000).

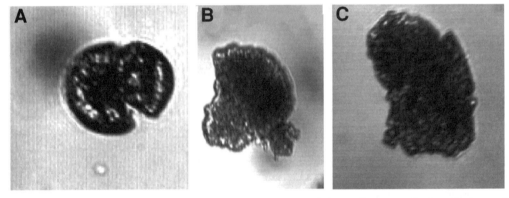

Fig. 8. Microscopic images of PLAGA microparticles containing 5-fluorouracil after 21 days of degradation in phosphate buffered saline. The relative ratios of 50:50 PLAGA (mol wt: 13,000) to 75:25 PLAGA (mol wt: 65,000) to PEG (mol wt: 6000) are (**A**) 2:5:0; (**B**) 2:5:0.5; and (**C**) 2:5:1.

approx 3.5% PEG (mol wt: 6000), the microparticles release 5-FU at a nearly constant rate for the entire profile. The hydrophilic PEG will release quickly (relative to hydrolysis rate of PLAGA) through diffusion, creating a more porous microparticle relative to those without PEG, enabling the encapsulated 5-FU to diffuse out of the microparticle at a higher rate. This combination of release behaviors then gives a monophasic release profile. Some microscopic images of these microparticles during degradation are shown in Fig. 8. These figures show that, while particles composed of PLAGA remain essentially spherical only until after all drug delivery has been completed, those microparticles containing PEG show significant physical changes and degradation during the drug delivery phase.

7.1.4. LEUTINIZING HORMONE RELEASING HORMONE (LHRH)

Proteins present a unique problem when being encapsulated in polymer matrices using the techniques described above. Leutinizing hormone releasing hormone (LHRH) is not only one of the best known peptides studied for controlled-release formulations from biodegradable microparticles but it also is one of the very few commercially available products using this technology (Lupron® Depot) *(54,55)*. LHRH in cancer treatment is used to suppress the production of sex hormones that lead to hormone-dependent cancers. Proteins in general are notorious for chemical instabilities, especially when exposed to organic solvents. Thus, proteins and peptides are almost always formulated into microparticles using a W/O/W emulsion. The use of an inner aqueous phase serves to protect the dissolved protein from the harsh environment of the organic solvent.

LHRH has been encapsulated in PLAGA microparticles using a W/O/W emulsion *(56)* and by cryogenic grinding of extruded PLG containing homogeneously distributed peptide *(57)*. Microparticles prepared using a W/O/W emulsion containing 75:25 PLAGA (mol wt: 14,000) and 5% LHRH released in vitro for several weeks (>4) with no initial burst of hormone. That a water-soluble drug could be efficiently entrapped in a PLAGA microparticle and display no initial burst using the W/O/W method is somewhat unusual and very encouraging for researchers in the field. For example, numerous research groups have used the W/O/W method to encapsulated various proteins (e.g., BSA) and the in vitro release typically displays a moderate to large burst. That LHRH has both high encapsulation efficiency and no initial burst has been attributed to the formation of a micelle-like structure between the PLAGA chains and the drug *(57)*. The release of the hormone is then strictly regulated by polymer degradation rather than diffusion.

7.2. Hydrophobic Drugs

Hydrophobic drugs often present less of a challenge to formulate in slowly degradable microparticle systems, relative to hydrophilic drugs, as they are often soluble in the organic solvents used, but are insoluble in water. Some hydrophobic anticancer agents that have been encapsulated in biodegradable microparticles include taxol, aclacinomycin, and camptothecin (water-insoluble forms) *(58–65)*.

Anticancer agents such as taxol, aclacinomycin, camptothecin, and related analogs have been successively encapsulated in PLAGA microparticles with high efficiency (> 90%) *(58,61,63)*. The maximum amount of drug encapsulated in the microparticles typically depends on its solubility in the organic solvent used in the formulation. Taxol is now a common anticancer agent used against a wide variety of solid tumors including breast and ovarian cancers. It is insoluble in water and has a limited solubility in ethanol. Therefore, commercial formulations of taxol use a 50:50 mixture of ethanol and Cremophor® EL (polyethoxylated castor oil) which are then designed to be diluted in saline or other intravenous infusion solutions. Alternative dosage forms are desired not only for the controlled release, but also to reduce adverse reactions to the relatively large amount of Cremophor EL used in the commercial formulation *(63)*.

Taxol has been encapsulated in PLAGA microparticles of varying LA/GA ratios using very simple O/W emulsions *(63)*. The authors used dichloromethane as the solvent for both PLAGA (mol wt: 10,000) and taxol. A 4% gelatin solution was used as the continuous phase with simple mechanical mixing. An encapsulation efficiency of

98% from microparticles with an average diameter of 30 µm was achieved using 75:25 PLAGA with no additional additives. The in vitro release displayed a slow-sustained release of taxol with no initial burst. In fact, the release was so slow that isopropyl myristate was added to change the microparticle matrix to allow the formation of channels that would allow for faster diffusion of taxol from the microparticle. These results are not unexpected considering the hydrophobic nature of the drug and the immiscible nature of the solvents used for both phases of the emulsion. Thermodynamically, taxol must remain solvated in the dichloromethane until which time the solvent is completely removed and, thus, the drug is homogeneously encapsulated in the newly formed microparticle. Because the release of taxol from PLGA microparticles is typically quite slow, the most significant obstacle in formulating these microparticles is obtaining a sustained release of therapeutic levels of drug. Thus, additives such as isopropyl myristate, sucrose, and the use of PLAGAs of varying molecular weight and hydrolytic degradation rates have been investigated as a means of accelerating the release of taxol *(63,64)*.

Camptothecin (CPT) is a promising anticancer agent being investigated in the treatment of a wide variety of tumors *(59)*. Because of the low solubility of camptothecin in water (3.8 µg/mL) and dichloromethane (10 µg/mL) the drug poses a somewhat different challenge with regard to formulating microparticles for controlled release. There are basically two options when formulating such compounds through the use of emulsions: encapsulate the drug in a solid form using a S/O/W emulsion or use a cosolvent system that will dissolve both polymer and drug to desired levels. Dimethlyformamide (DMF) is an excellent solvent for CPT and is also highly miscible with dichloromethane, therefore, it serves well as the second solvent component for the dispersed phase in a microparticle emulsion. However, DMF is also miscible with water, an undesirable property for any component of the dispersed-phase solvent. The authors' results are as expected: higher encapsulation efficiencies with decreased DMF volume and higher concentration of PLAGA in the dispersed-phase solvent. Drug release profiles are also consistent with expectations; the burst was minimized by decreasing the volume of DMF and increasing the concentration of PLAGA.

8. IN VIVO STUDIES

Although limited in terms of the number of studies reported in the public literature, data for the in vivo release of anticancer agents encapsulated in biodegradable microparticles demonstrates advantages over administration of the free drug. Doxorubicin, 5-FU, cisplatin, irinotecan (synthetic derivative of camptothecin), and LHRH have been administered into tumor-bearing rats and/or mice using biodegradable microparticles *(43,48,49,52,66–68)*.

Fibrinogen microparticles (average diameter, 2–3 µm) containing varying amounts of doxorubicin were injected into mice inoculated with Ehrlich ascites carcinoma cells, and survival times recorded versus those of mice treated with a doxorubicin solution *(43)*. Relative to the control animals, where half of the mice had died at 20 d (with no survivors at 29 d), the injection of doxorubicin solution decreased the lifespan of the mice, with half dead at 10 d (with no survivors at 28 d), whereas injection of fibrinogen microspheres containing doxorubicin significantly increased the lifespan of the mice, with more than half surviving longer than 60 d. These results were obtained for doxorubicin administered at a level of 13.7 mg/kg. The authors interpreted these results as an indication that biodegradable fibrinogen microspheres containing doxorubicin could be used to administer increased amounts of doxorubicin with decreased toxicity, thus reducing systemic side effects caused by the drug.

PLAGA microparticles containing 5-FU have been stereotactically implanted in the brains of rats with malignant gliomas to test their toxicity and efficacy (66). Similar microparticles (diameter, 3–6 μm) containing 5-FU were also injected into the tail veins of mice in order to measure the in vivo distribution of the drug particles (52). Stereotactically implanted microparticles effectively decreased the mortality of malignant tumor-bearing rats. However, the decreased mortality was found to be statistically significant only for the slow-releasing microspheres where the 5-FU was released over 18 d, as opposed to fast-releasing microspheres where the 5-FU was released over 3 d. Microparticles containing 5-FU, which were injected into the tail veins of mice, were found primarily in the lungs and liver within 24 h postinjection.

Microparticles containing cisplatin have been studied in vivo as a general aid to understanding the effect on surrounding muscle tissue in rabbits and mice as well as their ability to increase the survival time of tumor-bearing mice (48,49). For mice inoculated intraperitoneally with P815 mastocytoma cells, the mean survival times were compared to those mice injected with (1) cisplatin containing microspheres, (2) cisplatin solutions (free cisplatin), (3) blank microspheres, and (4) phosphate-buffered saline (PBS). Several different doses of cisplatin were also studied (49). All tumor-bearing mice injected with blank microspheres or PBS died within 20–30 d. At lower levels of cisplatin (<200 μg), the mice died from the tumors within 40–60 d and at higher levels of cisplatin (>350 μg), the mice died of drug toxicity in less than 7 d. For cisplatin-containing microspheres, the mice survived for an average as long as 140 d. From this study it seems clear that using a microparticle controlled-release formulation is advantageous in terms of relative toxicity and efficacy of the drug formulation.

The in vivo effectiveness of the release of irinotecan hydrochloride, a semisynthetic derivative of camptothecin, was also studied for microparticle formulations of PLA as well as 75:25 and 50:50 PLAGA (67). These studies, where mice were transplanted intraperitoneally with sarcoma 180 cells, showed a mean survival time for the control groups of approx 11 d. Treatment was begun 3 d after inoculation; irinotecan hydrochloride solutions at 50 mg eq/kg, 100 mg eq/kg, and 250 mg eq/kg showed mean survival times of 22, 16, and 16 d, respectively. Microparticle formulations prepared with PLA and at the same equivalent drug dosages showed mean survival times of 20, 16, and 32 d, respectively. Formulations at the 100 mg eq/kg level for 75:25 PLAGA and 50:50 PLAGA showed 20 and 24 d mean survival time. These studies demonstrated that, for the microparticle formulations to be significantly more effective in terms of survival time than the drug solution, the drug loading must be at least 250 mg eq/kg.

9. INDUSTRIAL EFFORTS, PRODUCTS, AND CLINICAL TRIALS

The one product currently on the market which uses microparticle formulations to treat cancer is the Lupron® Depot from TAP Pharmaceuticals (69). The Lupron® Depot is available in 4-, 3-, and 1-mo formulations which are approved in the United States for palliative treatment of advanced prostate cancer. These formulations contain 30, 22.5, and 7.5 mg of leuprolide acetate, respectively. In an open-label, noncomparative, multicenter clinical study of the 4-mo formulation, 49 patients with stage D2 prostatic adenocarcinoma (with no prior treatment) were enrolled. The objectives were to determine whether this 30 mg depot formulation, injected once every 16 wk, would reduce and maintain serum testosterone levels at castrate levels (less than or equal to 50 ng/dL). In the majority of patients, testosterone levels increased 50% or more above the baseline during the first week of treatment, however, these levels were subsequently suppressed to castrate levels within 30 d of the first injection in 94% of patients and within 43 d in all 49 patients during the initial 32-wk treatment period.

Lupron® Depot, available in formulations of 11.25 mg (3-mo dose) and 3.75 mg (1 mo dose), is also used with iron before surgery in the management of endometriosis and to treat anemia caused by fibroid tumors in the uterus when iron alone is not effective. For precocious puberty, the dosage is 7.5, 11.25, or 15 mg once per month, depending upon the weight of the child. Lupron® Depot has also been reported to have been used, quite effectively in some cases and questionably in others, in "off-label" situations such as infertility treatments for humans and adrenal tumor treatment in ferrets.

Although there are a vast number of clinical trials addressing cancer treatment at any time, very few of these are testing microencapsulated formulations. There are at least 1200 open clinical trials in the United States at any time and a recent review of those listed with the National Center Institute revealed only one to be testing a microparticulate delivery system for controlled drug delivery. Far more address the use of liposomal delivery systems, which are more widely used for cancer treatment than microparticulate systems. One clinical trial mentioned a study with PEGylated interferon, with a few underway with other pro-drug types of targeted delivery systems.

Although there are assuredly a number of clinical trials under way and not overly publicized, we will mention just a few here. The work that FeRx has done with magnetic targeted carriers has already been mentioned earlier in this chapter. The company also conducted a Phase I/II clinical trial in 1999 for delivery of doxorubicin for treatment of patients with primary liver cancer *(70)*. Paragon Medical introduced SIR-Spheres® in 1997, which are radioactive particles that are placed in liver cancers. The formulation is marketed in Australia, New Zealand, and Asia, with additional human studies being conducted in Hong Kong, Australia, and New Zealand *(71)*. Another set of clinical trials scheduled recently were to examine the treatment of human papillomavirus-associated cervical dysplasia, which can progress to cervical cancer. Zycos, Inc., and Chesapeake Biological Laboratories are collaborating on Biotope CD™, a PLAGA-based delivery system to deliver DNA-based drugs with increased potency *(72,73)*. Specifically for the cervical application, their plasmid DNA is encoded with disease-specific epitopes, which are designed to program cytotoxic Tcells to recognize and destroy the targeted disease.

10. FUTURE DIRECTIONS

Because it is clear that there is a great deal of potential for the use of microparticulate drug delivery formulations to treat cancer, only a few of these formulations have progressed enough in human studies to have proven their worth both in enhancing the efficacy of the drugs being delivered and in minimizing the undesirable side effects of traditional chemotherapy. Within the next 5–10 yr, we should certainly see some of the formulations currently in laboratories progress to the clinical setting and perhaps to a large number of cancer patients whose lives will be improved by using these advanced formulations. It should be emphasized that microparticulate formulations that provide controlled delivery can provide more than just a better-regulated chemotherapy regimen. They may also deliver cell-specific drugs, based on biotechnology and DNA, directly to the site of interest. This element of intelligent engineering is present to a smaller degree in liposomal formulations but, especially in biodegradable particles, its promise has yet to be realized or even understood.

REFERENCES

1. Schugens C, Laruelle N, Nihant N, Grandfils C, Jerome R, Teyssie P. Effect of the emulsion stability on the morphology and porosity of semicrystalline poly l-lactide microparticles prepared by W/O/W double emulsion-evaporation. *J Controlled Release* 1994; 32:161–176.
2. Tyle P. Sustained release growth hormone compositions for parenteral administration and their use, Europe Patent 0 278 103, assigned to American Cyanamid Co.
3. Tyle P. Sustained release growth hormone compositions for parenteral administration and their use, US Patent 4857506, assigned to American Cyanamid Co.
4. Viswanathan NB, Thomas PA, Pandit JK, Kulkarni MG, Mashelkar RA. Preparation of non-porous microspheres with high entrapment efficiency of proteins by a (water-in-oil)-in oil emulsion technique. *J Controlled Release* 1999; 58:9–20.
5. Yan C, Resau JH, Heweston J, West M, Rill WL, Kende M. Characterization and morphological analysis of protein-loaded poly(lactide-co-glycolide) microparticles prepared by water-in-oil-in-water emulsion technique. *J Controlled Release* 1994; 32:231–241.
6. Prankerd RJ, Stella VJ. The use of oil-in-water emulsions as a vehicle for parenteral administration. *J Parent Sci Technol* 1990; 44:139–149.
7. Malamataris S, Avgerinos A. Controlled release indomethacin microspheres prepared by using an emulsion solvent-diffusion technique. *Int J Pharmaceut* 1990; 62:105–111.
8. Kawashima Y, Niwa T, Handa T, Takeuchi H, Iwamoto T, Itoh K. Preparation of controlled-release microspheres of ibuprofen with acrylic polymers by a novel quasi-emulsion solvent diffusion method. *J Pharmaceut Sci* 1989; 78:68–72.
9. Grandfils C, Flandroy P, Nihant N, Barbette S, Jerome R, Teyssie P, Thibaut A. Preparation of Poly(D,L) lactide microspheres by emulsion-solvent evaporation, and their clinical applications as a convenient embolic material. *J Biomed Mater Res* 1992; 26:467–479.
10. Deng XM, Li XH, Yuan ML, Xiong CD, Huang ZT, Jia WX, Zhang YH. Optimization of preparative conditions for poly-dl-lactide-polyethylene glycol microspheres with entrapped vibrio cholera antigens. *J Controlled Release* 1999; 58:123–131.
11. Couvreur P, Blanco-Prieto MJ, Puisieux F, Roques B, Fattal E. Multiple emulsion technology for the design of microspheres containing peptides and oligopeptides. *Adv Drug Deliv Rev* 1997; 28:85–96.
12. Conway BR, Alpar HO. Double emulsion microencapsulation of proteins as model antigens using polymers: effect of emulsifier on the microsphere characteristics and release kinetics. *Europ J Pharmaceut Biopharmaceut* 1996; 42:42–48.
13. Candau F, Zekhnini Z, Heatley F, Franta E. Characterization of poly(acrylamide-co-acrylates) obtained by inverse microemulsion polymerization. *Colloid Polymer Sci* 1986; 264:676–682.
14. Ekman B, Sjoholm I. Improved stability of proteins immobilized in microparticles prepared by a modified emulsion polymerization technique. *J Pharmaceut Sci* 1978; 67:693–696.
15. Vert M, Schwach G, Engel R, Coudane J. Something new in the field of PLA/GA bioresorbable polymers? *J Controlled Release* 1998; 53:85–92.
16. Jeyanthi R, Thanoo BC, Metha RC, DeLuca PP. Effect of solvent removal technique on the matrix characteristics of polylactide/glycolide microspheres for peptide delivery. *J Controlled Release* 1996; 38:235–244.
17. Li W-I, Amderson KW, Mehta RC, DeLuca PP. Prediction of solvent removal profile and eeffect on properties for peptide-loaded PLGA microspheres prepared by solvent extraction/evaporation Method. *J Controlled Release* 1995; 37:199–214.
18. Thies C. Formulation of degradable drug-loaded microparticles by in-liquid drying processes, in *Microcapsules and Nanoparticles in Medicine and Pharmacy* (Dunbrow M, ed). CRC, Boca Raton, FL, 1992, pp 47–71.
19. Takakura Y, Hashida M. Macromolecular carrier systems for targeted drug delivery: pharmacokinetic considerations on biodistribution. *Pharmaceut Res* 1996; 13(6):820–831.
20. Chari RVJ. Targeted delivery of chemotherapeutics: tumor-activated prodrug therapy. *Adv Drug Deliv Rev* 1998; 31:89–104.
21. Kopecek J. Development of tailor-made polymeric prodrugs for systemic and oral delivery. *J Bioactive and Compatible Polymers* 1988; 3:16–26.

22. Mori A, Kennel SJ, Huang L. Immunotargeting of liposomes containing lipophilic antitumor prodrugs. *Pharmaceut Res* 1993; 10:507–514.

23. Nichifor M, Schacht EH. Cytotoxicity and anticancer activity of macromolecular prodrugs of 5-fluorouracil. *J Bioactive and Compatible Polymers* 1997; 12:265–281.

24. Nichifor M, Schacht EH, Seymour LW. Polymeric prodrugs of 5-fluorouracil. *J Controlled Release* 1997; 48:165–178.

25. Ranucci E, Spagnoli G, Latini R, Bernasconi R, Ferruti P. On the suitability of urethane bonds between the carrier and the drug moiety in the poly(ethyleneglycol)-based oligomeric prodrugs. *J Biomater Sci Polymer Edn* 1994; 6:133–139.

26. Ranucci E, Satore L, Peroni I, Latini R, Bernasconi R, Ferruti P. Pharmacokinetic results on naproxen prodrugs based on poly(ethyleneglycol)s. *J Biomater Sci Polymer Edn* 1994; 6:141–147.

27. Steyger PS, Baban DF, Brereton M, Ulbrich K, Seymour LW. Intratumoural distribution as a determinant of tumour responsiveness to therapy using polymer-based macromolecular prodrugs. *J Controlled Release* 1996; 39:35–46.

28. Subr V, Kopecek J, Pohl J, Baudys M, Kostka V. Cleavage of oligopeptide side- chains in n-(2-hydroxypropyl)methacrylamide copolymers by mixtures of lysosomal enzymes. *J Controlled Release* 1988; 8:133–140.

29. Dosio F, Brusa P, Crosasso P, Arpicco S, Cattel L. Preparation, characterization and properites in vitro and in vivo of a paclitaxel-albumin conjugate. *J Controlled Release* 1997; 47:293–304.

30. Yoo HS, Oh JE, Lee KH, Park TG. Biodegradable nanoparticles containing doxorubicin-PLGA conjugate for sustained release. *Pharmaceut Res* 1999; 16(7):1114–1118.

31. Yokoyama M, Fukushima S, Uehara R, Okamoto K, Kataoka K, Sakurai Y, Okano T. Characterization of physical entrapment and chemical conjugation of adriamycin in polymeric micelles and their design for in vivo delivery to a solid tumor. *J Controlled Release* 1998; 50:79–92.

32. Minko T, Kopeckova P, Kopecek J. Comparison of the anticancer effect of free and HPMA copolymer-boiund adriamycin in juman ovarian carcinoma cells. *Pharmaceut Res* 1999; 16(7):986–996.

33. Omelyanenko V, Kopeckova P, Prakash RK, Ebert CD, Kopecek J. Biorecognition of HPMA copolymer adriamycin conjugates by lymphocytes mediated by synthetic receptor binding epitopes. *Pharmaceut Res* 1999; 16(7):1010–1019.

34. Takeuchi H, Handa T, Kawashima Y. Controlled release theophylline tablet with acrylic polymers prepared by spray-drying technique in aqueous system. *Drug Develop Indust Pharm* 1989; 15:1999–2016.

35. Baras B, Benoit M-A, Youan C, Botti B, Gillard J. Spray-dried polylactide and poly(lactide-co-glycolide) microparticles in controlled oral vaccine delivery. *J Controlled Release* 1997; 48:289–363.

36. Bittner B, Mader K, Li YX, Kissel T. Evaluation of the microenvironment inside biodegradable microspheres from ABA triblock copolymers of poly(l-lactide-co- glycolide) and poly(ethylene oxide) prepared by spray drying. *Int Symp Control Rel Bioact Mater* 1997.

37. Bodmeier R, Chen H. Preparation of biodegradable poly(lactide) microparticles using a spray-drying technique. *J Pharm Pharmacol* 1988; 40:754–757.

38. Freitas C, Muller R. Spray-drying of solid lipid nanoparticles. *Europ J Pharmaceut Biopharmaceut* 1998; 46:145–151.

39. Gander B, Wehrli E, Alder R, Merkle HP. Quality improvement of spray-dried, protein-loaded D,L-PLA microspheres by appropriate polymer solvent selection. *J Microencapsul* 1995; 12:83–97.

40. Giunchedi P, Conte U. Spray-drying as a preparation method of microparticluate drug delivery systems: an overview. *STP Pharma Sci* 1995; 5:276–290.

41. Gupta PK, Hung CT, Perrier DG. Albumin microspheres. I. release characteristics of adriamycin. *Int J Pharmaceut* 1986; 33:137–146.

42. Chen Y, McCulloch RK, Gray BN. Synthesis of albumin-dextran sulfate microspheres possessing favourable loading and release characteristics for the anticancer drug doxorubicin. *J Controlled Release* 1994; 31:49–54.

43. Miyazaki S, Hasiguchi N, Hou WM, Yokouchi C, Takada M. Preparation and evaluation in vitro and in vivo fibrinogen microspheres containing adriamycin. *Chem Pharm Bull* 1986; 34:3384–3393.

44. Wada R, Tabata Y, Ikada Y. Preparation of poly(lactic acid) microspheres containing anti-cancer agents. *Bull Inst Chem Res* 1988; 66:241–250.

45. Spenlehauer G, Vert M, Benoit JP, Boddaert A. In vitro and in vivo degradation of poly(dl lactide/glycolide) type microspheres made by solvent evaporation method. *Biomaterials* 1989; 10:557–563.

46. Matsumoto A, Matsukawa Y, Suzuki T, Yoshino H, Kobayashi M. The polymer-alloys method as a new preparation method of biodegradable microspheres: principle and application to cisplatin-loaded microspheres. *J Controlled Release* 1997; 48:19–27.

47. Kyo M, Hyon S-H, Ikada Y. Effects of preparation conditions of cisplatin-loaded microspheres on the in vitro release. *J Controlled Release* 1995; 35:73–82.
48. Ike O, Shimizu Y, Wada R, Hyon S-H, Ikada Y. Controlled cisplatin delivery system using poly(d,l-lactic acid). *Biomaterials* 1992; 13:230–234.
49. Itoi K, et al. In vivo suppressive effects of copoly(glycolic/l-lactic acid) microspheres containing cddp on murine tumor cells. *J Controlled Release* 1996; 42:175–184.
50. Spenlehauer G, Vert M, Benoit J-P, Chabot F, Veillard M. Biodegradable cisplatin microspheres prepared by the solvent evaporation method:morphology and release characteristics. *J Controlled Release* 1988; 7:217–229.
51. Spenlehauer G, Veillard M, Benoit J-P. Formation and characterization of cisplatin loaded poly(d,d-lactide) microspheres for chemoembolization. *J Pharmaceut Sci* 1986; 75:750–755.
52. Ciftci K, Hincal AA, Kas HS, Ercan TM, Sungur A, Guven O, Ruacan S. Solid tumor chemotherapy and in vivo distribution of fluorouracil following administration in poly(l-lactic acid) microspheres. *Pharmaceut Develop Technol* 1997; 2:151–160.
53. Akbuga J, Bergisadi N. 5-fluorouracil-loaded chitosan microspheres:preparation and release characteristics. *J Microencapsulat* 1996; 13:161–168.
54. Sharifi R, Ratanawong C, Jung A, Wu Z, Browneller R, Lee M. Therapeutic effects of leuproelin microspheres in prostate cancer. *Adv Drug Deliv Rev* 1997; 28:121–138.
55. Schally AV, Comaru-Schally AM. Rational use of agonists and antagonists of luteinizing hormone-releasing hormone (lh-rh) in the treatment of hormone sensitive neoplasms and gynaecologic conditions. *Adv Drug Deliv Rev* 1997; 28:157–169.
56. Okada H, Yamamoto M, Heya T, Inoue Y, Kamei S, Ogawa Y, Toguchi H. Drug delivery using biodegradable microspheres. *J Controlled Release* 1994; 28:121–129.
57. Csernus VJ, Szende B, Schally AV. Release of peptides from sustained delivery systems (microcapsules and microparticles) in vivo. *Int J Peptide Protein Res* 1990; 35:557–565.
58. Wada R, Hyon S-H, Ikada Y. Lactic acid oligomer microspheres containing an anticancer agent for selective lymphatic delivery: I. In vitro studies. *J Bioactive and Compatible Polymers* 1988; 3:126–136.
59. Shenderova A, Burke TG, Schwendeman SP. The acidic microclimate in poly(lactide-co-glycolide) microspheres stabilizes campotothecins. *Pharmaceut Res* 1999; 16:241–248.
60. Yokoyama M, Satoh A, Sakurai Y, et al. Incorporation of water-insoluble anticancer drug into polymeric micelles and control of their particle size. *J Controlled Release* 1998; 55:219–229.
61. Shenderova A, Burke TG, Schwendeman SP. Stabilization of 10- hydroxycamptothecin in poly(lactide-co-glycolide) microsphere delivery vehicles. *Pharmaceut Res* 1997; 14:1406–1414.
62. Ertl B, Platzer P, Wirth M, Gabor F. Poly(d,l-lactic-co-glycolic acid) microspheres for sustained delivery and stabilization of camptothecin. *J Controlled Release* 1999; 61:305–317.
63. Wang YM, Sato H, Horkoshi I. In Vitro in vivo evaluation of taxol release from poly(lactic-co-glycolic acid) microspheres containing isopropyl myristate and degradation of the microspheres. *J Controlled Release* 1997; 49:157–166.
64. Vook N, et al. Taxol microencapsulation into biodegradable uncapped poly(lactide-co-glycolide) copolymers. *Int Symp Control Rel Bioact Mater* 1997; 24:881–882.
65. Ruiz JM, Benoit JP. In vivo peptide release from poly(dl-lactic-acid-co-glycolic acid) copolymer 50/50 microspheres. *J Controlled Release* 1991; 16:177–186.
66. Menei P, Boisdron-Celle M, Guy G. Effect of stereotactic implantation of biodegradable 5-fluorouracil-loaded microspheres in healthy and C6 glioma-bearing rats. *Neurosurgery* 1996; 39:117–124.
67. Machida Y, Onishi H, Morikawa A, Machida Y. Antitumour characteristics of irinotecan-containing microspheres of poly-d,l-lactic acid or poly(d,l-lactic acid-co-glycolic acid) copolymers. *STP Pharma Sciences* 1998; 8:175–181.
68. Hutchinson FG, Furr BJA. Biodegradable polymer systems for the sustained release of polypeptides. *J Controlled Release* 1990; 13:279–294.
69. Tap Pharmevauticals Urology, Lupron® Depot, 1999, http://www.tapurology.com/Html/lupron.htm.
70. FeRx Incorporated, FeRx Incorporated, 1999, http://www.ferx.com/home.htm.
71. Paragon Medical Limited, Publications on SIR-Spheres and Selective Internal Radiation Therapy, 1999; http://www.pml.com.au/corporate.hmtl.
72. Zycos, Breakthrough Cancer Drug Manufacturing Alliance, 1999; http://www.zycos.com/press/release15.html.
73. Hedley ML, Curley JM, Langer RS. Microparticles for delivery of nucleic acid, USA Patent 5 783 567, July 21, 1998; assigned to Pangaea Pharmaceuticals.

7

Polyethylene Glycol Conjugation of Protein and Small Molecule Drugs

Past, Present, and Future

Robert G. L. Shorr, PhD, Michael Bentley, PhD, Simon Zhsao, PhD, Richard Parker, PhD, and Brendan Whittle, PhD

Contents

From: *Drug Delivery Systems in Cancer Therapy*
Edited by: D. M. Brown © Humana Press Inc., Totowa, NJ

1. INTRODUCTION

Prior to the advent of biotechnology, use of protein drugs was largely limited to products isolated from human donor plasma such as serum albumin, immunoglobulin, and clotting factors. Use of these agents requires stringent protocols for collection, purification, and removal of infectious agents such as bacteria, virus, and, more recently, prions. Although for diabetics who require insulin, porcine sources were useful, use of animal or bacterial or other nonhuman-derived proteins was, and continues to be, complicated by the potential formation of antibodies that may rapidly clear the drug from the body or lead to anaphylactoid reactions and "allergic responses."

The ability to clone and express commercially useful quantities of recombinant human proteins in bacterial, insect cell, yeast fermentation systems, or transgenic animals has enabled the development and introduction into the marketplace of otherwise unavailable life-saving protein drugs. Numerous recombinant human protein and biotechnology products are in clinical trials or pending regulatory agency approval.

In addition to the cloning and expression of "normal or wild-type" human proteins in the aforementioned manner, the design and production of mutant forms of human and other proteins is possible. Such "muteins" include chimeric or "humanized" mouse antibodies and a variety of fragments such as single chains, Fab and Fab$_2$, fusion proteins, toxins, and enzymes. Human serum albumin fusion proteins are designed to have a more prolonged circulating life than the native protein product *(1)*. Human growth hormone and α-interferon human serum albumin fusions are being developed by Principia Pharmaceuticals, Inc. (Philadelphia, PA), recently acquired by Human Genome Sciences. Like nonhuman proteins, muteins may elicit an antibody or immune reaction that may or may not be clinically relevant.

With the sequencing of the human genome completed, the accelerated discovery of genes and gene products regulating growth and development, as well as disease, is likely to fuel the identification of novel protein therapeutics and drug targets. For each of the protein drugs seeking development, issues related to optimum circulating life, polyethylene glycol (PEG)ylation might address dosing levels and frequency of administration, as well as safety. However, not all that could are being pursued in this fashion; when and how to apply PEG technology is itself an emerging science.

To understand PEGylation, it is essential to understand what PEG does and does not do *vis-a-vis* drug performance, as well as proposed mechanisms of action.

2. WHAT IS PEG?

PEG is a polymer comprised of the repeating unit $(-CH_2CH_2O-)_n$ produced by polymerization of ethylene oxide. The polymer may be linear or be prepared as a branch chain or dendritic construct with varying numbers of branches. PEGs of different molecular weights and geometries have been used in pharmaceutical products.

For coupling reactions, PEG must be activated. Monomethoxy PEG [CH$_3$ (=O=CH$_2$=CH$_2$)$_n$=OH] has been activated by several methods including cyanuric chloride, 1,1′-carbonyldiimidazole, phenylchloroformate, or succidinimidyl active ester *(2–4)* to enable conjugation to proteins. The activating agent may also act as a linker between PEG and the protein. Multiple PEG strands may be attached to a protein or *bis* or multivalent activated PEGs may be used to "crosslink" or polymerize multiple protein molecules or subunits. Typically, pharmacokinetics and pharmacodynamics of any

PEG-protein conjugate are dependent on PEG molecular weight, the chemistry used for conjugation, the stability of any linker, the number of PEG strands per each molecule of protein, and the geometry of the PEG used. The PEG strands are capable of assuming some interactions with the protein surface as well as having certain surfactant-like properties *(5–7)*.

For many applications, linear methoxy PEG (blocked at one end) and activated at the other has been used to achieve the desired performance benefit. In general, activated PEGs nonselectively couple to such nucleophilic groups as amino, hydroxyl, and sulhydryl moieties available on the surface of the protein. The degree of PEGylation is dependent on reaction conditions such as pH and reagent concentrations. More recently, proteins have been modified at the level of the gene so as to insert groups suitable for conjugation or to remove those that might contribute to loss of activity or destabilization.

The rationale for selection of PEGylation chemistry and geometry is based on the structure of the protein to be PEGylated and the role that potential coupling sites play in any desired activity. The extent of PEGylation deemed optimal will also be driven by the need to prevent any potential allergic or immune reactions. For example, a nonhuman protein is likely to require more PEG substitution than a recombinant human one. The optimal PEG geometry and molecular weight to be selected is driven by the desired effect in terms of prolongation of circulating life.

The degree of PEGylation and the location of the PEGylation sites can have a dramatic impact on the desired activity of the PEGylated protein. In some cases, losses of activity of 20–95% have been reported *(2–8)*. The mechanism by which loss of activity occurs may vary. For an enzyme, it may be because of loss of key charged residues at or near an active site, or the blocking or prevention of interaction with substrate, or an allosteric regulator and important conformational changes. For receptor-directed ligands such as cytokines, PEGylation may interfere with ligand docking and site interactions that lead to receptor conformational changes and the activation of signal transduction cascades or effector proteins.

The PEGylation process may also contribute to loss of biological activity caused by adverse coupling conditions such as extremes of pH, temperature, or the presence of oxidizing or reducing agents, reaction byproducts, or side reactions *(2–10)*. Table 1 lists examples of "coupling chemistries" and conditions that may be used in the PEGylation of proteins and peptides.

Scientists at PolyMasc Inc. (London, UK) have proposed the use of tresyl chloride (2,2,2-trifluoroethanesulphonyl chloride) to attach PEG directly via a stable secondary amine bond to the NH2 groups of proteins under physiological conditions *(11–14)*. The authors have noted that the nitrogen atom to which the PEG chain is attached retains the ability to protonate conserving surface charges that may be essential for bioactivity.

The nature of the activation chemistry to be used in any PEGylation strategy requires special consideration both in terms of stability (in the vial and body) as well as potential for promotion of immune or allergic reaction.

The nature of activated PEG in terms of purity and polydispersity is also of critical importance to the control of reactions and the assurance of the most homogeneous product possible. In the absence of highly purified activated PEG, unwanted crosslinking, aggregation, and precipitation of protein may occur, reducing overall yield and activity.

Table 1
Examples of "Coupling Chemistries" and Conditions
That May Be Used in the PEGylation of Proteins and Peptides

Chemistry	Conditons
Cyanuric chloride	1 h, pH 9.2–9.8, RT
Phenychloroformate	1–5 h, pH 8.3–9.3, RT
PEG-acetaldehyde	pH 8.5, borohydride
PEG-acetaldehyde	18 h, pH 7, 37°C, cyanoborohydride
PEG-propionaldehyde	1 h, pH, RT, cyanoborohydride

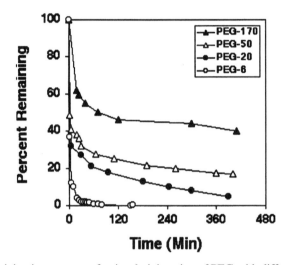

Fig. 1. Blood radioactivity time courses after iv administration of PEG with different molecular weights. Key: (▲) PEG-170,000; (△) PEG-50,000; (●) PEG-20,000; (○) PEG-6000. Adapted from *(16)*.

3. WHAT DOES PEG DO?

Plasma kinetics of PEG are likely to depend on molecular weight and geometry, as well as route of administration *(15–17)*. Yamaoka et al. *(16)* have described the circulating lifetimes of radiolabeled linear PEGs with molecular weights of 6000 (PEG-6), 20,000 (PEG-20), 50,000 (PEG-50), and 170,000 (PEG-170) after intravenous (iv) administration to mice (Fig. 1). Similar to other polymers such as dextrans, polyvinyl pyrrilidone, and similar materials *(18,19),* plasma concentrations and areas under the curve (AUCs) of the higher molecular weight PEGs are substantially greater than those of the lower molecular weight polymers (Table 2, Fig. 2). The half-lives of the polymers also progressively increase with molecular weight. The relationship between half-life and PEG molecular weight appears sigmoidal.

The most likely explanation for differences in plasma half-life of the tested PEGs may be differences in renal excretion rates. Chang et al. *(20)* reported that, in rats, renal elimination of "stiff" linear neutral dextrans with molecular weights of approx 10,000 occurred without any restriction. Excretion rates of dextrans with larger molecular weights progressively decreased and approached zero at molecular weights of approx

Table 2
Mean ± SD of AUC and Terminal Half-Life of PEGs
of Increasing Molecular Weight After iv Administration to Mice

Parameter	PEG-6	PEG-20	PEG-50	PEG-170
AUC, % dose/h/mL	6.17 ± 2.18	110 ± 7.17	600 ± 11.9	1110 ± 27.0
t1/2, min	17.6 ± 5.90	169 ± 20.0	987 ± 70.0	1390 ± 57.0

Adapted from (16).

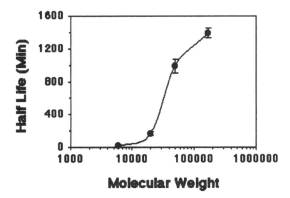

Fig. 2. Relationship between the plasma half-life of PEG and its molecular weight. Adapted from *(16)*.

40,000. PEG, unlike "stiff" dextran polymers, is flexible in its backbone and may be excreted through the kidney at even substantially higher molecular weights.

When attached to proteins and peptides, PEG has been shown to prolong circulation time. The increase in circulating lifetime being proportional to the number of attached PEG strands, their molecular weight, and geometry. The molecular weight of the PEGylated protein is also of importance, as is any protein specific uptake or metabolic events. In addition to the likelihood of decreased renal filtration, it is also likely PEGylation contributes to a decreased rate of degradation by protease and extravasation that might otherwise occur.

Increasing circulating lifetime and maintaining consistent drug levels that eliminate large "peak-to-trough" fluctuations can reduce the incidence and severity of peak-related side effects. PEG does not promote cellular uptake or necessarily improve protein stability, although some reports suggesting utility in the latter have been cited in the literature.

4. METABOLISM, TOXICITY, AND EXCRETION

There is limited information on the metabolism of PEG in the body. It may be that to some extent PEG undergoes cytochrome P-450 oxidation, resulting in the formation of ketone, ester, and aldehyde groups *(21,22)*.

In general, it has been shown that with iv, subcutaneous (sc), or intramuscular (im) administration, PEGs ranging in molecular weight from 6000 to 170,000 do not distribute significantly to heart, lung, liver, spleen, kidney, and thyroid gland, but rather distribute to the gastrointestinal tract via the bile *(21)*, and what is not excreted in the urine is excreted in the feces.

Table 3
Example of PEGylated Protein Preparations Showing
Blunted or Reduced, Immune or Allergic Reactions

PEG-Protein	Antigenicity	Test System	References
Asparaginase	blunted	precipitin	26,27
Adenosine deaminase	blunted	immunodiffusion	28
Uricase	blunted	immunodiffusion precipitin	29–31
Superoxide dismutase	reduced	immunodiffusion	32
Catalase	blunted reduced	immunodiffusion ELISA	33,34
Arginase	blunted	immunodiffusion	35
Streptokinase	reduced blunted	RIA neutralisation precipitin	36–38
β-Glucuronidase	reduced	immunodiffusion RIA	39
Trypsin	blunted	immunodiffusion	40
Phenylalanine ammonia-lyase	reduced	preciptin immunodiffusion	41
Bovine albumin	blunted	immunodiffusion	42

5. REDUCED ANTIGENICITY AND IMMUNE OR ALLERGIC REACTIONS

PEG itself is inert. PEGylation at or near sites on a protein or peptide surface possibly responsible for immune or allergic reactions may contribute to the masking of these sites and, therefore, to a reduced risk. The protective benefit of PEGylation to proteins, liposomes, or nanoparticles may be because of the high mobility of the PEG chains and the shrouding of much or all of the "offending" regions on the protein or liposomal particle (23–25) surface. It is also likely that PEGylation decreases uptake and recognition of "antigen" by cells of the immune surveillance system as well as interference with "antigen digestion" and processing. More specifically, PEGylation may alter the nature of peptides produced and presented by antigen presenting cells (APC) or even the ability of produced peptides to be recognized by the appropriate receptors.

The degree of reduction of immune or allergic reactions is likely to be a function of the degree of PEGylation, PEG molecular weight, geometry, chemistry of linkage and, more importantly, site of attachment. Empirical experimentation is the most likely approach to yield an optimized formulation.

Examples of PEGylated protein preparations showing blunted or reduced immune or allergic reactions are shown in Table 3.

6. PEG DRUGS: PAST AND PRESENT

Each year, approx 1.5 million Americans are newly diagnosed with cancer. About 1,220,000 cases were expected for the year 2000. Since 1990, nearly 13 million cases excluding skin and certain other cancers have been diagnosed. About 10 million Americans are presently living and coping with a cancer diagnosis and treatment history. Each year, approx 550,000 deaths or nearly one-quarter of disease-associated mortality in America is cancer-related. One in four Americans has been projected to experience cancer at some point during his or her lifetime. Cancer is the number two disease killer of Americans and will be the leading cause of death from disease in children ages 1–14. Nearly 90% of cases will be solid tumors with metastases distal to the primary tumor site.

Cancers causing the most deaths in the United States for both sexes are lung and colorectal, followed by breast and uterine cancer in women, and prostate cancer in men. Management of metastatic disease remains one of the most challenging aspects of oncology care to date.

The principal treatment modalities for cancer are surgery, radiation therapy, and the use of chemotherapeutic agents. Of these, surgery, if performed at an early stage of disease progression, offers the greatest chance for cure. Radiotherapy does not discriminate between normal and healthy tissue and must rely on external methods of targeting radiation beams to the desired location. Collateral damage to healthy organs and tissues can be high with devastating side effects. Chemotherapeutic agents, although capable of "killing" tumor cells, also kill healthy cells.

Most patients will experience chemotherapy and/or radiation treatments as well as surgery at some point during the course of their disease. Side effects will be so severe as to limit treatment. Surgery is likely to be disfiguring. Cancer-associated pain will be extreme and often require chronic, high doses of analgesics. Constipation, mental clouding, depression, respiratory depression, and distress may accompany analgesic use. For most, the prognosis will be poor.

Despite tremendous progress in understanding the underlying mechanisms of cancer generation and the emergence of biotechnology based therapeutics, chemotherapeutic agents designed to "kill" cancerous cells distributed systemically via im or sc injection, iv infusion, or oral administration remain the mainstay of anticancer therapy. Many of these cytotoxic agents are designed to affect rapidly dividing cells at the level of the DNA. Side-effect profiles reflecting the simultaneous "killing" of rapidly dividing "normal" cells and sensitive tissues, such as found in the bone marrow. Decreased platelet and blood cell formation are likely to contribute to patient death. Dose-limiting side effects may also curb an ability to "kill" tumors with higher concentration of drug, whereas suboptimal concentrations may favor the appearance of resistant clonogenic cells and disease.

While some progress has been made in the treatment of certain tumor types, nearly half of all patients will fail to respond or will relapse to metastatic disease. Despite the appearance of nearly 70 approved chemotherapeutic agents for the treatment of cancer, overall results have been disappointing. There is a desperate need for novel anticancer agents and ancillary treatment products.

7. THE PROBLEM

The primary problem in the treatment of cancer is that differences between normal cells of origin and malignant cells are subtle and difficult to identify, quantify, and translate to beneficial therapy. Shared properties between normal and tumor cells have confounded the development of tumor-specific agents.

7.1. Properties of Tumors and Malignant Cells

Normal tissues may be considered as those that are continuously renewing their cell populations (e.g., bone marrow, intestine), those that proliferate slowly but may regenerate in response to damage (e.g., liver, lung), or those that are relatively static (e.g., muscle and nerve).

Cancer can be defined as the emergence of cellular clusters resulting from continuous production of abnormal cells that invade and destroy normal tissues.

Human tumors often arise first in renewing tissues. The tumor cells are able to divide endlessly, without differentiating into a mature state and regardless of the function of the tissue they are in. As they begin to multiply, angiogenesis factors, growth factors, and cytokines to stimulate the formation of collateral blood vessels and other "support" tissues are released. Some tumors may increase in malignancy with time and shed clonogenic cells that will give rise to metastatic nodules and eventually additional tumor masses. Tumor cells are believed to be genetically unstable and subject to a high degree of random mutation during clonal expansion that gives rise to lethal or disadvantageous mutations, as well as greater autonomy and growth advantages to those cells that will go on to become tumor producers.

It is not surprising then, that tumors are heterogeneous in their origins and properties, extending to almost any property measured, including surface markers, karyotype, morphology, metastatic potential, and sensitivity to therapeutic agents. Nutritional heterogeneity may also occur and reflects the immature and (often) slower growing vasculature associated with tumors. Typically, nutritional and oxygen gradients appear as distance from the vascular tree increases. A dramatic influence on metabolic function and proliferation can be expected across cell layers. In some instances, regions of tumor necrosis may emerge. The development of subclones may be a key underlying mechanism for tumor progression and the emergence of resistance. Subclones with varying degrees of resistance may contribute to the "hitting a moving target" challenge for the cancer therapist.

It is the spread of cancerous cells and the appearance of metastases and resistance that represents the most difficult challenge to the oncologist. Routes and sites of metastases vary with different primary tumors. As cancers breakthrough the surface of the organ in which they originated, cells may shed, lodge, and begin to grow on the surface of adjacent organs. Tumor cells may also migrate into the lymphatic system and be carried to the lymph nodes and blood vessels. As malignant cells migrate through the blood stream, many die. Others become trapped in vessels too small to let them pass. Tumor cells originating in the GI tract may be stopped in the liver or eventually the lung. Other tumor cells originating in other parts of the body may be stopped first in the microvasculature of the lung. Smaller clusters of tumor cells, present as micrometastases, may remain relatively dormant and escape detection.

Four stages for cancer progression have been defined with increasing severity of disease and seriousness.

- **Stage 1:** Tumors are small and localized and, depending on location, may be removed surgically.
- **Stages 2 and 3:** Tumors are larger and may have broken through the initial organ to attach to additional surrounding organs and tissues; lymph node involvement is likely.
- **Stage 4:** Tumors are metastasized to other parts of the body, usually with nodal involvement.

Human tumors vary widely in their properties. They may arise in different parts of the body, and they vary in retention of normal differentiation pattern, grade, extent of expansion into surrounding normal tissue, and metastases or stage. It is likely that this variability reflects the different or individual initial genetic alterations at the root of the cancer emergence and the cells that ultimately will constitute the tumor mass. The collective biological properties of the tumor cells will determine the overall tumor phenotype. Cancer cells, even when spread throughout the body, are likely to retain at least some physical and biological characteristics of the tissue in which they originated. Tumors arising from endocrine tissue, for example, may continue to produce and release hormones. The more de-differentiated a tumor, the more aggressive its growth and ability to generate metastases.

Although the cause of cancer is not completely understood, a combination of hereditary factors, virus or environmental exposures, and lifestyle has been implicated. Linkage between cigarette smoking and lung cancer, for example, is widely accepted. Typically, more than 140,000 people each year will be newly diagnosed with lung cancer. Epidemiologists are predicting that even with cessation of smoking programs, these numbers are likely to continue for at least the next three decades.

Recently, specific genetic events have been implicated in the emergence of cancer and the control of cell growth. Use of agents to specifically turn these genes off or on has become the focus of intense preclinical and clinical research. It is likely that these agents will find use in conjunction with known cytotoxic agents and newer formulations as part of a "combination" or "cocktail" approach to cancer treatment.

Three major cancer subtypes have been described:

- **Sarcomas:** Arising from connective and supportive tissues, i.e., bone, cartilage, nerve, blood vessels, muscle, and fat.
- **Carcinomas:** Arising from epithelial tissue, i.e., skin, body cavity and organ linings, glandular tissue, breast, and prostate; squamous tumors resembling skin—adenocarcinomas resembling glandular tissue.
- **Leukemia and lymphomas:** Arising from blood cell-forming tissue and involving lymph nodes, spleen, and bone marrow with an overproduction of lymphocytes.

The ideal anticancer chemotherapy is one that is specific for cancer cells yet capable of diverse application to multiple tumor types and clonogenic lines while effectively, but safely, shrinking primary tumors, as well as preventing or eliminating metastatic nodules.

Present approaches in seeking to achieve this end include:

1. Tumor targeting and promotion of drug accumulation in solid tumor masses or nodules.
2. Tumor-specific or selectively acting agents based upon a unique feature of cancer cells.
3. Tumor-selective drugs using a cancer-specific activation mechanism or metabolic requirement.

In the latter regard, it has been shown earlier that certain tumors have essential requirements for amino acids such as asparagine, arginine, glutamine, and methionine. The targeting of these amino acids using metabolic enzymes from various sources has been one approach by which to "metabolically" select against tumor cells. Many of the enzymes that have been suggested to be useful are of nonhuman origin, and PEGylation has been explored for the reduction or blunting of any immune reaction, as well as for the prolongation of circulating life and minimizing of dosing frequency.

8. PEG ASPARAGINASE

Acute lymphoblastic leukemia (ALL) is a hematologic malignancy diagnosed in more than 3000 adults and children in the United States each year *(43)*. Substantial progress in treatment of acute lymphoblastic leukemia has been made. In the 1960s, the 5-yr survival rate was as low as 4% of patients. Today, more than 73% of pediatric patients are expected to survive 5 or more years. The response rate in adults, however, remains lower *(44)*.

In the early 1950s, the observation was made that a component in guinea pig serum had antitumor activity *(45,46)*. This component was later identified as the enzyme asparaginase which hydrolyses asparagine to aspartic acid and ammonia *(45,46)*. Up until that time, it had been thought that the nonessential amino acid asparagine played no critical role in tumor growth. Depletion of asparagine experiments in cell culture however, revealed the essential need for this amino acid in a number of neoplasms, most likely as a result of a lack of activity or presence of the enzyme asparagine synthase *(46,47)*. In 1964 *(46)*, asparaginase from *Escherichia coli* was found to be as effective as guinea pig serum in treating experimental tumors, and a supply of the enzyme in commercial quantities could be produced for human clinical trials. Active enzyme was also isolated from *Erwinia carotovora* and other sources *(48)*. With success in human trials, asparaginase entered the clinical setting for the treatment of acute lymphoblastic leukemia. Despite response to treatment, more than 50% of patients that obtain a complete remission have relapse *(49)*. Further, among those receiving asparaginase, more than 70% experience hypersensitivity reactions including life-threatening anaphylaxis *(50)*, an event that requires these patients to be closely monitored during treatment *(51)*. For those seeking reinduction of remission even years after time of diagnosis and initial treatment, hypersensitivity reactions still occur *(50)*.

Other limitations observed with asparaginase include a relatively short half-life of 20 h and a requirement for daily dosing for up to 14 d. Given the need for close monitoring, the repeated doses require a lengthy hospitalization or daily doctor office visits *(52)*. Other toxicities associated with the use of asparaginase include neurological disturbances and hepatic damage *(52)*. Nevertheless, asparaginase has been shown to be useful for prolonged use during consolidation and maintenance therapy for ALL; use of the drug for 20 wk after remission induction improved disease–free survival in children *(46)*.

To prevent the formation of antibodies and anaphylactoid reactions on repeated use of asparaginase, as well as to allow the use of enzyme where such antibodies had already been formed, PEGylated asparaginase was prepared and developed through the clinical trial process. Asparaginase, isolated from both *E. coli* and *Erwinia carotovora* was PEGylated. Several studies *(53–59)* have documented the usefulness of PEG asparaginase for the treatment of various cancers in both humans and animals. Ho et al. *(55,57)* showed that plasma half-life of the conjugated enzyme in humans *(55)* increased from 20 h (for native enzyme) to 357 h (for the conjugate). The increase in the plasma half-life was caused by a decrease in clearance of the enzyme *(55,57)*. Some improvements in toxicity and efficacy were reported *(53,59)*. PEGylated asparaginase (pegaspargase) has since been approved by the FDA and marketed for the treatment of ALL in patients who are hypersensitive to native forms of L-asparaginase.

Recently, Dr. Thomas C. Abshire of the Pediatric Oncology Group Operations Office in Chicago, IL, et al. evaluated remission rates and toxicity of treatment with PEGylated asparaginase in 144 children with B-precursor ALL in first relapse, with 95% of children having received native asparaginase during initial therapy *(60)*. In all cases, reinduction therapy included doxorubicin, prednisone, and vincristine. In addition, children were randomized to receive either weekly or biweekly doses of the PEGylated enzyme.

Complete remission occurred in 90% of cases overall, but occurred significantly more often in children given weekly, rather than biweekly, doses of PEGylated asparaginase. Low asparaginase levels were associated with high antibody titers to asparaginase, whereas high asparaginase levels were associated with a higher rate of complete remission. High-grade infectious toxicity occurred in half of the patients, although only four died of sepsis during treatment, and other toxicities were infrequent and hypersensitivity was rare.

9. PEG METHIONINASE

Many tumors have been shown to have a metabolic requirement for methionine. Colon, breast, prostate, ovary, kidney, larynx, melanoma, sarcoma, lung, brain, stomach, bladder, varieties of leukemia, and lymphomas have been studied and implicated. Methionine dependence has been defined as the lack of tumor growth when methionine is replaced with homocysteine in growth media (61,62). Methionine depletion has been suggested to synchronize tumor cells so that they become more sensitive to antimitotic agents (63,64). Hoffman et al. have proposed and are evaluating the use of methionase as an anticancer enzyme to "metabolically target" the elevated methionine dependency of tumors in conjunction with antimitotic agents. Tan et al. (65) have cloned the gene for methioninase (rMETase) from *Pseudomonas putida* and produced the protein in *E. coli*. The IC-50 for rMETase tested against breast, renal, colon, prostate, melanoma, and CNS tumor cells averaged 0.12 ± 0.06 U/mL whereas the observed IC-50 for normal cells tissues averaged 1.53 ± 1.39 U/mL. Depletion of methionine induced apoptosis.

The efficacy of recombinant rMETase alone and in combination with cisplatin (CDDP) was also examined in human colon cancer in nude mice (66). Results demonstrated growth arrest of human colon tumors in nude mice at doses of 100 or 200 U injected intraperitoneally every 8 h (T/C values were 23% and 20%, respectively, when compared with control; $p < 0.01$ in both groups). Cisplatin, given at 7 mg/kg intraperitoneally at day 1 of therapy in combination with the lower dose of rMETase, resulted in tumor regression (T/C value was 8% when compared with control; $p < 0.01$) with apparent cures in two of six animals. Neither CDDP nor the lower dose of rMETase alone caused tumor regression. Similar results have been observed with cotreatment using 5-FU (67).

A pilot Phase I clinical trial has been initiated in order to determine rMETase toxicity, rMETase pharmacokinetics, MET-depletion, and maximum tolerated dose (68,69). Results from 15 high-stage breast and other cancer patients have demonstrated thus far that doses up to 20,000 U are not toxic and can deplete serum methionine to levels shown to be therapeutic preclinically. However, it is likely that the bacterium-sourced enzyme will be antigenic.

Tan et al. (70) have thus also demonstrated that PEGylation of rMETase with PEG 5000 strands allows for retention of 70% of the enzyme activity while doubling the plasma half-life and quadrupling the time period in which methionine levels could be reduced in rats. Prolonged survival in tumor-bearing animals has also been shown. The utility of PEGylated rMETase in human clinical study warrants further investigation (71–74).

10. PEG ARGINASE AND PEG ARGININE DEIMINASE

Malignant melanoma and hepatoma kill approx 16,000 Americans each year. It has been suggested that arginine may be an "essential" amino acid for the growth and metastasis of malignant melanoma and certain hepatomas (75).

Arginase from a variety of sources has been identified and purified. A PEG with a conjugate of arginase (molecular weight, 5000) was shown to retain 65% of its activity and to possess a half-life prolonged from 1–12 h *(76)*. Some improvement in survival time of mice carrying Taper liver tumors was reported with no benefit seen for the non-PEGylated enzyme *(77)*.

Arginine deiminase (ADI: arginine dihydrolase, arginine desiminase, or guanidin-odesiminase) is an enzyme that hydrolyzes the guanidino group of L-arginine to release L-citrulline and ammonia. ADI has been obtained from mycoplasma, pseudomonas, and streptococcus. Each host strain produces a different structural form of the protein including variations in the active site.

Clark *(78,79)* and others have explored the utility of various PEGylated forms of ADI for the treatment of cancer. Phoenix Pharmaceuticals Inc., Kentucky developed a PEGylated ADI that recently was granted Orphan Drug Status by the FDA. Experiments in animals have shown that PEGylated ADI is likely to be useful in the treatment of human disease *(78,79)*.

Other PEG ADI conjugates have been suggested *(80)*, for example, ADI isolated from Mycoplasma arginini and conjugated with methoxy-polyethylene glycol 4,6-dichloro-1,3,5-triazine. Filpula and Wang *(81,82)* have suggested that the levels of retained ADI activity provided by this and other approaches have been too low to be useful in human disease, as shown in published growth inhibition studies. It has been postulated that certain lysine attachment points on the enzyme are intimately connected with the enzyme active site and that the protein would benefit from engineering. Therefore, highly modified conjugates that demonstrate higher levels of retained activity are being explored *(81,82)*.

11. PEG IL-2

An alternative approach to chemotherapy for the treatment of cancer has been the use of agents that stimulate the patient's own immune system to reject tumors or pathogens. Interleukin 2 (IL-2) is a lymphokine that stimulates the proliferation of T lymphocytes, stimulates B lymphocytes, and induces production and release of interferon-γ and activation of natural killer cells. Along with other cytokines, IL-2 serves as a regulator of immune function, amplifying a response to an antigen. Recombinant human IL-2 (rIL-2) when expressed in *E. coli* unlike the native protein is not glycosylated, has limited solubility and requires high and long-term dosing for optimal benefit (tumor regression or reconstituted immune function). Aggregation of protein may also occur. Antibodies to rIL-2 have been found in patients undergoing clinical trials or treatment. These antibodies could interfere with the effectiveness of the drug or lead to unwanted side effects.

The current standard of therapy for stage 4 and recurrent kidney cancer is based on IL-2. Kidney cancer patients were among the first to be treated with this form of immunotherapy. IL-2 under the trade name Proleukin® was approved by the FDA for use in patients with kidney cancer in 1992. In 1997, approx 30,600 people in the United States were diagnosed and 12,000 people died with kidney cancer.

The four stages of kidney cancer are:

- **Stage 1:** Cancer is found only in the kidney and is 7 cm or less in size.
- **Stage 2:** Cancer is found only in the kidney and is more than 7 cm in size.

- **Stage 3:** Cancer has spread to the fat around the kidney, or to the renal vein, inferior vena cava, or nearby lymph nodes.
- **Stage 4:** Cancer has spread to other organs including the bowel, pancreas, lungs, or bones.

The treatment for stages 1–3 kidney cancer is usually surgical removal of the kidney, with or without removal of the adjacent tissues and lymph nodes.

PEGylated IL-2 has been manufactured and tested in human clinical trials by the Chiron Corporation (Emeryville, CA). Earlier studies in animals (83,84) and humans (85) showed that PEG conjugation would increase stability, decrease clearance, and increase plasma half-life (>20-fold) of IL-2. Utility as an anticancer agent as well as immune system enhancer for treatment of HIV-AIDS has been explored (86–91).

In one study examining immune system enhancement, all patients demonstrated high levels of lymphokine-activated killer cell activity. Limiting dilution analysis revealed an increase in the frequency of IL-2-responsive cells starting from abnormally low levels and rising to above normal during the course of injections. In a subgroup of four patients with greater or equal to 400 CD4[+] T cells/μL at entry, there was a trend to sustained increases in CD4[+] T-cell numbers. However, this increase did not reach statistical significance. This subset of patients also exhibited higher proliferation responses to phytohemagglutinin as mitogen. Several of these effects persisted for 3–6 mo after cessation of therapy.

Goodson and Katre (92) have used a PEG maleimmide reagent to selectively PEGylate IL-2 at the glycosylation site found in the recombinant protein as expressed in an E.coli system. Full biological activity was maintained and a four-fold increase in circulating half-life was observed. In studies examining the correlation between PEGylated IL-2 administration and levels of predictive lymphokines in cancer therapy, responding patients did not show a consistent pattern (93).

12. PEG GMCSF AND PEG GCSF

Most anticancer agents that are cytotoxic and directed toward the cellular DNA of rapidly dividing cells have dose-limiting toxicities linked to destruction of the bone marrow and the ability to produce blood cells and platelets. One approach to overcome these "cytopenias" is to utilize agents that promote recovery of bone marrow function so as to restore blood cell and platelet levels but also to allow for a higher dosing of cytotoxic chemotherapeutic such that resistant tumors might be eradicated.

Growth and maturation of blood cells and platelets is under the control of a "cascade of cytokines." Both granulocyte-stimulating and granulocyte/macrophage-stimulating factors are important regulators of quantity and quality of white blood cell function.

Recombinant human granulocyte colony-stimulating factor has been prepared in *E. coli* (rhG-CSF) as a 156 amino acid protein (94). Recombinant human granulocyte/ macrophage colony-stimulating factor (rhGM-CSF) has been prepared in yeast as a 127 amino acid protein. Both proteins have a plasma half-life of approx 2–4 h and require frequent injections to achieve desired neutrophil levels in patients receiving chemotherapy.

Both molecules have been prepared in PEGylated form and studied in preclinical models (95–97). Tanaka et al. (95) reported that conjugation of rhG-CSF with PEG increased the plasma half-life from 1.8 h to 7 h in mice and increased observed neu-

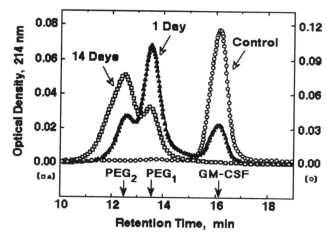

Fig. 3. Using PEG activation chemistries and reaction conditions designed to limit the degree of PEGylation the authors demonstrated (Fig. 3) that over a period of several days PEG GMCSF (murine) could be made with the desired properties.

trophil counts. Similar results (98) were obtained in neutropenic mice that had been treated with the anticancer agents, cyclophosphamide and 5-FU.

Satake-Ishikawa et al. (99) reported that G-CSF coupled to two or three strands of 10,000 molecular weight PEG, was more potent and longer acting in vivo than when coupled to five strands of 5000 molecular weight PEG.

The question of relationship between molecular weight and number of attachment sites, and potency and circulating life, has led to a number of studies examining PEG molecular weights of 20,000 and 40,000, linkage chemistry on preservation of activity, potency, and performance in animal models.

Thus, Malik et al. have prepared GMCSF (96,97) with a single linear strand with molecular weights of approx 20,000 or 40,000. From a circulating lifetime perspective, the authors predicted that this construct could be expected to have similar molecular radii and, hence, similar rates of renal clearance to conjugates containing an average of four or eight strands of PEG with a molecular weight of 5000.

Using PEG activation chemistries and reaction conditions designed to limit the degree of PEGylation the authors demonstrated (Fig. 3) that over a period of several days PEG GMCSF (murine) could be made with the desired properties. Analysis of PEG fractions was by size exclusion HPLC.

Injection of mice with a chromatographic pool containing PEG GMCSF with one or two strands of approx 40,000 molecular weight per molecule of GMCSF resulted in dose-dependent increases in numbers of eosinophils, neutrophils, and monocytes in peripheral blood (Fig. 4). Mice received two injections per day of the indicated doses for 6 d, and their blood was sampled on day 7. Increases in counts of each cell type were calculated relative to counts in mice injected with 100 ng GMCSF. Native GMCSF given at the same doses had negligible effects.

From the standpoints of both regulatory acceptability and cost-effectiveness, mono- or di-PEGylated conjugates may offer substantial advantages over the usual mixtures of a less homogenous PEGylated species with a larger range of lower molecular weight strands. Further, the attachment of fewer higher molecular weight strands may allow for greater retention of potency while preserving the increased circulating life benefit of "multiple" PEG attachments (100,101).

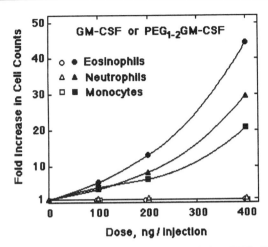

Fig. 4. Injection of mice with a chromatographic pool containing PEG GMCSF with one or two strands of approx 40,000 molecular weight per molecule of GMCSF resulted in dose-dependent increases in numbers of eosinophils, neutrophils, and monocytes in peripheral blood.

13. PEG HEMOGLOBIN

With periodic or seasonal shortages of blood cells and platelets for transfusion as well as with the discovery that virus, prions, and other infectious agents can be transmitted by transfusion, emphasis has been placed on the search for a blood substitute. Of the different blood cellular components that which lends itself toward substitution is the red blood cell. The red blood cell functions to deliver oxygen from the lungs to the tissues and return carbon dioxide from the tissues to the lung.

Oxygen-carrying perflourocarbon emulsions as well as various purified hemoglobin preparations are being explored in human clinical studies *(102,103)*. Aside from the potential use of hemoglobin as a "red blood cell substitute" the potential exists for the use of hemoglobin-based oxygen carriers for the treatment of cancer.

A characteristic of many human tumors is that as they grow various regions may become hypoxic because of an inability for mature vascularization to develop despite the release of angiogenic factors. Typically, a gradient of oxygenation is present, but with less oxygen available with increasing distance from the nearest blood vessel. The result is a metabolic gradient of activity within the tumor *(104)*.

Of the patients being treated for cancer, it has been estimated that at least 60% will receive radiation therapy sometime during the course of their disease. Since the 1950s, however, it has been known that oxygen is required to be present in the irradiated tissue for the radiation energy to generate oxygen-free radicals and destroy tumor cells. Studies in animals and humans have suggested that 10% to more than 50% of cells within a tumor mass may be hypoxic (oxygen pressure < 5–10 mmHg). Tumor hypoxia has been found to limit remission rates and decrease prospects for long-term survival or cure.

Among the more hypoxic tumors are breast, lung, colorectal, prostate, head-and-neck, bladder, brain, cervical, and fibrous histiocytoma *(105–109)*.

Several approaches to tumor sensitization to radiation have been proposed and explored using agents that produce free radicals in response to radiation or inhibit DNA repair after damage by ionizing radiation, but a comparatively simple possibility may be the raising of the degree of tumor oxygenation. Attempts to achieve this through the use of hyperbaric oxygen chambers, allosteric regulators of hemoglobin oxygen affinity *(110,111)*, and oxygen-delivering solutions have been reported and continue to be explored in clinical trials.

Use of hemoglobin-based solutions has also been explored. However, mammalian hemoglobins are multimeric and can readily dissociate from tetramers to dimers. Further, both dimers and tetramers can extravasate through the blood vessels into the "third space" and scavenge nitric oxide along the way.

The limited ability to be retained within the blood stream and the ability to scavenge nitric oxide of hemoglobin dimers and tetramers has been blamed for a variety of side effects ranging from elevated blood pressure, esophageal or gastric intestinal spasm and upset, to kidney damage. Further, for a red blood cell substitute to be useful, a relatively long circulating life (measured in days) is highly desirable *(102,103)*.

Attempts to crosslink by genetic means and produce "stabilized" or polymerized hemoglobin by recombinant means or to achieve such stabilization by use of chemical crosslinkers and polymerization agents has been reported *(103)*. Several such agents have been developed through the clinical trial regulatory process *(112–117)*.

An alternative to genetic or chemical crosslinking and/or polymerization for limiting the extravasation and side effects inherently associated with hemoglobin is PEGylation. A number of laboratories have pursued this approach and reported significant improvements over unmodified hemoglobin or genetic or chemically crosslinked preparations *(102,103)*. Human, bovine, and other sourced hemoglobins have been examined *(102,103,118)*.

An important consideration in the use of human-derived hemoglobin as a starting point for chemical modification or PEGylation is the removal of infectious disease agents from collected donor blood. Of special concern are strains of human immunodeficiency virus (HIV) and hepatitis (HBC, HCV). In addition to the benefit of protein purification protocols relative to infectious agent removal, specific virus inactivation steps such as sterilization and filtration have been adopted by those seeking to develop human hemoglobin-based products. These steps include rigorous screening of donor blood by a variety of diagnostic assays for infectious agents.

With respect to animal-derived hemoglobin, an important consideration has always been the removal of any adventitious viral or bacterial infectious agents that might transmit disease to humans. Most recent concerns have been prions. These have been identified as the likely causative agent in bovine spongiform encephalitis (BSE or "mad cow disease"). The corresponding disease in man is the rare disorder Creutzfeld Jacob disease (CJD). Recent increases in the number of CJD cases and, in particular, a modified strain of the disease appearing in young people in England and other parts of Europe has been linked to the consumption of beef or beef products obtained from infected cows. Transmittal of the culprit prion from cattle to man has been suggested and is strongly supported by recent experimental evidence. Public fears have emerged as a major barrier to the development of bovine-derived products *(119)*.

The risk of passage of infectious disease agents into final products derived from animal sources can be greatly diminished not only by the use of protein purification, sterilization, and filtration technology but also by limiting the collection of raw materials to those animals segregated in controlled herds. Such herds are maintained to be self propagating. Many consider this approach an essential component of any animal-derived product development plan. A process for purification of bovine hemoglobin from collected red blood cells and PEGylation has been described in the literature *(120–122)*.

Studies at Enzon, Inc. (Piscataway, NJ) have focussed in particular on the benefits of PEGylated hemoglobin (bovine-sourced) relative to tumor oxygenation *(104)*.

Researchers at Harvard's Dana-Farber Cancer Institute have examined the ability of PEG hemoglobin to oxygenate models of animal and human tumors in rodents. Oxygenation of hypoxic or near hypoxic tumors was found to increase from 100–300% after intravenous infusion of PEG hemoglobin. A detailed description of study materials, methods and results is given in *(104)*.

An increased response to radiation treatment consistent with increased oxygenation of tumors was also observed. In osteogenic sarcoma rodent models a greater than 80% response rate was seen compared with a 10% response rate seen in animals receiving radiation but no PEG hemoglobin *(123)*. In other studies, PEG hemoglobin was shown to oxygenate tumors to varying degrees dependent on animals breathing room air, or oxygen levels at 28% or 95%. A correlation between tumor oxygenation and increased tumor growth delay in radiation or chemotherapy treatment was shown *(124)*.

PEGylated bovine hemoglobin has been studied recently in a human clinical trial for the oxygenation of tumors as an adjunct to radiation therapy of cancer.

14. PEG URICASE

Increased levels of uric acid in blood (hyperuricemia) or urine (hyperuricosuria) *(125,126)* are associated with a number of diseases and disorders. Primary among these are lymphoid malignancies, severe gout, and certain patients receiving organ transplant. Whereas most hyperuricemia (gout) patients will respond to the drug of choice, allopurinol, a significant number do not. It has been estimated that approx 2% of patients respond poorly to allopurinol treatment *(127)*. It has also been reported that allopurinol may be contraindicated in patients undergoing therapy for leukemia or lymphoma or for organ graft rejection *(125,126,128)*. As a result, these patients may suffer from painful and disabling deposits of uric acid in their joints and connective tissues (tophi). Some are at risk for kidney failure.

Although most mammals possess urate oxidase (uricase) and metabolize uric acid to more readily excreted products, humans do not. Rather, humans possess two "nonsense mutations" in the gene for uricase *(129)*. Treatment of patients with injection of nonhuman uricase is complicated by the high risk of serious immune responses *(130)*.

Mountain View Pharmaceuticals, Inc. (Menlo Park, CA) is investigating PEG conjugates of genetically engineered mammalian uricase *(131–133)*. A product for human use (PURICASE) is being codeveloped with Biotechnology General, Inc. (Metro Park, NJ). The advantages of PEG-modified recombinant mammalian uricase over the fungal uricase that is currently used in a few European countries *(130)* are likely to include longer circulating lifetime and reduced immunogenicity.

15. PEG PHOSPHOLIPASE-ACTIVATING PROTEIN

PEGylation of peptides using the relatively non-site-directed chemistries that have been described for proteins can often result in the attachment of PEG strands to sites that are critical for biological activity. The disadvantage of the approach is especially acute with peptides of lower molecular weight where the probability of attachment to a critical site is proportionally increased.

One approach is to seek to attach PEG to either the amino or carboxyl end of the peptide during or postsynthesis *(134)*. The PEGylation of a fibrinectin related tripeptide *(arg-gly-asp)* in the latter manner has been described *(135)*. The tripeptide was coupled to amino PEG by activation of the aspartic acid side chain with dicyclohexylcarbodiimide and hydroxybenzotriazole. In mouse models of cancer reduction in tumor metastases, presumably through interference with cell–cell adhesion, was noted.

Mensi-Fattohi et al. *(136)* describe a process for synthesizing peptides with PEGylation of specifically predetermined sites in the peptide sequence. The authors report the preparation of PEGylated intermediates that can be inserted during peptide chain elongation.

More recently, PEGylated phospholipase activating protein (PLAP) derived peptides have been prepared and evaluated as novel anticancer agents. Phospholipase A_2 activating protein is an endogenous stimulator of phospholipase A_2 *(137,138)*. The enzyme cleaves the sn-2 fatty acid from phospholipids in eukaryotic cells. Frequently in mammalian cells the sn-2 fatty acid is arachidonic acid, which may go on to be oxygenated to form prostaglandins, leukotrienes, and other eicosinoid metabolites. The phospholipase-activating protein gene has been cloned and sequenced from human and animal sources. A peptide sequence responsible for the phospholipase enzyme activation has been identified *(137)*.

Interestingly, PLAP and the stimulatory domain peptide have been shown to activate infiltrating lymphocytes and on injection into rabbit knee joint to induce arthropathies that resemble rheumatoid arthritis *(139,140)*. PLAP and the stimulatory domain peptide have both been shown to increase eicosinoid and inflammatory cytokine production.

The notion that PLAP peptide might stimulate tumor-infiltrating lymphocytes and thus an immune response as an anticancer strategy has been explored *(141)*. In that study, PLAP peptide and a nonphospholipase-stimulating control peptide were each immobilized onto carrier beads and injected separately into rodent air pouches containing syngeneic tumors. Controls received nonactivating peptide; treated animals received activating peptide. Dramatic activation of tumor infiltrating lymphocytes was observed, with marked invasion of tumor tissue by NK cells and tumor shrinkage. Injection of peptide only without carrier bead immobilization showed no effect, suggesting the need for PEGylation to enhance circulating lifetime and systemic delivery.

PEGylated peptide (ESPLIAKVLTTEPPIITPVRRT) was prepared using linear methoxy PEG aldehyde (molecular weight, 5000) obtained from Shearwater Polymers, Inc. (Huntsville, AL). Mice bearing Lewis Lung tumors were evaluated in a study comparing equivalent doses of PEGylated peptide or paclitaxel. These results are summarized in Table 4.

16. PEG MEGAKARYOCYTE FACTOR

Platelets play an essential role in health and thrombosis. They are produced from bone marrow megakaryocytes. If the level of circulating platelets drops below a given threshold, thrombocytopenia occurs and the patient is at risk for hemorrhage.

Many cancer chemotherapeutics attack the bone marrow cells which produce the precursors for the blood cell components, including platelets. Patients who receive chemotherapy for cancer are often pancytopenic. The loss of immune protection and

Table 4
Comparison of PLAP and Paclitaxel Anticancer Activity

Dose mg/kg	PEGlated PLAP time to death (d)	Paclitaxel time to death (d)
none	17	17
0.5	21	
1.0	21	
5.0	23[a]	19
15	24[b]	22[a]
25	26[c]	7[d]

[a] $p < 0.5$
[b] $p < 0.05$
[c] $p < 0.001$ significantly improved survival vs untreated animals
[d] $p < 0.001$ significantly worsened survival vs untreated animals.
Animals were treated with 5000 MW PEG-PLAP peptide following development of an air pouch on the animals's backs that had been implanted with 101 Lewis Lung cancer cells. Survival was monitored. There were 20 animals in each group. Data are presented as the mean survival at each day examined; SD was less than 5%.

the propensity for hemorrhage are major contributors to mortality in the treatment of cancer.

Whereas erythropoietin and the granulocyte stimulatory factors have been developed for the treatment of anemia and leukopenia, little is available to stimulate platelet production or increase platelet count other than transfusion of donor-derived platelets. More than 7 million units of platelet concentrates are transfused annually in the United States.

It has been known for quite some time that a humoral factor present in the plasma of patients with severe thrombocytopenia could increase the platelet count when injected into animals. This factor has been named thrombopoietin or TPO. The isolation of this cytokine, however, proved to be difficult because of its low concentration in plasma and the lack of reliable assays. It was not until 1994 that TPO was cloned. Thrombopoietin moved from the laboratory to the clinic in less than 2 yr since its cloning. Two forms of recombinant TPO have been developed for clinical use. The full-length molecule (Genentech, Inc., San Francisco, CA) is referred to as recombinant human thrombopoietin, and a truncated version of the molecule (Amgen, Thousand Oaks, CA) is referred to as PEGylated recombinant human megakaryocyte growth and development factor or MGDF.

Proposed advantages of PEGylation include the reduction of antibody formation, which may limit the development of antibodies that could interfere with clinical treatments or cause unwanted side effects, and increased circulating life.

Both forms of TPO have been evaluated in human clinical trials. In a sample study, Fanucchi et al. (142) conducted a randomized, double-blind, placebo-controlled dose-escalation study of MGDF in 53 patients with lung cancer who were treated with carboplatin and paclitaxel. The patients were randomly assigned in blocks of four in a 1:3 ratio to receive by sc injection either placebo or MGDF (0.03, 0.1, 0.3, 1.0, 3.0, or 5.0 μg per kilogram of body weight per day). No other marrow-active cytokines were given.

In the 38 patients who received MGDF after chemotherapy, the median nadir platelet count was 188,000 per cubic millimeter (range, 68,000 to 373,000), compared to 111,000 per cubic millimeter (range, 21,000 to 307,000) in 12 patients receiving placebo ($p = 0.013$). The platelet count recovered to baseline levels in 14 d in the treated patients compared to more than 21 d in those receiving placebo ($p < 0.001$). Among all 40 patients treated with MGDF, one patient had deep venous thrombosis and pulmonary embolism, and another had superficial thrombophlebitis.

It was concluded that PEG MGDF has potent stimulatory effects on platelet production in patients with chemotherapy-induced thrombocytopenia.

In general, administration of TPO or MGDF elicits an increase in circulating platelet count by several-fold in patients who have normal hematopoiesis before chemotherapy. The response in platelets is accompanied by a significant increase in bone marrow megakaryocytes, an increase in frequency and the number of bone marrow progenitor cells of multiple cell lineages, and a marked mobilization of progenitor cells into the peripheral blood. The results of early trials suggest that TPO or MGDF attenuates thrombocytopenia and enhances platelet recovery after chemotherapy.

However, in 1998, Amgen announced that it was ceasing clinical development of PEG MGDF because of a follow-up onset of thrombocytopenia and the appearance of neutralizing antibodies in patients. Piacibello et al. *(143)* demonstrated that TPO may stimulate growth of human leukemic blasts and human leukemic progenitors. Concerns about widespread clinical use of TPO or PEG MDFK in the proposed treatment of thrombocytopenias of leukemic and preleukemic disorders have been raised.

17. PEG CONCANAVALIN A

Phytohemagglutinins, phytagglutinins, and lectins are proteins that are found in many mono- and dicotyledon plants, molds, and lichens. Lectins bind carbohydrates in a very specific manner. Lectins bind with free sugar or with sugar residues of polysaccharides, glycoproteins, or glycolipids in solution or bound to cell membranes.

The function of lectins in plants is the subject of considerable investigation. Lectins may be involved cell–cell recognition and regulation of physiological functions. Lectins may be multimeric with subunits with different binding sites. Specificity of binding sites implies the presence of endogenous saccharide receptors on other cells or glycoconjugates or in the tissues from which they are derived.

The biological activity of many lectins is dependant on the availability of metal ions. Lectins are well characterized as toxic molecules in animal models. The use of ribosome-inhibiting proteins such as ricin as fusion products or conjugates to antibodies directed against tumor selected antigens has been suggested. Understanding the binding specificity of lectins has been of great importance in elucidating the nature of mammalian glycoproteins as well as in their purification and in exploring the relationship between structure and function.

Glycoproteins or carbohydrate residues present on the surface of tumor cells have been suggested as targets for therapeutic purposes using lectins or antibodies. It has been found that treatment with antilectin antibodies can suppress growth of tumor cells in agarose and inhibit lung colonization in vivo. Lectins also have the potential use in cancer treatment strategies where lectins promote internalization by endocytosis.

Wheat germ lectin has been found to induce lectin-dependent macrophage-mediated cytotoxicity against human bladder cancer cells. Studies have also revealed that human alveolar macrophage tumoricidal activity can be induced by wheat germ lectin *(144–156)*.

Concanavalin is a protein with a molecular weight of 104,000 that at pH 4.5–5.6 exists as a single dimer. At pH > 7.0 it is predominantly tetrameric. Concanavalin A binds two transition metal ions per monomer. Both ions must be present for binding to nonreducing alpha-D-glucose and alpha-D-mannose residues.

Concanavalin A agglutinates red blood cells and forms complexes with blood group substances, immunoglobulin glycopeptides, and carcino-embryonic antigens. Concanavalin A exhibits mitogenic activity with lymphocytes. Cancer cells are readily aggregated by concanavalin A; normal cells are not.

For use of concanavalin A (or other lectins) as a therapeutic directly or via conjugation or fusion to other proteins and ligands, their plant origin should be considered as this raises the potential for immune or allergic reactions in humans.

Ueno et al. *(157)* have proposed the use of concanavalin A as an agent for the stimulation of antitumor cytotoxicity by lymphocytes. They prepared PEGylated concanavalin A (Con A) using 2,4-*bis*[*O*-methoxypoly(ethyleneglycol)]-6-chloro-s-triazine-activated PEG. The immunoreactivity of anti-Con A antibodies toward PEG-Con A was found to be dependant on the degree of PEGylation of amino groups. Circulating life in mice was also shown to be increased. Although the mitogenic activity of PEG Con A toward murine spleen cells was reduced by the conjugation, administration of PEG-Con A to mice enhanced the antitumor cytotoxicity of peripheral lymphocytes against melanoma B 16 cells.

18. PEG ANTIBODIES AND IMMUNOTOXINS

The discovery that antibodies could recognize antigens with a great deal of specificity contributed to the hope for "magic bullets" that could be used for the treatment of cancer. This hope was predicated on the identification of antigens that would be unique or at least highly selective for tumors and either of themselves therapeutic or able by some strategy to "bring" along a cytotoxic or other therapeutic agent or event. A major consideration for antibody-based therapy is whether or not binding is limited to the target cell surface or if postbinding internalization occurs.

To bring immunotherapy to human clinical trials has required the discovery of solutions to such problems as antigen identification, antibody production, chemical and genetic fusion approaches, and optimization of routes of delivery and dosing schedules. To date, substantial progress has been made and more than 200 antibody-based or combination agent human clinical trials are listed by the NIH (for latest update, see http://www.clinicaltrials.gov).

Advances in antigen identification and the ability to produce monoclonal antibodies as well as their fragments have enabled a variety of new approaches *(158–160)*.

Relative to the need for PEGylation, an important observation has been that antibodies produced by murine cells or in nonhuman species or cells, are themselves likely to promote an immune or allergic response. HAMAs (human antimouse antibodies) have been of particular concern, thus, considerable time and expense have been used to prepare the most promising antibodies in a humanized form.

For chimeric or mutein constructs as well as the use of antibody fragments the benefit of PEGylation relative to prolongation of circulating life has also been an attractive approach. For example, Kitamura et al. *(161)* have studied the PEGylation of the murine monoclonal antibody A7. This antibody has been suggested to be selective for colon and pancreatic tumors *(162,163)*. PEGylation of F(ab')2 fragments using activated linear strands of PEG of 5000 molecular weight has demonstrated longer circulating half-life and higher tumor accumulation when compared with non-conjugated

F(ab')2. However, the tumor:blood ratio of the free F(ab')2 fraction was higher than that for the conjugate.

Takashina et al. *(164)* compared conjugation of the A7 antibody or its fragments to linear strands of PEG (molecular weight, 5000) and dextran (molecular weight, 70,000). In vitro characterization showed retention of antigen binding activity. On iv administration the PEGylated antibody had twice the half-life of the nonconjugated antibody. Dextran conjugates showed a higher clearance rate and shorter half-life, when compared with nonconjugated and PEGylated antibody.

Eno-Amooquaye et al. *(165)* have also studied the benefits of PEGylation of antibody enzyme conjugates and report benefits to circulating lifetime as well as altered biodistribution. IgG, F(ab')2, and Fab' fragments of the anti-CEA antibody A5B7 have been PEGylated with activated linear strands of PEG with molecular weight of 5000, labeled with ^{125}I; the pharmacokinetics were compared with the unmodified forms in the LS174T colonic xenograft model in nude mice *(166)*. In this study, PEGylation of the intact antibody had little effect on biodistribution other than slight reduction of tumor accumulation.

In contrast, PEGylation of F(ab')2 and Fab'A5B7 significantly prolonged plasma half-life and increased labeled antibody accumulation in the tumor and to a lesser extent in normal tissues. Some reduction in tissue to blood ratios was also observed. Prior to PEGylation, Fab' A5B7 cleared more rapidly from the circulation than did F(ab')2. After PEGylation, their biodistribution and circulating lifetimes were more similar, whereas the tumor to blood ratios were reduced and resembled that of the intact antibody. The authors suggest that enhanced tumor accumulation, reduced normal tissue to blood ratios, and potentially reduced immunogenicity of fragments after PEGylation warrants further investigation.

As PEG modification of substances with anti-tumor activity was shown to enhance penetration into growing solid tumors and extend antitumor effects *(123)*, Hurvitz et al. *(167)* introduced as modifier two types of monoclonal antibodies (N12 and L26) specific to the ErbB2 (HER2) oncoprotein. These antibodies suppress the growth of tumors overexpressing *Erb*B2 (e.g., N87 human tumor) and the effect of PEG on their antitumor activity was evaluated. Methoxy-PEG-maleimmide conjugated to sulfhydryl groups at the hinge region of the antibodies, impaired their antibody binding to N87 tumor cells, and did not enhance the antitumor inhibitory activity in tumor-bearing mice.

A branched *N*-hydroxysuccinimide-activated PEG (PEG2), conjugated through amino groups of the protein, was used for binding to the whole antibody (Ab) or to its monomeric Fab' fragment. When tested against N87 cells in vitro, the binding activity and antitumor cytotoxic effects of Ab-PEG2 were mostly preserved. PEG2 modification did not seem to alter the tumor-inhibitory activity of the antibodies in vivo, and the same pattern of tumor development was observed during the first few weeks following administration. However, the stimulating effects of PEG were observed at later stages of tumor growth since tumor development was either slowed down or completely arrested. Furthermore, a second tumor implanted into these mice during the later stage was significantly or completely inhibited, contrasting with the results in mice injected with the unmodified antibody. The Fab'-PEG2 monomeric derivative was also shown to be effective in inhibiting the growth of a second tumor. The extended and prolonged enhancing effect of PEG on the antitumor activity of antibodies or Fab' fragments directed against *Erb*B2 may be of importance in the treatment of *Erb*B2-overexpressing neoplasms.

Mouse A33 antibody has been shown to target metastatic colon cancer and to be of some antitumor benefit (168,169). However, because of the development of human anti-mouse reactivity, only a single treatment was possible. A humanized version of mAb A33 (huA33) has been prepared and evaluated in patients who were treated in cycles of four weekly escalating iv doses. Significant toxicity was observed at the highest dose tested. However, partial responses were observed, although in some patients continued treatment in the presence of the humanized antibody resulted in the development of systemic reactions.

PEGylation of huA33 with linear methoxy-PEG (molecular weight, 5000 or 20,000) has been investigated. For the 5000 molecular weight PEG (32%–34% of primary amines conjugated) or the molecular weight 20,000 PEG (16%–18% conjugated) more than 50% of binding to SW1222 colon cancer cells could be preserved relative to non-conjugated antibody. In mice, after repeated immunization with PEGylated antibody, antiantibody titers occurred in less than 5% compared with titers of the non-PEGylated controls. Microdistribution of antibody uptake in xenograft models suggested that the PEGylated preparations reached the same peak staining intensity as native huA33, although more slowly. The authors suggest that PEGylation levels sufficient to suppress immunogenicity may be achieved (170).

With the availability of tumor-selective antibodies as well as the discovery of receptors and ligands that may be selective for tumors, the notion of the use of toxins as anti-cancer agents coupled to these targeting moieties has received considerable attention. Like antibodies themselves, issues that have emerged for the toxins as well as chimera include potential immune or allergic reactions to repeat administrations, short circulating lifetimes, and systemic effects.

Pseudomonas exotoxin A (PE) is composed of three structural and functional domains. Domain Ia is responsible for cell recognition, domain II for translocation of PE across the cell membrane, and domain III for ADP-ribosylation of elongation factor 2, thereby being toxic to cells. Pastan et al. (171) have investigated the role of the amino acids exposed on the surface of domain III and have determined conditions for PEGylation such that cytotoxic activity might be maintained but circulating lifetime increased and potential immune or allergic reactions blunted. The authors demonstrated that PEGs modified by a single linear PEG strand (molecular weight, 5000) via a disulfide or a thioether bond retained high levels of cytotoxic activity, but when a single linear strand (molecular weight, 20,000) was used activity was reduced.

Chimeric proteins or muteins have been explored to target *Pseudomonas exotoxin* to tumors. As aforementioned in such constructs the targeting moiety may be an antibody (or fragment) or receptor ligand directed to an antigen or receptor selective for tumors. Wang et al. (172) have constructed a chimera suitable for PEGylation, i.e., an engineered mutein composed of human transforming growth factor alpha (TGFα) fused to a fragment of Pseudomonas exotoxin (PE38) devoid of its cell-binding domain. The new protein, termed TGFα R29-L2-CH2-PE38QQ δ (TCP), has no lysine residues in the TGF α and PE38 portions. Human IgG4 constant region CH2 and a tetradecapeptide linker, L2, were inserted between TGF alpha and PE38. Together, L2 and CH2 contain 13 lysine residues that serve as potential PEGylation sites.

PEG conjugates of TCP (PEG-TCP) have been prepared and reaction products have been separated by ion exchange chromatography. Two PEG-TCP species termed B4 and B6 retained 15% and 4% of cytotoxicity, respectively, and 26% of their receptor binding activity when compared with unmodified TCP. Both B4 and B6 had prolonged circulation times in the blood and reduced toxicity in animals. The mean residence times of B4 and B6 were 37 and 68 min, respectively, compared to 7 min for TCP. When administered intraveneously to tumor-bearing mice, both B4 and B6 produced marked antitumor effects, whereas the unmodified TCP had none. The authors suggest that the prolonged circulating time and reduced toxicity of PEG-TCP compensate for a diminished cytotoxic activity and significantly enlarge the therapeutic window of this and other chimeric toxin or immunotoxin constructs. More recently, an SS1(dsFv)-PE38 immunotoxin construct has been studied in human clinical trials. SS1(dsFv) recognizes the antigen mesothelin, which is normally associated with cells lining cavities in the body but is also found associated with certain head-and-neck, lung, cervix, and ovarian cancers *(173–176)*.

Another recent preparation, PEGylated recombinant anti-Tac(Fv)-PE38 (LMB-2) is a recombinant immunotoxin composed of a single-chain Fv fragment of the antihuman Tac monoclonal antibody to the IL-2 receptor α-subunit fused to a 38-kDa fragment of *Pseudomonas exotoxin (177,178)*. For site-specific PEGylation with linear methoxy PEG (molecular weights of 5000 or 20,000), one cysteine residue was introduced into the peptide linker between the Fv and the toxin *(177)*. When compared with the non-PEGylated LMB-2, both PEGylated immunotoxins showed similar cytotoxic activities in vitro but a five- to eight-fold increase in plasma half-life in mice, and a three- to four-fold increase in anti-tumor activity. This was accompanied by a substantial decrease in animal toxicity and immunogenicity.

19. PEG PACLITAXEL

The biodistribution of anticancer agents has been shown to be altered by conjugation to polymers or by inclusion into various liposomal formulations *(123,179–185)*. In part, the change is a result of the hyperpermeability of tumors and the absence of a mature lymphatic drainage system *(186–188)*. This anatomic feature allows for the passive accumulation in tumors of various drug substances dependent on molecular weight, charge, and Stokes radius of any conjugates or liposomes. Murakami et al. *(184)* have characterized the relationship of PEG molecular weight (linear strands) and accumulation in rodent tumor models. As might be expected, the higher the molecular weight, the greater the degree of tumor accumulation.

Paclitaxel is an anticancer agent originally isolated from the bark of the Pacific yew tree *(Taxus brevifolia)*. It has been approved by the FDA to treat breast, ovarian, and lung cancers, as well as AIDS-related Kaposi's sarcoma. Numerous clinical trials are examining the use of paclitaxel alone or in combination with other therapies for the treatment of additional cancers (for latest updates, *see* http://www.clinicaltrials.gov).

Rather than function by intercalation or cutting of DNA as do many chemotherapeutic agents, paclitaxel affects microtubules. In normal cell growth microtubules are formed as cells begin dividing. When division stops microtubules are broken down or destroyed. Paclitaxel blocks microtubule breakdown, preventing further cell division. Like many anticancer agents, paclitaxel and related taxoids are poorly soluble in water.

Although paclitaxel was first evaluated in 1984, it was not until 1992 that the FDA approved the use of paclitaxel for refractory ovarian cancer. In 1994, the FDA approved paclitaxel for treating breast cancers that recur within 6 mo after adjuvant chemotherapy, as well as breast cancers that had not responded to combination chemotherapy. In 1997, paclitaxel was also approved by the FDA as a treatment for the AIDS-related cancer called Kaposi's sarcoma. In 1998, it was approved for first-line therapy for the treatment of ovarian cancer in combination with cisplatin and, in combination with other anticancer drugs, for the treatment of certain forms of advanced lung cancer.

Although operating through a different mechanism than many chemotherapeutics, the side effects associated with paclitaxel use are predominately the same, i.e., temporary damage to the bone marrow. In addition to altering biodistribution and promoting tumor accumulation, chemical conjugation of polymers to anticancer agents has been suggested to reduce side effects *(123)*. It is reasonable, then, to pursue polymeric conjugated forms of paclitaxel in an attempt to reduce dose-limiting side effects, and to use water-soluble polymers to help resolve solubility and formulation issues for this exciting drug.

Li et al. *(189)* have reported the conjugation of a linear strand of PEG with a molecular weight of 5000 to the 2' position of paclitaxel through a spacer succinyl group. The resultant PEGylated paclitaxel prodrug was highly water soluble (> 20 mg equiv. paclitaxel/mL). The rate of release of PEG from the paclitaxel conjugate was pH dependent with a half-life release rate of 7.6, 54, and 311 min at pH levels of 9.0, 7.4, and 6.0, respectively. The ability to inhibit growth of B16 melanoma cells in culture was similar for both the PEG conjugate and nonconjugated paclitaxel. In MCA-4 mammary tumor-bearing mice, a single dose of PEG-paclitaxel (40 mg equiv. paclitaxel/kg body weight) significantly delayed tumor growth.

Enzon, Inc. (Piscataway, NJ) has reported the preparation of water-soluble 2' taxol PEG esters as prodrugs *(190)*. The concept of a prodrug that would be activated by a tumor-selective mechanism or be released as conjugates that accumulate in tumors is an attractive approach to discovering safer and more effective anticancer compounds *(123,191,192)*. To optimize circulating lifetime with the rate of ester release, a 40,000 molecular weight linear PEG strand was used. Evaluation in rodent tumor models has suggested the PEG paclitaxel analogues are active against ovarian, colon, and lung tumors and possibly with less toxicity than with a non-PEGylated drug. This company has filed an IND with plans to pursue clinical development of PEGylated paclitaxel (December 2000). In addition to PEGylation, conjugation of paclitaxel to other polymers such as polyglutamic acid or its inclusion in a variety of foams, particles, and films has also been reported.

PG-TXL, a polyglutamate paclitaxel conjugate in preclinical animal studies, demonstrated fewer side effects and significantly improved tumor killing activity when compared with nonconjugated paclitaxel alone, including disappearance of tumors in established animal breast cancer models in which similar doses of paclitaxel merely slowed tumor growth. Paclitaxel is linked to the carboxylic residues of the polyglutamate backbone through an ester bond (about 10% of the carboxylic groups are conjugated). The highly charged glutamates help to make the complex highly water soluble. A total weight of 50,000 is believed to be optimal for tumor accumulation. PG-TXL remains inactive until paclitaxel is released within the tumor tissue by enzymatic action. Kinetic studies show that six times more PG-paclitaxel gets into tumors when compared with the nonconjugated drug *(193)*. Studies done on Lewis lung and melanoma models extended these results to a range of tumors *(194)*.

Cell Therapeutics, Inc. (Seattle, WA) in collaboration with The Cancer Research Campaign (CRC) sponsored a UK Phase I clinical trial of PG-TXL, and Phase II trials have been scheduled in the United States.

In addition to its use as an anticancer agent, paclitaxel has also found uses in the treatment of other diseases and conditions. The use of PEGylated or other polymeric conjugated forms of paclitaxel may warrant investigation here as well. In 1998, Angiotech Pharmaceuticals, Inc. (Vancouver, BC) announced encouraging preliminary results from the treatment extension phase of its Phase I/II clinical study of paclitaxel for the treatment of secondary progressive multiple sclerosis.

20. PEG DAUNORUBICIN/DOXORUBICIN

The anthracycline antibiotics doxorubicin and daunorubicin are among the most frequently prescribed anticancer agents. Their use is often as part of a cocktail of other agents. Doxorubicin hydrochloride is available for recommended use with leukopenia, thrombocytopenia, and anemia in a single, rapid iv infusion repeated after 21 d. Doxorubicin can extravasate causing local tissue necrosis. Doxorubicin is effective in acute leukemias, malignant lymphomas, breast cancer and—when combined with cyclophosphamide, vincristine, procarbazine, and other agents—in Hodgkin's disease and non-Hodgkin's lymphomas. Together with cyclophosphamide and cisplatin, it has been used for treatment of ovarian carcinoma; it has routinely been used for chemotherapy of small cell carcinoma of the lung, sarcomas, metastatic thyroid carcinoma, carcinomas of the endometrium, testes, prostate, cervix, head-and-neck, and for plasma cell myeloma.

As with most anticancer agents, myelosuppression is a major dose-limiting complication. Cardiomyopathy is an additional and unique complicating side effect of the anthracycline antibiotics. Cumulative dose-related toxicity may be manifested by congestive heart failure that is unresponsive to digitalis. Daunorubicin hydrochloride is also available for intravenous use. Daunorubicin is useful in the treatment of acute lymphocytic and acute granulocytic leukemias. Its activity against solid tumors in adults however appears to be minimal. Polymer conjugation with tumor accumulation benefits and alteration of biodistribution may enhance the safety and efficacy of the anthracycline antibiotics.

Greenwald et al. (195,196) have developed methods for the PEGylation of prodrugs containing amino groups based on the trimethyl block reaction. PEG-daunorubicin prodrugs, with a half-life of 2 h, were evaluated in an in vivo solid tumor model and found to be more efficacious against ovarian tumors than nonconjugated drug.

Rodrigues et al. (197) have prepared doxorubicin maleimmide derivatives containing an amide or acid-sensitive hydrazone linker coupled to alpha-methoxy-poly(ethylene glycol)-thiopropionic acid amide (molecular weight, 20,000), α, Ω-bis-thiopropionic acid amide poly(ethylene glycol) (molecular weight, 20,000) or α-tert-butoxy-poly(ethylene glycol)-thiopropionic acid amide (molecular weight, 70,000). Like many of the polymer conjugates, the previously described drug derivatives were designed to release doxorubicin within tumors. In this case, the PEG linkage cleaved by acid-catalysis of the hydrazone bond after uptake by endocytosis. PEG carboxylic hydrazone bonds exhibited in vitro activity against human BXF T24 bladder carcinoma and LXFL 529L lung cancer cells, resulting in IC70 values in the range of 0.02–1.5 μM. PEG amide doxorubicin conjugates showed no activity in vitro.

The use of PEGylated anticancer agents in combination with PEGylated antibody enzyme conjugates for activation of prodrug posttumor accumulation has attracted attention *(198–200)*. Cheng et al. *(198)* have modified *E. coli* β glucuronidase to improve stability and pharmacokinetics of antibody conjugates for activation of glucuronide prodrugs in tumor cells. Antibodies binding PEG have also been prepared to accelerate clearance of PEG-modified proteins using an IgM *(199,200)* and improving tumor blood ratios of activating enzyme.

To complement a prodrug-enzyme activation approach, 7-aminocephalosporin doxorubicin (AC-Dox) has also been prepared *(201)* by condensation with monomethoxy-poly(ethylene glycol)-propionic acid *N*-hydroxysuccinimide ester (5000 molecular weight PEG) or with a branched form of poly(ethylene glycol, 10,000 molecular weight)-propionic acid *N*-hydroxysuccinimide ester to form M-PEG-AC-Dox or B-PEG-AC-Dox, respectively. As part of a prodrug release strategy, PEG conjugates were designed so that doxorubicin would be released upon Enterobacter cloacae β-lactamase (bL)-catalyzed hydrolysis. Both M-PEG-AC-Dox and B-PEG-AC-Dox were found to be less toxic to human lung adenocarcinoma cells than native doxorubicin. In addition, the polymers were relatively stable in mouse plasma (< 26% hydrolysis after 24 h at 37°C) and were less toxic to mice (maximum tolerated dose > 52 μmol/kg) than doxorubicin (maximum tolerated dose = 13.8 μmol/kg). Pharmacokinetic studies were performed in mice bearing subcutaneous 3677 melanoma tumors. B-PEG-AC-Dox cleared from the blood more slowly than M-PEG-AC-Dox and was retained to a 2.1-fold greater extent in human 3677 melanoma tumor xenografts over a 4-h period. The intratumoral concentrations of both polymers far exceeded that of doxorubicin. As shown for other polymer conjugates, accumulation in tumors is achievable, and PEG-AC-Dox polymers offer the possibility of generating large intratumoral doxorubicin concentrations, reduced toxicities, and doxorubicin release upon β-lactam ring hydrolysis for localized tumor killing.

Like many anticancer agents, anthracycline antibiotics are subject to resistance via the P-glycoprotein multidrug resistance pathway. Stastny et al. *(202)* have examined *N*-(2-hydroxypropyl)methacrylamide (HPMA)-conjugated doxorubicin in models of drug resistance. In addition to HPMA polymers, various antibody conjugation strategies were used to promote active as well as passive targeting in vivo. Testing against mouse and human multiple drug resistant-cell lines (P388-MDR, CEM/VLB) suggested partially decreased resistance. HPMA-conjugated doxorubicin were studied in UK Phase II clinical trials and galactosamine-targeted HPMA-bound doxorubicin were studied in UK Phase I clinical trials. It is possible that PEGylation may also offer benefits to overcoming drug resistance.

Many anticancer drugs are hydrophobic and, depending on the nature of PEGylation or other polymer attachment chemistries and conditions, the formation of micelles could be favored. Such polymeric micelles may have desirable properties as drug carriers. Polymeric micelles based on AB block copolymers of polyethylene oxide (PEO) and poly(aspartic acid) [p*(Asp)*] with covalently bound adriamycin (ADR) have been prepared in radiolabeled form *(203,204)*. Long circulation times in blood for some compositions of PEO-p[*Asp*(ADR)] conjugates were evident in mice, a result the authors propose as atypical of colloidal drug carriers. This was attributed to the low interaction of the PEO corona region of the micelles with biocomponents (e.g., proteins, cells). The authors also report that biodistribution of the PEO-p[*Asp*(ADR)] conjugates is dependent on micelle stability, i.e., stable micelles maintain circulation in blood, whereas unstable micelles readily form free polymer chains which rapidly undergo renal excretion. Long circulation times in blood of PEO-p[*Asp*(ADR)] conjugates are thought to be the prerequisite for enhanced uptake at target sites (e.g., tumors).

21. PEG LIGNAN PODOPHYLLOTOXIN

Podophyllum species produce lignans that are among the natural plant products useful for the treatment of cancer. Although podophyllotoxin itself is cytotoxic and cannot be used directly, its modified forms, etoposide and teniposide, serve as effective treatments for various cancers and lymphomas *(205)*. A summary of the rationale and the evidence supporting lignan use in the treatment of cancer can be found in *(205–211)*.

As with the other anticancer agents already proposed and aforementioned, lignans may benefit from polymer conjugation strategies like PEGylation. Greenwald et al. *(212)* have prepared a series of PEG acyl derivatives of podophyllotoxin. Improved activity in a murine leukemia model over non-modified podophyllotoxin was observed. In a solid lung tumor (A549) model, some conjugated analogs were equivalent to a podophyllotoxin/intralipid emulsion, whereas others were more toxic. The authors suggest that evaluation of PEG lignan in leukemic models is warranted.

22. PEG 5-FU

5-Fluorouracil is a member of a class of agents that have in common the capacity to inhibit the biosynthesis of pyrimidine nucleotides or to mimic these natural metabolites to a point of interference in synthesis or function. Analogs of deoxycytidine and thymidine have been synthesized as inhibitors of DNA synthesis, and an analog of uracil, 5-FU, effectively inhibits both RNA function and/or processing and synthesis of thymidylate. 5-FU requires enzymatic ribosylation and phosphorylation to activate its cytotoxic activity.

5-FU has been used to treat metastatic carcinomas of the breast and the GI tract, hepatoma, carcinomas of the ovary, cervix, urinary bladder, prostate, pancreas, and oropharyngeal areas, as well as colorectal cancers. Improved response rates are seen when 5-FU is used in combination with other agents, such as cyclophosphamide and methotrexate (breast cancer), cisplatin (ovary and head-and-neck cancer), and leucovorin (colorectal cancer). As with most anticancer agents, a dose-limiting side effect is myelosuppression. Mucosal ulcerations throughout the GI tract that may lead to fulminant diarrhea, shock, and death have also been reported.

Ouchi et al. *(213)* have explored the preparation of a prodrug form of PEGylated 5-FU in an attempt to limit side effects while maintaining anticancer activity. PEGylation used a urethane or urea bond. Survival benefit was tested against p388 lymphocytic leukemia in female CDF1 mice by intraperitoneal injection. The release rate of 5-FU from the 5-FU-terminated PEG conjugates via urethane or urea bond was quick but dependent on PEG chain length and the addition or not of any hydrophobic spacer groups. PEGylated 5-FU analogs were shown to be effective anticancer agents in this model, with signs of acute toxicity seen at the highest doses tested.

23. PEG PHOTODYNAMIC THERAPY

Photodynamic therapy (PDT) is based upon the use of light of selected wavelength for the activation of specific compounds in the production of cytotoxic agents. Treatment starts with the iv injection of a photosensitizer; this subsequently binds to circulating low-density lipoproteins that are taken up into tumor cells to support rapid growth. After a sufficient concentration of drug has accumulated in the target cells, the drug is activated with (nonburning) light via fiber optic delivery to internal cavities (e.g., lung, esophagus) or via LEDs for skin cancer of a particular wavelength for the formation of single oxygen and, thus, tumor cell death.

Two levels of selectivity against tumors are available with this approach: first, directing the light source and, second, targeting the photodynamic therapeutic agent to tumors.

Photofrin (QLT, Inc., Vancouver, BC), using a combination of laser light of specific wavelength and fiber optic delivery devices to kill cancerous cells selectively with minimal side effects has been approved by the FDA for the treatment of esophageal cancer.

Krueger et al. prepared a tetra-substituted polyethylene glycol conjugate of meta-tetrahydroxyphenylchlorin (PEGylated mTHPC) for the treatment of malignant mesothelioma *(214)*. Intraoperative photodynamic therapy (PDT) following surgical tumor resection to enhance local tumor control has been proposed. Preclinical testing in nude mice bearing human mesothelioma xenografts and on intrathoracic tissues of minipigs has been described. Results demonstrate extensive PDT-related necrosis of mesothelioma xenografts using PEGylated mTHPC. The half-life of PEGylated mTHPC in pigs exceeds 90 h. The authors propose that PEGylated mTHPC may be used safely and effectively and may warrant further investigation. Evaluation of the safety and utility of PEG mTHPC in rat models by Hornung et al. *(215)* supports this notion.

In contrast, Rovers et al. *(216)* have examined the kinetics of a tetra-PEGylated derivative of meta-tetra(hydroxyphenyl)chlorin (mTHPC-PEG) in comparison to native meta-tetra(hydroxyphenyl)chlorin (mTHPC) in a rat liver tumor model. Both kinetics and bioactivity in normal liver tissue were determined. PEGylation of mTHPC resulted in a twofold increase in circulating half-life and a fivefold decrease in liver uptake with an increase in tumor selectivity at the early time points. However, PEG mTHPC levels in liver increased over time with a loss of tumor selectivity at all but the earliest time points. Native mTHPC tumor selectivity increased with time. For both drugs, the time course of bioactivity in the liver followed drug levels with extensive necrosis after irradiation of mTHPC-PEG-sensitized liver tissue up to drug–light intervals of 120 h. The authors conclude that PEG mTHPC offers no benefit over native mTHPC for the treatment of liver tumors.

Hornung et al. *(217,218)* also examined PEG mTHPC PDT as a minimally invasive procedure to debulk pelvic ovarian cancer in rats. The pelvic ovarian cancer model has been well characterized as a PDT model. PEG mTHPC was administered intravenously; 8 d later, laser light at 652 nm and optical doses ranging from 100–900 J cm(−1) diffuser-length were delivered by an interstitial cylindrical diffusing optical fiber inserted blindly into the pelvis. Three days following the light application, the volume of necrosis was measured and damage to pelvic organs was assessed histologically; the assessment of PDT-induced necrosis showed a nonlinear dose response for both the photosensitizer dose and the optical dose. The lowest drug dose activated with the highest optical dose did not induce more necrosis than that seen in the tumor-bearing control animals. Mean overall survival of untreated tumor-bearing rats was 25.0 ± 4.5 d compared to 38.4 ± 3.8 d and 40.0 ± 3.6 d for rats treated with 3 mg kg(−1) or 9 mg kg(−1) PEG mTHPC mediated PDT, respectively ($p < 0.05$). A comparison to non-PEGylated mTHPC was not included in the study.

24. PEG TRICOSANTHIN

Trichosanthin, also known as compound Q or GLQ233, is a 27,000 molecular weight, single-chain ribosome-inactivating protein. Trichosanthin isolated from the root tuber of the Chinese medicinal herb Trichosanthes kirilowii is the active ingredient of Tian Hua Fen. Trichosanthin has been used in China to induce abortion and to treat choriocarcinoma. Based on studies suggesting that the drug may selectively kill HIV-infected lymphocytes, trichosanthin has also been evaluated in clinical trials for HIV/AIDS treatment. Side effects associated with trichosanthin include allergic reactions, neurotoxicity, a flu-like syndrome, and anaphylactic shock.

PEGylation, as well as modification of the structure of tricosanthin, may maintain the therapeutic utility of the drug while making it safer to use. He et al. *(219)* have prepared tricosanthin mutants with site-directed cysteine insertion and PEGylated proteins using linear PEG 5000-maleimmide or PEG 20,000-maleimmide strands. Circulating lifetime increased as much 100-fold, however, ribosome-inactivating activity and cytotoxicity were decreased. The PEG 5000 had little effect on immunogenicity. PEGylation with the strand having a molecular weight of 20,000 reduced immunogenicity and showed a weaker systemic anaphylactic reaction in guinea pigs.

25. PEG TUMOR NECROSIS FACTOR (TNF)

TNF-α is a protein cytokine comprised of 185 amino acids glycosylated at positions 73 and 172. It is synthesized as a precursor protein of 212 amino acids. TNF has anticancer and proinflammatory activity. TNF-α is produced by many different cell types. Primary sources are stimulated monocytes, fibroblasts, and endothelial cells. Macrophages, T cells, and B lymphocytes, granulocytes, smooth muscle cells, eosinophils, chondrocytes, osteoblasts, mast cells, glial cells, and keratinocytes also produce TNF-α after stimulation. Monocytes express at least five different molecular forms of TNF-α with molecular weights of 21,500–28,000. They differ mainly by posttranslational alterations such as glycosylation and phosphorylation. The use of TNF in the treatment of cancer has been explored but has been complicated by side effects and toxicity.

The benefits of PEGylation relative to increased tumor accumulation, as well as increased circulating life make PEGylation of TNF an interesting strategy by which to increase antitumor activity and improve safety.

It has been reported *(220)* that PEGylated tumor necrosis factor-α (MPEG-TNF-α), in which 56% of the TNF-α-lysine amino groups are coupled with PEG, has about 100-fold greater antitumor effect than native TNF-α. Evaluation of MPEG-TNF-α as a systemic antitumor therapeutic drug, using B16-BL6 melanoma and colon-26 adenocarcinoma, compared with Meth-A fibrosarcoma has also been described. The authors report that MPEG-TNF-alpha markedly inhibits the growth of both tumors without causing any TNF-α-mediated side effects, whereas native TNF-α has no antitumor effects and caused adverse side effects under test conditions. In addition, MPEG-TNF-α drastically inhibited the metastatic colony formation of B16-BL6 melanoma when compared with native drug.

Tsunoda et al. *(221,222)* have explored in vitro the utility of PEGylated TNF using a novel pH-reversible amino-protective reagent, dimethylmaleic anhydride (DMMAn). PEGylated TNF-α, PEG-TNF-α(+), which was pretreated with DMMAn before PEGylation, had 20% to 40% higher specific activity than PEG-TNF-α(–) which was not treated with DMMAn. Moreover, PEG-TNF-α(+) more potently caused tumor necrosis in Meth-A solid tumors in mice than did PEG-TNF-α(–). Of the various PEG constructs tested, that considered by the authors to be optimal induced a 30-fold higher degree of tumor necrosis than the native TNF-α and twofold higher than the most potent MPEG-TNF-α(–), which was at a similar molecular weight. Significantly, improvements in antitumor activity in vivo were more marked than were the changes in specific activity. Furthermore, native TNF-α caused a dose-dependent body weight loss in mice, whereas no obvious side effects were observed in any PEG-TNF-α-treated mice. These results suggest that PEGylation using DMMAn is a useful approach for the clinical use of cytokines such as TNF.

26. PEG CAMPTOTHECIN

Camptothecin is a naturally occuring quinoline alkaloid found in the bark of the Chinese tree (*Camptotheca accuminata*). It and its close chemical relatives (aminocamptothecin, CPT-11 [irinotecan], DX-8951f, and topotecan) are the only known naturally occurring DNA topoisomerase I inhibitors.

In 1996, the FDA approved topotecan as a treatment for advanced resistant ovarian cancers. Topotecan, which worked as well as or better than paclitaxel in clinical trials, is sold under the trade name Hycamtin® (SmithKline Beecham Pharmeceuticals). In 1996, injectable irinotecan HC1 was approved as a treatment for metastatic cancer of the colon or rectum. The drug is available as a generic drug and under the trade name Camptosar® (Pharmacia & Upjohn)

Like other anticancer agents that attack certain aspects of the cellular reproductive machinery, camptothecin drugs and analogs can produce potentially severe diarrhea, nausea, damage to bone marrow, and leukopenia.

As for paclitaxel, 5-FU, and the anthracyclines, camptothecin and its analogs are excellent targets for PEGylation. Greenwald et al. at Enzon, Inc. *(223–229)* have explored a variety of PEGylation strategies and have investigated benefits in cell culture and animal models. PEG-camptothecin has been prepared as a water-soluble macromolecular prodrug and the rates of hydrolysis were studied in phosphate-buffered saline, as well as rat and human plasma. In vivo efficacy screens were performed against P388/0 murine leukemia and LS174T human colon solid-tumor xenograft models. Results showed that rates of hydrolysis varied in both rat and human plasma according to the nature of the amino acid spacer used. PEG-alanine camptothecin was evaluated across a range of solid tumor types (colon, ovarian, mammary, lung, pancreatic, and prostate) and the preparation demonstrated significant antitumor activity in all tested xenograft models.

Relative to PEG molecular weights, Greenwald et al. (Enzon, Inc.) have primarily focused on PEGs of higher molecular weights, in particular PEG 20,000 and PEG 40,000.

PEG 20,000-conjugated camptothecin-*O*-glycinate was examined in biodistribution studies in nude mice bearing colorectal carcinoma xenografts with tritium-labeled drug. A blood circulating half-life (α phase) of approx 6 min with a β phase of 10.2 h was observed. It was also found that more PEGylated-labeled drug than native drug accumulated in tumors.

PEG camptothecin has been studied in human clinical trials *(230)* under the trade name Prothecan®. In a Phase I study cohorts of 1–3 patients with advanced disease received iv drug once every 21 d. Doses ranged 600–4800 mg/m^2 with dose-limiting toxicity observed at 4800 mg/m^2. Preliminary pharmacokinetic data suggest a circulating half-life of 72 h. In November 2000, it was claimed by the company that one-third of patients receiving drug achieved stabilization and that one patient (subsequently terminal) had responded and had been receiving drug for more than 1 yr. Phase II clinical trials were then initiated.

27. THE FUTURE OF PEGYLATION

Important advances in biotechnology as well as combinatorial chemistry, gene mapping, and informatics are converging on the identification of the biochemical specifics of disease. Novel targets and drugs for treatment are expected to follow. It is likely that as a better understanding of gene regulation emerges, drugs that are designed to modify regulatory events will also be developed. In this scenario, drug delivery technology is likely to play an important role in the targeting of drugs to specific cells or organelles and tissue types. The need for sustained-release or optimized pharmacokinetics is also likely to increase. In combination with devices for regional delivery or more convenient dosing, considerable improvements in safety, efficacy, and patient compliance can be expected.

PEGylation has been demonstrated in numerous animal or human clinical studies to prolong the circulating lifetime of proteins. As most protein drugs are given by iv, im, or sc injection, decrease in frequency and number of injections will be an important patient benefit. Lowering or blunted potential for immune or allergic reactions has also been demonstrated for PEGylated proteins. This latter feature of PEGylation has enabled the use of bovine-derived adenosine deaminase for the treatment of adenosine deaminase deficiency linked immunodeficiency and the use of bacterial-derived asparaginase for the treatment of acute lymphoblastic leukemia. Although these drugs have been approved for some time, it has been FDA approval and demonstration of the clinical benefits of PEGylated α interferon that has truly fueled widespread acceptance and the increased practice of PEGylation. More specifically, PEGylation of α interferon has shown that increased circulating lifetime *can correlate* with improved safety and efficacy of protein drugs. This is an intriguing finding, and one that should be taken into consideration when selecting future PEGylation candidates. For some proteins, a prolonged circulating lifetime may not be desirable, as increased exposure may contribute to increased toxicity or tachyphylaxis.

The success of PEGylation has also sparked the exploration of alternative approaches by which to achieve similar or more prolonged circulating lifetimes. Chief among these competitive approaches are the development of technologies for production of proteins as fusions to serum albumin or other plasma proteins. Conjugation to polymers, both synthetic and natural is also being explored. Although not prolonging circulating lifetime *per se,* incorporation of proteins into sustained-release gels, foams, or pellets to achieve maintenance of a steady-state level of drug has also been explored.

Use of fusion proteins may be complicated by changes in activity of the fused protein, or the new mutein may be antigenic and lead to immune or allergic reactions. In the latter scenario, use of PEGylation to blunt such a response may be considered synergistic.

An exciting advance in the use of PEGylation has been the application of the technology to small molecule drugs. Anticancer therapies and other agents with limited solubility have been shown to be made soluble and to have altered and more favorable biodistribution patterns. Passive accumulation of drugs into a tumor mass, for example, may contribute to safer and more efficacious cancer chemotherapy.

An additional benefit of PEGylation has been the improvement of the circulating lifetime of various liposome and nanoparticle preparations. Use of PEG-lipids in the preparation of "stealth liposomes" has been enabling for some products. Use of PEG block copolymers for drug encapsulation is an intriguing possibility.

Based on expanded understanding of the benefits of PEGylation and its extension to small molecule drugs, liposomes, and nanoparticles, we can expect continued new developments not only in the practice of the technology but, with FDA approvals, the subsequent introduction of new PEGylated drugs as well.

REFERENCES

1. Yeh P, Landais D, Lermaitre M, et al. *Proc Natl Acad Sci U S A* 1992; 89(5):1904–1908.
2. Francis GE, Delgado C, Fisher D. PEG-modified proteins, in *Stability of Protein Pharmaceuticals: in vivo Pathways of Degradation and Strategies for Protein Stabilization* (Ahern TJ, Manning M, eds). (Pharmaceutical Biotechnology, Borchardt RT, Ed, vol 3). Plenum, New York, 1991, pp. 235–263.
3. Zalipsky S. *Adv Drug Deliv Rev* 1995; 16:157–182.
4. Zalipsky S, Gilon C, Zilkha A. *Eur Polym J* 1983; 19:1177–1183.
5. Israelachvilli J. *Proc Natl Acad Sci USA* 1997; 94:8378–8379.
6. Sheth SR, Leckband D. *Proc Natl Acad USA* 1997; 94:8399–8404.
7. Torchilin VP, Papisov MI. *J Liposome Res* 1994; 4:725–739.
8. Delgado C, Francis GE, Fisher D. Uses and properties of PEG-linked proteins, in *Critical Reviews in Therapeutic Drug Carrier Systems.* CRC, Boca Raton, FL, 1992, pp. 249–304.
9. McGoff P, Baziotis AC, Maskiewicz R. *Chem Pharm Bull Tokyo* 1988; 36:3079–3091.
10. Francis GE, Delgado C, Fisher D, Malik F, Agrawal AK. *J Drug Targeting* 1995; 3:321–340.
11. Nilsson K, Mosbach K. *Biochem Biophys Res Commun* 1981; 102:449–457.
12. Delgado C, Patel JN, Francis GE, Fisher D. *Biotechnol Appl Biochem* 1990; 12:119–128.
13. Knusli C, Delgado C, Malik F, et al. *Exp Hematol* 1990; 18:608.
14. Malik F, Delgado C, Knusli C, Irvine AE, Fisher D, Francis GE. *Exp Hematol* 1990; 18:624.
15. Delgado C, Francis GE, Fisher D. *Crit Rev Ther Drug Carrier Syst* 1992; 9:249–304.
16. Yamaoka T, Tabata Y, Ikada Y. *J Pharm Sci* 1994; 83:601–606.
17. Yamaoka T, Tabata Y, Ikada Y. *J Pharm Sci* 1995; 84:349–354.
18. Mehvar R, Shepard TL. *J Pharm Sci* 1992; 81:908–912.
19. Mehvar R, Robinson MA, Reynolds JM. *J Pharm Sci* 1994; 83:1495–1499.
20. Chang RLS, Ueki IF, Troy JL, Deen WM, Robertson CR, Brenner BM. *Biophys J* 1975; 15:887–906.
21. Friman S, Egestad B, Sjovall J, Svanvik J. *J Hepatol* 1993; 17:48–55.
22. Beranova M, Wasserbauer R, Vancurova D, Stifter M, Ocenaskova J, Mara M. *Biomaterials* 1990; 11:521–524.
23. Allen TM. *Adv Drug Deliv Rev* 1994; 13:285–309.
24. Senior JH, Delgado C, Fisher D, Tilcock C, Gregoriadis G. *Biochim Biophys Acta* 1991; 1062:77–82.
25. Woodle MC, Engbers CM, Zalipsky S. *Bioconj Chem* 1994; 5:493–496.
26. Kamisaki Y, Wada H, Yagura T, Matsushima A, Inada Y. *J Pharmacol Exp Ther* 1981; 216:410–414.
27. Ashihara Y, Kono T, Yamazaki S, Inada Y. *Biochem Biophys Res Commun* 1978; 83:385–391.
28. Davis S, Abuchowski A, Park YK, Davis FF. *Clin Exp Immunol* 1981; 46:649–652.
29. Chen RH, Abuchowski A, van Es T, Palczuk NC, Davis FF. *Biochim Biophys Acta* 1981; 660:293–298.
30. Nishimura H, Ashihara Y, Matsushima A, Inada Y. *Enzyme* 1979; 24:261–264.
31. Nishimura H, Matsushima A, Inada Y. *Enzyme* 1981; 26:49–53.
32. Veronese FM, Largajolli R, Boccu E, Benassi CA, Schiavon O. *Appl Biochem Biotechnol* 1985; 11:141–152.
33. Nucci ML, Olejarczyk J, Abuchowski A. *Free Radic Biol Med* 1986; 2:321–325.
34. Abuchowski A, McCoy JR, Palczuk NC, van Es T, Davis FF. *J Biol Chem* 1977; 252:3582–3586.

35. Savoca KV, Abuchowski A, van Es T, Davis FF, Palczuk NC. *Biochem Biophys Acta* 1979; 578:47–53.
36. Rajagopalan S, Gonias SL, Pizzo SV. *J Clin Invest* 1985; 75:413–419.
37. Tomiya N, Watanabe K, Awaya J, Kurono M, Fujii S. *FEBS Lett* 1985; 193:44–48.
38. Koide A, Suzuki S, Kobayashi S. *FEBS Lett* 1982; 143:73–76.
39. Lisi PL, van Es T, Abuchowski A, Palczuk NC, Davis FF. *J Appl Biochem* 1982; 4:19–33.
40. Abuchowski A, Davis FF. *Biochim Biophys Acta* 1979; 578:41–46.
41. Wieder KJ, Palczuk NC, van Es T, Davis FF. *J Biol Chem* 1979; 254:12,579–12,587.
42. Abuchowski A, van Es T, Palczuk NC, Davis FF. *J Biol Chem* 1977; 252:3578–3581.
43. Boring CC, Squires BA, Tong T. *Cancer Journal for Clinicians* 1993; 43:18.
44. Sheinberg DA, Golde DW. *Harrison's Principles of Internal Medicine* 13th Ed. (Isselbacher KJ, Braunwald E, Wilson JD, et al. eds). McGraw-Hill, New York, 1994, pp. 1764–1774.
45. Keating MJ, Estey E, Kantarjian H. *Cancer: Principles and Practice of Oncology* 4th Ed. (Devita VT Jr, Hellman S, Rosenberg SA, eds). Lippincott, Philadelphia PA, 1993, pp. 1938–1964.
46. Capizzi RL, Holcenberg JS. *Cancer Medicine* 3rd Ed. (Holland JF, Frei E III, Bast RC Jr, eds). Philadelphia PA Lea and Febiger, 1993, pp. 796–805.
47. Kidd JG. *J Exp Med* 1953; 98:565–581.
48. Asselin BL, Whitin JC, Coppola DJ, et al. *J Clin Oncol* 1993; 11:1780–1786.
49. Gulati SC. *Purging in Bone Marrow Transplantation.* RG Landes, Austin, TX, 1993, p. 50.
50. Weiss RB. *Seminars in Oncology* 1992; 19:458–477.
51. Evans WE, Tsiatis A, Rivera G, et al. *Cancer* 1982; 49:1378–1383.
52. Peters BG, Goeckner BJ, Ponzillo JJ, Velasquez WS, Wilson AL. Hospital Formulary 30: Number 7 (July) 1995; 388–393.
53. Park YK, Abuchowski A, Davis S, Davis F. *Anticancer Res* 1981; 1:373–376.
54. Abuchowski A, Kazo GM, Verhoest CR Jr, et al. *Cancer Biochem Biophys* 1984; 7:175–186.
55. Ho DH, Brown NS, Yen A, et al. *Drug Metab Dispos* 1986; 14:349–352.
56. MacEwen EG, Rosenthal R, Matus R, Viau AT, Abuchowski A. *Cancer* 1987; 59:2011–2015.
57. Ho DH, Wang CY, Lin JR, Brown N, Newman RA, Krakoff IH. *Drug Metab Dispos* 1988; 16:27–29.
58. Teske E, Rutteman GR, van Heerde P, Misdorp W. *Eur J Cancer* 1990; 26:891–895.
59. Aguayo A, Cortes J, Thomas D, Pierce S, Keating M, Kantarjian H. *Cancer* 1999; 86:1203–1209.
60. Abshire TC, Pollock BH, Billett AL, Bradley P, Buchanan GR. *Blood* 2000; 96:1709–1715.
61. Chello PL, Bertino JR. *Cancer Res* 1973; 33:1898–1904.
62. Hoffman RM. *Anticancer Res* 1985; 5:1–30.
63. Hoffman RM, Jacobson SJ. *Proc Natl Acad Sci USA* 1980; 77:7306–7310.
64. Stern PH, Hoffman RM. *J Natl Cancer Inst* 1986; 76:629–639.
65. Tan Y. (1999) US patent 5891704.
66. Tan Y, Sun X, Xu M, et al. *Clin Cancer Res* 1999; 5(8):2157–2163.
67. Yoshioka T, Wada T, Uchida N, et al. *Cancer Res* 1998; 58(12):2583–2587.
68. Tan Y, Zavala J, Xu M, Zavala J, Hoffman RM. *Anticancer Res* 1996; 16(6C):3937–3942.
69. Tan Y, Zavala J, Han Q, et al. *Anticancer Res* 1997; 17(5B):3857–3860.
70. Tan Y, Sun X, Xu M, et al. *Protein Expr Purif* 1998; 12(1):45–52.
71. Kokkinakis DM, Schold SC, Hori H, Nobori T. *Nutr Cancer* 1997; 29(3):195–204.
72. Schold CS, Kokkinakis DM. (2000) US patent 6017962.
73. Lishko V, Tan Y, Han Q, Xu M, Guo H. (1997) US patent 5690929.
74. Tan Y. (1999) US patent 5888506.
75. Jones JB. "The effect of arginine deiminase on murine leukemic lymphoblasts," Ph.D. dissertation, The University of Oklahoma, 1981, pp. 1–165.
76. Savoca KV, Abuchowski A, Van Es T, Davis FF, Palczuk NC. *Biochim Biophys Acta* 1979; 578:47–53.
77. Savoca KV, Davis FF, Van Es T, McCoy JR, Palczuk NC. *Cancer Biochem Biophys* 1984; 7:261–268.
78. Clark MA. (1998) International Patent Application WO 98/51784.
79. Clark MA. (2000) US patent 6183738.
80. Takaku H, Migawa S, Hayashi H, Miyazaki K. *Jpn J Cancer Res* 1993; 84:1195–1200.
81. Filpula DR, Wang M. (1999) US patent 5916793.
82. Filpula DR, Wang M. (1998) US patent 5804183.
83. Katre NV, Knauf MJ, Laird WJ. *Proc Natl Acad Sci USA* 1987; 84:1487–1491.
84. Yang JC, Schwarz SL, Perry-Lalley DM, Rosenberg SA. *Lymphokine Cytokine Res* 1991; 10:475–480.

85. Meyers FJ, Paradise C, Scudder SA, Goodman G, Konrad M. *Clin Pharmacol Ther* 1991; 49:307–313.
86. Mattijssen V, Balemans LT, Steerenberg PA, De Mulder PH. *Int J Cancer* 1992; 51:812–817.
87. Teppler H, Kaplan G, Smith KA, Montana AL, Meyn P, Cohn ZA. *J Exp Med* 1993; 177:483–492.
88. Carr A, Emert S, Lloyd A, et al. *J Infect Dis* 1998; 178:992–999.
89. Ramachandran R, Katzenstein DA, Winters MA, Kundu SK, Merigan TC. *J Infect Dis* 1996; 173:1005–1008.
90. Wood R, Montoya JG, Kundu SK, Schwartz DH, Merigan TC. *J Infect Dis* 1993; 167:519–525.
91. Teppler H, Kaplan G, Smith K, et al. *J Infect Dis* 1993; 167:291–298.
92. Goodson RJ, Katre NV. *Biotechnology* 1990; (84):343–346.
93. Shih Y, Konrad MW, Warren MK, et al. *Eur J Immunol* 1992; 22(3):727–733.
94. Hillman RS. Goodman and Gilman's The Pharmacological Basis of Therapeutics (Hardman JG, Limbird LE, Molinoff PB, Rudden RW, Goodman Gilman A, eds). McGraw-Hill, New York, 1996, pp. 1311–1340.
95. Tanaka H, Satake-Ishikawa R, Ishikawa M, Matsuki S, Asano K. *Cancer Res* 1991; 51:3710–3714.
96. Malik F, Delgado C, Knusli C, Irvine AE, Fisher D, Francis GE. *Exp Hematol* 1992; 20:1028–1035.
97. Knusli C, Delgado C, Malik F, et al. *J Haematol* 1992; 82:654–663.
98. Ishikawa M, Okada Y, Satake-Ishikawa R, et al. *Gen Pharmacol* 1994; 25:533–537.
99. Satake-Ishikawa R, Ishikawa M, Okada Y, et al. *Cell Struct Funct* 1992; 17:157–160.
100. Bowen S, Tare N, Inoue T, et al. 1999; 27:425–432.
101. Yamasaki M, Asano M, Yokoo Y, Okabe M. *Drugs Exp Clin Res* 1998; 24:191–196.
102. Winslow RM. *Hemoglobin-based Blood Substitutes.* John Hopkins University Press, 1992, Baltimore MD.
103. Chang TMS. (Ed.) *Blood Substitutes and Oxygen Carriers.* Marcel Dekker, New York, 1992.
104. Teicher BA, Gulshan A, Ying-nan C, et al. *Radiation Oncol Investigat* 1996; 4(5):200–210.
105. Gullino PM. *Adv Exp Med Biol* 1975; 75:521–536.
106. Siemann DW, Keng PC. *Br J Cancer* 1988; 58:296–300.
107. Vaupel P, Fortmeyer HP, Runkel S, Kallinowski F. *Cancer Res* 1987; 47:3496–3503.
108. Vaupel P, Frinak S, Bisher HI. *Cancer Res* 1981; 41:2008–2013.
109. Vaupel P. *Strahlenther Onkol* 1990; 166:377–386.
110. Ikebe M, Ara G, Teicher BA. *Proc 87th Meeting of Am Assoc Cancer Res* Abstract 4207, 1996, p. 613.
111. Kavanagh BD, Khandelwal SR, Schmidt-Ullrich RK, et al. *Int J Radiat Oncol Biol Phys* 1997; 39(2)S:330.
112. Carmichael FJL, et al. *Crit Care Med* 2000; 28:2283–2292.
113. Jacobs EE, et al. *Transfusion* 2000; 40:41S.
114. Kasper SM, et al. *Anesth Analg* 1998; 87:284–291.
115. Koenigsberg D, et al. *Acad Emerg Med* 1999; 6:379–380.
116. Creteur J, et al. *Crit Care Med* 2000; 28:3025–3034.
117. Remy B, et al. *Br Med Bull* 1999; 55:277–298.
118. Winslow RM. (2000) US patent 6054427.
119. Cowley G, et al. *Newsweek Mag Mar* 2001; 12 pp. 52–61.
120. Shorr RG, Gilbert C. US patents 5650388.
121. Shorr RG, Cho MK, Nho K. US patent 5478805.
122. Shorr RG, Cho MK, Nho K. US patent 5312808.
123. Shorr RG. *Encyclopedia for Drug Delivery* (Mathiowitz E, ed). Wiley, New York, 1999, pp. 143–161.
124. Teicher BA, Gulshan A, Herbst R, Hideya T, Keyes S, Northey D. *In vivi* 1997; 11:301–312.
125. Fam AG. *Bailliere's Clin Rheumatol* 1990; 4:177–192.
126. Kelley WN, Wortmann RL. In *Textbook of Rheumatology* (Kelley WN, Ruddy S, Harris ED Jr, Sledge CB, eds). Fifth Edition, Vol. 2. Saunders WB, Philadelphia, 1997, pp. 1313–1351.
127. McInnes GT, Lawson DH, Jick H. *Ann Rheum Dis* 1981; 40:245–249.
128. Arrelano F, Sacristán JA. *Ann Pharmacother* 1993; 27:337–343.
129. Wu X, Muzny DM, Lee CC, Caskey CT. *J Mol Evol* 1992; 34:78–84.
130. Pui C-H, Relling MV, Lascombes F, et al. *Leukemia* 1997; 11:1813–1816.
131. Wu X, Wakamiya M, Vaishnav S, et al. *Proc Natl Acad Sci USA* 1994; 91:742–746.
132. Saifer MGP, Williams LD, Sherman MR, et al. *Polymer Preprints* 1997; 38:576–577, (http://www.mvpharm.com/PGGM_ART.html).
133. Sherman MR, Williams LD, Saifer MGP, et al. In *Poly(ethylene glycol) Chemistry and Biological Application* (Harris JM, Zalipsky S, eds). ACS Symposium Series 680, 1997, pp. 155–169. Washington, D.C., American Chemical Society.

134. Atassi MZ, Manshouri T. *J Protein Chem* 1991; 10(6):623–627.
135. Kawasaki K, Namikawa M, Yamashiro Y, Hama T, Mayumi T. *Chem Pharm Bull (Tokyo)* 1991; 39(12):3373–3375.
136. Mensi-Fattoh N, Molineaux CJ, Shorr RG. (1995) US patent 5428128.
137. Bomalaski JS, Clark MA, Shorr RG. (1998) US patent 5786154.
138. Clark MA, et al. *J Biol Chem* 1987; 262:(9)4402–4406.
139. Clark MA, Ozgur LE, Conway TM, et al. *Proc Natl Acad Sci USA* 1991; 88:5418–5422.
140. Bomalaski JS, Fallon M, Turner RA, et al. *J Lab Clin Med* 1990; 116:814–825.
141. Goddard DH, Bomalaski JS, Lipper S, Shorr RG, Clark MA. *Cancer Lett* 1996; 102:1–6.
142. Fanucchi M, Glaspy J, Crawford J, et al. *N Engl J Med* 1997; 336(6):404–409.
143. Piacibello W, Sanavio F, Severino A, et al. *Cancer Detection and Prevention* 1996; 20(5).
144. Barondes SH. *Ann Rev Biochem* 1981; 50:207–231.
145. Brownlee M, Cerami A. *Ann Rev Biochem* 1981; 50:385–432.
146. Cooper-Driver GA. In *Handbook of Naturally Occurring Food Toxicants* (Miloslav Rechcigl, ed). CRC, Boca Raton, FL, 1983, pp. 213–240.
147. Etzler M. Introduction, in *Chemical taxonomy, molecular biology, and function of plant lectins* (Goldstein I, Etzler M, eds). *Progress in Clinical and Biological Research*, Vol. 138. Alan R Liss, New York, 1983, pp. 1–5.
148. Jaffe WG. In *Toxic Constituents of Plant Foodstuffs* (Liener I, ed). Academic, New York, 1969, pp. 69–101.
149. Jaffe W. Handbook of Naturally Occurring Food Toxicology. In *Handbook of Naturally Occurring Food Toxicants* (Rechcigl M, ed). CRC, Boca Raton, FL, 1983, pp. 31–38.
150. Lotan R. In *Lectins and Cancer* (Gabius H, Gabius S, eds). Springer-Verlag, Berlin, 1983, pp. 153–169.
151. Nachbar M, Oppenheim J. *Am J Clin Nutr* 1980; 33, 11:2338–2345.
152. Ogawara M, Utsugi M, Yamazaki M, Sone S. *Jpn J Cancer Res (Gann)* 1985; 76, 11:1107–1114.
153. Ogawara M, Sone S, Ogura T. *Jpn J Cancer Res (Gann)* 1987; 78, 3:288–295.
154. Peumans W, Nsimba-Lubaki M, Broekaert W, Van Damme E. In *Molecular biology of seed storage proteins and lectins* (Shannon L, Chrispeels M, eds). *The Am Soc Plant Physiol* 1986, pp. 53–63.
155. Pusztai A. *Plant lectins*. Cambridge University Press, Cambridge, UK, 1991.
156. Suddath F, Parks E, Suguna K, Subramanian E, Einspahr H. In *Molecular biology of seed storage proteins and lectins* (Shannon L, Chrispeels M, eds). *The Am Soc Plant Physiol* 1986, pp. 29–43.
157. Ueno T, Ohtawa K, Kimoto Y, et al. *Cancer Prevention and Detection* 2000; 24(1):100–106.
158. Goel A, Batra SK. *Teratog carcinog mutagen* 2001; 21(1):45–57.
159. Wu AM, Yazaki PJ. *Q J Nucl Med* 2000; 44(3):268–283.
160. Merluzzi S, Figini M, Colombatti A, Canevari S, Pucillo C. *Adv Clin Path* 2000; 4(2):77–85.
161. Kitamura K, Takahashi T, Takashina K, et al. *Biochem Biophys Res Commun* 1990; 171:1387–1394.
162. Kitamuar K, Takahashi T, Yamaguchi T, Kitai S, Amagai T, Imanishi J. *Jpn J Clin Oncol* 1990; 20(2):139–144.
163. Otsujji E, Yamaguchi T, Yamaoka N, Yamaguchi N, Imanishii J, Tkahashi T. *J Surg Oncl* 1992; 50(3):173–178.
164. Takashina K, Kitamura K, Yamaguchi T, Noguchi A, Tsurumi H, Takahashi T. *Jpn J Cancer Res* 1991; 82:1145–1150.
165. Eno-Amooquaye EA, Searle F, Boden JA, Sharma SK, Burke PJ. *Br J Cancer* 1996; 73(11):1323–1327.
166. Pedley RB, Boden JA, Begent RH, Turner A, Haines AM, King DJ. *Br J Cancer* 1994; 70(6):1126–1130.
167. Hurvitz E, Klapper LN, Wilchek M, Yarden Y, Sela M. *Cancer Immunol Immunother* 2000; 49(4–5):226–234.
168. Welt S, Divgi CR, Real FX, et al. *J Clin Oncol* 1990; 8(11):1894–1906.
169. Welt S, Divgi CR, Kemeny N, et al. *J Clin Oncol* 1994; 12(8):1561–1571.
170. Deckert PM, Jungbluth A, Montalto N, et al. *Int J Cancer* 2000; 87(3):382–390.
171. Benhar I, Wang QC, FitzGerald D, Pastan I. *J Biol Chem* 1994; 269:13,398–13,404.
172. Wang QC, Pai LH, Debinski W, FitzGerald DJ, Pastan I. *Cancer Res* 1993; 53:4588–4594.
173. Choudhury PS. Pastan I. *Nat Biotechnology* 1999; 17:568–572.
174. Choudhury PS, Viner JL, Beers R, Pastan I. *Proc Natl Acad Sci USA* 1998; 95(2):669–674.
175. Chang K, Pai LH, Batra JK, Pastan I, Willingham MC. *Cancer Res* 1992; 52(1):181–186.

176. Chang K, Pastan I, Willingham MC. *Int J Cancer* 1992; 50(3):373–381.
177. Tsutsummi Y, Onda M, Nagata S, Lee B, Kreitman RJ, Pastan I. *Proc Natl Acad Sci USA* 2000; 97(15):8548–8553.
178. Kreitman RJ, Wilson WH, White JD, et al. *J Clin Oncol* 2000; 18(8):1622–1636.
179. Kaneo Y, Tanaka T, Fujihara Y, Mori H, Iguchi S. *Int J Pharm* 1988; 44:265–267.
180. Melton RG, Wiblin CN, Foster RL, Sherwood RF. *Biochem Pharmacol* 1987; 36:105–112.
181. Takakura Y, Takagi A, Hashida M, Sezaki H. *Pharm Res* 1987; 4:223–230.
182. Hashida M, Atsumi R, Nishida K, Nakane S, Takakura Y, Sezaki H. *J Pharmacobiodyn* 1990; 13:441–447.
183. Yoshimoto T, Nishimura H, Saito Y, et al. *Jpn J Cancer Res (Gann)* 1986; 77:1264–1270.
184. Murakami Y, Tabata Y, Ikada Y. *Drug Delivery* 1997; 4:23–31.
185. Yamaoka T, Tabata Y, Ikada Y. 1995; 47:470–486.
186. Jain RH. *Cancer Res* 1987; 47:3039–3051.
187. Maeda H, Matsumura Y. *Crit Rev Ther Drug Carrier Syst* 1989; 6:193–210.
188. Seymour LW. *Ther Drug Carrier Syst* 1992; 9:135–187.
189. Li C, Yu D, Inoue T, et al. *Anticancer Drugs* 1996; 7(6):642–648.
190. Greenwald RB. *Exp Opin Ther Patents* 1997; 7(6):601–609.
191. Senter PD, Pearce WE, Greenfield RS. 1990; 55:2975–2978.
192. Nicolaou KC, et al. *Angew Chem Int Ed Engl* 1991; 30:1032–1036.
193. Li C, Yu DF, Newman RA, et al. *Cancer Res* 1998; 58(11):2404–2409.
194. Li C, Price JE, Milas L, et al. *Clin Cancer Res* 1999; 5(4):891–897.
195. Greenwald RB, Choe YH, Conover CD, Shum K, Wu D, Royzen M. *J Med Chem* 2000; 43(3):475–487.
196. Greenwald RB, Pendri A, Conover CD, et al. *J Med Chem* 1999; 42(18):3657–3667.
197. Rodrigues PC, Beyer U, Schumacher P, et al. *Biorg Med Chem* 1999; 7(11):2517–2524.
198. Cheng TL, Chen BM, Chan LY, Wu PY, Chern JW, Roffler SR. *Cancer Immunol Immunother* 1997; 44(6):305–315.
199. Cheng TL, Wu PY, Wu MF, Chern JW, Roffler SR. *Bioconjug Chem* 1999; 10(3):520–528.
200. Cheng TL, Chen BM, Chern JW, Wu MF, Roffler SR. *Bioconjug Chem* 2000; 11(2):258–266.
201. Senter PD, Svensson HP, Schreiber GJ, Rodriguez JL, Vrudhula VM. *Bioconjug Chem* 1995; 6(4):389–394.
202. Stastn_ M, Jelínkovà M, Strohalm J, et al. *Cancer Detection and Prevention* 1998; 22(supplement 1).
203. Kwon GS, Yokoyama M, Okano T, Sakurai Y, Kataoka K. *Pharm Res* 1993; 10(7):970–974.
204. Yokoyama M, Kwon GS, Okano T, Sakurai Y, Seto T, Kataoka K. *Bioconjug Chem* 1992; 3(4)295–301.
205. Ayres DC, Loike JD. Lignans: Chemical, biological and clinical properties. Chemistry and Pharmacology of Natural Products, ed. Phillipson JD, Ayres DC, Baxter H. Cambridge University Press, Cambridge, UK, 1990.
206. Thompson LU. Flaxseed, Lignans and Cancer, in *Flaxseed in Human Nutrition* (Cunnane SC, Thompson LU, eds). AOCS, Champaign, IL, 1995, pp. 219–236.
207. Adlercreutz H, et al. *J Steroid Biochem* 1986; 25:791–797.
208. Adlercreutz H, et al. *Clin Chim Acta* 1986; 158:147–154.
209. Setchell KDR, Adlercreutz H. In *Role of the gut flora in toxicity and cancer* (Rowland IR, ed). Academic, New York, 1988, pp. 315–345.
210. Hartwell JL. *Cancer Treat Reports* 1976; 60:1031–1067.
211. Adlercreutz H. *Environmental Health Perspectives* 1995; 103:103–112.
212. Greenwald RB, Conover CD, Pendri A, et al. *J Control Release* 1999; 61(3):281–294.
213. Ouchi T, Hagihara Y, Takahashi K, Takano Y, Igarashi I. *Drug Des Discov* 1992; 9(1):93–105.
214. Ris HB, Kruegre T, Giger A, et al. *Br J Cancer* 1999; 79(7–8):1061–1066.
215. Hornung R, Fehr MK, Walt H, Wyss P, Berns MW, Tadir Y. *Photochem Photobiol* 2000; 72(5):696–700.
216. Rovers JP, Saarnak AE, de Jode M, Sterenborg HJ, Terpstra OT, Grahn MF. *Photochem Photobiol* 2000; 71(2):211–217.
217. Hornung R, Fehr MK, Monti-Frayne J, Tromberg BJ, Berns MW, Tadir Y. *Br J Cancer* 1999; 81(4):631–637.
218. Hornung R, Fehr MK, Monti-Frayne J, et al. *Photochem Photobiol* 1999; 70(4):624–629.
219. He XH, Shaw PC, Tam SC. *Life Sci* 1999; 65(4):355–368.

220. Tsutsumi Y, Tsunoda S, Kaneda Y, et al. *Jpn J Cancer Res* 1996; 87(10):1078–1085.
221. Tsunoda S, Ishikawa T, Yamamoto Y, et al. *J Pharmacol Exp Ther* 1999; 290(1):368–372.
222. Tsutsumi Y, Tsunoda S, Kaneda Y, et al. 1996; 87(10):1078–1085.
223. Zhao H, Lee C, Sai P, et al. *J Org Chem* 2000; 65(15):4601–4606.
224. Conover CD, Greenwald RB, Pendri A, Shum KL. *Anticancer Drug Des* 1999; 14(6):499–506.
225. Greenwald RB, Conover CD, Choe YH. *Crit Rev Ther Drug Carrier Syst* 2000; 17(2):101–161.
226. Conover CD, Greenwald RB, Pendri A, Gilbert CW, Shum K. *Cancer Chemother Pharmacol* 1998;
     42(5):407–414.
227. Greenwald RB, Pendri A, Conover CD, et al. *Bioorg Med Chem* 1998; 6(5):551–562.
228. Conover CD, Pendri A, Lee C, Gilbert CW, Shum KL, Greenwald RB. *Anticancer Res* 1997;
     17(5A):3361–3368
229. Greenwald RB, Pendri A, Conover CD, Gilbert C, Yang R, Xia J. *J Med Chem* 1996; 39(10):
     1938–1940.
230. Ochoa L, Tolcher AW, Rizzo J, et al. Abstract 770 NCI-EORTC-AARC Symposia Amsterdam 2000.

8 Emulsions As Anticancer Delivery Systems

S. Esmail Tabibi, PhD

CONTENTS

1. INTRODUCTION

Anticancer agents are typically hydrophobic and unstable in water, making formulation development a major undertaking. For this reason emulsion, the semihomogeneous mixture of two immiscible liquids, is an attractive dosage form for anticancer drugs. However, because of processing difficulties, lack of physiologically safe ingredients, and thermodynamic instability of the emulsion system, development of injectable emulsion formulations, particularly those containing anticancer drugs, has not been very successful. However, an intravenous (iv) emulsion containing a water insoluble and heat labile anticancer agent, penclomedine, was successfully developed and tested in clinical trials *(1–3)*.

This chapter will explore advances in and problems associated with development of emulsions as viable dosage forms for anticancer drugs. The first section will review the emulsion as a dosage form and the second section will focus on research related to emulsions as delivery systems for anticancer drugs.

2. EMULSION AS A DOSAGE FORM

2.1. Definitions

Generally, *emulsions* are heterogeneous, or "semi-homogenous" as stated in the foregoing: liquid-dispersed formulations with two distinct and immiscible liquid phases separated by interfacial boundaries. The *continuous phase* is the medium in which no boundaries among the phase ingredients exist, and the *discontinuous* or *disperse phase* is the other liquid that has been distributed throughout the continuous phase as small droplets with discrete boundaries separating each from the other. Disperse phase droplets suspend within the structure of the continuous phase by means of one or more *dispersants*. A dispersant, also called a *surfactant, emulsifying agent,* or *surface active agent,* is

From: *Drug Delivery Systems in Cancer Therapy*
Edited by: D. M. Brown © Humana Press Inc., Totowa, NJ

Table 1
Description of Different Types of Emulsions

Type of Emulsion	Description	Known as
Oil in Water	Oil dispersed in water	O/W
Water in Oil	Water dispersed in oil	W/O
Oil in Oil	Oil dispersed in oil	O/O
Water in Oil in Water	Water dispersed in oil and the formed W/O emulsion dispersed in water again	W/O/W
Oil in Water in Oil	Oil dispersed in water and the formed O/W emulsion dispersed in oil again	O/W/O

an amphiphilic molecule, a molecule with both hydrophilic and lipophilic moieties, that aids dispersion by situating itself in the interfacial boundaries, hence, preventing the coalescence of the dispersed droplets and giving physical stability to the emulsion.

Emulsions have been used in various industries and most of the scientific disciplines. However, it is beyond the scope of this chapter to cover all of these delivery systems and their processing within the pharmaceutical industry. Rather, this chapter will focus on the emulsions used to deliver anticancer agents because the lack of sufficient aqueous solubility makes the emulsion an ideal dosage form.

Emulsions and self-emulsifying systems may also be used to enhance the oral bioavailability of anticancer agents. This chapter will review emulsions for oral as well as parenteral administration of anticancer drugs.

2.2. Types of Emulsions

There are several different types of emulsions, and Table 1 provides a list and description of these varieties. Among these various emulsion types, only oil-in-water (O/W) and water-in-oil-in-water (W/O/W) emulsions have been used directly in delivery of anticancer medications. On the other hand, oil-in-oil (O/O) emulsions have been used indirectly in developing microencapsulated forms of anticancer agents (4–6).

Emulsions are thermodynamically unstable systems, and formulating a physically stable emulsion is always a challenge. This thermodynamic instability is generally exacerbated when preparing multiple emulsions. Various stabilization approaches have been suggested, but Kawashima (7) used an innovative method to stabilize a multiple emulsion by simply increasing the concentration of the solutes in the inner aqueous phase. Various types are schematically presented in Fig. 1.

2.3. Formulation Development

When a parenteral emulsion, based on preformulation work or based on a deliberate decision, appears to be an optimum approach for a specific anticancer agent, the pharmaceutical scientist responsible for development will need to consider various factors associated with designing, developing, and manufacturing the final product.

Besides the active ingredient(s) and water, two major components of emulsion formulations are oil and dispersant(s). These components play a major role in the toxicity, elegance, and stability of the final product, and we will provide some relevant examples.

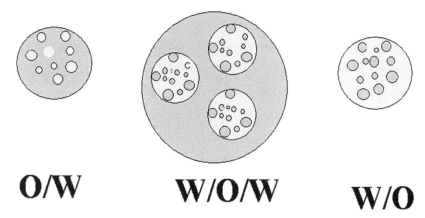

Fig. 1. Schematic presentation of the emulsion types.

2.3.1. SELECTION OF THE OIL PHASE

Oil is generally composed of various mono-, di-, and triglycerides. The fatty acid moieties of the oil are not only a caloric energy source but also play a role in various physiological and biological processes. For example, Mousa et al. *(8)* have demonstrated that the oleic acid component of an O/W emulsion has activated lymphocytes in rats. In addition, Waitzberg et al. *(9)* showed a moderate decrease in bactericidal function of human neutrophils after injection of a lipid emulsion composed of long chain fatty acids. However, Lavoie and Chessex *(10)* have shown that an imbalance in the production of vasoconstricting and vasodilating prostanoids after injection of lipid emulsions is related to hydroperoxide contamination in oils used in the lipid emulsions. Fatty acid composition of the oil is also important. For example, the manufacturer of a parenteral emulsion containing safflower oil claims that its product can be used to treat essential fatty acid deficiency.

Vegetable oils such as soybean oil, safflower oil, and cottonseed oil were the first oils used in parenteral emulsions to provide caloric requirements. The oil should be highly purified, and free from hydrogenation and naturally saturated fatty acids and glycerides. This purification is generally achieved by a process called *winterization,* i.e., storing the oil at a cold temperature for a long period of time to allow the precipitation of fatty materials and waxes before filtration. The oil should also be free of pesticides and herbicides. The American manufacturer of an emulsion containing cottonseed oil withdrew its product from the market based on reports of toxic side effects owing to the contamination of the oil with a trace amount of gossypol *(11).*

Chemical stability of the oil and the solubility of the drug in the oil are other important aspects to consider. For the emulsion to be stable and pharmaceutically elegant, with a small droplet size for iv administration, the amount of oil in the emulsion should not exceed 20% of the total volume.

2.3.2. SELECTION OF DISPERSANTS

Two immiscible phases separate naturally from each other because the cohesive force on the molecules within each phase is greater than the adhesive force on the molecules between the two phases. By situating itself on the oil–water interface, the dispersant generates a monomolecular layer causing a reduced interfacial tension, hence, avoiding separation of the two immiscible phases.

Physical stability of an emulsion generally depends on the molecular structure of the dispersant and its hydrophilic-lipophilic balance (HLB) value, a measure set forth by Griffith *(12)*. A high HLB value means that the dispersant is more water soluble and hence more suitable for stabilizing O/W emulsions. Conversely, a dispersant with a low HLB value is used to stabilize W/O emulsions. Two or more emulsifying agents are commonly used to further stabilization of the emulsion systems or impart different characteristics to the emulsions *(13)*.

Naturally occurring phospholipids, commercially called lecithins, are common emulsifying agents in parenteral emulsions. Tabibi et al. *(14–15)* have shown that the size of the oil droplets of the emulsions will not be further reduced by increasing the concentration of the phospholipids. The type of natural phospholipid used varies from supplier to supplier and may affect the overall physical stability of the emulsion. Degradation by hydrolysis of the phospholipids (phosphatidylcholine and phosphatidylethanolamine) may affect the long-term storage stability of emulsions. Lundberg *(16)* studied the stabilization effect of other dispersants in combination with phosphatidylcholine and found that polysorbate 80 provided superior results when compared with other surface-active agents including block copolymers (Pluronic® or Poloxamer® series).

Dispersants are used as detergents in various industries and, as such, they have both pharmacologic and toxicologic effects *(17–21)*. However, such effects are beyond the scope of this review.

2.3.3. OTHER INGREDIENTS

Emulsions generally have a low osmotic pressure and are made iso-osmotic by the addition of inert compounds. Reducing sugars or electrolytes are commonly used to make parenteral products isotonic, but are incompatible with phospholipids. Polyalcohols such as glycerin are widely used for this purpose. Sorbitol and xylitol have also been used. To prevent the oxidation of unsaturated fatty acid moieties of the oil and phospholipids, antioxidants such as vitamin E or vitamin E acetate may be added.

2.3.4. PARTICLE SIZE

Monodispersity, or uniformity in particle size, helps maintain the stability of an emulsion. Nakashima et al. *(22)* designed a membrane emulsification apparatus to control the droplet size and were able to obtain monodispersed multiple emulsions.

2.4. Preparation

Figure 2 briefly outlines the steps involved in preparing an emulsion. A detailed account would be too involved for this review, however, a few aspects of the preparation process should be emphasized for those who may want to use contemporaneous emulsion formulations for proof of principle in their research. To ensure a low level of bioburden, it is recommended that both phases of the emulsion be filtered through suitably sized and compatible filters (i.e., hydrophilic filters for the aqueous phase and hydrophobic filters for the oil phase). For iv O/W emulsions, the droplet size of the dispersed phase should be at least similar to or smaller than the smallest particles in the blood stream, preferably in the range of less than 200 nm *(23–24)*. For this reason, homogenization of the crude emulsion to reduce droplet size is an important step *(25–26)*.

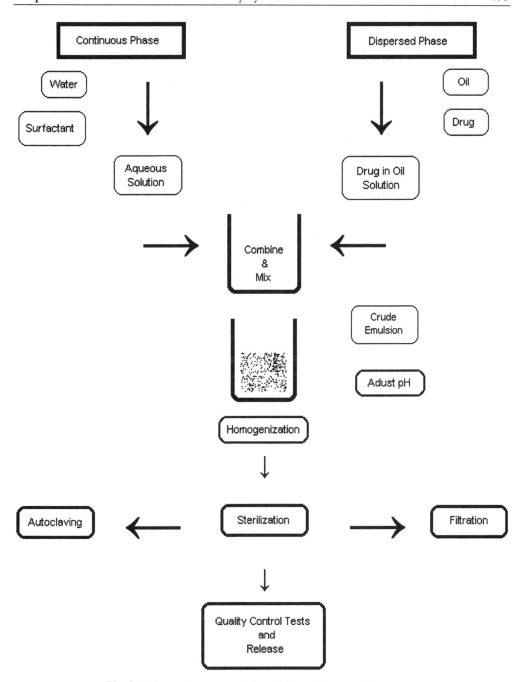

Fig. 2. Schematic representation of the various emulsion types.

3. EMULSIONS IN CANCER THERAPY

3.1. Locoregional Therapy

3.1.1. TARGETING THE LYMPHATIC SYSTEM

When an emulsion is injected into tissue, it is rarely taken up by the vasculature, and thus it remains in the tissue for a relatively extended period, slowly distributing to the surrounding tissues and regional lymph nodes. This phenomenon prompted Taka-hashi et al. *(27)* to test the ability of three types of emulsions, O/W, W/O, and W/O/W, to deliver the anticancer agent 5-fluourouracil (5-FU) to the lymph nodes. They injected the formulation into rat testes and followed the presence of both the oil droplets by a fat-staining method and ^{3}H 5-FU by radioactivity count in lumbar and/or renal lymph nodes. Although it was a crude test using emulsifying agents not approved for human use, the results indicated that, in contrast to intravenous administration, intratesticular administration of the W/O/W emulsion, and the W/O emulsion to a lesser extent, yielded high radioactivity counts in the lymph nodes, with a maximum attained at 3 h.

In a series of experiments, Nakamoto et al. *(28–29)* attempted to prevent metastasis formation in rats by delivering mitomycin C and bleomycin C to the lymph nodes using both W/O and O/W emulsions. Both intraperitoneal and intramuscular injections of the W/O emulsion delivered more drug to the lymph nodes than either the O/W emulsion or aqueous solution via these routes. Results also showed that gelatin served as a better emulsifier than polysorbate 80. Both mitomycin C and bleomycin C showed similar lymphatic delivery, the latter being more lipophilic than the former. Bleomycin showed better results with the W/O emulsion when compared with the mitomycin C in the same system.

Takahashi et al. *(30)* also evaluated the use of a fat emulsion to deliver bleomycin C in rats and humans. Compared to systemic or intratumoral administration of aqueous solution, intratumoral injection of the emulsion resulted in a significantly higher con-centration of bleomycin C in the tumor tissue of rats. In a clinical setting, six of eight patients with either local recurrence breast adenocarcinoma or squamous cell carci-noma of the skin responded favorably to treatment using an emulsion system.

In a clinical trial, Hanaue et al. *(31)* evaluated the effectiveness of oral administra-tion of tegafur, 1-(2-tetrahydrofuryl)-5-fluorouracil, in W/O and O/W emulsions in eight postoperative patients with gastric cancer. The concentrations of 5-FU in thoracic lymph and peripheral blood were determined. The results indicated that the concentra-tions of the drug in both lymph and plasma were much higher when the W/O emulsion was used when compared with those obtained with the use of the O/W emulsion. The study clearly showed that the W/O emulsion could reduce the unwanted toxicity to the nervous system caused by tegafur by reducing its circulating concentration, but could not improve tegafur's rate of conversion to 5-FU.

Yarkoni et al. *(32)* administered the emulsified mycobacterial glycolipid, trehalose-6,6'-dimycolate, into established fibrosarcomas of mice. This resulted in dose-depen-dent antitumor activity with complete regression in some animals.

3.1.2. CHEMOEMBOLIZATION

Chemoembolization is a palliative treatment for cancer whereby a mixture of chemotherapeutic drugs and oil are delivered directly to a tumor via the artery that sup-plies its blood. The artery is blocked, thereby depriving the tumor of nutrients and oxy-gen, preventing chemotherapeutic agents from being washed out of the tumor, and limiting the side effects of these agents in other organ systems.

Iodized poppy-seed oil has been used in various emulsions for treatment of hepatic cancer. This compound has good solvent action and, when administered via the hepatic artery, selectively accumulates in hepatocellular carcinomas. Novell et al. *(33–34)* has used this compound for locoregional targeting. However, because of rapid separation of the drug from the oil at the site of action, the usefulness of this technique has been limited. Various types of emulsions have been tested and have provided better results when compared with the oily solution currently used in chemoembolization. The following is a brief description of the methodology with some important comparative results.

Higashi et al. *(35)* prepared by extrusion through a fine-pore glass membrane a W/O/W multiple emulsion containing epirubicin, the water-soluble anticancer drug, and evaluated the physicochemical properties of the preparation. Median droplet size of the inner emulsion, W/O, was 0.55 ± 0.43 µm, and the median droplet size of the outer emulsion, O/W, was 30.1 ± 0.71 µm. The emulsion was stable for at least 40 d at room temperature. The in vitro drug release from the multiple emulsion in the presence of lipase at 37°C after 7 d was 3% of the initial amount. They reported no critical side effects after 24 arterial infusions for 21 patients, but a rise in body temperature above 37.5°C was observed in all patients. Based on the deposition of the multiple emulsion in the tumors, the antitumor effect, determined by the reduction in tumor size, was 13% (i.e., 1/8) for low-dose patients and 86% (i.e., 6/8) for high-dose patients. These results demonstrated that an anticancer agent formulated as a W/O/W emulsion and injected into the liver could remain in the hepatocellular carcinoma without separating from the oil phase droplets.

In other trials, Higashi et al. *(36–38)* studied the effect of droplet size of the outer emulsion. They used 30 and 70 µm W/O/W emulsions containing 60 mg epirubicin in the inner aqueous phase. They randomly assigned 16 patients to each group and measured the amount of α-fetoprotein (AFP), a surrogate marker for hepatocellular carcinoma, immediately before and 7 d after intraarterial administration of the multiple emulsion. The decline in AFP was significantly greater in the group receiving the large-droplet-size emulsion. From the results, they concluded that optimizing the droplet size of the outer emulsion in multiple emulsions played a major role in the outcome of the treatment of hepatocarcinoma by hepatic artery embolism. The effect of droplet size on the efficacy of the emulsion in chemoembolization has also been studied by Nakanishi *(22)* with similar results.

Kanematsu *(39)* compared the effects of iodized oil and the W/O emulsion in patients with single nodular HCC who were candidates for hepatectomy. The aqueous phase of the W/O emulsion contained epirubicin HCl and mitomycin C dissolved in iohexol, a nonionic aqueous contrast medium. Three different water-to-oil ratios were evaluated: 1:1, 1:2, and 1:3. In vitro release rates presented in Table 2 indicate that the emulsion with the lowest water content has a considerably slower release rate. Because the 1:3 emulsion yielded longer retention of the iodized oil in the HCC, no significant therapeutic effect was observed. This lack of therapeutic effect is due to the slower release rate of the drug from the thicker oil wall of the O/W emulsion, which provides lower than efficacious concentration in the site of action.

De Baere et al. *(40)* studied the effect of droplet size of W/O and O/W emulsions containing doxorubicin HCl in the aqueous phase and pure iodized oil as the oil phase. The droplet size of each emulsion was either 10–40 µm (small) or 30–120 µm (large). The emulsions were injected in vitro into a silicon macroscopic model of the artery tree and in vivo into the iliac arteries of rabbits. Their properties were evaluated by means of Doppler flow and their microvascular behavior in the arterial tree of the rabbit cremaster muscle using video microscopy. The results showed that O/W emulsions were mixed well in the in vitro model with the glycerin solution while the W/O emulsions were not.

Table 2
In Vitro Drug Release from Various W:O Ratio Emulsions

Water: Oil Ratio	%Drug Release			
	Epirubicin HCl		Mitomycin C	
	10 h	24 h	10 h	24 h
1:3	5	6	7.5	10
1:2	62.5	62.5	67.5	67.5
1:1	87.5	87.5	85	85

The results of this study clearly demonstrate that the formulation of the emulsion with respect to type and characteristics of size play a major role in the effectiveness of the therapy. Because changes in the droplet size of the emulsions containing the same proportions of drug and iodized oil will change the distribution of iodized oil in the arterial tree, the location at which the drug will be released to produce effect, and the better distribution of the oil droplet in O/W type emulsions, reduces the embolic action.

3.1.3. ADJUVANT THERAPY

Realizing that solid tumors are hypoxic, which would impede the activity of anticancer agents, Teicher et al. *(41–48)* studied the effect of oxygenation in combination with chemotherapy on tumor growth. They used perfluorochemical emulsions as an oxygen supply and showed that the level of cellular oxygenation plays an important role in the efficacy of many anticancer agents. Although this formulation was not used to treat cancer, the solubilizing power of perfluorochemicals suggests that it would be an effective delivery system.

Sadtler et al. *(49),* however, used the marker carboxyfluorescein to study its diffusion from the internal water phase of fluorocarbon emulsions. Using a fluorinated surfactant, they obtained very good emulsion stability with a particle size of less than 0.22 μm. The results indicated that fluorocarbon emulsions could be used as a promising potential drug delivery system through the pulmonary route with the possibility of regulating drug release. Another type of adjuvant therapy in which emulsions are used is anticancer vaccine. Holmerg et al. *(50)* studied the effectiveness of emulsified THERATOPE® STn-KLH vaccine in developing anti-STn lytic cells in breast and ovarian cancer patients following stem cell transplant. They concluded that the vaccine was well tolerated by the patients but the treatment effects were not statistically significant. However, their data suggest that the THERATOPE vaccine might decrease the risk of relapse and death, which warrants further study.

3.1.4. SYSTEMIC DELIVERY

Ames and Kovach *(51)* studied an emulsion formulation of hexamethylmelamine, a water-insoluble anticancer agent, in the rabbit. To prepare the intravenous emulsion, they dissolved the drug in either ethanol or dimethylacetamide and then added the drug solution to a 20% fat emulsion (Intralipid®). The drug disposition from emulsion was similar to that of an acidic solution of the compound. Tabibi and Siciliano *(52)* prepared without organic solvent containing 4 mg of hexamethylmelamine an emulsion formulation that can be scaled up and sterilized either by heat or by filtration.

Yalkowsky *(53)* formulated an O/W emulsion for parenteral administration consisting of paclitaxel with triacetin used for the oil phase and found that it was stable for at least 3 months. In another attempt, Tabibi and Yalkowsky *(54)* prepared an intravenous emulsion that could be used in combination therapy consisting of paclitaxel in tributyrin, which had a better stability profile than emulsion containing triacetin. Chu et al. *(55)* used a mixed emulsifying system consisting of a nonionic surfactant and phospholipid to prepare an O/W emulsion containing paclitaxel. After 3 mo of treatment in tumor-bearing mice, the emulsion was stable and effective in blocking the proliferation of HeLa cells with a marked improvement in survival time of the tumor-bearing mice.

Flavopiridol was formulated as an emulsion to overcome the potential gelling problem of high concentration of drug in the presence of its current excipients *(56)*. Maranhao et al. *(57)* studied the removal rate of an O/W emulsion prepared to resemble a low-density lipoprotein (LDL) in patients with acute myeloid leukemia. The preparation contained ^{14}C-labeled cholesteryl oleate, phospholipids, cholesteryl oleate, nonesterified cholesterol, and triglycerides. Results showed that the removal rate of the emulsions resembled that of LDL in these patients, suggesting that microemulsions resembling LDL could be used to deliver anticancer drugs to neoplastic cells, thus avoiding the toxic effects of these drugs to normal tissues.

Lundberg *(58)* assembled a complex of prednimustine, a lipophylic anticancer agent, and a model LDL to evaluate its cytotoxicity in vitro against T-47D breast cancer cells and normal 3T3 fibroblasts. The model LDL was prepared by emulsification of the oily composition containing prednimustine, and the delipidated apolipoprotein B was added to the microemulsion to form the complex. The complex was dialyzed against phosphate-buffered saline (PBS) and filtered through a 0.22 μm filter prior to use. The surfactant system of this emulsion, which seems very harsh for any in vivo system, consisted of egg phosphatidylcholine, Pluronic F68, and Triton X-100. This study indicated that the activity of prednimustine-lipoprotein complex was higher than that of free drug.

Fukui et al. *(59)* found that trioctanoylglyceride improves the stability of α-linolenic acid emulsified with cholesterol-bearing pullulan. They then investigated the selective cytotoxicity of α-linolenic acid in an O/W emulsion. Intraperitoneal administration of the emulsion effectively prolonged the survival of mice bearing peritoneally transplanted MM46 mammary tumor cells. In mice bearing subcutaneously transplanted MM46, iv injection of the emulsion resulted in tumor suppression without loss of body weight.

Lundberg *(60)* solubilized lipophilic derivatives of podophyllotoxins in lipid emulsions and studied their cytotoxic effects in cell culture against T-47D breast cancer and K562 erythroleukemic cells. Both etoposide oleate and teniposide oleate accumulated in these cells with a high cell kill value. In another study, Lundberg *(61)* prepared a very fine lipid emulsion containing paclitaxel. The emulsion had a droplet size of about 40 nm and was physico-chemically stable for several months at refrigerated conditions (4°C). The emulsion was also freeze-dried in the presence of glucose and was able to be reconstituted to its original state with distilled water. The cytotoxicity of the drug in emulsion against the T-47D cell line was retained and its 50% inhibitory dose (ID_{50}) was 7 n*M* compared to 35 n*M* using Diluent 12 and 10 n*M* using a liposomal formulation.

Versluis et al. *(62)* prepared a lipophylic prodrug of daunorubicin (LAD) by coupling it to a cholesteryl oleate analog through a degradable peptidic spacer. They formulated this compound in a lipid emulsion containing apolipoprotein E for LDL receptor mediated tumor targeting. They showed that the LAD was not separated from the emulsion droplets, indicating a strong association with the surface of the lipid droplets. In subsequent studies *(63–64)*, they used liposomal formulation in cell culture and tumor-bearing mice and showed that the LAD accumulates in tumor cells that express elevated levels of LDL receptors.

Lundberg *(65)* prepared oleic acid esters of the DNA topoisomerase I inhibitor camptothecin (CPT) and its analogs and incorporated them into liposomes and microemulsions. He showed that these lipophylic molecules of CPT were intercalated into the lipid layers of the delivery system, hence chemically protecting the hydroxy-lactone ring of the CPT and preventing its loss of activity by hydrolytic degradation. He also showed that the in vitro cytotoxic activity of these formulations against T-47D, Caco 2, and Raji cells was equal to or higher than that of the parent drugs. This would suggest that drug-lipid carrier complexes could be suitable formulations for intra-venous or intramuscular administration of lipophilic CPT analogs by providing a higher concentration of the active lactone form of the drugs in the circulation.

Lundberg et al. have coupled an antibody with a long-circulating lipid emulsion to enhance the efficacy of the LL2 monoclonal antibody. The conjugation efficiency was approx 85%, which was independent of the emulsion particle size and concentration of surface-bound polyethylene glycol modified phosphatidylethanolamine. Using various immunoreactivity tests, they showed that the binding of the conjugates to anti-idiotype antibody was increased by increasing the surface density of LL2, indi-cating that this type of emulsion can be a useful tool in delivering biotechnologic drugs into the target *(66)*.

In a review article, Fukushima et al. *(67)* examined, and eloquently explained, the progression of development of an O/W emulsion for the antitumor agent prostaglandin from preclinical experimentation, process development, and selection of the optimal formulation for clinical trials.

Ravichandran et al. *(68)* tested an emulsion to treat pancreatic tumors where the oil phase, consisting of essential fatty acids (EFAs), was the active ingredient. The emul-sion allowed a larger dose of EFA into the circulation while reducing or eliminating the unwanted side effects of these medicaments. By means of a validated microcul-ture tetrazolium in vitro assay, they showed that the EFA emulsion had antitumor activity in vitro. Concentrations of 25 and 68 μM resulted in a 50% growth inhibition of human pancreatic cancer cell lines MIA PaCa-2 and Pane-1, whereas the con-trolled lipid emulsion had no effect on these cell lines. However, no antitumor effect was observed in mice.

To overcome short circulation half-life and severe side effects of 6-mercaptopurine, Khopade and Jain *(69)* developed stealth multiple emulsions with a mean particle size of 150 nm. The W/O/W emulsion was prepared by a two-step method. First, the oil phase containing corn oil, palmitic acid, and phosphatydil choline was dispersed in internal water phase containing the active ingredient to make the W/O emulsion. Then this was further emulsified in phosphate buffer by the aid of taurodeoxycholate and butyric acid. The multiple emulsions were then coated by sphingomyelins (SM), monosialogangliosides (GM1), or polyethylene-glycol-grafted phosphatidylcholine lipid (PEG-PC). The third compound provided stealth characteristics, whereas the first two provided a solid-like coating on the droplet surface, preventing rupture and coales-cence. The stealth W/O/W multiple emulsion provided better tissue distribution than the emulsions coated with SM or GM1. Because there was no difference between the emulsions containing SM and GM1, they provided a better tissue distribution than the control W/O/W emulsion.

In conclusion, one should consider emulsions as useful drug delivery systems when low aqueous solubility is a major concern.

REFERENCES

1. O'Reilly S, Grochow LB, Donehower RC, et al. Phase I and pharmacologic study of penclomedine, a novel alkylating agent, in patients with solid tumors. *J Clin Oncol* 1997; 15:1974–1984.
2. Jodrell DI, Bowman A, Stewart M, et al. Dose limiting neurotoxicity in a phase I study of penclomedine (NSC 388720, CRC 88–04), a synthetic alpha-picoline derivative, administered intravenously. *Brit J Cancer* 1998; 77:808–811.
3. Berlin J, Stewart JA, Storer B, et al. Phase I clinical and pharmacokinetic trial of penclomedine using a novel, two-stage trial design for patients with advanced malignancy. *J Clin Oncol* 1998; 16:1142–1149.
4. Wang YM, Sato H, Adachi I, Horikoshi I. Optimization of the formulation design of chitosan microspheres containing cisplatin. *J Pharm Sci* 1996; 85:1204–1210.
5. Kyo M, Hyon SH, Ikada Y. Effects of preparation conditions of cisplatin loaded microspheres on the in vitro release. *J Control Rel* 1995; 35:73–82.
6. Sakakura C, Takahashi T, Hagiwara A, et al. Controlled release of cisplatin from lactic acid oligomer microspheres incorporating cisplatin: in vitro studies. *J Control Rel* 1992; 22:69–73.
7. Kawashima Y, Hino T, Takeuchi H, Niwa T. Stabilization of water oil-water multiple emulsion with hypertonic inner aqueous phase. *Chem Pharm Bull* 1992; 40:1240–1246.
8. Moussa M, Le Boucher J, Garcia J, et al. In vivo effects of olive oil-based lipid emulsion on lymphocyte activation in rats. *Clin Nutr* 2000; 19:49–54.
9. Waitzberg DL, BellinatiPires R, Salgado MM, et al. Effect of total parenteral nutrition with different lipid emulsions on human monocyte and neutrophil functions. *Nutrition* 1997; 13:128–132.
10. Lavoie JC, Chessex P. The increase in vasomotor tone induced by a parenteral lipid emulsion is linked to an inhibition of prostacyclin production. *Free Radical Biol Med* 1994; 16:795–799.
11. Pelham LD. Rational use of intravenous fat emulsions. *Am J Hosp Pharm* 1981; 38:198–208.
12. Griffin WC, Soc J. *Cosmetic Chem* 1949; 1:311, through [Griffin WC, in Kirk-Othamer Encyclopedia of Chemical Technology, 3rd ed., Vol. 8, Wiley-Interscience, New York 1978; pp 913–916].
13. Rossof M. Specialized Pharmaceutical Emulsions in *Pharmaceutical Dosage Forms: Disperse Systems* (Lieberman HA, Reiger MM, Banker GS, eds). Marcel Dekker, New York, 1998, Vol. 3, 2nd ed. pp 1–42.
14. Siciliano AA, Tabibi SE. Effect of microfluidizer processing and formulation on the droplet size of parenteral emulsions. *J Pharm Sci* 1987; 76:S298.
15. Tabibi SE, Siciliano AA. Effect of Composition and Processing on the Particle Size of Liposomes. *Pharm Res* 1989; 6:S76.
16. Lundberg B. Preparation of drug-carrier emulsions stabilized with phosphatidylcholine-surfactant mixtures. *J Pharm Sci* 1994; 83:72–75.
17. Anonymous. Cremophor EL: Toxicity Report, BASF Tech. Inform. No. CCE/PK 008, Dec. 1977 (HH).
18. Wang Y-C J, Kowal RR. Review of excipients and pH's for parenteral products used in the United States. *J Pareteral Drug Assoc* 1980; 34:452–462.
19. Gough WB, Zeiler RH, Barreca P, El-Sherif N. Hypotensive action of commercial intravenous amiodarone and polysorbate 80 in dogs. *J Cardvasc Pharmacol* 1982; 4:375–380.
20. Varma RK, Kaushal R, Junnarkar AY, et al. Polysorbate 80: A pharmacological study. *Arzneim Forsch/Drug Res* 1985; 35:804–808.
21. Platou ES, Refsum H. Acute electrophysiologic and blood pressure effect of amiodarone and its solvent in the dog. *Acta Pharmacol Toxicol* 1986; 58:163–168.
22. Nakashima T, Shimizu M, Kukizaki M. Particle control of emulsion by membrane emulsification and its applications. *Adv Drug Deliver Rev* 2000; 45:47–56.
23. Washington C, Koosha F, Davis SS. Physicochemical properties of parenteral fat emulsions containing 20-percent triglyceride – intralipid and ivelip. *J Clin Pharm Ther* 1993; 18:123–131.

24. Collins-Gold L, Feichtinger N, Warnheim T. Are lipid emulsions the drug delivery solutions? *Modern Drug Discovery* Apr. 2000; 44–48.
25. Tabibi SE. Production of disperse drug delivery systems in *Specialized Drug Delivery Systems: Manufacturing and Production Technology* (Tyle P, ed), Marcel Dekker, New York, 1990, pp 317–332.
26. Scott RR, Tabibi SE. A practical guide to equipment selection and operating techniques in *Pharmaceutical Dosage Forms: Disperse Systems* (Lieberman HA, Reiger MM, Banker GS eds). Marcel Dekker, New York, 1998, vol. 3, 2nd edition, pp 291–362.
27. Takahashi T, Mizuno M, Fujita Y, Ueda S, Nishioka B. Increased concentration of anticancer agents in regional lymph nodes by fat emulsions, with special reference to chemotherapy of metastasis. *Gann* 1973; 64:345–350.
28. Nakamoto Y, Hashida M, Muranishi S, Sezaki H. Studies on pharmaceutical modification of anticancer agents. II. Enhanced delivery of bleomycin into lymph by emulsions and drying emulsions. *Chem Pharm Bull (Tokyo)* 1975; 23:3125–3131.
29. Nakamoto Y, Fujiwara M, Noguchi T, Kimura T, Muranishi S, Sezaki H. Studies on pharmaceutical modification of anticancer agents. I. Enhancement of lymphatic transport of mitomycin C by parenteral emulsions. *Chem Pharm Bull (Tokyo)* 1975; 23:2232–2238.
30. Takahashi T, Ueda S, Kono K, Majima S. Attempt at local administration of anticancer agents in the form of fat emulsion. *Cancer* 1976; 38:1507–1514.
31. Hanaue H, Kurosawa T, Kitano Y, Miyakawa S, Horie F, Nemoto A, Shikata J. N1-(2 tetrahydrofuryl)-5-fluorouracil (FT-207) in the postoperative adjuvant chemotherapy of gastric cancer. Delivery of a fat-emulsified agent to the lymph. *Cancer* 1986; 57:693–698.
32. Yarkoni E, Meltzer MS, Rapp HJ. Tumor regression after intralesional injection of emulsified trehalose-6,6′-dimycolate (cord factor): efficacy increases with oil concentration. *Int J Cance* 1977; 19:818–821.
33. Novell R, Hilson A, Hobbs K. Ablation of recurrent primary liver cancer using ^{131}I-Lipiodol. *Postgrad Med J* 1991; 67:393–395.
34. Novell JR. Targeted therapy for recurrent breast carcinoma with regional lipiodol′/epirubicin infusion. *Lancet* 1990; 336:1383.
35. Higashi S, Shimizu M, Nakashima T, et al. Arterial-injection chemotherapy for hepatocellular-carcinoma using monodispersed poppy-seed oil microdroplets containing fine aqueous vesicles of epirubicin—initial medical application of a membrane-emulsification technique. *Cancer* 1995; 75:1245–1254.
36. Higashi S, Tabata N, Kondo KH, et al. Size of lipid microdroplets effects results of hepatic arterial chemotherapy with an anticancer agent in water-in-oil-in-water emulsion to hepatocellular carcinoma. *J Pharmacol Exp Ther* 1999; 289:816–819.
37. Tabata N, Higashi S, Kondo KH, Shimizu M, Nakashima T, Setoguchi T. Size of lipid microdroplets effects results of hepatic arterial chemotherapy with an anticancer agent in water-in-oil-in-water emulsion to hepatocellular carcinoma. *Hepatology* 1998; 28:2400, Pt 2, Suppl. S.
38. Higashi S, Setoguchi T. Hepatic arterial injection chemotherapy for hepatocellular carcinoma with epirubicin aqueous solution as numerous vesicles in iodinated poppy-seed oil microdroplets: clinical application of water-in-oil-in-water emulsion prepared using a membrane emulsification technique. *Adv Drug Deliver Rev* 2000; 45:57–64.
39. Kanematsu M. Transcatheter arterial chemoembolization therapy with epirubicin hydrochloride, mitomycin c, iohexol lipidol emulsion (EMILE) for hepatocellular carcinoma. *J Gastroenterol* 1995; 30:215–223.
40. De Baere T, Dufaux J, Roche A, et al. Circulatory alterations induced by intraarterial injection of iodized oil and emulsions of iodized oil and doxorubicin: experimental-study. *Radiology* 1995; 194:165–170.
41. Teicher BA, Rose CM. Enhancement of anticancer drug efficacy by a perfluorocarbon emulsion (Pfc). *Proc AACR* 1984; 25:316–316.
42. Teicher BA, Holden SA, Ara G, Ha CS, Herman TS, Northey D. A new concentrated perfluorochemical emulsion and carbogen breathing as an adjuvant to treatment with antitumor alkylating-agents. *J Cancer Res Clin Oncol* 1992; 118:509–514.
43. Holden SA, Teicher BA, Ha C, Ara G, Herman TS. Enhancement by perflusion emulsion (Oxygent®) and carbogen breathing of the tumor-growth delay of the fsaiic fibrosarcoma after treatment with antitumor alkylating-agents. *Biomat Artif Cells Immobil Biotechnol* 1992; 20:895–898.
44. Teicher BA, Holden SA, Northey D, Dewhirst MW, Herman TS. Therapeutic effect of infused fluosol-da carbogen with ephedrine, flunarizine, or nitroprusside. *Int J Radiat Oncol* 1993; 26:103–109.

45. Teicher BA. Combination of perfluorochemical emulsions and carbogen breathing with cancer chemotherapy. *Artif Cells Blood Substit Immobil Biotechnol* 1994; 22:1109–1120.
46. Dupuis NP, Kusumoto T, Robinson MF, Liu F, Menon K, Teicher BA. Restoration of tumor oxygenation after cytotoxic therapy by a perflubron emulsion carbogen breathing. *Artif Cells Blood Substit Immobil Biotechnol* 1995; 23:423–429.
47. Teicher BA, Holden SA, Ara G, et al. Influence of an anti-angiogenic treatment on 9l gliosarcoma—oxygenation and response to cytotoxic therapy. *Int J Cancer* 1995; 61:732–737.
48. Teicher BA, Ara G, Takeuchi H, Coleman CN. Tumor oxygenation after hyperthermia in the rat 13762 mammary carcinoma and the Du-145 human prostate carcinoma. *Int J Oncol* 1997; 10:437–442.
49. Sadtler VM, Krafft MP, Riess Jg. Reverse water-in-fluorocarbon emulsions as a drug delivery system: an in vitro study. colloids surfaces A. *Physicochem Eng Aspects* 1999; 147:309–315.
50. Holmberg LA, Oparin DV, Gooley T, et al. Clinical outcome of breast and ovarian cancer patients treated with high-dose chemotherapy, autologous stem cell rescue and THERATOPE (R) STn-KLH cancer vaccine. *Bone Marrow Transplant* 2000; 25:1233–1241.
51. Ames MM, Kovach JS. Parenteral formulation of hexamethylmelamine potentially suitable for use in man. *Cancer Treat Rep* 1982; 66:1579–1581.
52. Tabibi SE, Siciliano AA. Hexamethylmelamine containing parenteral emulsions. U.S. Pat. 5 039 527, Aug. 13, 1991.
53. Tarr BD, Sambandan TG, Yalkowsky SH. New parenteral emulsion for the administration of taxol. *Pharm Res* 1987; 4:162–165.
54. Simamora P, Dannenfelser R-M, Tabibi SE, Yalkowsky S. Emulsion formulations for the administration of paclitaxel. *PDA J Pharm Sci Tech* 1998; 52:170–172.
55. Kan P, Chen Z-B, Lee C-J, Chu I-M. Development of nonionic surfactant/ phospholipid o/w emulsion a paclitaxel delivery system. *J Control Rel* 1999; 58:271–278.
56. Dannenfelser RM, Surakibanharn Y, Tabibi SE, Yalkowsky SH. Parenteral formulation of flavopiridol (NSC-649890). *PDA J Pharm Sci Tech* 1996; 50:356–359.
57. Maranhao RC, Garicochea B, Silva EL, Llacer PD, Pileggi FJC, Chamone DAF. Increased plasma removal of microemulsions resembling the lipid phase of low-density lipoproteins (LDL) in patients with acute myeloid-leukemia—a possible new strategy for the treatment of the disease. *Braz J Med Biol Res* 1992; 25:1003–1007.
58. Lundberg B. Assembly of prednimustine low-density-lipoprotein complexes and their cytotoxic activity in tissue-culture. *Cancer Chemo Pharmacol* 1992; 29:241–247.
59. Fukui H, Akiyoshi K, Sato T, Sunamoto J, Yamaguchi S, Numata M. Anticancer activity of polyunsaturated fatty-acid emulsion stabilized by hydrophobized polysaccharide. *J Bioact Compat Polymers* 1993; 8:305–316.
60. Lundberg B. The solubilization of lipophilic derivatives of podophyllotoxins in submicron sized lipid emulsions and their cytotoxic activity against cancer cells in culture. *Int J Pharm* 1994; 109:73–81.
61. Lundberg BB. A submicron lipid emulsion coated with amphipathic polyethylene glycol for parenteral administration of paclitaxel (Taxol). *J Pharm Pharmacol* 1997; 49:16–21.
62. Versluis AJ, Rump ET, Rensen PC, Van Berkel TJ, Bijsterbosch MK. Synthesis of a lipophilic daunorubicin derivative and its Incorporation into lipidic carriers developed for LDL receptor-mediated tumor therapy. *Pharm Res* 1998; 15:531–537.
63. Versluis AJ, Rensen PC, Rump ET, Van Berkel TJ, Bijsterbosch MK. Low-density lipoprotein receptor-mediated delivery of a lipophilic daunorubicin derivative to B16 tumours in mice using apolipoprotein E-enriched liposomes. *Br J Cancer* 1998; 78:1607–1614.
64. Versluis AJ, Rump ET, Rensen PC, van Berkel TJ, Bijsterbosch MK. Stable incorporation of a lipophilic daunorubicin prodrug into apolipoprotein E-exposing liposomes induces uptake of prodrug via low-density lipoprotein receptor in vivo. *J Pharmacol Exp Ther* 1999; 289:1–7.
65. Lundberg BB. Biologically active camptothecin derivatives for incorporation into liposome bilayers and lipid emulsions. *Anti-Cancer Drug Design* 1998; 13:453–461.
66. Lundberg BB, Griffiths G, Hansen HJ. Conjugation of an anti-B-cell lymphoma monoclonal antibody, LL2, to long-circulating drug-carrier lipid emulsions. *J Pharm Pharmacol* 1999; 51:1099–1105.
67. Fukushima S, Kishimoto S, Takeuchi Y, Fukushima M. Preparation and evaluation of O/W type emulsions containing antitumor prostaglandin. *Adv Drug Delivery Rev* 2000; 45:65–75.
68. Ravichandran D, Cooper A, Johnson CD. Effect of 1-gamma linolenyl-3-eicosapentaenoyl propane diol on the growth of human pancreatic carcinoma in vitro and in vivo. *Eur J Cancer* 2000; 36:423–427.
69. Khopade AJ, Jain NK. Long-circulating multiple-emulsion system for improved delivery of an anticancer agent. *Drug Delivery* 1999; 6:107–110.

III

CURRENT APPLICATIONS
PRODUCTS APPROVED OR IN ADVANCED CLINICAL DEVELOPMENT

9

Liposomal Drug Delivery Systems for Cancer Therapy

Daryl C. Drummond, PhD,
Dmitri Kirpotin, PhD, Christopher C. Benz, MD,
John W. Park, MD, and Keelung Hong, PhD

CONTENTS

1. INTRODUCTION

Liposomes are currently one of the most well-studied drug delivery systems used in the treatment of cancer. They are being employed in the treatment of a wide variety of human malignancies *(1–4)*. Their large size relative to the gaps in the vasculature of healthy tissues inhibits their uptake by these tissues, thus avoiding certain nonspecific toxicities. However, the "leaky" microvasculature supporting solid tumors allows for the uptake of these large (~ 100 nm) drug carriers *(5–8)* and their subsequent interaction with cancer cells *(9)*, or release of the encapsulated drug specifically near the tumor, where it can diffuse into the tumor in its free form *(10,11)*. Liposomes have many other potential advantages over the corresponding free drugs, including favorable pharmacokinetic properties, where encapsulation of a usually rapidly cleared drug results in a considerable increase in the circulation lifetime for the drug *(12–14)*. In addition, encapsulation or complexation of a normally labile therapeutic agent, such as DNA, antisense oligonucleotides, or the lactone ring of camptothecins, can protect the agent from premature degradation by enzymes in the plasma or from simple hydrolysis. The result of liposome formulation can thus be a substantial increase in antitumor efficacy when compared to the free drug or standard chemotherapy regimens *(15–17)*.

From: *Drug Delivery Systems in Cancer Therapy*
Edited by: D. M. Brown © Humana Press Inc., Totowa, NJ

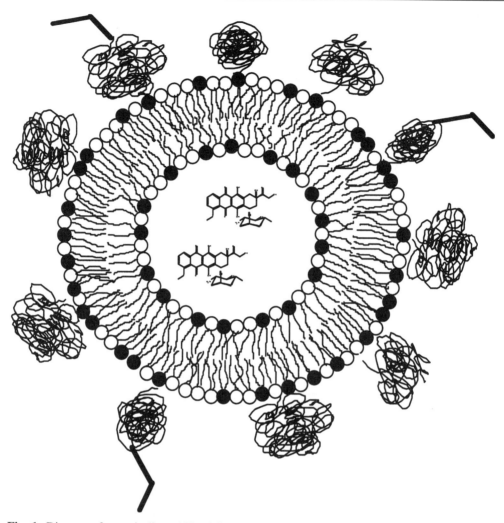

Fig. 1. Diagram of a sterically stabilized liposome containing the antineoplastic drug, doxorubicin. Liposomes are composed of a lipid membrane that encloses an internal aqueous space. This aqueous space can be used to entrap drugs following passive loading of the agent by its inclusion in the hydration media or remote-loading using ion- or pH-gradients. The lipids used to compose the liposomal membrane can be both phospholipids, such as phosphatidylcholine, and neutral lipids, such as cholesterol. In addition sterically stabilized liposomes contain a lipid-anchored PEG-coating that reduces its uptake by macrophages. Finally, targeting ligands, such as single-chain antibody fragments, can be attached to the terminal ends of PEG and used to actively direct the liposomal carriers to tumor-specific antigens.

A diagram of a liposome is given in Fig. 1. Liposomes are composed of a lipid bilayer that may contain both phospholipids, such as phosphatidylcholine, and neutral lipids, such as cholesterol. The lipid bilayer encloses an internal aqueous space that can be utilized to carry antineoplastic drugs, imaging agents, proteins, and even genes. The surface of the liposome can be modified with hydrophilic polymers, such as polyethlene glycol (PEG), to reduce interactions with reticuloendothelial cells responsible for their elimination from the systemic circulation *(13,18–21)*. The pharmacological properties of liposomes can be widely varied by modifying the lipid composition of the liposome, the therapeutic agent to be encapsulated, the method of drug encapsulation, the surface

Table 1
Important Considerations in the Design of Liposome-Formulated Therapeutics

Component	Considerations for optimum design
Liposome	*Stability*
	Stable as intact construct in vivo
	Lipid components chemically stable during storage
	Pharmacokinetics
	Long circulating (small diameter, steric stabilization, charge optimization)
	Tumor penetration
	Capable of extravasation in solid tumors
	Small diameter improves penetration into tumor tissue
Drug	*Encapsulation*
	Efficient, high capacity (remote loading or passive entrapment)
	Encapsulated drug resists leakage during storage and minimizes leakage in systemic circulation
	Bystander Effect
	Agent affects tumor cells not directly targeted (bystander cells)
	Interaction with Tumor Cells
	Effective against target cell population
	If internalized, therapeutic agent capable of escaping internal organelles and/or stable to degradative environment in lysosomes

charge density, the presence or absence of steric stabilization, the size of the carrier, the presence of a targeting ligand on the liposome surface, the dose to be administered, and the route of administration. Thus, it is essential that the cancer researcher understand how these various properties affect the pharmacokinetics, biodistribution, and the bioavailability of the entrapped therapeutic agent to maximize the therapeutic index. Several additional reviews discuss in detail how these different characteristics act to modify the pharmacological properties of liposomes and liposomal drugs (3,12,13,22–26).

2. FORMULATION ISSUES

2.1. Effects of Liposome Physical Properties on Pharmacokinetics and Tissue Distribution

There are many formulation issues to consider when designing a liposomal or lipid-based carrier system for a particular therapeutic agent. The various properties of the carrier have to be considered when taking into account the interactions of liposomes with the biological milieu. Many of the optimal properties for design of a liposome-based therapeutic are given in Table 1. For example, relatively small unilamellar liposomes (70–150 nm) are often desirable when treating solid tumors because they are taken up less readily by reticuloendothelial system (RES) macrophages (12,26,27) and able to extravasate more readily into solid tumors (5,28). However, large multilamellar vesicles have been used when the drug was administered at a peripheral site and effectively acted as a slow release depot for the drug from that site (29), or where the drug was targeted to the RES, as is the case for some infectious diseases (30). Surface charge is another important and often misunderstood property of liposomal carriers that affects their disposition in vivo (3,26,31,32). Although certain anionic phospholipid components have been shown to increase liposome clearance in vivo *(26,33)*, other sterically shielded anionic lipids have been shown to substantially increase circulation half-lives of liposomal carriers *(19,31,34,35)*. In addition, surface charge density and the presence of gel phase phospholipid components may also play a role in the magnitude of the charge effect on liposome clearance *(3,32,36)*.

Along with surface charge and size, other physical characteristics of the carrier such as membrane fluidity play a role in liposome and drug circulation lifetimes. In the absence of steric stabilization, liposomes that contain fluid-phase lipid components, such as unsaturated phospholipids, are cleared more rapidly from the circulation than liposomes containing gel-phase phospholipids *(26,37)*. This is presumably due to the increased potential for binding of serum opsonins to liposomes that, in turn, bind macrophages and result in more rapid uptake of the carrier by macrophages *(38–40)*. The presence of cholesterol in the formulation also prevents disintegration of the carrier by lipoproteins in the blood and, thus, is thought to be essential in maintaining a stable liposome formulation in vivo *(41,42)*. Steric stabilization of liposomal carriers, by addition of polymer-coated lipid conjugates, is thought to both reduce the binding of serum opsonins to the liposome surface and reduce interactions of bound opsonins with receptors on the surface of RES macrophages, thus reducing clearance *(43–47)*. Depending on the nature of the ligand attached, ligands such as antibodies, used for specific targeting of receptor-overexpressing cancer cells, can also alter the pharmacokinetics of liposomes (Subheading 5.). The importance of understanding the interactions of these relative physical properties, and their effect on liposome disposition in vivo, cannot be emphasized enough.

2.2. Formulation Stability

There are other formulation issues, such as in vivo formulation stability, degree of drug entrapment, and ability to make the agent bioavailable at the site of action, that determine the degree of success of a delivery-specific approach to treating cancer. In order to carry a cytotoxic agent specifically to solid tumors while avoiding healthy tissues, the drug must be stably encapsulated in the liposome interior when in the general circulation. Drugs vary in their ability to be stably entrapped depending on the physicochemical properties of the drug, the method of drug entrapment, and the lipid composition of the carrier *(3,23,48)*. In general, amphipathic drugs such as doxorubicin and vincristine are the most ideal for delivery via liposomes. These drugs can be entrapped inside liposomes at concentrations exceeding their aqueous solubility by using remote-loading techniques involving pH or ion gradients across the membrane surface *(49–54)*. Using one of these methods, the degree of entrapment can approach 100% for certain drugs. The presence of cholesterol and high-phase transition phospholipids, such as sphingomyelin (SM) and highly saturated phospholipids, enhance the stability of these formulations *(55,56)*. Hydrophobic drugs, such as paclitaxel, are carried in the lipid bilayer rather than the aqueous interior *(57–59)*. However, they usually require a large excess of lipid to completely solubilize the drug and prevent their recrystallization. In addition, this class of drugs/therapeutic agents is often rapidly redistributed to extraliposomal sites including plasma lipoproteins *(57,60,61)*. A third class of compounds, the highly hydrophilic class, are able to be stably entrapped in liposomes by passive entrapment, although at low yields (< 33%) relative to active loading. However, release of the drug from the liposome may be slow and require an external trigger such as pH *(62–65)* or temperature *(66–68)* to release the drug from the carrier.

2.3. Release of Therapeutic Agents from Liposomal Carriers

Another important, yet often neglected parameter in designing liposomal carriers is the rate of release of drug from the liposome. In order to be effective in treating a particular malignancy, liposomes must be able to make their drug bioavailable, preferably at the site of the tumor. Upon release, the drug can subsequently diffuse into the target cell by passive diffusion or be taken up by membrane transporters, such as nucleoside transporters *(69,70)* or the reduced folate carrier *(71,72)*. The majority of drugs studied thus far have been amphipathic in nature and thus able to passively diffuse from the liposomal carrier with a rate that depends on the lipid composition of the carrier, the mode of drug entrapment, the osmolarity of the entrapped species, and the effects of local stimuli *(3,50,68,73–76)*. These liposomal drugs can either be released rapidly ($t_{1/2}$ = minutes to hours), where an important fraction of the drug is released from the carrier while in the circulation, or slowly ($t_{1/2}$ = hours to days), where the liposome accumulates in the tumor at a rate more rapid than the rate for drug release. More complicated liposome systems are also being developed that rely on programmed loss of a protective PEG coating *(77–79)*, temperature-mediated *(67,68)* or pH-mediated *(62,64)* membrane destabilization, or specific enzymatic destabilization of liposomes *(80)*. Continued optimization of drug leakage rates is needed to more fully take advantage of the increased tumor accumulation of drug afforded by liposome encapsulation.

3. ANIMAL PHARMACOLOGY

3.1. Pharacokinetics and Biodistribution of Liposomal Drugs

The half-life of sterically-stabilized liposomal doxorubicin (SSL-DOX) in the systemic circulation ($t_{1/2}$) is approx 22–24 h in rats *(81,82)*, and 45 h in humans *(15)*. For SSL-DOX, the $t_{1/2}$ is relatively independent of dose *(15)*, while for conventional formulations without the steric PEG coat, the $T_{1/2}$ increases rapidly with increasing dose. This increase in circulation lifetimes with increasing dose is thought to be because of either saturation of RES macrophages with liposomal lipid *(12,26,27)* or drug-induced toxicity of RES macrophages *(55,83)*, with either mechanism resulting in reduced clearance. Drug-induced toxicity has been observed with SSL-DOX as well, but only at relatively high doses *(2)*. The rate of clearance for SSL-DOX in rats is approx 60-fold lower than free doxorubicin in rats *(82)*. This translates into a similar increase in the area under the curve (AUC) for concentration versus time for SSL-DOX when compared to free doxorubicin. The significant increases in plasma AUCs and reductions in clearance following liposome encapsulation were also observed in humans *(15,84,85)*, although the relative difference was considerably less for conventional formulations *(84,85)* than for a sterically stabilized formulation *(15)*. As mentioned earlier, these effects are likely due to the ability of the steric PEG coat to reduce recognition of liposomes by RES macrophages. Fig. 2A shows the effect of liposome encapsulation on clearance of vincristine (VCR) from the circulation of SCID mice bearing A431 tumors *(73)*. This figure emphasizes the importance of formulation stability on liposome clearance. When 1,2-distearoyl-3-*sn*-phosphatidylcholine (DSPC) is replaced with sphingomyelin, the liposome is able to more readily retain vincristine when in the circulation, and this translates into reduced drug clearance. For doxorubicin, DSPC/Chol liposomes are sufficient to hold the drug while in the circulation and, thus, the importance of tailoring the liposomal carrier to the drug to be encapsulated is demonstrated (Subheading 2.2.). The increased circulation

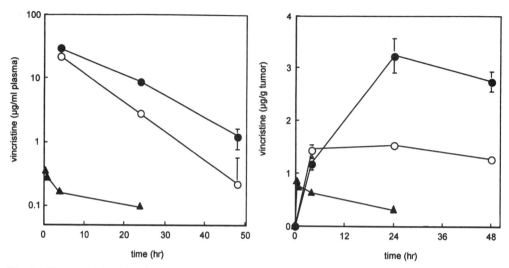

Fig. 2. Pharmacokinetics of free and liposome-encapsulated vincristine. Plasma (**A**) and tumor (**B**) levels of vincristine were determined after administration of free vincristine (▲), or vincristine entrapped in DSPC/Chol (○) or SM/Chol (●) liposomes. The tumor model used was that of a squamous cell carcinoma (A431 tumors) in SCID mice. The dose of vincristine was 2 mg/kg for all samples and the lipid dose for the liposome formulations was 20 mg/kg. (This figure was taken from Webb et al. *Br J Cancer* 1995; 72:896–904, with permission.)

lifetime of liposomal drugs also helps translate into increased tumor accumulation of drug *(36,86–88)*. As can be seen in Fig. 2B, the more stable SM/Chol liposomal vincristine formulation shows considerably greater levels of vincristine accumulation in the tumor.

The biodistribution of liposomal and free drugs are determined by a variety of factors, including circulation lifetimes, the presence of phagocytic cells, and the vascular barrier of the particular tissue. Most free drugs redistribute rapidly to tissues due to their small size and membrane-permeable amphipathic nature, and they are often rapidly excreted by the kidneys. The result is a large volume of distribution for the free drug. Stable liposomal formulations, on the other hand, have a relatively small volume of distribution that is not much greater than the volume of the central compartment *(15,82,85)*. This is because of the inability of liposomes to pass through the vasculature and accumulate in these tissues as a result of their prohibitively large size (~100 nm). Liposomes distribute primarily to the liver and spleen owing to the high number of phagocytic macrophages in these tissues that are responsible for their elimination *(33,89,90)*. The presence of a steric coat reduces the rate of liposome accumulation in these organs, although the spleen and liver remain the major sites for their disposition in vivo *(21,43,89)*. The ability to avoid uptake by these two major tissues allows for a greater probability of their accumulation in other target tissues, such as sites of inflammation *(91–93)* or various malignancies *(15,19,36,87–89)*.

Accumulation of liposomal drugs in solid tumors occurs as a result of extravasation through a discontinuous microvasculature supporting the tumor and the absence of functioning lymphatics *(6–8,94–97)*. The average size of the discontinuities varies greatly depending on the tumor microenvironment but, in general, are much greater (100–780 nm) than the size of the most commonly employed liposomes (~100 nm) *(5,7)*. Factors that control the rate of accumulation of liposomal drugs in tumors are not

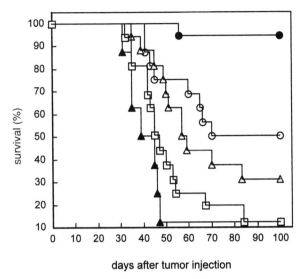

Fig. 3. Antitumor efficacy of free DOX (●) and SSL-DOX (○ ●), either alone (●, ○) or in combination with liposomal IL-2 (●), in the treatment of M109 pulmonary metastases. Control animals treated with saline (□) or liposomal IL-2 alone (▲) are also shown. BALB/c mice were inoculated intravenously (iv) with M109 tumor cells (10^6 cells) and DOX or SSL-DOX was administered on Day 7 after tumor inoculation at a dose of 8 mg/kg and IL-2 at a dose of 50,000 Cetus U/dose on Days 10, 13, and 16. (This figure was modified from Cabanes et al. *Clin Cancer Res* 1999; 5:687–693, with permission.)

fully understood at this time. Factors such as the size of the liposome relative to the gaps in the microvasculature, the stability of the formulation, the tumor microenvironment, and the presence of a PEG coat are likely involved in determining how rapidly liposomes extravasate across the tumor vasculature *(3,5,7,36,98–100)*. In general, the accumulation of free drug in tumor is relatively fast, reaching maximal levels within 1 hour. However, liposomal accumulation is much slower, with maximal accumulation in tumors varying from 8–48 h, depending on the formulation *(11,36,88,98,101–103)*. Total drug levels in the tumor can peak much earlier if the formulation at least partially leaks its contents while in the circulation, as is the case for rapid-release systems such as phosphatidylcholine derived from egg (eggPC:Chol) liposomes *(100,103)*, although the overall tumor AUC is considerably lower than for long-circulating slow-release formulations. The ability to manipulate vascular permeability, pharmacokinetic parameters, and the biodistribution of liposomal drugs for increased specificity of delivery to malignant tissues is extremely important in the design of more efficacious and less toxic liposomal drug delivery systems.

3.2. Antitumor Efficacy of Liposomal Drugs

Both sterically stabilized liposomal (SSL-) and conventional liposomal (CL-) drugs have been examined for antitumor efficacy in a wide variety of different tumor models *(9,19,20,59,81,87,98,101,104–107)*. Liposomal anthracycline formulations have been by far the most widely studied, although in recent years other liposomal drugs and combinations of drugs have been increasingly developed *(59,73,105,106,108)*. Many of these studies demonstrated a considerable survival advantage or reduction in tumor size following treatment with liposomal therapeutics when compared to free drug controls. When conventional and sterically stabilized formulations were compared directly at clinically relevant doses, the sterically stabilized formulations showed superior efficacy in most instances *(36,89,103,109)*. In a few studies, where exceedingly high and nonrelevant doses were used *(83,98)* or where the tumor was localized to either the liver or spleen (the major depots for liposomes in vivo) *(110)*, conventional formulations were shown to have similar efficacy to SSL formulations. Combinations of liposomal drugs with other therapeutic agents, such as interleukin 2 (IL-2) have been shown to increase therapeutic efficacy even further (Fig. 3) *(106)*. The use of drug combinations employing liposomal drugs will help increase the effectiveness of anticancer treatments by allowing drugs with different modes of action and drug resistance to be administered with a reduction in many of their dose-limiting toxicities. These studies give rise to significant hope that liposomal drugs will provide considerable improvements in therapeutic efficacy in addition to their well-documented reductions in many common toxicities (Subheading 4.2.).

4. CLINICAL RESULTS

There are presently many liposomal agents for the treatment of cancer that are already approved, awaiting approval by the appropriate drug regulatory agencies, in clinical trials, or in development by an everincreasing number of liposome or lipid-based formulation companies. A list of these products and their current status of development is given in Table 2. The most developed of liposome-formulated products are those containing anthracyclines. Anthracyclines are good candidates for liposome encapsulation due to their broad activity against a wide variety of human malignancies *(111,112)* and the physicochemical properties that facilitate their stable entrapment inside liposomes *(3,23,48)*. However, other drugs such as vincristine *(4,113)* and lurtotecan *(114,115)* are beginning to show considerable promise in early clinical studies.

4.1. Efficacy of Liposomal Drugs

Encapsulation of a therapeutic agent inside liposomes can result in a reduction in the grade of certain important toxicities, an increase in efficacy due to preferential accumulation in tumors or active targeting, a better quality of life owing to the mode of delivery or shift in toxicities, or a combination of these outcomes. Until recently, AIDS-related Kaposi's sarcoma had been the most commonly treated neoplasm in clinical trials using liposomal agents *(16,17,85,86,116–119)*. Single agent therapy using standard chemotherapy was ineffective in treating Kaposi's sarcoma and combination regimens including doxorubicin (DOX), bleomycin, and VCR (ABV regimens), or simply bleomycin and VCR (BV regimens), have been used in the clinical setting. However, both SSL-DOX and CL-daunorubicin have shown significant activity against Kaposi's sarcoma in various clinical trials *(16,17,85,86,116–119)*. Response rates varied considerably depending on the trial design and patient characteristics, but these approached 70–75% as a single agent in some trials *(116,118,120,121)* and was more effective than either free doxorubicin or the standard chemotherapy regimens *(16,17)*.

SSL-DOX was also effective in the treatment of breast *(122)* and ovarian cancers *(123,124)*. In addition, there were fewer problems with patient compliance because of the moderate degree of most toxicities (Subheading 4.2.; *125*). SSL-DOX was shown to accumulate in bone metastases from patients with breast carcinomas *(126)*. Rapid-

Table 2
Liposome- or Lipid-Based Therapeutics for the Treatment of Cancer

Company	Product	Progress
Alza Corporation (Palo Alto, CA)	Doxil: sterically stabilized (Stealth®) liposome formulation of doxorubicin	Approved for the treatment of ovarian cancer and Kaposi's sarcoma
Elan Pharmaceuticals (Dublin, Ireland)	Myocet: eggPC/Chol liposome formulation of doxorubicin	Approved in Europe
	TLC ELL-12: liposomal ether lipid	
Gilead Sciences (Foster City, CA)	DaunoXome: DSPC/Chol liposome formulation of daunorubicin	Approved for the treatment of Kaposi's sarcoma
	NX 211: Liposomal lurtotecan	Phase I: solid tumors, hematological malignancies
Inex Pharmaceuticals (Vancouver, BC, Canada)	Onco TCS: SM/Chol formulation of vincristine	Phase III: relapsed lymphoma Phase II: small cell lung cancer and first line lymphoma
	INXC-6295: liposomal mitoxantrone	In development
	INCX-3001: liposomal camptothecins	In development
Hermes Biosciences, Inc. (San Francisco, CA)	Anti-HER2 directed immunoliposome containing doxorubicin	Scale-up for phase I clinical trials (HER2 breast cancers)
Endovasc Ltd., Inc. (Montgomery, TX)	Liprostin TM: liposomal PGE1 formulation	In development
DepoTech (San Diego, CA)/Skye Pharma PLC (London, UK)	DepoCyt: a sustained-release multivesicular lipid-based formulation of cytosine arabinoside	Approved in US for lymphomatous meningitis
Biomira Inc. (Edmonton, AB, Canada)	Theratope®: MUC1-specific vaccine	Phase III: metastatic breast cancer
Valentis, Inc. (Burlingame, CA)	Cationic lipid-DNA complexes of IL-12 gene	Phase I/II: head and neck tumors
	Cationic lipid-DNA complexes of IL-2 gene	Phase IIa: malignant melanoma (w/superantigen) Phase IIb: head and neck (w/chemotherapy)
Aronex Pharmaceuticals, Inc. (The Woodlands, TX)	Platar (Aroplatin™): liposomal form of cis-Bis-neodecanoato-trans-R,R-1,2-diaminocyclohexane plantinum(II)	Phase II: mesothelioma (lung cancer) Phase II: renal cell carcinoma
	Atragen: liposomal form of all-trans retinoic acid	Phase II: Promyelocytic leukemia Phase II: Prostate cancer Phase I/II: Renal cell carcinoma Phase I/II: Bladder cancer

(Continued)

Table 2
(Continued)

Company	Product	Progress
	Annamycin: lipid-based anthra-cycline formulation (not recognized by MDR transporter)	Phase II: breast cancer
NeoPharm, Inc. (Bannockburn, IL) / Pharmacia (Peapack, NJ)	LEP: liposome-encapsulated paclitaxel	Phase II: various neoplasms
	LED: liposome-encapsulated doxorubicin	Phase II: prostate and breast cancer

release CL-DOX had similar efficacy against metastatic breast cancer but was administered at almost twice the dose (75 mg/m^2) as that used for SSL-DOX *(127)*. Elevation to even greater doses (135 mg/m^2 every 3 wk) was not associated with any additional clinical benefit *(128)*. In another study, CL-DOX was combined with cyclophosphamide and 5-fluorouracil to achieve a response rate of 73%, and a median duration of response of approx 11 mo in the treatment of metastatic breast cancer *(129)*. Other combinations are also being enthusiastically explored. A Phase I study combining SSL-DOX with vinorelbine for the treatment of metastatic breast cancer has been completed with relatively few toxicities observed *(130)*. SSL-DOX is also currently being combined with paclitaxel *(131,132)* or cyclophosphamide *(133)* for the treatment of metastatic breast cancer in different clinical trials. Combinations of CL-DOX with docetaxel or Herceptin® in clinical trials are also planned. Although both CL-DOX and SSL-DOX have been shown to be effective in treating ovarian and metastatic breast cancer when used as single agents, combinations with drugs having nonoverlapping modes of action or drug resistance may give rise to greater response rates and milder toxicities when compared to standard chemotherapy regimens.

Liposomal doxorubicin (L-DOX) and L-Daunorubicin are being studied in clinical trials in a number of other cancers as well. SSL-DOX was found to be ineffective for the treatment of soft tissue sarcomas *(134)* or advanced hepatocellular carcinoma *(135)*, despite the mild toxicity profile. Both of these studies were completed with patients who had advanced disease and a poor prognosis. CL-daunorubicin was also ineffective against hepatocellular carcinomas using doses of 100 mg/m^2 every 3 wk *(136)*. CL-daunorubicin is being studied for the treatment of tumors of the central nervous system *(137,138)*, with some effectiveness being noted in early trial results. SSL-DOX is being studied in combination with conventionally fractionated radiotherapy for the treatment of both head-and-neck cancer and non-small cell lung cancer *(139)*. This approach was shown to be feasible, although further study was suggested to determine the exact role of such a combination in the treatment of these cancers.

One of the most promising nonanthracycline liposome formulations is CL-vincristine. Liposomes in this formulation are composed of SM and Chol, and are loaded with vincristine using a pH-gradient method *(4,73)*. Phase I trials have been completed and have shown the liposomal formulation to be considerably less neurotoxic than the free drug *(4)*. In addition, preliminary Phase II trial results for the treatment of non-Hodgin's lymphomas (NHL) have shown CL-vincristine to be effective against transformed or aggressive NHL, but relatively ineffective in treating indolent NHL *(113)*.

Some preclinical studies have been completed with a SSL-vinorelbine as well, but clinical studies with these or similar formulations have not yet been performed *(108,140)*. A number of other liposomal drugs are also in clinical trials and continue to show promise in the treatment of cancer (Table 2). The full potential of liposomes in increasing the efficacy of antineoplastic agents has yet to be fully realized and further improvements in carrier design and treatment approach should lead to even greater advances in the future.

4.2. Toxicity Profiles of Liposomal Drugs

Liposome encapsulation results in a substantial shift in the toxicity profile of antineoplastic agents. For example, many of the common toxicities associated with free doxorubicin are considerably milder upon encapsulation of the drug inside liposomes *(82,90,122,141)*. These include cardiotoxicity, alopecia, nausea, vomiting, and local tissue necrosis at the site of injection due to extravasation of the drug. Cardiotoxicity is the therapy-limiting toxicity of many anthracyclines *(111,142)*, whereas myelosuppression is often the dose-limiting toxicity *(111,143,144)* of the free drug. The reduced ability of liposomal drugs to pass through the healthy endothelium into healthy tissues, such as cardiac muscle *(145)*, reduces considerably these toxicities *(90,117,141,146,147)*. Myelosuppression remains the dose-limiting toxicity for the two CL-anthracycline formulations in the clinical setting *(84,117,146,148)*, although at reduced levels when compared to free drug; this toxicity can be partially controlled through the addition of colony-stimulating factors *(146)*. The severity of many of the common toxicities are dependent on the rate of leakage from the liposomal carrier *(90,149,150)*. Liposomes that leak their contents more readily while in the circulation, for example, fast-release systems such as eggPC:Chol, usually have higher degrees of these toxicities. Liposome encapsulation of vincristine was shown to reduce the severity of neurotoxicity observed with the free drug *(4)* and the association of antitumor ether lipids with liposomes reduces the incidence of hemolytic anemia seen with other formulations of these lipids *(151,152)*.

However, depending on the mode of liposome encapsulation, certain other toxicities may be amplified. For example, with CL formulations, there is a greater risk of acquiring opportunistic infections *(153)* owing to localization of the drug in RES macrophages and the resulting macrophage toxicity *(154–156)*. This problem is accentuated in immune deficient patients, such as AIDS patients with Kaposi's sarcoma. In patients treated with SSL-DOX, palmar-plantar erythrodysesthesia syndrome, or hand and foot syndrome (H-F syndrome), they become dose limiting *(122,157,158)*. This painful desquamation of the skin on the hands and feet can be overcome by modifying the dose intensity *(122,159)*. In addition, mucositis is also slightly elevated in patients receiving SSL-DOX *(15,125,158)*. However, similar to H-F syndrome, this toxicity can be controlled by simple dose reduction. It is interesting to note that both of these toxicities are also seen in patients treated with prolonged infusions of certain chemotherapeutic drugs, such as doxorubicin *(125,160,161)*. Thus, the increase in these toxicities may result from either increased accumulation of long-circulating SSL in skin or because of the slow release of free doxorubicin from the liposomal carrier over an extended duration of time while in the circulation. Thus, although many of the commonly observed toxicities for free anthracyclines are reduced upon liposome encapsulation, the presence of alternative toxicities prevents dose intensification to achieve greater efficacy.

5. ACTIVE TARGETING OF LIPOSOMES

Thus far, we have been concerned primarily with liposomes that are passively targeted to solid tumors owing to their favorable pharmacokinetic parameters and the enhanced permeability of the tumor microvasculature. However, an additional increase in anti-cancer cytotoxicity or antitumor efficacy has been observed in cancers treated with lig-and-directed liposomes to tumor-specific antigens located on the surface of cancer cells *(9,24,162–167)*. An important criteria for their enhanced effectiveness is internalization of the bound liposome; this allows the liposomal drug access to the interior of the cancer cell, limits diffusion of the active agent away from the site of action, and results in the degradation of the carrier and, thus, release of the active agent from the confines of its carrier *(3,162)*. Vitamin and growth factor receptors are some of the more attractive targets because of their elevated levels of expression on neoplastic tissues and their ability to be internalized following binding to certain epitopes *(24,25,168–170)*. These types of targets have been the most commonly exploited in our laboratories.

There are many additional barriers to be overcome when actively targeting lipo-somes in vivo. Some preferable characteristics of ligand-targeted liposomal therapeu-tics and their targeted receptors are given in Table 3. These should be considered in addition to the properties of the carrier described in Table 1 for nontargeted liposomal therapeutics. For example, if liposomal drug formulations were unable to retain their drug while in the circulation, then little clinical benefit would result from active target-ing owing to loss of the active agent before reaching the target site. Ligands can be covalently bound to liposomes using a variety of different chemical linkages *(171–178)*. To ensure binding to cell surface receptors, ligands have been placed at the ends of PEG spacers to place them at a significant distance from the liposome surface and thus prevent steric hindrance of binding due to other moieties *(44,177)*, such as the PEG-DSPE used to increase circulation lifetimes in vivo. A very important characteristic of the targeting ligand is that it should be relatively nonimmunogenic. The attachment of antibodies to the surface of liposomes, either directly *(179)*, or via a PEG spacer *(180–184)*, has been shown to result in increased clearance and greater accumulation in RES organs. This effect is even more pronounced after repeated administration *(180)*. Fab' fragments can be attached to liposomes in an orientation-specific manner *(177,185,186)*, and are less immunogenic due to their lack of an Fc region which can cause recognition by the Fc receptor on macrophages *(187,188)*. In addition, "human-ized" antibody fragments have been conjugated to liposomes in an attempt to further reduce the immunogenicity *(9,25,165,177,189)*. Repeated administration of these lipo-somes resulted in no observed differences in pharmacokinetic parameters *(190)*. Another important characteristic is the nature of the hydrophobic anchor. As was men-tioned above, PEG is often used as a spacer to prevent steric hindrance of the attached ligand to its receptor. However, this spacer can also result in the conjugate being more hydrophilic and thus more readily extracted from the liposome while in the circulation. The conjugate should have a minimum of a distearoylglycero-based lipid anchor to prevent its extraction *(191)*. These characteristics of the liposomal carrier control the disposition in vivo and will ultimately help determine its effectiveness as a drug deliv-ery vehicle. Thus, while valuable, the addition of targeting ligands to the liposome for-mulation results in a considerable increase in the complexity of drug delivery with a significant number of new in vivo barriers to overcome.

Table 3
Desirable Ligand-Targeted Liposomal Therapeutics

Component	Considerations for optimum design
Target antigen	*Expression:*
	Highly and homogenously overexpressed in target tissue
	Function:
	Vital to tumor progression, so that down-modulation does not occur or is associated with therapeutic benefit
	Shedding of antigen:
	Limited, to avoid binding to soluble antigen and accelerated clearance
Targeting ligand	
	Affinity:
	High enough to ensure binding at low liposome concentrations
	Low enough to avoid "binding-site barrier" effect (Weinstein)
	Immunogenicity:
	Humanized MAb, to remove murine sequences. Use fragments without Fc portion (Fab', scFv) to avoid interaction with Fc receptor
	Small molecular weight ligands should not be immunogenic; may act as haptens
	Internalization:
	Efficient endocytosis by target cells is desirable for increasing drug release from the carrier
	Drug should be stable following internalization or able to efficiently escape the endosomal and lysosomal compartments (e.g., pH-sensitive liposomes)
	Production:
	Easy and economical scale-up, e.g., by efficient bacterial expression system
	Stable during storage
Membrane anchor	
	Stability:
	Covalent attachment to hydrophobic anchor, stable in blood
	Protein ligands are stable during storage
	Attachment site
	Away from the binding site, to ensure correct orientation of antibody or ligand molecule.
	Well-defined, to ensure reproducibility and uniformity of coupling
	Avoids steric hindrance (e.g., from PEG) of ligand binding and internalization
	Potential for being inserted into preformed and drug-loaded liposomes
	Chemical nature of the linker
	Non-toxic, non-immunogenic, and avoids opsonization
	Does not affect drug loading or membrane stability
	Excess linker may be quenched to avoid non-specific coupling to bio molecules
	Good availability, economical manufacturing process

The antigen being targeted should be located on the cell surface, be overexpressed on tumors and minimally expressed on healthy tissues having access to the vasculature, preferably be endocytosed following liposome binding, be vital to tumor progression so that the targeted antigen is not completely downmodulated, and have limited shedding. The accessibility of the targeted receptor is also a serious consideration. Targets that are readily accessible, such as those having direct exposure to the vasculature are in theory more attractive for active targeting. Small metastases, hematological cancers, and endothelial cells are examples of this class of targets and have been targeted using ligand-directed liposomes *(163,164,182,192–194)*. However, when considering targets such as small metastases or hematological cancers, the heterogeneity of expression becomes very important. The failure of a certain subset of tumor cells or metastases to express the desired receptor may result in a population of resistant tumors.

Solid tumors are thought to be relatively more difficult to treat because of the poor penetration of liposomes into the tumor mass *(95)* and owing to the binding site barrier *(195–197)* whereby targeted liposomes are localized to target receptors on the surface of the tumor mass. However, by using small molecular weight and low-affinity ligands to target receptors on the tumor surface liposomes are able to partially bypass the binding site barrier and distribute more uniformly within the tumor (Kirpotin et al., unpublished observations) *(3,24)*. The enhanced activity in solid tumors may be because of an enhanced bioavailability of the drug following degradation in the lysosomes of cancer cells and the reduced diffusion of released drug from the tumor. Solid tumors will likely suffer less from receptor heterogeneity because neighboring nonoverexpressing cancer cells may be killed by drug released from adjacent or dying cells: the bystander effect. One important consideration when targeting internalizing receptors is the stability of the drug to be encapsulated. Because endocytosis often results in accumulation of liposomes in the degradative and acidic environment of late endosomes and lysosomes, a therapeutic agent labile under these conditions may be ineffective *(198)*. It should be noted that, unlike targeting more accessible antigens, liposomes targeted to receptors on solid tumors do not accumulate in these tumors to an extent greater than for similar nontargeted formulations *(102,189)*. This suggests that accumulation of targeted liposomes in solid tumors is limited not by specific binding to cell surface receptors, but by the rate of extravasation across the tumor microvasculature and the degree of trapping in these tumors owing to the lack of a functioning lymphatics. It also suggests that the observed increases in efficacy are caused by differences in the bioavailability and distribution of the drug in the tumor following extravasation. These results with solid tumors are encouraging and suggest that, using optimized liposome constructs, other solid tumors may be effectively targeted in the future.

6. CONCLUSIONS

Great progress has been and is continuing to be made in the development of liposomal drugs for treating human malignancies. Greater optimization of physical properties controlling both pharmacokinetic parameters of liposomal drugs and drug release rates from liposomal carriers are still needed and could yield even greater increases in the therapeutic index of these drugs. Combinations of liposomal drugs or conventional free drugs with liposomal drugs need to be explored further in the clinical setting, and many of these studies are currently underway with the anthracycline formulations Doxil® or Evacet™. Tremendous opportunities also remain in increasing the specificity of delivery by ligand-directed targeting of liposomes to tumor-specific antigens located on tumor cell surfaces. The mechanisms affecting their delivery in vivo have yet to be fully explored and continued study in this area is needed. Finally, advances in the development of delivery systems for therapeutic genes and antisense oligonucleotides using cationic lipid-based formulations are beginning to offer promise for the development of complimentary therapies. The considerable achievements in the liposome field over the past several decades, and the excitement of the yet unknown, provide significant promise and opportunity that drug delivery systems such as liposomes will provide unprecedented increases in the therapeutic index of anticancer drugs and give rise to great improvements in the overall quality of life for cancer patients.

ACKNOWLEDGMENTS

This work was supported in part by grants from the NIH (1RO1CA72452 & 1R01-CA71653-01) and the California Breast Cancer Research Program (2CB-0004). The work of Daryl C. Drummond is supported by a postdoctoral fellowship from the Breast Cancer Research Program of the University of California, Grant Number 4FB-0154.

REFERENCES

1. Gabizon AA. Clinical trials of liposomes as carriers of chemotherapeutic agents: synopsis and perspective, in *Medical Applications of Liposomes* (Lasic DD, Papahadjopoulos D, eds). Elsevier Science B.V., New York, 1998, pp 625–634.
2. Martin FJ. Clinical pharmacology and antitumor efficacy of DOXIL (pegylated liposomal doxorubicin), in *Medical Applications of Liposomes* (Lasic DD, Papahadjopoulos D, eds). Elsevier Science B.V., New York, 1998, pp 635–688.
3. Drummond DC, Meyer OM, Hong K, Kirpotin DB, Papahadjopoulos D. Optimizing liposomes for delivery of chemotherapeutic agents to solid tumors. *Pharmacol Rev* 1999; 51:691–743.
4. Gelmon KA, Tolcher A, Diab AR, et al. Phase I study of liposomal vincristine. *J Clin Oncol* 1999; 17:697–705.
5. Hobbs SK, Monsky WL, Yuan F, et al. Regulation of transport pathways in tumor vessels: role of tumor type and microenvironment. *Proc Natl Acad Sci USA* 1998; 95:4607–4612.
6. Huang SK, Martin FJ, Jay G, Vogel J, Papahadjopoulos D, Friend DS. Extravasation and transcytosis of liposomes in Kaposi's sarcoma-like dermal lesions of transgenic mice bearing the HIV Tat gene. *Am J Path* 1993; 143:10–14.
7. Yuan F, Lwunig M, Huang SK, Berk DA, Papahadjopoulos D, Jain RK. Microvascular permeability and interstitial penetration of sterically stabilized (stealth) liposomes in a human tumor xenograft. *Cancer Res* 1994; 54:3352–3356.
8. Yuan F, Dellian M, Fukumura D, et al. Vascular permeability in a human tumor xenograft: molecular size dependence and cutoff size. *Cancer Res* 1995; 55:3752–3756.
9. Park JW, Hong K, Kirpotin DB, Meyer O, Papahadjopoulos D, Benz CC. Anti-HER2 immunoliposomes for targeted therapy of human tumors. *Cancer Lett* 1997; 118:153–160.
10. Horowitz AR, Barenholz Y, Gabizon AA. In vitro cytotoxicity of liposome-encapsulated doxorubicin: dependence on liposome composition and drug release. *Biochim Biophys Acta* 1992; 1109:203–209.
11. Vaage J, Donovan D, Working P, Uster P. Cellular distribution of DOXIL® within selected tissues, assessed by confocal laser scanning microscopy, in *Medical Applications of Liposomes* (Lasic D, Papahadjopoulos D, ed). Elsevier Science B.V., New York, 1998, pp 275–282.
12. Hwang KJ, Liposome pharmacokinetics, in *Liposomes: from biophysics to therapeutics* (Ostro MJ, ed). Marcel Dekker, New York, 1987, pp 109–156.
13. Allen TM, Hansen CB, Lopes de Menezes DE. Pharmacokinetics of long-circulating liposomes. *Adv Drug Del Rev* 1995; 16:267–284.
14. Allen TM, Stuart DD. Liposome pharmacokinetics. Classical, sterically-stabilized, cationic liposomes and immunoliposomes, in *Liposomes: Rational Design* (Janoff AS, ed). Marcel Dekker, New York, 1999, pp 63–87.

15. Gabizon A, Catane R, Uziely B, Kaufman B, Safra T. Prolonged circulation time and enhanced accumulation in malignant exudates of doxorubicin encapsulated in polyethylene-glycol coated liposomes. *Cancer Res* 1994; 54:987–992.

16. Northfelt DW, Dezube BJ, Thommes JA, et al. Pegylated-liposomal doxorubicin versus doxorubicin, bleomycin, and vincristine in the treatment of AIDS-related Kaposi's sarcoma: results of a randomized phase III clinical trial. *J Clin Oncol* 1998; 16:2445–2551.

17. Stewart S, Jablonowski H, Goebel FD, et al. Randomized comparative trial of pegylated liposomal doxorubicin versus bleomycin and vincristine in the treatment of AIDS-related Kaposi's sarcoma. *J Clin Oncol* 1998; 16:683–691.

18. Klibanov AL, Maruyama K, Torchilin VP, Huang L. Amphipathic polyethyleneglycols effectively prolong the circulation time of liposomes. *FEBS Lett* 1990; 268:235–237.

19. Papahadjopoulos D, Allen TM, Gabizon A, et al. Sterically stabilized liposomes: improvements in pharmacokinetics and antitumor therapeutic efficacy. *Proc Natl Acad Sci USA* 1991; 88:11,460–11,464.

20. Allen TM, Newman MS, Woodle MC, Mayhew E, Uster PS. Pharmacokinetics and anti-tumor activity of vincristine encapsulated in sterically stabilized liposomes. *Int J Cancer* 1995; 62:199–204.

21. Woodle MC. Controlling liposome blood clearance by surface-grafted polymers. *Adv Drug Del Rev* 1998; 32:139–152.

22. Bally MB, Lim H, Cullis PR, Mayer LD. Controlling the drug delivery attributes of lipid-based drug formulations. *J Liposome Res* 1998; 8:299–335.

23. Barenholz Y. Design of liposome-based drug carriers: from basic research to application as approved drugs, in *Medical Applications of Liposomes* (Lasic DD, Papahadjopoulos D, eds). Elsevier Science B.V., New York, 1998, pp 545–565.

24. Kirpotin DB, Park JW, Hong K, et al. Targeting of liposomes to solid tumors: the case of sterically stabilized anti-HER2 immunoliposomes. *J Liposome Res* 1997; 7:391–417.

25. Park JW, Hong K, Kirpotin DB, Papahadjopoulos D, Benz CC. Immunoliposomes for cancer treatment. *Adv Pharmacol* 1997; 40:399–435.

26. Senior JH. Fate and behaviour of liposomes in vivo: a review of controlling factors. *CRC Crit Rev Therap Drug Carrier System* 1987; 3:123–193.

27. Abra RM, Hunt CA. Liposome disposition in vivo. III. Dose and vesicle-size effects. *Biochim Biophys Acta* 1981; 666:493–503.

28. Ishida O, Maruyama K, Sasaki K, Iwatsuru M. Size-dependent extravasation and interstitial localization of polyethyleneglycol liposomes in solid tumor-bearing mice. *Int J Pharmaceut* 1999; 190:49–56.

29. Senior JH. Medical applications of multivesicular lipid-based particles: DepoFoam™ encapsulated drugs, in *Medical Applications of Liposomes* (Lasic DD, Papahadjopoulos D, eds). Elsevier Science B.V., New York, 1998, pp 733–750.

30. Johnson EM, Ojwang JO, Szekely A, Wallace TL, Warnock DW. Comparison of in vitro antifungal activities of free and liposome-encapsulated nystatin with those of four amphotericin B formulations. *Antimicrob Agents Chemother* 1998; 42:1412–1416.

31. Woodle MC, Matthay KK, Newman MS, et al. Versatility in lipid compositions showing prolonged circulation with sterically stabilized liposomes. *Biochim Biophys Acta* 1992; 1105:193–200.

32. Ahl PL, Bhatia SK, Meers P, et al. Enhancement of the in vivo circulation lifetime of L-alpha-distearoylphosphatidylcholine liposomes: importance of liposomal aggregation versus complement opsonization. *Biochim Biophys Acta* 1997; 1329:370–382.

33. Senior J, Crawley JCW, Gregoriadis G. Tissue distribution of liposomes exhibiting long half-lives in the circulation after intravenous injection. *Biochim Biophys Acta* 1985; 839:1–8.

34. Gabizon A, Papahadjopoulos D. Liposome formulations with prolonged circulation time in blood and enhanced uptake in tumors. *Proc Natl Acad Sci USA* 1988; 85:6949–6953.

35. Allen TM, Hansen C, Martin F, Redemann C, Yau-Young A. Liposomes containing synthetic lipid derivatives of poly(ethylene glycol) show prolonged circulation half-lives in vivo. *Biochim Biophys Acta* 1991; 1066:29–36.

36. Gabizon A, Chemla M, Tzemach D, Horowitz AT, Goren D. Liposome longevity and stability in circulation: effects on the in vivo delivery to tumors and therapeutic efficacy of encapsulated anthracyclines. *J Drug Target* 1996; 3:391–398.

37. Gregoriadis G, Senior J. The phospholipid component of small unilamellar liposomes controls the rate of clearance of entrapped solutes from the circulation. *FEBS Lett* 1980; 119:43–46.

38. Patel HM. Serum opsonins and liposomes: their interaction and opsonophagocytosis. *CRC Crit Rev Therap Drug Carrier System* 1992; 9:39–90.

39. Semple SC, Chonn A. Liposome-blood protein interactions in relation to liposome clearance. *J Liposome Res* 1996; 6:33–60.
40. Moghimi SM, Patel HM. Serum opsonins and phagocytosis of saturated and unsaturated phospholipid liposomes. *Biochim Biophys Acta* 1989; 984:384–387.
41. Allen TM. A study of phospholipid interactions between high-density lipoproteins and small unilamellar vesicles. *Biochim Biophys Acta* 1981; 640:385–397.
42. Damen J, Regts J, Scherphof G. Transfer and exchange of phospholipid between small unilamellar liposomes and rat plasma high density lipoproteins: dependence on cholesterol content and phospholipid composition. *Biochim Biophys Acta* 1981; 665:538–545.
43. Allen TM. The use of glycolipids and hydrophilic polymers in avoiding rapid uptake of liposomes by the mononuclear phagocyte system. *Adv Drug Del Rev* 1994; 13:285–309.
44. Klibanov AL, Maruyama K, Beckerleg AM, Torchilin VP, Huang L. Activity of amphipathic poly(ethylene glycol) 5000 to prolong the circulation time of liposomes depends on the liposome size and is unfavorable for immunoliposomes binding to target. *Biochim Biophys Acta* 1991; 1062:142–148.
45. Lasic DD, Martin FJ, Gabizon A, Huang SK, Papahadjopoulos D. Sterically stabilized liposomes: a hypothesis on the molecular origin of the extended circulation times. *Biochim Biophys Acta* 1991; 1070:187–192.
46. Needham DKH, McIntosh TJ, Dewhirst M, Lasic DD. Polymer-grafted liposome: physical basis for the "stealth" property. *J Liposome Res* 1992; 2:411–430.
47. Needham D, Zhelev DV, McIntosh TJ. Surface chemistry of the sterically stabilized PEG-liposome, in *Liposomes: Rational Design* (Janoff AS, ed). Marcel Dekker, New York, 1999, pp 13–62.
48. Barenholz Y, Cohen R. Rational design of amphiphile-based drug carriers and sterically stabilized carriers. *J Liposome Res* 1995; 5:905–932.
49. Lasic DD, Ceh B, Stuart MCA, Guo L, Frederik PM, Barenholz Y. Transmembrane gradient driven phase transitions within vesicles: lessons for drug delivery. *Biochim Biophys Acta* 1995; 1239:145–156.
50. Haran G, Cohen R, Bar LK, Barenholz Y. Transmembrane ammonium sulfate gradients in liposomes produce efficient and stable entrapment of amphiphathic weak bases. *Biochim Biophys Acta* 1993; 1151:201–215.
51. Fenske DB, Wong KF, Maurer E, et al. Ionophore-mediated uptake of ciprofloxacin and vincristine into large unilamellar vesicles exhibiting transmembrane ion gradients. *Biochim Biophys Acta* 1998; 1414:188–204.
52. Cullis PR, Hope MJ, Bally MB, Madden TD, Mayer LD, Fenske DB. Influence of pH gradients on the transbilayer transport of drugs, lipids, peptides and metal ions into large unilamellar vesicles. *Biochim Biophys Acta* 1997; 1331:187–211.
53. Madden TD, Harrigan PR, Tai LCL, et al. The accumulation of drugs within large unilamellar vesicles exhibiting a proton gradient: a survey. *Chem Phys Lipids* 1990; 53:37–46.
54. Mayer LD, Bally MB, Hope MJ, Cullis PR. Uptake of antineoplastic agents into large unilamellar vesicles in response to a membrane potential. *Biochim Biophys Acta* 1985; 816:294–302.
55. Bally MB, Nayar R, Masin D, Hope MJ, Cullis PR, Mayer L. Liposomes with entrapped doxorubicin exhibit extended blood residence times. *Biochim Biophys Acta* 1990; 1023:133–139.
56. Gabizon AA, Barenholz Y, Bialer M. Prolongation of the circulation time of doxorubicin encapsulated in liposomes containing polyethylene glycol-derivatized phospholipid: pharmacokinetic studies in rodents and dogs. *Pharm Res* 1993; 10:703–708.
57. Allison BA, Pritchard PH, Richter AM, Levy JG. The plasma distribution of benzoporphyrin derivative and the effects of plasma lipoproteins on its biodistribution. *Photochem Photobiol* 1990; 52:501–507.
58. Sharma A, Sharma US, Straubinger RM. Paclitaxel-liposomes for intracavitary therapy of intraperitoneal P388 leukemia. *Cancer Lett* 1996; 107:265–272.
59. Sharma A, Mayhew E, Bolcsak L, Cavanaugh C, Harmon P. Activity of paclitaxel liposome formulations against human ovarian tumor xenografts. *Int J Cancer* 1997; 71:103–107.
60. Reddi E. Role of delivery vehicles for photosensitizers in the photodynamic therapy of tumors. *J Photochem Photobiol B: Biol* 1997; 37:189–95.
61. Ramaswamy M, Wallace TL, Cossum PA, Wasan KM. Species differences in the proportion of plasma lipoprotein lipid carried by high-density lipoproteins influence the distribution of free and liposomal nystatin in human, dog, and rat plasma. *Antimicrob Agents Chemother* 1999; 43:1424–1428.

62. Zignani M, Drummond DC, Meyer O, Hong K, Leroux JC. In vitro characterization of a novel polymeric-based pH-sensitive liposome system. *Biochim Biophys Acta* 2000; 1463:383–394.

63. Düzgünes N, Straubinger RM, Baldwin PA, Papahadjopoulos D. pH-Sensitive Liposomes: Introduction of foreign substances into cells, in *Membrane Fusion* (Wilschut J, Hoekstra D, eds). Marcel Dekker, New York, 1991, pp 713–730.

64. Litzinger DC, Huang L. Phosphatidylethanolamine liposomes: drug delivery, gene transfer, and immunodiagnostic applications. *Biochim Biophys Acta* 1992; 1113:201–227.

65. Torchilin VP, Zhou F, Huang L. pH-Sensitive liposomes. *J Liposome Res* 1993; 3:201–255.

66. Huang SK, Stauffer PR, Hong K, et al. Liposomes and hyperthermia in mice: increased tumor uptake and therapeutic efficacy of doxorubicin in sterically stabilized liposomes. *Cancer Res* 1994; 54:2186–2191.

67. Gaber MH, Wu NZ, Hong K, Huang SK, Dewhirst MW, Papahadjopoulos D. Thermosensitive liposomes: extravasation and release of contents in tumor microvascular networks. *Int J Radiat Oncol Biol Phys* 1996; 36:1177–1187.

68. Gaber MH, Hong K, Huang SK, Papahadjopoulos D. Thermosensitive sterically stabilized liposomes: formulation and in vitro studies on the mechanism of doxorubicin release by bovine serum and human plasma. *Pharm Res* 1995; 12:1407–1416.

69. Wiley JS, Jones SP, Sawyer WH, Paterson ARP. Cytosine arabinoside influx and nucleoside transport sites in acute leukemia. *J Clin Invest* 1982; 69:479–489.

70. Plageman PGW, Marz R, Wohlhueter RM. Transport and metabolism of deoxycytidine and 1-β-D-arabinofuranosyl-cytosine into cultured Novikoff rap hepatoma cells, relationship to phosphorylation, and regulation of triphosphate synthesis. *Cancer Res* 1978; 38:978–989.

71. Westerhof GR, Rijnboutt S, Schornagel JH, Pinedo HM, Peters GJ, Jansen G. Functional activity of the reduced folate carrier in KB, MA104, and IGROV-I cells expressing folate binding protein. *Cancer Res* 1995; 55:3795–3802.

72. Westerhof GR, Jansen G, van Emmerik N, et al. Membrane transport of natural folates and antifolate compounds in murine L1210 Leukemia cells: role of carrier- and receptor-mediated transport systems *Cancer Res* 1991; 51:5507–5513.

73. Webb MS, Harasym TO, Masin D, Bally MB, Mayer LD. Sphingomyelin-cholesterol liposomes significantly enhance the pharmacokinetic and therapeutic properties of vincristine in murine and human tumour models. *Br J Cancer* 1995; 72:896–904.

74. Li X, Cabral-Lilly D, Janoff AS, Perkins WR. Complexation of internalized doxorubicin into fiber bundles affects its release rate from liposomes. *J Liposome Res* 2000; 10:15–27.

75. Maurer-Spurej E, Wong KF, Maurer N, Fenske DB, Cullis PR. Factors influencing uptake and retention of amino-containing drugs in large unilamellar vesicles exhibiting transmembrane pH gradients. *Biochim Biophys Acta* 1999; 1416:1–10.

76. Mui BL-S, Cullis PR, Pritchard PH, Madden TD. Influence of plasma on the osmotic sensitivity of large unilamellar vesicles prepared by extrusion. *J Biol Chem* 1994; 269:7364–7370.

77. Adlakha-Hutcheon G, Bally MB, Shew CR, Madden TD. Controlled destabilization of a liposomal drug delivery system enhances mitoxantrone antitumor activity. *Nature Biotech* 1999; 17:775–779.

78. Kirpotin D, Hong K, Mullah N, Papahadjopoulos D, Zalipsky S. Liposomes with detachable polymer coating: destabilization and fusion of dioleoylphosphatidylethanolamine vesicles triggered by cleavage of surface-grafted poly(ethylene glycol). *FEBS Lett* 1996; 388:115–118.

79. Zalipsky S, Qazen M, Walker JA, 2nd, Mullah N, Quinn YP, Huang SK. New detachable poly(ethylene glycol) conjugates: cysteine-cleavable lipopolymers regenerating natural phospholipid, diacyl phosphatidylethanolamine. *Bioconj Chem* 1999; 10:703–707.

80. Pak CC, Erukulla RK, Ahl PL, Janoff AS, Meers P. Elastase activated liposomal delivery to nucleated cells. *Biochim Biophys Acta* 1999; 1419:111–126.

81. Mayhew EG, Lasic D, Babbar S, Martin FJ. Pharmacokinetics and antitumor activity of epirubicin encapsulated in long-circulating liposomes incorporating a polyethlene glycol-derivatized phospholipid. *Int J Cancer* 1992; 51:302–309.

82. Working PK, Dayan AD. Pharmacological-toxicological expert report – Caelyx™. (Stealth® liposomal doxorubicin HCl) – Foreword. *Hum Exp Toxicol* 1996; 15:751–785.

83. Parr MJ, Masin D, Cullis PR, Bally MB. Accumulation of liposomal lipid and encapsulated doxorubicin in murine lewis lung carcinoma: the lack of beneficial effects of coating liposomes with poly(ethylene glycol). *J Pharmacol Exp Therapeut* 1997; 280:1319–1327.

84. Cowens JW, Creaven PJ, Greco WR, et al. Initial clinical (phase I) trial of TLC D-99 (doxorubicin encapsulated in liposomes). *Cancer Res* 1993; 53:2796–2802.

85. Gill PS, Espina BM, Muggia F, Cabriales S, Tulpule A, Esplin JA, Phase I/II clinical and pharmacokinetic evaluation of liposomal daunorubicin. *J Clin Oncol* 1995; 13:996–1003.

86. Northfelt DW, Martin FJ, Working P, et al. Doxorubicin encapsulated in liposomes containing surface-bound polyethylene glycol: pharmacokinetics, tumor localization, and safety in patients with AIDS-related Kaposi's Sarcoma. *J Clin Pharmacol* 1996; 36:55–63.

87. Gabizon A, Goren D, Horowitz AT, Tzemach D, Lossos A, Siegal T. Long-circulating liposomes for drug delivery in cancer therapy: A review of biodistribution studies in tumor-bearing animals. *Adv Drug Del Rev* 1997; 24:337–344.

88. Forssen EA, Coulter DM, Proffitt RT. Selective in vivo localization of daunorubicin small unilamellar vesicles in solid tumors. *Cancer Res* 1992; 52:3255–3261.

89. Huang SK, Mayhew E, Gilani S, Lasic DD, Martin FJ, Papahadjopoulos D. Pharmacokinetics and therapeutics of sterically stabilized liposomes in mice bearing C-26 colon carcinoma. *Cancer Res* 1992; 52:6774–6781.

90. Mayer LD, Tai LCL, Ko DSC, et al. Influence of vesicle size, lipid composition, and drug-to-lipid ratio on the biological activity of liposomal doxorubicin in mice. *Cancer Res* 1989; 49:5922–5930.

91. Laverman P, Boerman OC, Oyen, WJG, Dams ETM, Storm G, Corstens FHM. Liposomes for scintigraphic detection of infection and inflammation. *Adv Drug Del Rev* 1999; 37:225–235.

92. Bakker-Woudenberg IAJM, Lokerse AF, Kate MTt, Storm G. Enhanced localization of liposomes with prolonged blood circulation time in infected lung tissue. *Biochim Biophys Acta* 1992; 1138:318–326.

93. Oyen WJG, Boerman OC, Storm G, et al. Detecting infection and inflammation with technetium-99m-labeled Stealth® liposomes. *J Nucl Med* 1996; 37:1392–1397.

94. Jain RK. Delivery of molecular medicine to solid tumors. *Science* 1996; 271:1079–1080.

95. Huang SK, Lee K-D, Hong K, Friend DS, Papahadjopoulos D. Microscopic localization of sterically stabilized liposomes in colon carcinoma-bearing mice. *Cancer Res* 1992; 52:5135–5143.

96. Matsumura Y, Maeda H. A new concept for macromolecular therapeutics in cancer chemotherapy: mechanism of tumoritropic accumulation of proteins and the antitumor agent. SMANCS *Cancer Res* 1986; 46:6387–6392.

97. Maeda H, Matsumura Y. Tumoritropic and lymphotropic principles of macromolecular drugs. *CRC Crit Rev Therap Drug Carrier Syst* 1989; 6:193–210.

98. Mayer LD, Dougherty G, Harasym TO, Bally MB. The role of tumor-associated macrophages in the delivery of liposomal doxorubicin to solid murine fibroscarcoma tumors. *J Pharmacol Exp Therapeut* 1997; 280:1406–1414.

99. Mayer LD, Cullis PR, Bally MB. Designing therapeutically optimized liposomal anticancer delivery systems: lessons from conventional liposomes, in *Medical Applications of Liposomes* (Papahadjopoulos LA, ed). Elsevier Science B.V., New York, 1998.

100. Harasym TO, Cullis PR, Bally MB. Intratumor distribution of doxorubicin following i.v. administration of drug encapsulated in egg phophatidylcholine/cholesterol liposomes. *Cancer Chemother Pharmacol* 1997; 40:309–317.

101. Siegal T, Horowitz A, Gabizon A. Doxorubicin encapsulated in sterically stabilized liposomes for the treatment of a brain tumor model: biodistribution and therapeutic efficacy. *J Neurosurg* 1995; 83:1029–1037.

102. Goren D, Horowitz AT, Zalipsky S, Woodle MC, Yarden Y, Gabizon A. Targeting of stealth liposomes to erbB-2 (Her/2) receptor: In vitro and in vivo studies. *Br J Cancer* 1996; 74:1749–1756.

103. Krishna R, St-Louis M, Mayer LD. Increased intracellular drug accumulation and complete chemosensitization achieved in multidrug-resistant solid tumors by co-administering valspodar (PSC 833) with sterically stabilized liposomal doxorubicin. *Int J Cancer* 2000; 85:131–141.

104. Allen TM, Mehra T, Hansen C, Chin YC. Stealth liposomes: an improved sustained release system for 1-β-D-arabinofuranosylcytosine. *Cancer Res* 1992; 52:2431–2439.

105. Colbern GT, Dykes DJ, Engbers C, et al. Encapsulation of the topoisomerase I inhibitor GL147211C in pegylated (STEALTH) liposomes: pharmacokinetics and antitumor activity in HT29 colon tumor xenografts. *Clin Cancer Res* 1998; 4:3077–3082.

106. Cabanes A, Even-Chen S, Zimberoff J, Barenholz Y, Kedar E, Gabizon A. Enhancement of antitumor activity of polyethylene glycol-coated liposomal doxorubicin with soluble and liposomal interleukin 2. *Clin Cancer Res* 1999; 5:687–693.

107. Newman MS, Colbern GT, Working PK, Engbers C, Amantea M. Comparative pharmacokinetics, tissue distribution, and therapeutic effectiveness of cisplatin encapsulated in long-circulating, pegylated liposomes (SPI-077) in tumor-bearing mice. *Cancer Chemother Pharmacol* 1999; 43:1–7.

108. Colbern G, Vaage J, Donovan D, Uster P, Working P, Tumor uptake and therapeutic effects of drugs encapsulated in long-circulating pegylated STEALTH® liposomes. *J Liposome Res* 2000; 10:81–92.

109. Unezaki S, Mauryama K, Ishida O, Suginaka A, Jun-ichi H, Iwatsuru M. Enhanced tumor targeting and improved antitumor activity of doxorubicin by long-circulating liposomes containing amphipathic poly(ethylene glycol). *Int J Pharmaceut* 1995; 126:41–48.

110. Chang CW, Barber L, Ouyang C, Masin D, Bally MB, Madden TD. Plasma clearance, biodistribution and therapeutic properties of mitoxantrone encapsulated in conventional and sterically stabilized liposomes after intravenous administration in BDF1 mice. *Br J Cancer* 1997; 75:169–177.

111. Doroshaw JH, Anthracyclines and antracenediones, in *Cancer chemotherapy and biotherapy: principles and practice* (Chabner BA, Longo DL, eds). Lippincott-Raven, Philadelphia, 1996, pp 409–433.

112. Young RC, Ozols RF, Myers CE. The anthracycline antineoplastic drugs. *N Engl J Med* 1981; 305:139–153.

113. Sarris AH, Hagemeister F, Romaguera J, et al. Liposomal vincristine in relapsed non-Hodgkin's lymphomas: early results of an ongoing phase II trial. *Ann Oncol* 2000; 11:69–72.

114. Kruszewski S, Chavan AS, Grycynski I, Lakowicz JR, Burke TG. Comparison of the human blood chemistry of free versus liposomal forms of the clinically-relevant topoisomerase I inhibitor lurtotecan (GI147221). *Am Assoc Cancer Res* 2000; 41:A2056.

115. Gelmon KA, Eisenhauer E, Renyo L, et al. Phase I study of NX211 (liposomal lurtotecan) given as an intravenous infusion on days 1 2 &3 every 3 weeks in patients with solid tumors- and NCIC Clinical Trials Group study. *Am Assoc Cancer Res* 2000; 41:A3879.

116. Amantea MA, Forrest A, Northfelt DW, Mamelok R. Population pharmacokinetics and pharmacodynamics of pegylated-liposomal doxorubicin in patients with AIDS-related Kaposi's sarcoma. *Clin Pharmacol Therap* 1997; 61:301–311.

117. Gill PS, Wernz J, Scadden DT, et al. Randomized phase III trial of liposomal daunorubicin versus doxorubicin, bleomycin, and vincristine in AIDS-related Kaposi's sarcoma. *J Clin Oncol* 1996; 14:2353–2364.

118. Girard PM, Bouchaud O, Goetschel A, Mukwaya G, Eestermans G, Ross M. Phase II study of liposomal encapsulated daunorubicin in the treatment of AIDS-associated mucocutaneous Kaposi's sarcoma. *Aids* 1996; 10:753–757.

119. Presant CA, Scolaro M, Kennedy P, et al. Liposomal daunorubicin treatment of HIV-associated Kaposi's sarcoma. *Lancet* 1993; 341:1242–1243.

120. Tulpule A, Yung RC, Wernz J, et al. Phase II trial of liposomal daunorubicin in the treatment of AIDS-related pulmonary Kaposi's sarcoma. *J Clin Oncol* 1998; 16:3369–3374.

121. Harrison M, Tomlinson D, Stewart S. Liposomal-entrapped doxorubicin: an active agent in AIDS-related Kaposi's sarcoma. *J Clin Oncol* 1995; 13:914–920.

122. Ranson MR, Carmichael J, O'Byrne K, Stewart S, Smith D, Howell A. Treatment of advanced breast cancer with sterically stabilized liposomal doxorubicin: results of a multicenter phase II trial. *J Clin Oncol* 1997; 15:3185–3191.

123. Muggia FM. Clinical efficacy and prospects for use of pegylated liposomal doxorubicin in the treatment of ovarian and breast cancers. *Drugs* 1997; 54:22–29.

124. Muggia FM, Hainsworth JD, Jeffers S, et al. Phase II study of liposomal doxorubicin in refactory ovarian cancer: antitumor activity and toxicity modification by liposomal encapsulation. *J Clin Oncol* 1997; 15:987–993.

125. Alberts DS, Garcia DJ. Safety aspects of pegylated liposomal doxorubicin in patients with cancer. *Drugs* 1997; 54 Suppl. 4:30–35.

126. Symon Z, Peyser A, Tzemach D, et al. Selective delivery of doxorubicin to patients with breast carcinoma metastases by stealth liposomes. *Cancer* 1999; 86:72–78.

127. Harris L, Winer E, Batist G, Rovira D, Navaria R, Lee L. Phase III study of TLC D-99 (liposome encapsulated doxorubicin) vs. free doxorubicin (DOX) in patients with metastatic breast carcinoma (MBC). *Proc Am Soc Clin Oncol* 1998; 17:124a.

128. Shapiro CL, Ervin T, Welles L, Azarnia N, Keating J, Hayes DF. Phase II trial of high-dose liposome-encapsulated doxorubicin with granulocyte colony-stimulating factor in metastic breast cancer. *J Clin Oncol* 1999; 17:1435–1441.

129. Valero V, Buzdar AU, Theriault RL, et al. Phase II trial of liposome-encapsulated doxorubicin cyclophosphamide, and fluorouracil as first-line therapy in patients with metastatic breast cancer. *J Clin Oncol* 1999; 17:1425–1434.

130. Burstein HJ, Ramirez MJ, Petros WP, et al. Phase I study of Doxil and vinorelbine in metastatic breast cancer. *Ann Oncol* 1999; 10:1113–1116.

131. Woll PJ, Carmichael J, Chan S, Howell A, Ranson M, Miles D, Welbank H. Phase II study results on safety and tolerability of caelyx® (Doxil®) in combination with paclitaxel in the treatment of metastatic breast cancer. *Proc Am Soc Clin Oncol* 1999; 18:A442.

132. Modiano M, Taylor C, Sharpington R, Ng M, Martinez A. Phase I study of Doxil® (pegylated liposomal doxorubicin) plus escalating doses of taxol® in the treatment of patients with advanced breast or gynecologic malignancies. *Proc Am Soc Clin Oncol* 1999; 18:A848.

133. Silverman P, Overmoyer B, Holder L, Tripathy D, Marrs N, Sharpington T. Doxil® and intravenous cyclophosphamide as first-line therapy for patients with metastatic breast cancer (MBC): interim results of an ongoing pilot trial. *Proc Am Soc Clin Oncol* 1999; 18:A435.

134. Garcia AA, Kempf RA, Rogers M, Muggia FM. A phase II study of Doxil (liposomal doxorubicin): lack of activity in poor prognosis soft tissue sarcomas. *Ann Oncol* 1998; 9:1131–1133.

135. Halm U, Etzrodt G, Schiefke I, et al. A phase II study of pegylated liposomal doxorubicin for treatment of advanced hepatocellular carcinoma. *Ann Oncol* 2000; 11:113–114.

136. Yeo W, Chan KK, Mukwaya G, et al. Phase II studies with DaunoXome in patients with nonresectable hepatocellular carcinoma: clinical and pharmacokinetic outcomes. *Cancer Chemother Pharmacol* 1999; 44:124–130.

137. Boiardi A, Pozzi A, Salmaggi A, Eoli M, Zucchetti M, Silvani A. Safety and potential effectiveness of daunorubicin-containing liposomes in patients with advanced recurrent malignant CNS tumors. *Cancer Chemother Pharmacol* 1999; 43:178–179.

138. Zucchetti M, Boiardi A, Silvani A, Parisi I, Piccolrovazzi S, D'Incalci M. Distribution of daunorubicin and daunorubicinol in human glioma tumors after administration of liposomal daunorubicin. *Cancer Chemother Pharmacol* 1999; 44:173–176.

139. Koukourakis MI, Koukouraki S, Giatromanolaki A, et al. Liposomal doxorubicin and conventionally fractionated radiotherapy in the treatment of locally advanced non-small-cell lung cancer and head and neck cancer. *J Clin Oncol* 1999; 17:3512–3521.

140. Kirpotin DB, Park JW, Demetzos K, et al. Stealth® liposomal vinorelbine: synthesis stability and antitumor activity against human breast and lung cancer xenografts. *Proc Am Assoc Cancer Res* 1999a; 40:417.

141. Working PK, Newman MS, Sullivan T, Yarrington J. Reduction of the cardiotoxicity of doxorubicin in rabbits and dogs by encapsulation in long-circulating, pegylated liposomes. *J Pharmacol Exp Therap* 1999; 289:1128–1133.

142. Von Hoff DD, Layard MW, Basa P, et al. Risk factors for doxorubicin-induced congestive heart failure. *Ann Intern Medicine* 1979; 91:710–717.

143. Legha SS, Hortobagyi GN, Benjamin RS. Anthracyclines, in *Cancer Chemotherapy by Infusion* (Lokich JJ, ed). 1 Ed. Precept Press, Inc. Chicago, 1987, pp 130–144.

144. Speth PAJ, van Hoesel QGCM, Haanen C. Clinical pharmacokinetics of doxorubicin. *Clin Pharmacokin* 1988; 15:15–31.

145. Working PK, Newman MS, Huang SK, Mayhew E, Vaage J, Lasic DD. Pharmacokinetics, biodistribution, and therapeutic efficacy of doxorubicin encapsulated in Stealth® liposomes (Doxil®). *J Liposome Res* 1994; 4:667–687.

146. Casper ES, Schwartz GK, Sugarman A, Leung D, Brennan MF. Phase I trial of dose-intense liposome-encapsulated doxorubicin in patients with advanced sarcoma. *J Clin Oncol* 1997; 15:2111–2117.

147. Kanter PM, Bullard GA, Ginsberg RA, et al. Comparison of the cardiotoxic effects of liposomal doxorubicin (TLC D-99) versus free doxorubicin in beagle dogs In vivo. 1993; 7:17–26.

148. Conley BA, Egorin MJ, Whitacre MY, Carter DC, Zuhowski EG. Phase I and pharmacokinetic trial of liposome-encapsulated doxorubicin. *Cancer Chemother Pharmacol* 1993; 33:107–112.

149. Bally MB, Nayar R, Masin D, Cullis PR, Mayer LD. Studies on the myelosuppresive activity of doxorubicin entrapped in liposomes. *Cancer Chemother Pharmacol* 1990; 27:13–19.

150. Oussoren C, Eling WMC, Crommelin DJA, Storm G, Zuidema J. The influence of the route of administration and liposome composition on the potential of liposomes to protect tissue against local toxicity of two antitumor drugs. *Biochim Biophys Acta* 1998; 1369:159–172.

151. Perkins WR, Dause RB, Li X, et al. Combination of antitumor ether lipid with lipids of complementary molecular shapes reduces its hemolytic activity. *Biochim Biophys Acta* 1997; 1327:61–68.

152. Ahmad I, Filep JJ, Franklin JC, et al. Enhanced therapeutic effects of liposome-associated 1-*O*-Octadecyl-2-*O*-methyl-sn-glycero-3-phosphocholine. *Cancer Res* 1997; 57:1915–1921.

153. White RM. Liposomal daunorubicin is not recommended in patients with less than advanced HIV-related Kaposi's sarcoma. *Aids* 1997; 11:1412–1413.

154. Allen TM, Murray L, MacKeigan S, Shah M. Chronic liposome administration in mice: effects on reticuloendothelial function and tissue distribution. *J Pharmacol Exp Therap* 1984; 229:267–275.

155. Daemen T, Hofstede G, Kate MTT, Bakker-Woudenberg IAJM, Scherphof G. Liposomal doxoru-
     bicin-induced toxicity: depletion and impairment of phagocytic activity of liver macrophages. *Int J
     Cancer* 1995; 61:716–721.
156. Daemen T, Regts J, Meesters M, Ten Kate MT, Bakker-Woudenberg IAJM, Scherphof GL. Toxicity
     of doxorubicin entrapped within long-circulating liposomes. *J Controlled Release* 1997; 44:1–9.
157. Gabizon A, Isacson R, Libson E, et al. Clinical studies of liposome-encapsulated doxorubicin. *Acta
     Oncol* 1994; 33:779–786.
158. Uziely B, Jeffers S, Isacson R, et al. Liposomal doxorubicin: antitumor activity and unique toxicities
     during two complementary phase I studies. *J Clin Oncol* 1995; 13:1777–1785.
159. Amantea M, Newman MS, Sullivan TM, Forrest A, Working PK. Relationship of dose intensity to the
     induction of palmar-plantar erythrodysesthia by pegylated doxorubicin in dogs. *Hum Exp Toxicol*
     1999; 18:17–26.
160. Lokich JJ, Moore C. Chemotherapy-associated palmar-plantar erythrodysesthesia syndrome. *Ann
     Intern Med* 1984; 101:798–800.
161. Vogelzang NJ, Ratain MJ. Cancer chemotherapy and skin changes. *Ann Intern Med* 1985;
     103:303–304.
162. Allen TM, Hansen CB, Stuart DD. Targeted sterically stabilized liposomal drug delivery, in *Medical
     Applications of Liposomes* (Lasic DD, Papahadjopoulos D, eds). Elsevier Science B.V., New York,
     1998, pp 545–565.
163. Ahmad I, Longenecker M, Samuel J, Allen TM. Antibody-targeted delivery of doxorubicin
     entrapped in sterically stabilized liposomes can eradicate lung cancer in mice. *Cancer Res* 1993;
     53:1484–1488.
164. Lopes de Menezes DE, Pilarski LM, Allen TM. In vitro and in vivo targeting of immunoliposomal
     doxorubicin to human B-cell lymphoma. *Cancer Res* 1998; 58:3320–3330.
165. Park JW, Hong K, Carter P, et al. Development of anti-p185[HER2] immunoliposomes for cancer ther-
     apy. *Proc Natl Acad Sci USA* 1995; 92:1327–1331.
166. Tseng Y-L, Hong R-L, Tao M-H, Chang F-H. Sterically stabilized anti-idiotype immunoliposomes
     improve the therapeutic efficacy of doxorubicin in a murine B-cell lymphoma model. *Int J Cancer*
     1999; 80:723–730.
167. Lee RJ, Low PS. Folate-mediated tumor cell targeting of liposome-entrapped doxorubicin in vitro.
     Biochim Biophys Acta 1995; 1233:134–144.
168. Wang S, Low PS. Folate-mediated targeting of antineoplastic drugs, imaging agents, and nucleic
     acids to cancer cells. *J Control Rel* 1998; 53:39–48.
169. Lee RJ, Low PS. Folate-targeted liposome for drug delivery. *J Liposome Res* 1997; 7:455–466.
170. Drummond DC, Hong K, Park JW, Benz CC, Kirpotin DB. (2000) *Liposome Targeting to Tumors
     Using Vitamin and Growth Factor Receptors.* Vitamins and Hormones. Edited by Litwack G., in press.
171. Hansen CB, Kao GY, Moase EH, Zalipsky S, Allen TM. Attachment of antibodies to sterically stabi-
     lized liposomes: evaluation comparison and optimization of coupling procedures. *Biochimica et Bio-
     physica Acta* 1995; 1239:133–144.
172. Zalipsky S, Gittelman J, Mullah N, Qazen MM, Harding JA. Biologically active ligand-bearing poly-
     mer-grafted liposomes, in *Targeting of drugs 6: strategies for stealth therapeutic systems* (Gregori-
     adis, G., McCormack B. eds). Plenum, New York, 1998, pp 131–138.
173. Zalipsky S, Mullah N, Harding JA, Gittelman J, Guo L, DeFrees SA. Poly(ethylene glycol)-grafted
     liposomes with oligopeptide or oligosaccharide ligands appended to the termini of the polymer
     chains. *Bioconj Chem* 1997; 8:111–118.
174. Zalipsky S, Puntambekar B, Boulikas P, Engbers CM, Woodle MC. Peptide attachment to extremities
     of liposomal surface grafted PEG chains: preparation of the long-circulating form of laminin pen-
     tapeptide, YIGSR. *Bioconj Chem* 1995; 6:705–708.
175. Zalipsky S, Functionalized poly(ethlene glycol) for preparation of biologically relevant conjugates.
     Bioconj Chem 1995; 6:150–165.
176. Zalipsky S. Synthesis of an end-group functionalized polyethylene glycol-lipid conjugate for prepara-
     tion of polymer-grafted liposomes. *Bioconj Chem* 1993; 4:296–299.
177. Kirpotin D, Park JW, Hong K, et al. Sterically stabilized anti-HER2 immunoliposomes: design and
     targeting to human breast cancer cells in vitro. *Biochemistry* 1997; 36:66–75.
178. Lee RJ, Low PS. Delivery of liposomes into cultured KB cells via folate receptor-mediated endocyto-
     sis. *J Biol Chem* 1994; 269:3198–3204.
179. Debs RJ, Heath TD, Papahadjopoulos D. Targeting of anti-Thy 1.1 monoclonal antibody conjugated
     liposomes in Thy 1.1 mice after intravenous administration. *Biochim Biophys Acta* 1987; 901:183–190.

180. Harding JA, Engbers CM, Newman MS, Goldstein NI, Zalipsky S. Immunogenicity and pharmacokinetic attributes of poly(ethyleneglycol)-grafted immunoliposomes. *Biochim Biophys Acta* 1997; 1327:181–192.

181. Allen TM, Agrawal AK, Ahmad I, Hansen CB, Zalipsky S. Antibody-mediated targeting of long-circulating (Stealth®) liposomes. *J Liposome Res* 1994; 4:1–25.

182. Allen TM, Ahmad I, Lopes de Menezes DE, Moase EH. Immunoliposome-mediated targeting of anticancer drugs in vivo. *Biochem Soc Trans* 1995; 23:1073–1079.

183. Mori A, Klibanov AL, Torchilin VP, Huang L. Influence of the steric barrier activity of amphipathic poly(ethyleneglycol) and ganglioside GM1 on the circulation time of liposomes and on the target binding of immunoliposomes in vivo. *FEBS Lett* 1991; 284:263–266.

184. Zalipsky S, Hansen CB, de Menezes DEL, Allen TM. Long-circulating, polyethylene glycol-grafted immunoliposomes. *J Controlled Release* 1996; 39:153–161.

185. Martin FJ, Hubbell WL, Papahadjopoulos D. Immunospecific targeting of liposomes to cells: a novel and efficient method for covalent attachment of Fab' fragments via disulfide bonds. *Biochemistry* 1981; 20:4229–4238.

186. Martin FJ, Papahadjopoulos D. Irreversible coupling of immunoglobulin fragments to preformed vesicles. An improved method for liposome targeting. *J Biol Chem* 1982; 257:286–288.

187. Derksen JTP, Morselt HWM, Scherphof GL. Uptake and processing of immunoglobulin-coated liposomes by subpopulations of rat liver macrophages. *Biochim Biophys Acta* 1988; 971:127–136.

188. Aragnol D, Leserman LD. Immune clearance of liposomes inhibited by an anti-Fc receptor antibody in vivo. *Proc Natl Acad Sci USA* 1986; 83:2699–2703.

189. Kirpotin DB, Park JW, Hong K, et al. Targeting of sterically stabilized liposomes to cancers overexpressing HER2/neu proto-oncogene, in *Medical Applications of Liposomes* (Lasic DD, Papahadjopoulos D, eds). Elsevier Science B.V., New York, 1998, pp 325–345.

190. Park JW, Hong K, Kirpotin DB, et al. Anti-HER2 immunoliposomes: enhanced efficacy attributable to targeted delivery. *Clin Cancer Res* 2002; 8:1172–1181.

191. Parr MJ, Ansell SM, Choi LS, Cullis PR. Factors influencing the retention and chemical stability of poly(ethylene glycol)-lipid conjugates incorporated into large unilamellar vesicles. *Biochim Biophys Acta* 1994; 1195:21–30.

192. Scherphof GL, Kamps JAAM, Koning GA. In vivo targeting of surface-modified liposomes to metastatically growing carcinoma cells and sinusoidal endothelial cells in the rat liver. *J Liposome Res* 1997; 7:419–432.

193. Mori A, Kennel SJ, Waalkes MvB, Scherphof GL, Huang L. Characterization of organ-specific immunoliposomes for delivery of 3',5'-*O*-dipalmitoyl-5-fluoro-2'-deoxyuridine in a mouse lung-metastasis model. *Cancer Chemother Pharmacol* 1995; 35:447–456.

194. Oku N, Tokudome Y, Koike C, et al. Liposomal Arg-Gly-Asp analogs effectively inhibit metastatic B16 melanoma colonization in murine lungs. *Life Sci* 1996; 58:2263–2270.

195. Fujimori K, Covell DG, Fletcher JE, Weinstein JN. A modeling analysis of monoclonal antibody percolation through tumors: a binding site barrier. *J Nucl Med* 1990; 31:1191–1198.

196. Weinstein JN, Eger RR, Covell DG, et al. The pharmacology of monoclonal antibodies. *Ann N Y Acad Sci* 1987; 507:199–210.

197. Jain RK. Delivery of novel therapeutic agents in tumors: physiological barriers and strategies. *J Natl Cancer Inst* 1989; 81:570–576.

198. Huang A, Kennel SJ, Huang L. Interactions of immunoliposomes with target cells. *J Biol Chem* 1983; 258:14,034–14,040.

10 Gliadel®
A New Method for the Treatment of Malignant Brain Tumors

Francesco DiMeco, MD, Henry Brem, MD, Jon D. Weingart, MD, and Alessandro Olivi, MD

CONTENTS

INTRODUCTION
SELECTION OF CONTROLLED-RELEASE POLYMER
SELECTION OF CHEMOTHERAPEUTIC AGENT
PRECLINICAL STUDIES
CLINICAL STUDIES
LESSONS LEARNED FROM GLIADEL® AND FUTURE DIRECTIONS
CONCLUSIONS
ACKNOWLEDGMENT
REFERENCES

1. INTRODUCTION

Designing effective therapies for patients with malignant brain tumors represents a major challenge. Despite significant advances in neuroimaging, microsurgery, and radiation therapy, the prognosis of patients harboring malignant gliomas still remains poor *(1)*. The addition of systemic chemotherapy does not provide significant impact on survival of patients *(1,2)*. One of the reasons for such failure is that systemic chemotherapy has several limitations that reduce its effectiveness in fighting the progressive nature of central nervous system (CNS) malignancies. First, the blood–brain barrier keeps a large number of chemotherapeutic agents from reaching the brain parenchyma. Second, the amount of drug administered is limited by variable systemic toxicities. Because the goals of chemotherapy for brain tumors should be achieving and sustaining cytotoxic concentrations of drug in the brain with minimal systemic concentrations, local delivery of these agents could result in a more effective treatment. Moreover, the notions that 80% of malignant gliomas recur within 2 cm of the original tumor site, and that extra CNS metastases are exceedingly rare *(3)* strengthen the rationale for strategies aiming at controlling local disease.

From: *Drug Delivery Systems in Cancer Therapy*
Edited by: D. M. Brown © Humana Press Inc., Totowa, NJ

One approach for intratumoral delivery of chemotherapy is the development of polymer systems capable of sustained release of drugs to be surgically placed at the tumor site. Direct implant of drug-embedded polymers makes it possible to overcome the limitations imposed by the blood–brain barrier and to achieve high local concentrations of anticancer agents while greatly decreasing systemic toxicity. Additionally, polymer-mediated delivery of drugs provides continuous release of active drugs which, systemically, would often have a short half-life. Finally, this technology has opened the door to the testing of new therapeutic agents that, in the past, could not be used because of their systemic toxicity for the treatment of brain tumors. In this chapter, we describe the steps necessary to develop this novel approach: from the selection of a physiologically and biologically promising biodegradable polymer system; to the preclinical studies demonstrating the safety and efficacy of polymer drug delivery to the brain; to the clinical trials that finally lead to the FDA approval of BCNU (carmustine) loaded polymer (Gliadel®) for the treatment of malignant glial tumors. Finally, we discuss potential applications of controlled-release polymers, providing an insight into future development of local delivery of antineoplastic agents.

2. SELECTION OF CONTROLLED-RELEASE POLYMER

Although many types of polymers are available for local delivery of drugs *(4)*, only a few meet the criteria required for their use in clinical settings, such as absence of toxicity, and sustained releasing of drug with both high and low molecular weight. Polymers that have been investigated belong to two different categories identified by their mechanism of release: diffusion-regulated and degradation-regulated polymers. Nonbiodegradable polymers are an example of compounds that release the drug by means of diffusion at the interface of polymer/tissue. These polymers were first described by Langer and Folkman who discovered that macromolecules could be incorporated into a nonbiodegradable ethylene-vinyl acetate co-polymer (EVAc) capable of highly predictable and reproducible drug-release profile *(4,5)*. The major disadvantage of this system, however, is that the empty polymer matrix remains at the site of implantation indefinitely, thus, theoretically necessitating a follow-up surgery to remove the foreign body. Conversely, biodegradable polymer systems provide controlled drug delivery through the surface erosion, over time, of the matrix itself *(6)*. Because these polymers degrade as they release the drug, surgical removal is not necessary. Based on these observations we thought that a biodegradable polymer would be more suitable for implantation into the brain.

The polyanhydride poly[1,3-*bis* (carboxyphenoxy) propane-co-sebacic-acid] (PCPP-SA) matrix is an example of a biodegradable polymer. Polyanhydride copolymers react with water to form dicarboxylic acids leading to the sustained release of the incorporated drug. In addition, polyanhydride copolymers are extremely hydrophobic, thus protecting chemotherapeutic agents incorporated into the matrix from hydrolysis and enzymatic degradation. Therefore, as the matrix degrades at a steady rate, drugs that would last only a few minutes when systemically administered can be released in a biologically active form, over a period of weeks, at a relatively steady concentration. Moreover, the time period of polymer breakdown, and therefore of drug release, can be modulated by modifying the ratio of carboxyphenoxypropane (PCPP) to sebacic acid (SA) in the polymer formulation. Indeed, the rate of degradation can be increased significantly with increasing percentages of SA. Thus, considering that a 1-mm disk of pure PCPP (without sebacic acid) degrades in approx 3 yr, it has been estimated that altering the CPP-to-SA ratio could achieve nearly any degradation rate between 1 d and several years *(7)*. The 20:80 PCPP-SA copolymer, obtained by mixing the two monomeres in a 1:4 ratio, degrades over 5 wk *(8)*. The process of manufacturing the copolymers PCPP-SA has been established. Drugs are incorporated into the matrix at low temperature (below 37°C) and compressed under high pressure. The solid polymeric matrix can then be shaped into any configuration, including wafers, rods, sheets, and microspheres *(9)*.

The fatty acid dimer-sebacic acid (FAD-SA) copolymer, is another example of a biodegradable polymer that shares with the PCPP-SA system both the mechanism of release and the possibility to vary the release kinetic by varying the ratio of the two monomers. However, whereas PCPP-SA copolymers are designed to release hydrophobic molecules, the FAD-SA copolymers have been specifically developed to deliver hydrophilic compounds *(10)*.

3. SELECTION OF CHEMOTHERAPEUTIC AGENT

We chose the chemotherapeutic alkylating agent 1,3-*bis*(2-chloroethyl)-1-nitrosourea (BCNU, carmustine) as the first candidate for our polymer-based treatment strategy because of its known activity against both experimental and human malignant gliomas and the extensive pharmacological experience with this drug. BCNU is a lipid-soluble nitrosourea that alkylates the nitrogen bases of DNA, e.g., the alkylation of O-6 position of guanine. The accumulation of DNA damage results in mutagenesis, carcinogenesis, and cytotoxicity. Being lipophilic, BCNU is capable of some degree of penetration through the blood–brain barrier and has been the most widely used chemotherapeutic agent for the treatment of brain tumors to date. However, BCNU systemic administration has significant toxicity, including bone marrow suppression and pulmonary fibrosis. Furthermore, BCNU's systemic activity is limited by its serum half-life of approx 15 min *(11)*. Therefore, we postulated that delivering BCNU interstitially via a biodegradable polymer would clinically improve its efficacy.

4. PRECLINICAL STUDIES

4.1. Biocompatibility Studies

The safety of implantation of the PCPP-SA was studied in rabbit cornea, and in rat, rabbit, and monkey brains. The implantation of the polymers in the rabbit cornea did not show signs of inflammation over a 6-wk period after surgery. Specifically, there was no evidence of neovascularization or edema or inflammatory infiltrates on histological examination *(12,13)*. The polymers were also well tolerated after implantation into the brain of rats and rabbits. Animals were followed over 5 wk (rats) and 9 wk (rabbits) and serially sacrificed at specified time points. All animals survived to their scheduled date of sacrifice without showing any signs of behavioral changes or neurological deficits indicative of significant toxicity from the polymer implant. The histological evaluation of the site of implant revealed transient and minimal inflammatory signs similar to the reactions elicited by common hemostatic implants such as oxidized cellulose (Surgicel®) and gelatin sponges (Gelfoam®) *(8,14)*. PCPP-SA polymers were finally implanted into the frontal lobe of Cynomolgus monkeys. No signs of behavioral or neurological deterioration or hematological changes have been detected in these animals after the implantation of polymers with or without carmustine. Post-mortem analysis of brain tissue from these animals showed only a localized reaction at the site of implantation. Additionally, in this study, the safety of combining local BCNU with radiotherapy was demonstrated *(15)*.

4.2. In Vivo Kinetics of Drug Release from the Polymers

The release of the BCNU in vivo from the PCPP-SA polymers was determined in rabbit and monkey brains using radiolabeled markers. Autoradiography-radiolabeled BCNU delivered to the rabbit brain, either by direct injection or by BCNU-impregnated polymers, demonstrated that drug released from the polymers was extensively distributed for a longer period of time. In fact, tissue concentrations of BCNU, two standard deviations above background, were detected in the polymer-implanted hemisphere 21 d after the implant. By contrast, no detectable levels of drug were present 72 h after direct injection *(16)*. Further kinetic studies have been carried out in monkeys demonstrating that brain concentrations of BCNU released by intracerebrally implanted 20%-loaded polymers were 1200 times higher than that achieved by intravenous (iv) infusion of the drug. Moreover, using quantititative autoradiography and thin-layer chromatography, this study demonstrated that tumoricidal concentrations of BCNU were detectable at the following: at 4 cm of distance from the site of polymer implantation 1 d after surgery, at 2 cm on day 7, and at 1.3 cm on day 30 *(17)*.

4.3. Efficacy Studies

The efficacy of local delivery of BCNU by means of PCPP-SA copolymers or EVAc polymers, was investigated against 9L gliosarcoma tumors implanted either subcutaneously (sc) or orthotopically into the brain of Fisher 344 rats. These studies consistently and clearly demonstrated the superior effectiveness of local delivery of BCNU by polymers when compared with systemic administration. Animals bearing established intracranial tumors and treated locally by intratumoral implantation of BCNU–impregnated polymers showed a statistically significant improvement of survival when compared with the group treated with empty polymer or intraperitoneal (ip) administration of BCNU. Moreover, local delivery of BCNU resulted in 17% of long-term survivors whereas no long-term survivors were seen among systemically treated animals (Fig. 1) *(18)*.

5. CLINICAL STUDIES

The aforementioned preclinical studies aimed at assessing the biocompatibility, biodistribution, and efficacy of BNCU-loaded PCPP-SA polymers constituted the basis for the subsequent translation into the clinical field. Several clinical trials were designed in order to test the safety and efficacy of this new approach.

5.1. Gliadel for the Treatment of Recurrent Malignant Gliomas

The safety of the PCPP-SA copolymer (20:80 formulation) has been assessed first with a Phase I–II multicentric trial. A total of 21 patients affected by recurrent malignant gliomas were enrolled in this study *(19)*. Eligibility criteria included the following: histologic diagnosis of malignant glioma, previous external radiotherapy, radiographic evidence of single focus of recurrence of 1.5 cm or greater, KPS >60, indication for surgical reoperation, no chemotherapy within 1 mo, and no nitrosoureas within 6 wk before enrollment. These patients underwent surgical debulking of their lesions followed by the placement of BCNU-impregnated wafers in the resection cavity (Fig. 2). Three different formulations of wafers with increasing concentrations of

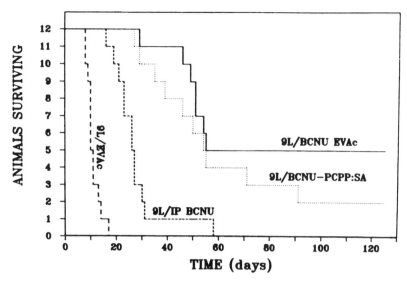

Fig. 1. Survival curves of animals bearing brain tumors treated with either systemic (9L/IP BCNU) or interstitial (9L-BCNU-EVAc and 9L-BCNU-PCPP:SA) BCNU. Reprinted with permission from AACR (*Can Res* 1993; 53:331).

BCNU were studied: 1.93%, 3.85%, and 6.35%; these yielded 3.85, 7.7, and 12.7 mg of carmustine, respectively. Five patients received wafers with the lowest concentration of drug, and another five patients received wafers with the intermediate concentration; 11 patients received the highest BCNU-wafer formulation. A maximum of eight wafers were implanted for each patient, therefore, the final dose of BCNU per each group was 31, 62, and 102 mg. No evidence of systemic toxicity and no signs of neurological deterioration were observed in any of the treatment groups. Blood cell count, chemistries, and urinalysis did not show changes accounting for bone marrow, hepatic, or renal injury. Postoperative imaging with CT scan and MRI revealed, in most cases, the presence of a thin layer of contrast-enhancing ring surrounding the wafers. These changes were detectable only in the first 7 wk from time of surgery. The quality of the MRI was not affected by the presence of the wafers, which are, instead, clearly visible as areas of markedly decreased signal on T1-weighted sequences. The average survival period after reoperation for the lowest, intermediate, and highest dose group was, respectively, 65, 64, and 32 wk. The overall mean survival time was 48 wk from reoperation, and 94 wk from the original operation. Eighteen (86%) of 21 patients lived more than 1 yr from the time of their initial diagnosis and eight (38%) of 21 patients lived more than 1 yr after intracranial implantation of the polymer. The results of the trial indicated that the BCNU-PCPP-SA polymer was safe when implanted intracranially into patients and prompted the start of a placebo-controlled clinical trial.

The encouraging results obtained with the safety studies motivated us to evaluate the efficacy of local delivery of BCNU by polymers for the treatment of malignant gliomas. The study was carried out using 3.8% BCNU-loaded wafers in patients with recurrent malignant gliomas who had failed standard therapy. A total of 222 patients from 27 medical centers in the United States and Canada were entered into this randomized, placebo-controlled double-blinded prospective, Phase III clinical trial. The enrollment criteria for this study were similar to those in a Phase I–II study. Patients

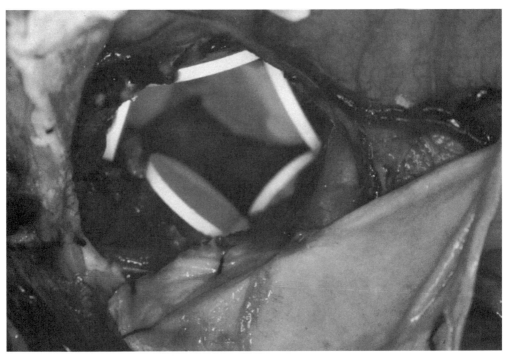

Fig. 2. Intraoperative photograph showing the resection cavity lined with Gliadel wafers. (Courtesy of Dr. Henry Brem.)

were divided into two groups equally distributed for all known prognostic factors (e.g., median age, neurologic performance, prior treatment, time from previous surgical operation, and histologic grade). One group of 110 patients received BCNU wafer and the other (112 patients) empty polymers. Overall median survival was 31 wk for the BCNU group and 23 wk for the placebo group (hazard ratio=0.67, p=0.006, after accounting for the effects of prognostic factors) (Fig. 3). Moreover, 6 mo survival for patients with glioblastoma was 50% greater in the active group than in the placebo group (mortality=32 of 72 [42%] vs 47 of 73 [64%], p=0.02). No deleterious effects occurred as a result of wafer implants. There were no statistically significant differences between active and placebo group regarding the incidence of either seizures or intracranial infections, which both occurred within the range of the expected rate of postcraniotomy complications. KPS was not affected by the wafer implants and no signs of systemic side effects were detected *(20)*. This study demonstrated that BCNU delivered via polyanhydride polymers is a safe, effective treatment for patients with recurrent malignant gliomas. This trial, together with the others previously mentioned, also provided the basis of the FDA approval of BCNU-loaded polymer (Gliadel) as a treatment for patients with recurrent glioblastoma. To date, Gliadel has received clinical approval in more than 20 countries.

5.2. Treatment of Newly Diagnosed Malignant Gliomas

Once demonstrated that BCNU wafer implants were safe and effective for the palliative therapy of recurrent gliomas, our attention turned to evaluating the safety and efficacy of such an approach for the initial treatment of malignant gliomas. A Phase I trial with 22 patients newly diagnosed with malignant glioma was conducted to evaluate the overall

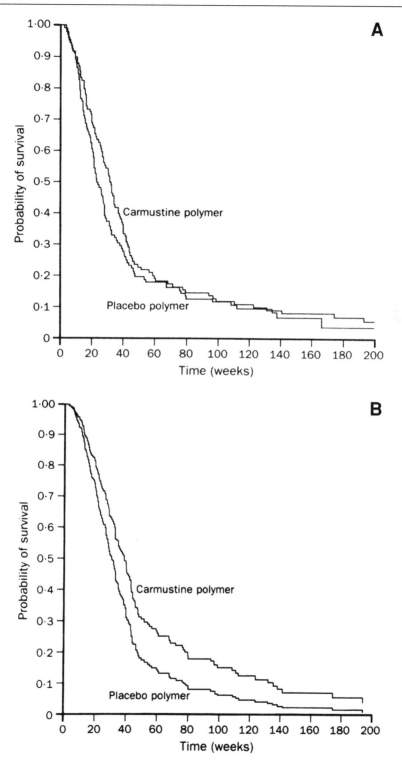

Fig. 3. Kaplan-Meier survival curves for patients with recurrent malignant gliomas treated with either Gliadel™ or empty wafers. (**A**) Overall survival by treatment group; (**B**) Overall survival by treatment group after adjustment for prognostic factors. Reprinted with permission from Elsevier Science (*Lancet* 1995; 345:1011).

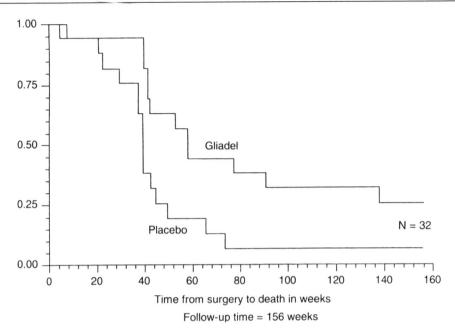

Fig. 4. Kaplan-Meier survival curves for patients with newly diagnosed malignant gliomas treated with Gliadel or empty polymers. Reprinted with permission from Lippincott Williams & Wilkins (*Neurosurg* 1997; 41:47).

safety of BCNU-loaded wafers and also the safety of concurrent standard external beam radiation therapy. Eligibility criteria included the following: age of 18 or older, unilateral single focus of disease greater than 1 cm in diameter, and KPS above 60. Twenty-one patients had a diagnosis of glioblastoma multiforme and one patient had an anaplastic astrocytoma. Each patient received gross removal of the lesion followed by the implantation of seven or eight 3.85% BCNU-loaded wafers (PCPP-SA, 20–80). All patients received adjuvant standard postsurgical radiation therapy averaging 50 Gy. No evidence of systemic or neurological toxicity was detected. This study not only demonstrated the safety of BCNU-polymers as initial therapy for malignant gliomas, but also established the safety of combining local chemotherapy with conventional radiotherapy *(21)*.

Subsequently, a prospective, randomized, placebo-controlled Phase III trial was conducted in Scandinavia by Valtonen et al. aiming at assessing safety and efficacy of BCNU wafers as an adjunctive therapy with surgery and radiation in newly diagnosed patients. Thirty-two patients, 27 with glioblastoma and 5 with other malignant gliomas, were enrolled in this study and randomized to receive either BCNU wafers or empty polymers. All patients had subsequent radiation therapy. Median survival was 58 wk for the active arm vs 40 wk for the placebo arm (*p*=0.001) (Fig. 4). Patients bearing glioblastoma had a median survival of 53 wk when treated with local BCNU compared to 40 wk when treated with placebo (*p*=0.0083). One-year survival in patients receiving BCNU wafers was 63% compared to 19% for those receiving empty polymers. For treated group vs placebo group, 2-yr survival was 31% vs 6%, and 3-yr survival was 25% vs 6%, respectively. Also, no signs of either systemic or local toxicity were recorded *(22)*.

Recently, Westphal et al. have repeated a subsequent Phase III randomized, prospective, placebo-controlled study of Gliadel as the initial treatment. This 240-patient study showed a similar, statistically significant prolongation of survival in patients treated with Gliadel (23). In February 2003, the FDA approved the use of Gliadel as initial treatment for malignant gliomas in the United States.

6. LESSONS LEARNED FROM GLIADEL® AND FUTURE DIRECTIONS

6.1. Future Applications for Interstitial Chemotherapy

Recent laboratory studies have demonstrated that increasing concentrations of up to 20% of BCNU are safe and more effective than lower doses in prolonging survival of rats bearing 9L gliosarcoma tumors. Therefore, a study was performed in monkeys which has shown that 20% BCNU polymers are well-tolerated and yield effective sustained distribution of BCNU throughout the brain (24). In view of these observations, we have completed, through the NABTT CNS Consortium, a Phase I multicenter, multilabeled clinical trial of escalating doses in patients with recurrent glioma. Gliadel wafers containing 6.5%, 10%, 14.5%, 20%, and 28% concentrations of BCNU have been tested in patients undergoing surgery for recurrent gliomas. No major drug-related toxicity has been identified in the first four groups, although three of four patients receiving the 28% polymers experienced serious adverse events (seizures and brain edema). This study demonstrated that wafers containing BCNU concentrations up to 20% can be safely administered to patients with recurrent gliomas (25). Based on these results, additional Phase III studies are planned to evaluate the added efficacy of BCNU wafers at the established maximum tolerated dose (20% BCNU).

6.2. Future Developments

The results achieved with BCNU-loaded polymers have opened the door to use of biodegradable polymers as a vehicle for a variety of other chemotherapeutic drugs. In particular, this approach has renewed interest in experimentally promising agents that have been not utilized clinically because of brain barrier impermeability or systemic toxicity. For example, the microtubule stabilizator paclitaxel (Taxol®) has been shown to possess potent antitumor action against glioma cell cultures (26). Its utility is limited, however, because it does not penetrate the blood–brain barrier (27). As a consequence, despite its potency against gliomas in vitro, clinical trials in which it was administered systemically have failed to show benefit. This makes it an ideal drug for local delivery to the brain tumor with sustained-release polymers. Therefore, paclitaxel has been incorporated into PCPP-SA polymers where it is released in a sustained fashion for up to 1000 h. Local deliveries of paclitaxel by 40%- and 20%-loaded polymers were capable of doubling and tripling survival times of rats bearing 9L gliosarcomas when compared with controls treated with empty polymers (mean survival: 38 d with 40% paclitaxel, 61.5 d with 20% paclitaxel, 19.5 d with placebo) (28). Moreover, in studies conducted in primates, tumoricidal concentrations of paclitaxel were measured up to 5 cm from the site of the implant of paclitaxel-loaded polymers for as long as 30 d after implantation.

The topoisomerase I inhibitor camptothecin is another ideal candidate for antitumor local therapy owing to its poor bioavailability and high systemic toxicity. We showed that camptothecin released by the nonbiodegradable polymer EVAc significantly extends survival of rats bearing intracranial 9L gliosarcomas. More specifically, local delivery of camptothecin resulted in 59% long-term survivors, whereas none of the control animals survived longer than 32 d *(29)*. A variety of potent camptothecin derivatives are being prepared for future clinical trials *(30)*.

Platinum drugs are another class of agents that also have shown promise in the treatment of CNS tumors including malignant glioma, medulloblastoma, optic pathway glioma, brainstem glioma, and ependymoma *(31–36)*. Unfortunately, the systemic use of platinum-based drugs is limited by marked toxicity, particularly hematological toxicity *(37)*. Furthermore, being water soluble, these drugs barely cross the blood–brain barrier. Hence, controlled-release polymers constitute an ideal tool to overcome those limitations and exploit the antitumor potential of platinum drugs. Carboplatin is potently effective in vitro against CNS tumors *(32)* and, when delivered directly to the CNS, it is less neurotoxic than other platinum-based compounds *(38)*. Therefore, we have optimized the delivery of carboplatin by incorporating it into both the FAD:SA and PCPP:SA biodegradable polymers *(39)*. We also developed a method to encapsulate carboplatin into ethylcellulose microcapsules *(40)* that offer the possibility to be injected stereotactically when surgical resection is not indicated. We found that local delivery of carboplatin via either polymers or microcapsules is safe and highly effective against F98 gliomas in rats *(39)*. Based on these promising findings, studies are underway to assess safety and toxicity of carboplatin-based polymers in primates.

Cyclophosphamide (Cytoxan®) is an alkylating agent not suitable for systemic treatment of brain tumors because its active metabolite, 4-hydroxy-cyclophosphamide (4-HC), does not cross the blood–brain barrier. We developed a process to incorporate 4-hydroperoxy-cyclophosphamide (a hydrophilic derivative of cyclophosphamide which spontaneously converts to the active form 4-HC) into FAD-SA polymers. We demonstrated that controlled release of 4-HC by polymers extend median survival of animals intracranially challenged with F98 glioma cells from 14 d (placebo controls) to 77 d (treated animals) *(41)*.

The use of polymers to treat brain tumors has largely focused on the delivery of chemotherapeutic drugs. Advances in basic and clinical research in brain tumor biology and immunology, however, have led to new therapeutic strategies that could potentially benefit controlled-release biodegradable polymer technology. Local delivery of minocycline, a semisynthetic derivative of tetracycline, by controlled-release polymers has been shown to be effective in inhibiting tumor-induced neovascularization in rabbit corneas *(42)*, as well as in extending the survival of rats challenged intracranially with 9L gliosarcoma cells *(43)*. Local treatment with minocyline also showed synergistic properties with the systemic administration of BCNU *(43)*.

Cytokines have been increasingly used in cancer therapy and one of them, interleukin 2 (IL-2), is currently FDA approved for systemic administration to treat patients with metastatic renal cancer. Given the rationale for using local chemotherapy to treat brain tumors, as well as considering the idea that cytokines exert their immunomodulatory activity in a paracrine fashion, we hypothesized that local cytokine-based immunotherapy could be utilized to control tumor growth in the brain. The delivery of a cytokine by genetically modified cells directly to the brain, bypassing the blood barrier, has proven to be highly effective in treating established brain tumors in animals in our laboratory *(44–46)*. Although efficacious in animal models, many practical considerations may limit the translation of this strategy into the clinical setting for treatment of human brain tumors. We reasoned that, by incorporating controlled-release technology, we could develop a simpler strategy to achieve paracrine cytokine production at the tumor site as a more practical alternative to genetically modified cells. Thus, we tested the ability of IL-2- and IL-12-containing microspheres to act against metastatic and primary brain tumor models. IL-2 microspheres were highly effective in the treatment of metastatic B16-melanoma brain tumors in mice and 9L gliosarcomas in rats *(47,48)*. In addition to IL-2, we recently developed a similar process to encapsulate interleukin 12 (IL-12) into microspheres. IL-12 loaded microspheres have been shown to be as effective against 9L glioma tumors in rats as 9L cells engineered to secrete IL-12 *(49)*. Thus, we demonstrated that polymers can be used to locally deliver sustained cytokine concentrations for the safe and effective treatment of experimental brain tumors. Because of its ease of use and reproducibility compared to genetically modified cells, this polymeric system may be the ideal candidate for the delivery of cytokine-based immunotherapy to human brain tumors.

Finally, promising results have been achieved by the combination of local chemo- and immunotherapy. Given the theoretical and experimental evidence of increased antigenicity of tumors after exposure to cytotoxic drugs *(50,51)*, we hypothesized that the combination of paracrine immunotherapy and local delivery of chemotherapy by biodegradable polymers may act synergistically against brain tumor models. We initially established the validity of this hypothesis using cells genetically engineered to secrete IL-2 in combination with either BCNU- or carboplatin-loaded polymers against a metastatic murine brain tumor *(52)*. We then tested the efficacy of the combination of IL-2 microspheres and either BCNU, carboplatin, or adriamycin incorporated in polymers against rat primary malignant brain tumor models (9L gliosarcomas and F98 gliomas). Our results clearly confirmed the effectiveness of this novel, promising strategy.

7. CONCLUSIONS

The use of biodegradable polymers to deliver high concentrations of drugs locally at the tumor site is a powerful tool which has been added to the neurosurgical armamentarium against brain tumors. Controlled interstitial drug delivery to brain tumors represents an effective means of bypassing the limits imposed by the blood–brain barrier, thus achieving elevated local concentrations of drug while minimizing systemic exposure and toxicity. The success achieved in the preclinical and clinical fields with Gliadel validates the concept that biodegradable polymers could represent an effective vehicle for several other drugs that are otherwise ineffective against brain tumors. Moreover, the concept of local delivery of chemotherapeutic drugs can be broadened to include other classes of antitumor agents such as inhibitors of neovascularization or immunotherapeutic agents that, alone or in combination with chemotherapeutic drugs, offer promising perspectives.

Although the prognosis of patients affected by brain tumors remains poor, the further development and expansion of the concept of utilizing biodegradable polymers to deliver antineoplastic agents and biologically active agents to the brain holds considerable promise for the treatment of these patients.

ACKNOWLEDGMENT

Under a licensing agreement between Guilford Pharmaceuticals and the Johns Hopkins University, Dr. Brem is entitled to a share of royalty received by the University on sales of products described in this work. Dr. Brem and the University own Guilford Pharmaceuticals stock, which is subject to certain restrictions under University policy. Dr. Brem also is a paid consultant to Guilford Pharmaceuticals. The terms of this arrangement are being managed by the Johns Hopkins University in accordance with its conflict of interest policies.

REFERENCES

1. Parker S, Tong T, Bolden S, et al. Cancer Statistics. *Ca Cancer J Clin* 1996; 46:5–27.
2. Black P. Brain tumors – part I. *New Engl J Med* 1991; 324:1471–1476.
3. Hochberg F, Pruitt A. Assumptions in the radiotherapy of glioblastoma. *Neurology* 1980; 30:907–911.
4. Langer R. New methods in drug delivery. *Science* 1990; 249:1527–1533.
5. Langer R, Folkman J. Polymers for the sustained release of proteins and other macromolecules. *Nature* 1976; 263:797–800.
6. Tamargo R, Brem H. Drug delivery to the central nervous system: A review. *Neurosurg Quart* 1992; 2(4):259–279.
7. Chasin M, Domb A, Ron E, et al. Polyanhydrides as drug delivery systems, in *Biodegradable Polymers as Drug Delivery Systems* (Langer MCaR, ed). Marcel Dekker, New York, 1990, pp 43–70.
8. Tamargo R, Epstein J, Reinhard C, Chasin M, Brem H. Brain biocompatibility of a biodegradable, controlled-release polymer in rats. *J Biomed Mater Res* 1989; 23:253–266.
9. Leong KW, Brott BC, Langer R. Bioerodible polyanhydrides as drug-carrier matrices. I: Characterization, degradation, and release characteristics. *J Biomed Mater Res* 1985; 19:941–955.
10. Domb A, Bogdansky S, Olivi A, et al. Controlled delivery of water soluble and hydrolytically unstable anti-cancer drugs for polymeric implants. *Polymer Preprints* 1991; 32(2):219–220.
11. Loo T, Dion R, Dixon R, et al. The antitumor agent 1,3-*bis*(2-chloroethyl)-1-nitrosourea. *J Pharm Sci* 1966; 55:492–497.
12. Langer R, Wise D. *Medical Application of Controlled Release,* vol. I and vol. II. CRC, Boca Raton, FL: 1986.
13. Leong K, D'Amore P, Marletta M, et al. Bioerodable polyanhydrides as drug-carrier matrices: II. Biocompatibility and chemical reactivity. *J Biomed Mater Res* 1986; 20:51–64.
14. Brem H, Kader A, Epstein J, et al. Biocompatibility of a biodegradable, controlled-release polymer in the rabbit brain. *Sel Cancer Ther* 1989; 5:55–65.
15. Brem H, Tamargo R, Olivi A, et al. Biodegradable polymers for controlled delivery of chemotherapy with and without radiation therapy in the monkey brain. *J Neurosurg* 1994; 80:283–290.
16. Grossman S, Reinhard C, Colvin O, et al. The intracerebral distribution of BCNU delivered by surgically implanted biodegradable polymers. *J Neurosurg* 1992; 76:640–647.
17. Fung L, Ewend M, Sills A, et al. Pharmacokinetics of interstitial delivery of carmustine, 4-hydroperoxycyclophosphamide, and paclitaxel from a biodegradable polymer implant in the monkey brain. *Cancer Res* 1998; 58:672–684.
18. Tamargo R, Myseros J, Epstein J, Yang M, Chasin M, Brem H. Interstitial chemotherapy of the 9L gliosarcoma: controlled release polymers for drug delivery in the brain. *Cancer Res* 1993; 53:329–333.
19. Brem H, Mahaley MJ, Vick N, et al. Interstitial chemotherapy with drug polymer implants for the treatment of recurrent gliomas. *J Neurosurg* 1991; 74:441–446.
20. Brem H, Piantadosi S, Burger P, et al. Placebo-controlled trial of safety and efficacy of intraoperative controlled delivery by biodegradable polymers of chemotherapy for recurrent gliomas. The Polymer-brain Tumor Treatment Group. *Lancet* 1995; 345:1008–1012.
21. Brem H, Ewend M, Piantadosi S, Greenhoot J, Burger P, Sisti M. The safety of interstitial chemotherapy with BCNU-loaded polymer followed by radiation therapy in the treatment of newly diagnosed malignant gliomas: phase I trial. *J Neuro-Oncol* 1995; 26:111–123.
22. Valtonen S, Timonen U, Toivanen P, et al. Interstitial chemotherapy with carmustine-loaded polymers for high-grade gliomas: a randomized double-blind study. *Neurosurgery* 1997; 41:44–48; discussion 48, 49.
23. Westphal M, Delavault P, Hilt D, Olivares R, Belin V, Daumas-Duport C. Placebo controlled multicenter double-blind randomized prospective phase III trial of local chemotherapy with biodegradable carmustine implants (Gliadel) in 240 patients with malignant gliomas: final results. *Neuro-Oncology* 2000; 2:3.
24. Sipos E, Tyler B, Piantadosi S, Burger P, Brem H. Optimizing interstitial delivery of BCNU from controlled release polymers for the treatment of brain tumors. *Cancer Chemother Pharmacol* 1997; 39:383–389.

25. Olivi A, Barker F, DiMeco F, et al. Results of a multicenter Phase I dose escalation study of interstitial BCNU administered via wafers to patients with recurrent malignant glioma, in 2001 AANS Annual Meeting, Toronto, Ont., Canada, Apr. 21–26, 2001, p 238.

26. Cahan M, Walter K, Colvin O, Brem H. Cytotoxicity of taxol in vitro against human and rat malignant brain tumors. *Cancer Chemother Pharmacol* 1994; 33:441–444.

27. Klecker R, Jamis-Dow C, Egorin M, Erkmen K, Parker R, Collins J. Distribution and metabolism of 3H-Taxol in the rat. *Proc Am Assoc Cancer Res* 1993; 34:A381.

28. Walter K, Cahan M, Gur A, et al. Interstitial taxol delivered from a biodegradable polymer implant against experimental malignant glioma. *Cancer Res* 1994; 54:2207–2212.

29. Weingart J, Thompson R, Tyler B, Colvin O, Brem H. Local delivery of the topoisomerase I inhibitor camptothecin sodium prolongs survival in the rat intracranial 9L gliosarcoma model. *Int J Cancer* 1995; 62:605–609.

30. Sampath P, Davis JD, Wall M, Brem H. Campothecin analogs effects in vitro against glioma lines, in Society of Neuro-Oncologysts Conference (SNO) Oct. 28–Nov. 1, 1997.

31. Gaynon P, Ettinger L, Baum E, Siegel S, Krailo M, Hammond G. Carboplatin in childhood brain tumors. A Children's Cancer Study Group Phase II Trial. *Cancer* 1990; 66:2465–2469.

32. Doz F, Berens M, Dougherty D, Rosenblum M. Comparison of the cytotoxic activities of cisplatin and carboplatin against glioma cell lines at pharmacologically relevant drug exposures. *J Neuro-Oncol* 1991; 11:27–35.

33. Poisson M, Pereon Y, Chiras J, Delattre J. Treatment of recurrent malignant supratentorial gliomas with carboplatin (CBDCA). *J Neuro-Oncol* 1991; 10:139–144.

34. Zeltzer P, Epport K, Nelson M, Huff K, Gaynon P. Prolonged response to carboplatin in an infant with brain stem glioma. *Cancer* 1991; 67:43–47.

35. Charrow J, Listernik R, Greenwald M, Das L, Radkowski M. Carboplatin-induced regression of an optic pathway tumor in a child with neurofibromatosis. *Med Pediatr Oncol* 1993; 21:680–684.

36. Williams P, Henner W, Roman-Goldstein S, et al. Toxicity and efficacy of carboplatin and etoposide in conjunction with disruption of the blood-brain tumor barrier in the treatment of intracranial neoplasms. *Neurosurgery* 1995; 37:17–27.

37. Hannigan E, Green S, Alberts D, O'Toole R, Surwit E. Results of a Southwest Oncology Group Phase II Trial of carboplatin plus cyclophosphamide versus cisplatin plus cyclophosphamide in advanced ovarian cancer. *Oncology* 1993; 50 Supp 2:2–9.

38. Olivi A, Gilbert M, Duncan K, Corden B, Lenartz D, Brem H. Direct delivery of platinum-based antineoplastics to the central nervous system: a toxicity and ultrastructural study. *Cancer Chemother Pharmacol* 1993; 31:449–454.

39. Olivi A, Ewend M, Utsuki T, et al. Interstitial delivery of carboplatin via biodegradable polymers is effective against experimental glioma in the rat. *Cancer Chemother Pharmacol* 1996; 39:90–96.

40. Utsuki T, Brem H, Pitha J, et al. Potentiation of anticancer effects of microencapsulated carboplatin by hydroxypropyl α-cyclodextrin. *J Controlled Release* 1996; 40:251–260.

41. Judy K, Olivi A, Buahin K, et al. Effectiveness of controlled release of a cyclophosphamide derivative with polymers against rat gliomas. *J Neurosurg* 1995; 82:481–486.

42. Tamargo R, Bok R, Brem H. Angiogenesis inhibition by minocycline. *Cancer Res* 1991; 51:672–675.

43. Weingart J, Sipos E, Brem H. The role of minocycline in the treatment of intracranial 9L glioma. *J Neurosurg* 1995; 82:635–640.

44. Thompson R, Pardoll D, Jaffee E, et al. Systemic and local paracrine cytokine therapies using transduced tumor cells are synergistic in treating intracranial tumors. *J Immunother* 1997; 19:405–413.

45. Ewend M, Thompson R, Anderson R, et al. Intracranial paracrine interleukin-2 therapy stimulates prolonged antitumor immunity which extends outside the central nervous system. *J Immunother* 2000; 23:438–448.

46. DiMeco F, Rhines LD, Hanes J, et al. Paracrine delivery of IL-12 against intracranial 9L gliosarcoma in rats. *J Neurosurg* 2000; 92:419–427.

47. Hanes J, Suh K, Tyler B, et al. Local interleukin-2 delivery eradicates brain and liver tumors, Proc. Int Symp. Control. Rel. Bioact. Mater., Las Vegas, NV, June 21–26, 1998.

48. Hanes J, Sills A, Zhao Z, et al. Controlled local delivery of interleukin-2 by biodegradable polymers protects animals from experimental brain tumors and liver tumors. *Pharm Res* 2001; 18:899–906.

49. DiMeco F, Rhines L, Hanes J, et al. Local delivery of IL-12 microspheres (IL-12MS) against experimental brain tumors. *Congress of Neurolog Surg* 1999; Boston, MA.

50. Nigam A, Yacavone F, Zahurak M, et al. Immunomodulatory properties of antineoplastic drugs administered in conjunction with GM-CSF secreting cancer cell vaccines. *Int J Oncol* 1998; 12:161–170.

51. Tsung K, Meko J, Tsung Y, Peplinski G, Norton J. Immune response against large tumors aradicated by treatment with cyclophospamide and IL-12. *J Immunol* 1998; 160:1369–1377.
52. Sampath P, Hanes J, DiMeco F, et al. Paracrine immunotherapy with interleukin-2 and local chemotherapy is synergistic in the treatment of experimental brain tumors. *Cancer Res* 1999; 59:2107–2114.

11 Intralesional Chemotherapy with Injectable Collagen Gel Formulations

Elaine K. Orenberg, PhD

1. INTRODUCTION

Management of solid tumors continues to be a major challenge in cancer therapy. Two traditional approaches for local disease are surgical excision and radiation therapy, although treatment of metastatic disease requires systemic chemotherapy. Researchers have explored the concept of intratumoral chemotherapy via simple injection of drugs directly into tumors as an additional option along with surgery or radiation to manage locally confined malignant tumors. However, intratumoral injection of aqueous solutions of cytotoxic agents has had only marginal success. The heterogenous blood supply and interstitial pressure in solid tumors can limit drug penetration and dispersion throughout the tumor *(1)*. Moreover, aqueous drugs are rapidly cleared from the tumor mass. Thus, inclusion of drugs into slow-release systems provides an attractive alternative.

Novel drug systems developed by Matrix Pharmaceutical Inc.* have been specially designed to treat local tumors with the goal of achieving high, sustained, and homogenous intratumoral drug concentrations without the toxicities typically observed with systemically administered agents. The injectable drug systems use a carrier matrix that can be formulated with a variety of hydrophilic drugs. Two examples of this approach for therapy of solid tumors and cutaneous epitheliomas are the cisplatin/epinephrine gel (CDDP/epi) gel and the fluorouracil/epinephrine (5-FU/epi) gel that have been extensively evaluated experimentally in clinical trials with veterinary and human patients.

---

* Technology now owned by Biomedicines, Inc.

From: *Drug Delivery Systems in Cancer Therapy*
Edited by: D. M. Brown © Humana Press Inc., Totowa, NJ

The injectable gels are composed of a uniform suspension of CDDP or 5-FU and epinephrine in an aqueous collagen matrix. The major active drugs are antineoplastic agents with a long history of proven effectiveness. The gel matrix entraps and provides a uniform suspension of the drug, and is believed to provide enhanced drug retention by inhibiting fluid flow, thus slowing drug clearance from the tumor. The second active component, epinephrine, acts as a vasoconstrictor to further inhibit clearance of the cytotoxic drug from the injection site. These localized delivery systems also produce slowed and reduced entry of the drug into the systemic circulation, resulting in minimal exposure of distant tissues to the drug and a lower incidence of systemic side effects. The efficacy in terms of tumor response can be achieved with a total drug dose substantially lower than those administered systemically.

The pharmacology of the active drugs, CDDP and 5-FU, and epinephrine has been well-characterized. Preclinical studies in various tumor models with intratumorally administered CDDP/epi gel and 5-FU/epi gel have shown the gels to be efficacious and superior to aqueous solutions of these cytotoxic drugs administered either intratumorally or systemically. Epinephrine was documented as essential to optimize the antitumor effect.

This chapter will summarize the scope of clinical studies that have been conducted with CDDP/epi injectable gel and 5-FU/epi-injectable gel for local tumor control.

2. INTRALESIONAL CHEMOTHERAPY WITH COLLAGEN GELS FOR TREATMENT OF SPONTANEOUS TUMORS IN VETERINARY PATIENTS

2.1. Overview of Drugs and Regimens

The protein carrier matrix system comprised of bovine collagen gel combined with chemotherapeutics such as fluorouracil (5-FU) and cisplatin (CDDP) had been initially validated in experimental mouse tumor models. Compared with a free drug, collagen gel drug delivery enhanced drug concentration of 5-FU and CDDP and retention time in tumor tissue (2–4), delayed tumor regrowth, and resulted in lower systemic side effects (5). To advance these therapeutic opportunities a pilot study was conducted to assess technical feasibility, local and systemic adverse reactions, and tumor responses of intralesional chemotherapy of collagen gels in veterinary patients with spontaneously occurring skin and subcutaneous tumors (6).

A total of 247 patients including small domestic companion animals, horses, and a variety of other animals were involved in studies conducted in university and private veterinary clinics. A total of 638 cutaneous tumors were evaluated including 23 histologically distinct tumor types; the majority (85%) of patients had squamous cell carcinoma (SCC), equine sarcoid, canine oral melanoma, equine and feline fibrosarcoma, and feline eosinophilic granuloma. Therapeutic regimens in open-label drug protocols consisted of either a single drug delivered in a collagen gel or up to three drugs given sequentially in a series of gels. Specific regimens were based on sensitivity and the clinical response of the diseased tissue. The investigational agents were comprised of the carrier protein (purified bovine collagen), epinephrine (epi; 0.1 mg/mL of gel) and a chemotherapeutic drug including one of the following seven agents: 5-FU (30 mg/mL); CDDP (1–3 mg/mL); methotrexate (6 mg/mL); vinblastine (0.5–1.0 mg/mL); bleomycin (15 U/mL); carmustine (BCNU, 32 mg/mL); or triamcinolone (1–8 mg/mL). Each chemotherapeutic agent had been previously character-ized by in vitro and in vivo pharmacokinetic drug-release studies in mouse tumor models.

Small animals were treated under anesthesia; large animals were restrained prior to treatment and anesthetized when necessary. Up to three collagen gel treatments were administered intralesionally (1–3 mL) in a 1- to 2-wk period. For tumors with less than 50% reduction in tumor volume, subsequent treatments were with a second drug in a collagen gel. Feasibility of delivery of the seven different therapeutic agents was demonstrated. Of all tumors in cats, dogs, and horses treated with the collagen gel for-mulations, 72% had a 50% or greater reduction in tumor size, and 45% of these had complete clinical regressions. An average of three treatments with a single drug elicited these responses. The drug regimen of two drugs given sequentially, 5-FU/epi gel fol-lowed by CDDP/epi gel, resulted in 82% of all SCCs in all species to have a partial response (50% tumor reduction) with 62% of these having a complete response. Recur-rent canine oral melanoma was treated effectively with CDDP/epi gel alone; 10 of 11 tumors (91%) had partial or better responses and 55% had complete responses. These animals had had previous therapy with surgical debulking or cryotherapy. Fibrosarco-mas in horses were effectively treated with a multiple-drug regimen of 5-FU/epi gel, methotrexate/epi gel, and CDDP/epi gel, whereas feline fibrosarcoma was responsive to CDDP/epi gel followed by methotrexate/epi gel.

2.2. Use for Canine Squamous Cell Carcinoma

SCC is the most frequently reported malignant epithelial tumor in dogs. As in humans, chronic sun exposure causes actinic damage, which ultimately results in SCC. Several breeds of dogs with lightly pigmented skin or sparsely haired regions of the abdomen and inner thighs are at increased risk. They sunbathe lying on their backs exposing the abdomen to ultraviolet radiation, which eventually results in premalignant and malignant skin changes. The sun-induced SCC is typically well-differentiated and has a low metastatic potential. Thus, the dog serves as a useful model to investigate new therapeutic approaches for similar human malignant epitheliomas. Traditional therapy for SCC in dogs has included surgical excision and radiation therapy, or cryosurgery and topical or systemic 5-FU.

Dogs with large, single SCC or fields of multiple SCC were treated with sustained-retention collagen gels containing either 5-FU (30 mg in the 5-FU/epi gel) or cisplatin (3.3 mg in the CDDP/epi gel) (7). Treatments were given while dogs were under general anesthesia. The drug was injected intralesionally using a fanning pattern to ensure uni-form distribution of the gel throughout the lesion. Treatments began with 5-FU/epi gel given for a minimum of three treatments at weekly intervals. Dogs who did not achieve a complete response (no clinical evidence of disease at the treated site) were then treated with CDDP/epi gel for a minimum of three injections or until a complete response. The rationale for using 5-FU as the initial treatment agent followed by CDDP was based on the increased efficacy of this drug sequence reported in murine tumors (8).

From one to 11 primary, recurrent, or refractory SCCs were treated per dog (tumor size 0.2–92.4 cm^2, mean cumulative tumor area of 40.7 cm^2 per dog). All animals had at least a 50% reduction in cumulative tumor area with 5-FU/epi gel. More than half (7 of 13) had a complete response after treatment with the 5-FU and CDDP gels. The mean disease-free interval for dogs with complete response was 153 wk (range,

9–461). Three dogs with partial response had residual tumor excised and remained alive from 87 to 268 wk. The injectable gel therapy was well tolerated. Local necrosis, limited to the treatment site, occurred in most tumors (17 of 20), and was an expected reaction associated with tumor response. Systemic adverse events were minimal. None of the owners reported clinical signs associated with the toxicity often reported for CDDP given systemically. CDDP toxicity was not expected because the small dose of CDDP (mean dose, 5.3 mg/cm^3 of tumor) used in the study represented a substantially lower dose than that used for intravenous (iv) CDDP for the treatment of disseminated disease (50–70 mg/m^2 of body surface area). The study demonstrated the feasibility, safety, and efficacy of collagen gel chemotherapy for spontaneous sun-induced SCC, and the potential application of this local therapy for human cutaneous cancers.

2.3. Use for Malignant Melanoma in Horses and Dogs

Regional chemotherapy with CDDP/epi gel has been investigated as adjuvant or primary therapeutic approach for malignant melanoma. The first report involved use of the injectable collagen gel containing CDDP (5 mg) and epinephrine (0.375 mg) to treat residual tumor margins after excision of melanoma in the foot of a horse (9). The surgical defect healed with granulation and the horse remained clinically free of disease for 2 yr before disease recurrence. This form of local chemotherapy was advocated for future use in clinical situations where surgery is only moderately successful and there is the need to reduce the number of residual, viable tumor cells.

The CDDP/epi gel was evaluated for treatment of primary oral malignant melanoma in dogs (10). Twenty dogs were treated including 16 with advanced local disease (Stage II, III, or IV) with a primary tumor > 2 cm diameter; 13 of the tumors were recurrent. One dog had multiple primary nodules and was treated to palliate local oral disease only. Mean tumor volume was 7.0 cm^3 (range, 0.19–35 cm^3). Animals were treated at weekly intervals for a mean of 5.2 treatments with CDDP/epi gel only (17 dogs); empirically, one was treated with a methotrexate/epi gel after the CDDP/epi gel, and two dogs received methotrexate/epi gel and BCNU/epi gel after the CDDP/epi gel.

Melanomas in 14 (70%) of the 20 dogs had a 50% decrease in tumor volume; 11 (55%) of these had a complete tumor response. The median survival of 51 wk in the dogs with complete responses was substantially greater than that of dogs without local tumor control, median of 10.5 wk. The survival duration exceeded that reported for mandibular melanomas treated with surgery, radiation therapy, or radiation therapy plus hyperthermia. This observation was considered pertinent because most of the tumors in the study were recurrent after previous surgery and had a poor prognosis for further local control.

3. CISPLATIN/EPINEPHRINE INJECTABLE GEL

Introduced three decades ago, cisplatin (CDDP) as a single agent or in combination with other cytotoxic drugs, administered intravenously (iv), has shown significant activity in the treatment of a variety of primary and metastatic tumors including head and neck squamous cell carcinoma (HNSCC) (11,12). Cisplatin plus 5-FU is one of the standard regimens for recurrent or metastatic HNSCC, with an overall response rate of 30% and a 5% complete response rate (13). There is evidence to support a dose-response relationship for CDDP in sensitive tumors. Attempts to increase dose intensity have been limited by toxicity, commonly nephrotoxicity, peripheral neuropathy, ototoxicity, myelosuppression, and electrolyte and magnesium wasting *(14)*. Nausea and vomiting can be severe, necessitating the use of potent antiemetics *(15)*.

To improve the efficacy of CDDP chemotherapy, the drug system, cisplatin/epi injectable gel (CDDP/epi gel), was designed for direct intratumoral injection in order to achieve high, sustained concentrations of CDDP within the tumor and to minimize systemic exposure. The injectable gel is comprised of CDDP (4 mg/mL) and the vasoconstrictor epinephrine (0.1 mg/mL) in a purified bovine dermal collagen as the carrier matrix.

In the initial clinical experience with CDDP/epi gel (a multicenter dose-escalation pilot study including 45 patients with 82 solid tumors) it was shown that the adverse effects typical of systemically administered cisplatin were rare and mild *(16)*. Objective tumor responses, complete or partial, were achieved in half (41 of 82) of the tumors, of which 33 were complete responses.

The CDDP/epi gel was used in a number of Phase II and III trials to further evaluate the safety and efficacy of local chemotherapy in patients with a variety of solid tumors. Most patients had generally undergone extensive prior therapy with surgery or chemotherapy, or had received near-maximum tolerated radiation. Many tumors were considered inoperable having recurred or having not responded to previous treatment. Many patients with advanced disease were often poor candidates for aggressive combination therapy, or had refused further therapy. Therefore, CDDP/epi gel was used in an attempt to provide effective local or regional control of the tumor or to palliate symptoms associated with the tumor.

The Phase II studies in patients with metastatic breast cancer, cutaneous and soft tissue metastases of malignant melanoma, and esophageal and gastric cancers used a dose of 0.5 mL/cm^3 (equivalent to CDDP 2 mg/cm^3) of tumor volume. Doses of 0.25 mL/cm^3 (equivalent to CDDP 1 mg/cm^3) of tumor volume were used in the Phase III placebo-controlled trials for patients with HNSCC. A maximum of 10 mL injectable gel was permitted for each treatment visit. Intratumoral injections of the drug were given at weekly intervals for up to six treatments in an 8-wk period. In the Phase II studies of primary hepatocellular carcinoma (HCC) and colorectal metastases to the liver, the maximum dose was 10 mL of CDDP/epi gel administered percutaneously into liver lesions under ultrasound or computed tomography (CT) guidance. From four to eight injections were given at weekly intervals.

Objective tumor responses were based on the responses of individual tumors treated for local control. A complete response was defined as a 100% reduction in tumor volume (no detectable tumor); partial response was defined as 50% to <100% reduction in tumor volume, both sustained for at least 28 d. In some studies the "patient benefit" (also referred to a "clinical benefit") was assessed. A new quality of life instrument, the Treatment Goals Questionnaire© (TGQ) was designed and used to evaluate patient benefit achieved during treatment of local or regional disease *(17)*. Patient benefit was based on patient's progress toward achieving prospectively selected primary treatment goals by patient and investigator for the most troublesome (symptomatic) tumor. From the TGQ patients selected one of eight palliative goals: wound care, pain control, ability to see, ability to hear, ability to smell, physical appearance, obstructive symptoms, or mobility. The investigator could select one of the eight palliative goals but also had the option of selecting one of three preventative goals: prevention of invasion, obstruction, or subcutaneous tumor breakthrough. All benefits had to be sustained for at least 28 d. The association between tumor response and achievement of patient benefit was also assessed.

3.1. Use in Head and Neck Cancer

HNSCC is diagnosed yearly in more than 600,000 persons worldwide and in about 40,000 Americans. The majority of patients present with locally or regionally advanced disease, invasion of local structures, nodal metastases, and/or distant metastases. Despite aggressive therapy about 60% of patients have recurrences *(18)*. Recurrent tumors are often symptomatic and impair function. Therapeutic options for these patients with advanced disease are limited. Local-regional therapies are frequently associated with significant toxicity or morbidity, as is systemic chemotherapy, which is characterized by brief durations of remission but has little effect on survival *(13)*.

Intratumoral chemotherapy with CDDP/epi gel was evaluated as a new local therapy in patients with advanced HNSCC who had problematic tumors that might benefit from a form of local intervention. Two prospective, randomized, double-blind, placebo-controlled Phase III studies of similar design were conducted in North American and in Europe/Israel involving a total of 178 intensely pretreated patients with recurrent or refractory head and neck cancer *(19)*. The comprehensive results from the individual studies have also been reported *(20,21)*. A crossover from the blinded phase to open-label phase of study was permitted for patients with disease progression.

Combined results from the two trials (178 evaluable patients by intent to treat analysis) confirmed objective tumor responses in 35 of 119 (29%) including 33 tumors (19%) with complete responses achieved with CDDP/epi gel, vs only 1 of 59 (2%) for placebo ($p < 0.001$). Stable disease was maintained in 29 of 119 (24%) of patients. Tumor responses generally occurred within 2–3 wk of the first treatment. The median duration of response was 78 d (range, 30–554+). Many patients with responses were unable to extend participation in the study beyond a few months owing to the advanced stage of their disease with subsequent systemic disease progression, general physical debilitation, or death.

The response rates for patients who rolled over from placebo to active drug treatment were similar to those patients treated with active drug during the blinded phase: 27% (11 of 41). These responses were notable because between the times of the first placebo treatment in the blinded phase until the first treatment with CDDP/epi gel, median tumor sizes had almost doubled from 5.7 cm^3 to 10.8 cm^3. Similar response rates were also attained in patients who had previously received systemic cisplatin or carboplatin treatment (29%, 14 of 48) and in patients who were "platinum naïve" (30%, 2 of 7).

Patient benefit was evaluated using the validated Treatment Goals Questionnaire®. The most frequently selected goals were improved pain control, improved wound care, relief of obstructive symptoms, and improved physical appearance. The patients treated with CDDP/epi gel achieved significant palliative clinical benefits when compared with patients treated with placebo gel: 27% vs 12% ($p < 0.05$). There was a significant and positive association between tumor response and attainment of patient benefit compared to patients without tumor responses ($p = 0.006$). Patients with tumor responses were three times more likely to benefit from treatment than nonresponders (47% vs 15%, respectively).

Pain during injection was the most common side effect of the treatment procedure: 24% (29 of 119) patients treated with CDDP/epi gel reported immediate injection pain (within –20 min) as did 17% (10 of 60) of the placebo patients. Local cytotoxic effects at the treatment site were expected including inflammation, bleeding, erosion, ulceration, necrosis, and eschar observed in 88% of the treated tumors treated with active drug versus 63% in the placebo group. As tumor necrosis proceeds, the diseased tissues are replaced by normal healing and reepithelialization. Four cases of cerebrovascular events occurred early in the North American Phase III study; none occurred after protocols were modified to exclude tumors directly invading or in immediate proximity to that carotid artery. The CDDP/epi gel treatment had a favorable adverse event profile in comparison to iv cisplatin with a markedly lower incidence of chemotherapy-related systemic events.

Intratumoral CDDP/epi-injectable gel may find a role in the current treatments regimens for patients with HNSCC who can benefit from local tumor control and who cannot be managed with surgery or radiation alone, or as an alternative to systemic chemotherapy. Preclinical investigations in support of further explorations of combination therapy include a report on the use of CDDP/epi gel to prevent local tumor growth after margin-positive resection *(22)* and reports on radiosensitization by intratumoral CDDP/epi gel in combination with radiation *(3,23,24)*.

3.2. Use in Metastatic and Recurrent Breast Cancer

Breast cancer is the second most common cause of cancer death in American women. When diagnosed early, the disease is often curable with surgical excision alone or surgery and adjuvant therapy (i.e., hormonal, chemo-, and/or radiation therapy). However, advanced disease is rarely curable. Treatment for these patients focuses on prolongation of life when possible, and management of the disease, both the metastatic and local symptoms caused by tumor masses.

CDDP/epi injectable gel was evaluated in patients with advanced disease to provide palliation of tumor symptoms, and local tumor control with higher local drug concentrations and much milder toxicity than possible with systemically administered cisplatin chemotherapy.

Patients with recurrent or metastatic, histologically confirmed breast cancer were enrolled in a multicenter, open-label Phase II trial *(25,26)*. All 27 evaluable patients had previously undergone surgery, chemotherapy, hormonal or radiation therapy; 78% had been treated with all three modalities. Seventy percent of tumors were in previously irradiated fields. The 27 patients presented with 72 tumors that were treated at the first visit; a total of 89 tumors, including newly emergent lesions, were treated during the course of study. One tumor per patient was identified as the most troublesome; this target tumor was monitored for objective tumor response and used to assess patient benefit. Median baseline tumor volume for target tumors *(27)* was 3.4 cm^3 (range, 0.4–413 cm^3); for all 89 tumors treated, the median was 0.65 cm^3.

Overall, 52% (14 of 27) target tumors had objective responses, 6 complete and 8 partial responses, after a median of three *(1–7)* treatments. The median duration of response was 82 d (range, 29–211), although some patients retained responses for more than 2 yr, as reported anecdotally after study completion. Many patients discontinued follow-up beyond 28 d as a result of progressive systemic disease. For all tumors treated, 40% (36 of 89) had objective responses, 26 complete and 10 partial responses.

This therapy provided clinical benefit (e.g., pain control, improved wound care) for 11 (41%) of the patients as assessed by the validated Treatment Goals Questionnaire *(17)*. Response of the target tumor and attainment of patient benefit were strongly associated; patients who had tumor responses were four times more likely to gain benefit (64%) than nonresponding patients (15%).

As expected with this local treatment, almost all patients experienced necrosis at the treatment sites. Other related tissue conditions included eythema and swelling, as well as ulceration/eosion and eschar formation. No systemic toxicities typically associated with intravenous cisplatin administration (nephrotoxicity, ototoxicity, myelosupression) were reported.

The CDDP/epi-injectable gel provides a new treatment option for local tumor control and palliation in patients with advanced breast cancer. It may be complementary to systemic chemotherapy and/or radiation. A preliminary study combining radiation and intratumoral 5-FU gel, as a radiopotentiator *(27)*, supports further exploration of the potential of CDDP/epi gel as a potentiator of standard radiotherapy.

3.3. Use in Malignant Melanoma

The primary treatment goal for metastatic melanoma is palliation because the use of immunomodulatory treatment modalities and systemic chemotherapy has been ineffective in improving survival. Local-regional therapies have provided the most effective means of managing this disease. Surgery is the standard therapy for Stage I and II melanoma, can be curative for Stage III melanoma, and can provide considerable palliative benefits (relief of obstruction, perforation, bleeding). Both radiotherapy and isolated limb profusion have been used, however, these are often associated with significant toxicity or morbidity as is systemic chemotherapy. Less invasive local therapies for cutaneous metastases have been explored in order to provide improved quality of life, including CO_2 laser therapy, photodynamic therapy, and intralesional injections of dinitrochlorobenzene and bacilli Calmette-Guerin, with varying degrees of success *(28)*.

The feasibility of treating refractory or recurrent cutaneous and soft tissue melanoma metastases with CDDP/epi injectable gel was evaluated in an open-label, multicenter Phase II trial *(29)*. The primary consideration was local tumor control and palliation of symptoms especially in a group of patients with a poor prognosis for long-term survival. The opportunity to limit toxicity typical of intravenous chemotherapy was important to maximize or maintain their quality of life.

Treatments were usually performed as an outpatient procedure. The gel (0.5 mL/cm^3 of tumor volume) was injected directly into tumors which were located by direct visual examination or palpation. Up to six weekly treatments with CDDP/epi gel were given or until a complete response was achieved. Additional cycles of therapy were given if patients developed a new tumor(s) during the follow-up period or if a treated tumor recurred or regressed less than 100%.

A total of 25 patients with 244 lesions were treated during the study, with one patient receiving treatment for 72 tumors. Median baseline tumor volume of all tumors treated was 0.02 cm^3 (range, 0.001–201 cm^3). Objective tumor responses were attained in 53% (130 of 244 tumors); complete responses occurred in 114 (47%) and partial responses in 16 tumors (7%). The median duration of response was 347 d (range, 30 783 d).

The CDDP/epi gel produced significant but expected local cytotoxic reactions (erosion, ulceration, eschar, bleeding) that are associated with the therapeutic effect of the agent. These effects were managed by delaying the treatment or by ordinary supportive care.

Additional studies are warranted to determine how best to utilize CDDP/epi injectable gel to treat metastatic melanoma; therapy appears appropriate to treating multiple, recurrent, cutaneous, and subcutaneous metastases. Because of the localized nature of this intratumoral chemotherapy and generally mild systemic toxicity profile, the drug may serve as an additive therapy to surgery and radiation.

3.4. Use in Malignant Dysphagia in Esophageal Cancer

Therapy for advanced esophageal cancer aims to relieve dysphagia with minimal treatment-related morbidity. Most patients with this cancer present when the disease is too far advanced for any prospect of cure, although many can be treated for palliation of dysphagia that plagues them for the duration of their illness. A minimum number of interventions and minimal morbidity are mandatory. Established palliative techniques for patients not suitable for surgery or radiotherapy and/or chemotherapy are endoscopic insertion of prostheses (stents), alcohol injection, and laser therapy. Each modality has limitations regarding functional outcome, requirement of expensive equipment, and specialized skills, and safety, respectively.

The CDDP/epi gel was evaluated in a Phase II, multicenter, open-label trial as a potential alternative palliative treatment for malignant dysphagia *(30)*. Patients had inoperable esophageal cancer (adenocarcinoma and SCC) and dysphagia caused by exophytic tumor in the esophagus, accessible for direct endoscopic injection, and with an estimated tumor volume of 0.5–20 cm^3.

Tumors were injected through an endoscope using a 23- or 25-gauge, 5-mm sclerotherapy needle attached to a Luer-lock syringe containing the drug. The procedure was performed under mild sedation; number of injection sites and volume of gel injected (typically 0.1 mL to 0.5 mL) depended on size of the tumor nodule and ease of access to inject the calculated dose of 0.5 mL/cm^3.

Twenty-four patients were enrolled in the study; 18 patients were evaluable for response and all 24 were included in the safety assessment. Patients received a median of three treatments (range, 1–6), usually at weekly intervals. Dysphagia grade improved in four (duration, 30–45 d), stabilized in 11; lumen patency improved in six (duration, 29–111 d), stabilized in 10; and exophytic tumor volume decreased in eight (duration, 29–114 d). Eight of 18 (44%) of patients judged their ability to swallow as improved. The length of response in these patients was short, which was unfortunately similar to the duration of response of all palliative treatments. However, the improved or stable dysphagia is encouraging, especially in this advanced group of patients who were less likely to demonstrate a clinical benefit.

The endoscopic administration of CDDP/epi gel was generally well tolerated and involved none of the medically significant toxicities typically associated with systemic cisplatin, particularly nephrotoxicity, severe nausea and vomiting, or electrolyte abnormalities. One patient with intramural and exophytic tumor injected with CDDP/epi gel developed a tracheoesophageal fistula, possibly related to treatment.

Injecting CDDP/epi gel endoscopically was feasible and tolerable as confirmed by others for both esophageal *(31)* and gastric carcinomas *(32)*. This therapy has the potential to serve in the palliation of endoscopically accessible tumors in the upper and lower gastrointestinal tract where debulking of exophytic tumor is needed to relieve obstruction. It may be used either alone or as an adjunct to stent insertion with or without concomitant radiation therapy.

3.5. Use in Unresectable Primary and Metastatic Liver Cancer

The worldwide incidence of HCC is reported to be approx 500,000 cases per year; overall, the median survival after diagnosis is less than 1 yr. HCC often develops secondary to cirrhosis and chronic viral hepatitis. This highly malignant disease is a major health problem throughout Asia, Africa, southern Europe, and increasingly in the United States. Surgical resection or orthotopic liver transplantation (OLT) offer the only possibility for long-term survival, but is applicable in only 10–20% of cases. The majority of patients are not candidates for resection, either because of the presence of advanced disease, inadequate liver function as a result of underlying cirrhosis, or both. Nonsurgical treatments for patients with unresectable HCC include systemic chemotherapy, chemoembolization, and radiation therapy. The overall treatment results are poor.

Patients with small tumors confined to the liver, but considered unresectable with surgery, may be considered candidates for OLT or local ablative therapies such as radiofrequency ablation, ethanol injection, or microwave coagulation. These local modalities are typically only appropriate for patients with small tumors (5 cm diameter) and with few (3) lesions. The goal of these ablative procedures is to produce a high degree of necrosis in the tumor and tumor margins without toxicity to surrounding liver parenchyma and structures.

CDDP/epi injectable gel was evaluated in a multicenter, open-label Phase II trial in patients with localized unresectable HCC who had no more than three tumors, each with a maximum diameter of 7 cm, and a total tumor volume up to 200 cm^3 *(33,34)*. A separate pharmacokinetic study on a subset of six patients who received intratumoral CDDP/epi gel has been reported *(35)*. Patients were treated percutaneously with CDDP/epi gel under ultrasound or CT guidance, delivering up to 10 mL of agent per treatment; four weekly treatments over a 6-wk period for a maximum of two cycles. The primary endpoint was tumor response defined as percent change in total viable tumor volume (total lesion volume minus total necrotic tumor volume) based on repeated CT imaging. The appearance of any new tumors in an untreated site was not considered a treatment failure.

A total of 51 patients with histologically confirmed, unresectable HCC with no extrahepatic or major vascular involvement, and no prior therapy other than surgical resection were evaluable for response. The objective response rate was 53% (27 of 51 patients) including 16 complete and 11 partial responses after a median of four treatments (range, 1–8). Of the 27 responders, 14 (52%) subsequently developed progressive disease, but only one patient (7%) developed new tumor at a previously treated liver site. The median survival for responders was 22.5 mo compared to 11.4 mo for nonresponders; these patients were similarly matched prior to treatment for Child-Pugh liver function and levels of α-fetoprotein.

The pathology of six treated lesions in three patients was examined histologically; two patients received OLT after completion of treatment with CDDP/epi gel, and the third had an autopsy. Histological examination of the livers revealed extensive necrosis for lesions treated with CDDP/epi gel; there was a good correlation in four of five lesions between the CT scan assessment of degree of necrosis and the microscopic examination *(36)*.

The percutaneous treatment procedure was well tolerated with only minor side effects, including immediate injection-associated pain, transient hypertension, and tachycardia. Nausea and vomiting, common cisplatin-related side effects, were observed in 22% and 24% of patients, respectively, and were easily managed. Two deaths, considered related to treatment, occurred during study.

Intrahepatic colorectal cancer metastases result in significant cancer-related mortality worldwide, accounting for more that 50% of deaths in newly diagnosed patients. Only 10–20% of these patients are candidates for surgical resection, which still remains the only potentially curative regional therapy. However, the option for surgical resection is often limited due to multiple tumors involving both lobes, location of metastases close to major vessels, poor liver reserve, or comorbid conditions.

CDDP/epi injectable gel has also been evaluated in 31 patients with colorectal cancer metastatic to the liver. The Phase II, multicenter, open-label study used the same study design, dosing schedule, and tumor response evaluation criteria as the trial for HCC *(34,37)*. Many (61%) patients had received previous therapy for their primary or metastatic disease with multiple *(2–4)* modalities. The hepatic metastases were considered unresectable primarily because of location/difficulty to resect (15 of 31), prior lobectomy/hepatectomy (6), both lobes involved (5), patient refused resection (3), and poor surgical risk (2). Median total viable tumor treated was 60 cm^3 (range, 4–776 cm^3; 1–3 tumors per patient).

The overall response rate was 29% (9 of 31 patients) including six complete responses and three partial responses; 10 (32%) had stable disease. The median duration of response was 10.2 mo; median time to progression in all patients was 8.1 mo. The group of patients who had previously received systemic chemotherapy had an objective response rate of 25% (6 of 24) suggesting that this local therapy may be useful in liver-limited metastases in patients for whom chemotherapy is no longer an option.

Progression or relapse was seen frequently at new sites not treated with CDDP/epi gel. Twenty-one patients (4 responders, 17 nonresponders) subsequently had progressive disease; in 81% (17 of 21) progression was limited to the liver. No further treatment had been permitted in these patients by protocol design. Results of this study suggest that the efficacy of CDDP/epi gel for colorectal cancer metastases could be further enhanced by treating new tumors or tumors that progress after the initial course of therapy, or by using the drug in combination with systemic chemotherapy.

In conclusion, percutaneous intratumoral injection of CDDP/epi gel is efficacious for localized treatment of unresectable HCC and intrahepatic metastases of colorectal cancer. Side effects are tolerable. Owing to the echogenic nature of the drug, it is readily visible under ultrasound or real-time CT scan. This property is unique among all the local ablative therapies and can facilitate proper placement and distribution of the drug in the tumor. The extent of drug infiltration is clearly visible, thus allowing the physician to inject the drug close to tumor margins and avoid irritation of the liver capsule. This results in less pain than with other ablative therapies.

Based on the safety profile of CDDP/epi gel, it is a potential treatment for new, emerging, or recurrent tumors. It could be used to manage HCC in patients awaiting liver transplantation, and should be evaluated in combination with systemic chemotherapy for unresectable metastatic tumors in the liver.

4. FLUOROURACIL/EPINEPHRINE INJECTABLE GEL

4.1. Human Clinical Trials: Treatment of Cutaneous Malignancies and Benign Hyperplasia

Local chemotherapy has been used for decades for treatment of various cutaneous premalignant, malignant, and virally induced lesions, sometimes with limited success but frequently limitations in safety and efficacy. A drug formulation comprised of fluorouracil and epinephrine in a collagen gel as a carrier matrix, administered intralesionally, has been extensively evaluated clinically as a site-specific means of achieving uniform drug concentrations at target lesion sites that are not possible with topical 5-FU cream or intratumoral injection of aqueous 5-FU alone.

The cytotoxic drug 5-FU has a long history of use as an antiproliferative agent, applied topically for treatment of actinic keratosis, Bowen's disease, superficial basal cell carcinoma (BCC) (38,39), and condylomata acuminata (genital warts) (40–42). The highest success has been for multiple, small, nonkeratinizing genital warts. Inadequate drug penetration, low cure rates, and high recurrence rates make topical 5-FU unsuitable for nodular BCC. Some improvements in efficacy have been reported when an intralesional injection of the aqueous 5-FU was used for nodular BCC (43,44) and keratoacanthoma (43,45).

4.2. Use for SCC and BCC

Cutaneous neoplasms are usually treated with ablative procedures such as surgical excision, curettage and electrosurgery, cryosurgery, or irradiation (46). A nonsurgical treatment alternative to conserve tissue and obtain better cosmetic outcome would be of value in selected patients with an aversion to surgery or who are not good surgical candidates.

The safety and efficacy of 5-FU/epi gel was evaluated in an open-label, multicenter pilot study of 25 patients with histologically proven SCC on sun-exposed skin of the face, head, neck, trunk, or extremities (47). A single well-defined tumor of 0.6–3.0 cm diameter was selected per patient. Each lesion was confined to the upper half of the reticular dermis with the absence of nodular involvement or metastases. Each tumor site was treated with up to 1.0 mL of 5-FU/epi gel at weekly intervals for up to 6 wk. The tumor and surrounding tumor margins of at least 0.5 cm were injected intradermally using a 30-gauge needle on a Luer-Lok syringe by fanning or multiple injections to provide uniform drug distribution. After at least 4 wk of follow-up and assessment of cosmetic outcome, the tumor site was completely excised, then step-sectioned for histological examination. The absence of tumor in all sections was defined as a complete response.

Twenty-two of the 23 SCCs (96%) in patients who completed treatment had a histologically confirmed complete tumor clearing. Only one SCC did not respond completely, but this lesion had focal Bowen's disease at the surgical margin and no evidence of invasive malignancy. Evaluations of the cosmetic appearance of treated sites were rated as good to excellent by both clinical investigators and patients, and these were generally in close agreement.

BCCs are the most common form of skin cancer primarily resulting from actinic damage. About 85% of all BCCs occur on the face, head, and neck. As with SCC, the treatment goal focuses on complete tumor removal and tissue sparing to minimize cosmetic and functional defects. A total of 20 patients, each with biopsy-proven nodular BCC of 0.6–1.5 cm diameter with clinically well-defined margins were evaluated in an open-label pilot study *(48)*. Patients were randomly assigned to one of two doses of 5-FU/epi gel, either 0.25 mL (7.5 mg 5-FU) or 0.5 mL (15 mg 5-FU) and treated weekly by intralesional injections for up to 6 wk. To maintain a double-blind study, one investigator at each site prepared and administered the drug and the second investigator, not informed about dose, assessed the tissue conditions and determined the percent improvement of the test sites on the basis of overall response related to size and appearance before and after treatment. After 18 wk, the entire treatment site was excised and serial sections of tissue examined histologically for residual tumor.

Eight (80%) of the 10 patients treated with 0.5 mL of 5-FU/epi gel showed histologically confirmed elimination of tumor as did six (60%) of the 10 patients who received the lower dose. There was no statistical difference in responses between the two treatment groups. Before excision, most lesions had disappeared clinically. In two cases with an apparent clinical cure, the excision specimens showed residual tumor. Prior to excision at 18 wk, most tissue conditions had disappeared, with the exception of mild erythema and/or induration in a few patients. The treatment was well tolerated and no clinically significant side effects were reported. The doses of 5-FU in the 5-FU/epi gel were approximately one-third to one-twelfth less than doses reported for intralesional injection of aqueous drug in the treatment of BCC *(43,44)*.

To optimize the dose and treatment schedule for 5-FU/epi gel in patients with BCC, a second open-label, randomized study was conducted with 122 patients with biopsy-proven superficial and nodular BCC *(49)*. Two doses (0.5 mL and 1.0 mL) were examined in six different treatment regimens including: once weekly for 6 wk, twice weekly for 3 wk, twice weekly for 4 wk, or three times weekly for 2 wk (0.5 mL). Injections were intradermally at the base of the lesion, infiltrating the lesion and margins. Overall, 91% of evaluable treated tumors (106 of 116) in all regimens had histologically confirmed complete responses. The best response rate, tolerance, and patient compliance were in patients receiving 0.5 mL three times weekly for 2 wk. In this group, the histological response was 100%. The 5-FU/epi gel was both safe and efficacious, resulting in complete response rates comparable to surgery, thus providing a potential nonsurgical treatment alternative in selected patients.

4.3. Use in Psoriatic Plaques

Both topical 5-FU cream and intralesional aqueous 5-FU have been used on a limited basis for treatment of psoriasis, a benign hyperproliferative skin disease. The primary mechanism of action of 5-FU as an antimetabolite is thought to inhibit DNA synthesis by competitive inhibition of thymidylate synthesis and, thus, in psoriasis the intent of use is to attenuate the hyperproliferation of the epidermal keratinocytes characteristic of this skin disease.

A pilot study with 5-FU/epi gel represented the first application of this form of local chemotherapy for treatment of psoriatic plaques *(50)*. Fifty-three plaques (2.5 cm diameter) in 11 patients were randomly assigned to one of five treatment groups including 0.1, 0.33, or 1.0 mL 5-FU/epi gel injectable gel, an epinephrine gel without 5-FU (0.33 mL) and untreated control. A single treatment produced responses in 20 of 33 (60%) of plaques receiving 5-FU/epi gel. Responses were characterized by 50% or greater improvement in clinical appearance and complete clearing in four of 33 plaques. Qualitative responses were comparable with all three doses; no responses occurred with the two controls. The area of plaque response was related to dose volume, presumably because the dose increments from 0.1 to 1.0 mL permitted greater distribution of the drug in the plaques. These plaque responses after the single treatment were comparable to results produced with topical psoriasis therapies where twice daily applications for up to 2 wk are usually required. The intralesional gel increased the therapeutic index by increasing drug exposure within the diseased tissue, and thereby limiting the cutaneous reactions typically seen with topical 5-FU preparations or injection of 5-FU aqueous solution. The plaque responses observed in this single dose study suggest that 5-FU/epi gel would be clinically useful to treat chronic recalcitrant plaque psoriasis that is nonresponsive to other therapies.

4.4. Use for Condylomata Acuminata

Condylomata acuminata, highly contagious warts in the genital and perianal region, represent a common sexually transmitted disease that is a therapeutic challenge because current topical and ablative treatments yield low response rates and may lead to adverse events *(51)*. Although genital warts are usually benign growths, patients are concerned about the cosmetic appearance of warts, the psychosocial issues of having a sexually transmitted disease, the risk of transmission to a sexual partner, and fears of the association of human papillomavirus infection with cervical cancer.

The 5-FU/epi gel was evaluated in two Phase II, randomized, double-blind placebo-controlled studies involving 324 men and women with new, recurrent, or recalcitrant genital warts *(52)*. The purpose of the study was to evaluate the contribution of each component of the formulation and consisted of eight treatment groups. Up to six injections were administered intralesionally to each wart. Patients treated with the 5-FU/epi gel had a significantly higher ($p < 0.05$) complete response rate of 65% and a lower cumulative 90-d recurrence rate than those lesions treated with 5-FU gel without epinephrine or with individual or various combinations of components.

In a subsequent Phase III randomized, double-blind study of the safety and efficacy of 5-FU/epi gel was compared with 5-FU gel (without epinephrine) and placebo *(53)*. A total of 359 patients with 1926 condylomata underwent evaluation. Each lesion was injected once a week for up to 6 wk, and patients were followed for 3 mo. The minimum dose administered per wart (1 to <30 mm^2) was 0.25 mL with a maximum weekly dose of 150 mg 5-FU delivered in up to 5 mL of gel. The complete response rate for all lesions treated with 5-FU/epi gel was 77%, which was significantly ($p < 0.002$) more effective than 5-FU gel without epinephrine (complete response rate, 43%); both were superior to placebo (complete response rate, 5%). The treatment was well tolerated and no clinically significant drug-related systemic reactions occurred. Thus, intralesional chemotherapy with 5-FU/epi gel provides a new safe and effective treatment modality for condylomata acuminata.

5. CONCLUSION

Extensive experience in human clinical trials has demonstrated the safety and efficacy of local chemotherapy using novel drug systems designed to deliver cisplatin, CDDP/cpi gel, and fluorouracil, 5-FU/epi gel, using purified bovine collagen as the carrier matrix. These formulations are injected directly into tumors with the goal of achieving high, sustained, and homogeneous intralesional drug concentrations for extended periods of time, but without the atttendent toxicities typically observed with systemically administered CDDP or 5-FU.

The 5-FU/pei gel was used to treat almost 900 patients with cutaneous diseases including malignant epitheliomas (BCC and SCC) and benign, hyperproliferative lesions (psoriasis and genital warts). The injectable gel provided the opportunity to overcome the limitations of inadequate drug penetration and low cure rates of topical 5-FU and intralesional aqueous 5-FU, often used for decades to treat these skin diseases. For cutaneous neoplasms, the drug has shown potential as a nonsurgical treatment alternative to conserve tissue and to obtain a better cosmetic outcome in selected patients who are not good surgical candidates or have an aversion to surgery. No clinically significant drug-related systemic side effects were reported. Tissue reactions at the site of injection occurred in many patients as an expected event associated with the cytotoxic or antiproliferative activity of the drug. In the experimental arena of the clinical studies, strict adherence to protocols often required up to six treatments given at weekly intervals, thus not allowing attenuation of dosing to potentially reduce tissue reactions. Determination of the minimum number of treatments would be warranted in order to produce response and a better concomitant cutaneous reaction profile.

CDDP/epi injectable gel was evaluated as a single drug in more than 450 patients with a variety of solid tumors, primarily those with recurrent, local-regional carcinomas, who could benefit from local tumor control and palliation of tumor-related symptoms. All patients involved in the clinical studies had advanced disease, especially those with head and neck cancers, and had experienced local tumor recurrences after primary therapy with conventional surgery, radiation, or multiple modalities. Recurrent tumors can be painful and can invade vital structures, resulting in impaired function and curtailment of normal activities. Patients with recurrent tumors are often not candidates for repeated irradiation or resection because these tumors occur in previously irradiated fields and surgical excision is associated with excessive morbidity, slow recovery, and cost. Many patients are too fragile to tolerate the additional high-dose systemic chemotherapy that would be required to achieve substantial rates of local tumor control. For these patients, CDDP/epi gel can have a substantial impact.

The CDDP/epi injectable gel is easy to administer, although treatment is not without some toxicity. Local pain during and following intratumoral injection was the most common problem. This was rarely severe and could be controlled as needed with appropriate administration of pain medications and/or local anesthetics. Necrosis and skin breakdown are frequent consequences of progressing tumors. These manifestations were necessarily increased by treatment with CDDP/epi gel which caused rapid tumor killing; necrosis was found to occur and had a positive association with tumor response. Finally, the systemic side effects typically associated with iv administration of CDDP were milder or much reduced in the clinical setting of local intratumoral treatment. No nephrotoxicity, ototoxicity, or neurotoxicity were reported. Most important, however, is that treatment with CDDP/epi gel did not affect patients adversely to preclude additional treatment with other therapies as needed.

In all tumors treated with CDDP/epi injectable gel, the tumor responses were of high quality and patients had appreciable palliative clinical benefits. Efficacy is clearly demonstrated, even in patients with advanced disease, and suggests that the drug could be used in patients with earlier stage disease as a promising therapeutic option, either as a single agent, or added to the armamentarium of therapies in combination with radiation and /or systemic chemotherapy.

REFERENCES

1. Jain RK. Barriers to drug delivery in solid tumors. *Sci Am* 1994; 271:58–65.
2. Yu N, Conley F, Luck E, Brown D. Response of murine tumors to matrix-associated cisplatin intratumoral implants. *NCI Monogr* 1988; 6:137–140.
3. Howes A, Herman T, Montoya V, Luck EE, Brown DM. Effect of matrix-associated chemotherapy in combination with irradiation *in vivo. NCI Monog* 1988; 6:141–143.
4. Yu NY, Orenberg EK, Luck EE, Brown DB. Antitumor effect of intratumoral administration of fluorouracil/epinephrine injectable gel in C3H mice. *Cancer Chemother Pharmacol* 1995; 36:27–34.
5. Begg AC, Bartelink H, Stewart FA, Brown DM, Luck EE. Improvement of differential toxicity between tumor and normal tissues using intratumoral injection with or without a slow-drug-release matrix system. *NCI Monogr* 1988; 6:133–136.
6. Orenberg EK, Luck EE, Brown DM, Kitchell BE. Implant delivery system. Intralesional delivery of chemotherapeutic agents for treatment of spontaneous skin tumors in veterinary patients. *Clin Dermatol* 1992; 9:561–568.
7. Kitchell BE, Orenberg EK, Brown DM, et al. Intralesional sustained-release chemotherapy with therapeutic implants for treatment of canine sun-induced squamous cell carcinoma. *Euro J Cancer* 1995; 31:2093–2098.
8. Yu NY, Patawaran MB, Chen JY, Orenberg EK, Brown DM, Luck EE. Influence of treatment sequence on efficacy of fluorouracil and cisplatin intratumoral drug delivery in vivo. *Cancer J Sci Am* 1995; 1:215–221.
9. Honnas CM, Liskey CC, Meagher DM, Brown D, Luck EE. Malignant melanoma in the foot of a sorrel horse. *J Am Vet Med Assoc* 1990; 197:756–758.
10. Kitchell BE, Brown DM, Luck EE, Woods L, Orenberg EK, Bloch DA. Intralesional implant for treatment of primary oral malignant melanoma in dogs. *J Am Vet Med Assoc* 1994; 204:229–236.
11. Vokes EE, Weichselbaum RR, Lippman SM, Hong WK. Head and neck cancer. *N Engl J Med* 1993; 328:184–194.
12. Clayman GL, Dreiling LK. Injectable modalities as local and regional strategies for head and neck cancer. *Hematol Oncol Clin North Am* 1999; 13:787–810.
13. Posner MR, Colevas AD, Tishler RB. The role of induction chemotherapy in the curative treatment of squamous cell cancer of the head and neck. *Semin Oncol* 2000; 27 (suppl 8):13–24.
14. Robbins KT, Storniolo AM, Kerber C, et al. Phase I study of highly selective supradose cisplatin infusions for advanced head and neck cancer. *J Clin Oncol* 1994; 12:2113–2120.
15. Dorr RT, Von Hoff DD. Cisplatin. *Cancer Chemotherapy Handbook.* 2nd ed. Appleton & Lange Norwalk, CT, 1994, pp 286–298.
16. Burris H, Vogel C, Castro D, et al. Intratumoral cisplatin/epinephrine injectable gel as a palliative treatment for accessible solid tumors: A multicenter pilot study. *Otolaryngol Head Neck Surg* 1998; 118:496–503.
17. Mackowiak J, Stewart M, Leavitt R, Burris H III. Validation of the Treatment Goals Questionnaire© (TGQ): a new instrument to assess patient benefit following treatment of squamous cell carcinoma of the head and neck (HNSCC) with intratumoral cisplatin/epinephrine injectable gel. *Proc Am Soc Clin Oncol* 2001; 20:232.
18. Khuri FR, Shin DM, Glisson BS, Lippman SM, Hong WK. Treatment of patients with recurrent or metastatic squamous cell carcinoma of the head and neck: current status and future directions. *Semin Oncol* 2000; 27 (suppl 8):25–33.
19. Wenig BL, Werner JA, Castro DJ, et al. The role of intratumoral therapy with cisplatin/epinephrine injectable gel in the management of advanced squamous cell carcinoma of the head and neck. *Arch Otolaryngol Head Neck Surg* 2002; 128:880–885.
20. Castro DJ, Shridhar KS, Garewal HS, et al. Intratumoral cisplatin/epinephrine gel in recurrent or metastatic head and neck cancer: A randomized Phase III study in North America. *Head and Neck,* in press.
21. Werner JA, Kehrl W, Pluzanska A, et al. A phase III placebo-controlled study in advanced head and neck cancer using intratumoral cisplatin/epinephrine gel. *Br J Cancer* 2002; 87:938–944.
22. Davidson BS, Izzo F, Cromeens DM, Stephens LC, Siddik ZH, Curley SA. Collagen matrix cisplatin prevents local tumor growth after margin-positive resection. *J Surg Res* 1995; 58:618–624.
23. Theon AP, Madewell BR, Ryu J, Castro J. Concurrent irradiation and intratumoral chemotherapy with cisplatin: A pilot study in dogs with spontaneous tumors. *Int J Radiat Oncol Biol Phys* 1994; 29:1027–1034.

24. Ning S, Yu N, Brown DM, Kanekal S, Knox SJ. Radiosensitization by intratumoral administration of cisplatin in a sustained-release drug delivery system. *Radiother Oncol* 1999; 50:215–223.

25. Fernando I, Eisenberg PD, Roshon S, Mansi J, Mills G, de Vries E. Intratumoral focused chemotherapy with cisplatin/epinephrine injectable gel for palliative treatment of metastatic breast cancer. *Eur J Cancer* 1999; 35 (suppl 4):S318.

26. Roshon S, Fernando I, Mansi J, Jäger W, Kennedy P, and the Clinical Trials Group. Intratumoral cisplatin/epinephrine injectable gel for local control of recurrent breast cancer. 3rd Annual Lynn Sage Breast Cancer Symp Chicago, IL, Oct. 19–21, 2001.

27. Kuske RR, Gage I, Solin L, McCormick B. Intratumoral fluorouracil injectable gel (5-FU gel) as a potentiator of standard radiotherapy in patients with locally recurrent breast cancer: Preliminary experience in a phase I/II trial. *Breast Cancer Res Treat* 1998; 50:287.

28. Shapiro RL, Oratz R, Roses DF. Treatment of regionally recurrent malignant melanoma. *Arch Oncol* 1999; 15:15–21.

29. Oratz R, Hauschild A, Sebastian G, et al. Intratumoral cisplatin/epinephrine injectable gel for treatment of patients with cutaneous and soft tissue metastases of malignant melanoma. *Melanoma Res* 2003; 13:1–8.

30. Harbord M, Dawes RFH, Giovannini M, et al. Palliation of dysphagia in advanced esophageal cancer by endoscopic injection of cisplatin/epinephrine injectable gel. *Gastrointest Endosc* 2002; 56:644–651.

31. Monga DK, Mishra L. Intratumoral therapy of cisplatin/epinephrine injectable gel for palliation in patients with obstructive esophageal cancer. *Am J Clin Oncol* 2000; 23:386–392.

32. Monga SPS, Wadleigh R, Adib H, Harmon JW, Berlin M, Mishra L. Endoscopic treatment of gastric cancer with intratumoral cisplatin/epinephrine injectable gel: A case report. *Gastrointest Endosc* 1998; 48:415–417.

33. Leung TWT, Johnson PJ, Yu S, et al. A phase II study of the safety and efficacy of cisplatin/epinephrine injectable gel administered to patients with unresectable hepatocellular carcinoma. *J Clin Oncol* 2003; 21:652–658.

34. Vogl TJ, Engelmann K, Mack MG, et al. CT-guided intratumoral administration of cisplatin/epinephrine gel for treatment of malignant liver tumors. *Brit J Cancer* 2002; 86:524–529.

35. Mok TSK, Kanekal S, Lin XR, et al. Pharmacokinetic study of intralesional cisplatin for the treatment of hepatocellular carcinoma. *Cancer* 2001; 91:2369–2377.

36. Thuluvath PJ, Geschwind JF, Johnson PJ, Heneghan MA, O'Grady J. Management of hepatoma using cisplatin/epinephrine gel in patients awaiting orthotopic liver transplantation. *Transplant Proc* 2001; 33:1359.

37. Vogl T, Lipton A, Abramson N, Benson AB, Kemeny M. Percutaneous cisplatin/epinephrine (CDDP/epi) injectable gel for treatment of unresectable intrahepatic metastases of colorectal adenocarcinoma. *Proc Am Soc Clin Oncol* 2001; 20:137a.

38. Sturm HM. Bowen's disease and 5-fluorouracil. *J Am Acad Dermatol* 1979; 1:513–522.

39. Goette DK. Topical chemotherapy with 5-fluorouracil. *J Am Acad Dermatol* 1981; 4:633–649.

40. Von Krogh G. 5-Fluorouracil cream in the successful treatment of therapeutically refractory condylomata of the urinary meatus. *Acta Derm Venereol (Stockh)* 1976; 56:297–301.

41. Ferenczy A. Comparison of 5-fluorouracil and CO_2 laser for treatment of vaginal condylomata. *Obstet Gynecol* 1984; 64:773–778.

42. Krebs HB. The use of topical 5-fluorouracil in the treatment of genital condylomas. *Obstet Gynecol Clin North Am* 1987; 14:559–568.

43. Kurtis B, Rosen T. Treatment of cutaneous neoplasms by intralesional injections of 5-fluorouracil (5-FU). *J Dermatol Surg Oncol* 1980; 6:122–127.

44. Avant WH, Huff RC. Intradermal 5-fluorouracil in the treatment of basal cell carcinoma of the face. *South Med J* 1976; 69:561–563.

45. Goette DK, Odom RB. Successful treatment of keratoacanthoma with intralesional fluorouracil. *J Am Acad Dermatol* 1980; 2:212–216.

46. Miller SJ. Biology of basal cell carcinoma (Part II). *J Am Acad Dermatol* 1991; 24:161–175.

47. Kraus S, Miller BH, Swinehart JM, et al. Intratumoral chemotherapy with fluorouracil/epinephrine injectable gel: A nonsurgical treatment of cutaneous squamous cell carcinoma. *J Am Acad Dermatol* 1998; 38:438–442.

48. Orenberg EK, Miller BH, Greenway HT, et al. The effect of intralesional 5-fluorouracil therapeutic implant (MPI 5003) for treatment of basal cell carcinoma. *J Am Acad Dermatol* 1992; 27:723–728.

49. Miller BH, Shavin JS, Cognetta A, et al. Nonsurgical treatment of basal cell carcinomas with intralesional fluorouracil/epinephrine injectable gel. *J Am Acad Dermatol* 1997; 36:72–77.

50. Lowe NJ, Orenberg EK, Nychay S, Korey A. Intradermal fluorouracil/epinephrine injectable gel for treatment of psoriatic plaques. *Arch Dermatol* 1995; 131:1340–1341.
51. Parmer JB, Basiliere EJ, Orenberg EK. Genital wart management: A partnership between physician and patient. *The Female Patient* 1997; 22:53–66.
52. Swinehart JM, Skinner RB, McCarty JM, et al. Development of intralesional therapy with fluorouracil/adrenaline injectable gel for management of condylomata acuminata: Two phase II clinical studies. *Genitourin Med* 1997; 73:481–487.
53. Swinehart JM, Sperling M, Phillips S, et al. Intralesional fluorouracil/epinephrine injectable gel for treatment of condylomata acuminata: A phase III clinical study. *Arch Dermatol* 1997; 133:67–73.

12 Sustained-Release Drug Delivery with DepoFoam

Sankaram B. Mantripragada, PhD
and Stephen B. Howell, MD

Contents

1. SUSTAINED-RELEASE DRUG DELIVERY

Sustained-release drug delivery systems, which meter out the encapsulated drug over a long period of time, augment the effectiveness of therapy in several ways. An ideal sustained-release drug delivery system prolongs the half-life of the drug while maintaining the concentration of the released drug in the therapeutic range during the entire duration of drug release (Fig. 1). For cell-cycle phase-specific drugs in particular, prolonging the half-life of the administered drug has a profound effect on its efficacy by increasing the area under the "exposure vs time" curve for a given amount of drug while, at the same time, decreasing toxicity by reducing the high concentration peak of drug which otherwise occurs immediately after injection. Tissue distribution of the drug is often altered, resulting in higher concentrations and greater efficacy at the desired site, and lower exposure and toxicity elsewhere. Sustained-release formulations are an effective tool in cases where patient compliance is a problem. The feasibility of delivering treatment with fewer injections may enable outpatient treatment that can markedly improve the patient's quality of life. There are, of course, economic incentives. For parenteral products that require administration and monitoring by medical personnel, decreasing the number of injections may reduce overall treatment cost. Proprietary sustained-release formulations can extend the economic viability of a compound beyond the termination of its patent life.

2. DEPOFOAM TECHNOLOGY

The DepoFoam® drug delivery system was developed to permit sustained release of drugs from a depot after direct injection into a body compartment or a tissue. The

From: *Drug Delivery Systems in Cancer Therapy*
Edited by: D. M. Brown © Humana Press Inc., Totowa, NJ

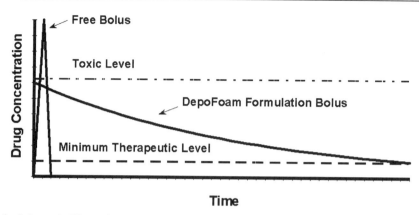

Fig. 1. Schematic illustrating the objective of an ideal sustained-release drug delivery system.

DepoFoam particles are made up of synthetic cognates of lipids that occur naturally in the human body, such as phospholipids, cholesterol, and triglycerides. Unlike many types of microspheres, there are no foreign chemical entities in DepoFoam, and the delivery system itself completely disintegrates over time. When the particles are suspended in physiologic saline, the final product has the appearance and consistency of skim milk. During storage at 4–8°C, the drug remains inside the chambers of the Depo-Foam particle. However, when the particle is injected into the patient, gradual reorganization of the structure of the particle occurs with the intermittent rupture of individual chambers and the sequential release of increments of drug. The duration of release can be up to 6–8 wk, which is a significantly longer duration than that obtained with current commercial lipid-based delivery systems. Appropriate injection routes include subcutaneous (sc), intramuscular (im), intrathecal, intraarticular, intraocular, intraperitoneal (ip), intrapleural, and epidural injections. The name DepoFoam reflects the foam-like appearance of the particles comprising the delivery system and the fact that, upon injection, they act as a depot for releasing the drug over time. DepoFoam particles are also known, as shown in the literature cited in this chapter, as multivesicular liposomes or multivesicular lipid particles. The technology is versatile, in that both small organic molecules and large macromolecules such as proteins and nucleic acids can be encapsulated in and released from DepoFoam particles.

2.1. Structure

Structurally, DepoFoam particles consist of microscopic spherical particles (average diameter 10–20 μm) composed of nonconcentric chambers, each separated from adjacent chambers by a bilayer lipid membrane *(1,2)*. In contrast to unilamellar vesicles with a single spherical membranous shell, or multilamellar vesicles with multiple concentric membranes arranged like the layers of an onion, the lipids of a multivesicular liposome particle are arranged in a structure possessing hundreds of contiguous nonconcentric chambers (Fig. 2). Each chamber sequesters a small amount of the drug to be delivered. The individual internal compartments within a DepoFoam particle are typically on the order of a micron in diameter, whereas the diameter of the particle as a whole is on the order of tens of microns. The characteristic nonconcentric nature of a DepoFoam particle results in a higher aqueous-to-lipid ratio than for a concentric struc-

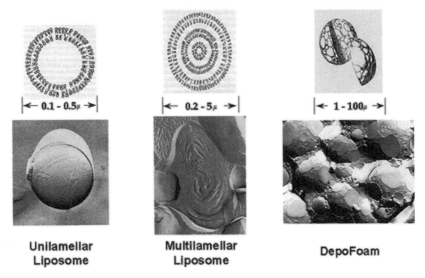

Unilamellar
Liposome

Multilamellar
Liposome

DepoFoam

Fig. 2. Structural differences between conventional liposomes and DepoFoam.

ture such as a multivesicular liposome, resulting in greater encapsulation efficiency for water-soluble drugs. The large size of a DepoFoam particle relative to unilamellar liposomes further increases the encapsulation efficiency, because the internal volume scales as the cube of the radius of the particle.

Although a DepoFoam particle resembles a simple aggregate of separate and individual large unilamellar liposomes, there is a profound structural difference. The membranes of the internal compartments of a DepoFoam particle are interconnected *(1,2)*. A single bilayer lipid membrane separates any two adjacent aqueous compartments (Fig. 3). Where three internal compartments meet, there is an intersection of membranes called a "plateau border:" this is a topological feature commonly observed with the watery films of soap bubble aggregates *(1)*. The multiple chambers with intersecting membranes give DepoFoam particles a greater mechanical strength and stability than possessed by traditional liposomes of equivalent size and aqueous content.

2.2. Methods of Preparation

In order to obtain the unique multivesicular structure of DepoFoam particles, there are two requirements *(2–4)*. The first is that, in addition to the phospholipids and cholesterol, a triglyceride or other biodegradable oil must be present to hold the individual chambers together in an organized structure *(2,3)*. In the absence of such oil, the structures obtained are a combination of multi-, oligo-, or unilamellar liposomes (Fig. 2). The second is that a double-emulsification process must be used *(2,4)*. In this process, an aqueous solution of the drug is emulsified with a solution of lipids in an immiscible solvent phase to produce a water-in-oil emulsion. The water-in-oil emulsion is then broken up into solvent spherules by mixing it in an excess of a second aqueous solution, typically an isotonic solution of dextrose and lysine, resulting in a water-in-oil-in-water double emulsion. The solvent is stripped from the spherules resulting in the formation of DepoFoam particles (Fig. 4). The suspending aqueous medium can then be exchanged for a solution suitable for injection, such as normal saline.

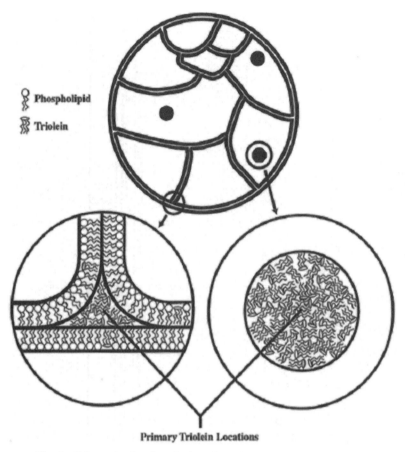

Fig. 3. Schematic showing the location of triglycerides in DepoFoam.

2.3. Formulation Variables

A number of parameters can be varied to obtain the desired rate of drug release from DepoFoam formulations. Increasing the acyl chain length of the phospholipids results in an increase in encapsulation efficiency, as well as slower rates of release *(5,6)*. Use of higher molecular weight triglycerides leads to slower rates of release when compared with the use of shorter chain lower molecular weight oils. Blends of triglycerides give rise to intermediate rates of release *(7)*. Acids and osmotic spacers dissolved in the first aqueous solution containing the drug also act as release rate modifiers *(8,9)*. Although the system works best with hydrophilic drugs, hydrophobic and amphipathic compounds may also be encapsulated, as long as they do not disrupt the membranes. In some cases, it is possible to solubilize hydrophobic compounds by forming complexes with cyclodextrins *(10)* or by conversion into soluble salts. Although there is concern that exposure to the solvent may denature proteins during encapsulation, this has not been a problem, possibly because of the presence of phospholipids and cholesterol at the interface between solvent and water. Whereas chemical stability is a function of the individual polypeptide involved, DepoFoam encapsulation has been shown with numerous proteins not to lead to aggregation, oxidation of sulfhydryls or methionines, deamidation, or diminished bioactivity *(11)*.

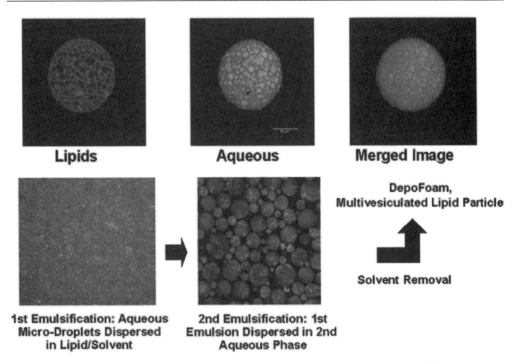

Fig. 4. Confocal micrographs of DepoFoam and its precursors, the first emulsion (oil-in-water) and the second emulsion (water-in-oil-in-water). The distribution of lipids and aqueous phases are visualized by use of a phospholipid or an aqueous fluorescent probe.

The formulation variables aforementioned have been successfully used to encapsulate into DepoFoam a variety of molecules including cytarabine *(3,12–15)*, methotrexate *(16,17)*, amikacin *(18,19)*, gentamycin *(20)*, bleomycin *(21)*, tobramycin *(22,23)*, morphine *(7, 24–27)*, bupivacaine, 5-fluorouridine-5′-monophosphate *(15,28–30)*, 2-nor-cyclic-GMP *(31)*, interferon-alpha (α) *(32)*, interleukin-2 (IL-2) *(11)*, granulocyte colony stimulating factor *(7)*, granulocyte-macrophage colony stimulating factor *(7)*, insulin *(7)*, leutinizing hormone releasing hormone *(11)*, insulin-like growth factor I (IGF-1) *(33)*, antisense oligonucleotides, and DNA *(7,9)*.

2.4. Pharmacokinetics

The ability of DepoFoam encapsulation to prolong in vivo half-life has been demonstrated for a large number of drugs (Table 1). For injections of DepoFoam formulations into a body cavity (e.g., intrathecal, intraventricular, intraperitoneal, epidural), the pharmacokinetics typically show a biphasic profile, with an initial distribution phase followed by an elimination phase. In the case of sc and im injections, the pharmacokinetic profile may be either mono- or biphasic, depending on the drug.

Because the drug is released slowly, it is possible to inject a larger total amount of the drug at a single time with a DepoFoam formulation than with the unencapsulated drug. For example, the maximum tolerated dose of epidurally injected morphine sulfate in dogs is approx 5 mg, whereas with a DepoFoam formulation of morphine, doses as high as 30 mg can be safely injected by the epidural route without producing severe

Table 1

Comparison of Elimination Half-Life Values Obtained for a Single Bolus Injection of DepoFoam Formulations with Those Obtained for a Single Bolus Injection of Unencapsulated Drugs

Drug	Dose	Species	Elimination Half-Life, $T_{1/2}$ (h)[a]		Route of Administration	Reference
			DepoFoam	Unencapsulated		
Cytarabine	2 mg	Monkey	156	0.74	Intrathecal	36
Cytarabine	1 mg	Mouse	21	0.26	ip	42
Cytarabine	1 mg[b]	Mouse	165	0.26	ip	37
Cytarabine	1 mg	Rat	148	2.7	Intrathecal	38
Cytarabine	1.1 mg	Mouse	96	0.16	sc	43
Cytarabine	6 mg	Rabbit	52.5	0.2	Subconjuctival	14
Methotrexate	100 µg	Rat	96	7.2	Intrathecal	17
Methotrexate	100 µg[f]	Rat	216	0.72	Intrathecal	17
Methotrexate	10 mg/kg	Mouse	50.4	0.16	sc	44
Methotrexate	10 mg/kg	Mouse	45.6	0.54	ip	44
Methotrexate	10 mg/kg[f]	Mouse	62.4	0.45	ip	44
Morphine	250µg	Rat	82	2.6	Epidural	25
Morphine	10 mg	Dog	7.5±0.4	3.5±0.2[c]	Epidural	26
Morphine	30 mg	Dog	10.0±0.6	3.5±0.2[c]	Epidural	26
Morphine	1 mg	Mouse	62.16±3.84	11.04±0.96	sc	24
IGF-1[d]	20 mg/kg	Rat	26	4	sc	33
Interferon α-2b	30,000 IU	Mouse	20	1.5	ip	32
Interferon α-2b	30,000 IU[f]	Mouse	13	1.3	ip	32
Bleomycin	2 mg	Mouse	31.8	0.13	sc	21
2'3'Deoxycytidine	50 µg	Rat	23	1.1	Intraventricular	45
5-FUMP[e]	1 mg	Rabbit	124	4.5	Intravitreal	15

[a] For intracavitary delivery (intrathecal, intraventricular, intravitreal, and epidural), the pharmacokinetic profile shows an initial distribution and a later elimination phase. Only elimination half-life values are reported here. Unless noted otherwise, T1/2 values were calculated using the concentration of drug vs time profiles;
[b] With a predose of blank DepoFoam;
[c] With a 5-mg dose of unencapsulated morphine sulfate;
[d] IGF-1;
[e] 5-fluorouridine-5′-monophosphate;
[f] Half-life values were calculated using the amount of drug vs time profiles.

opiate side effects *(26)*. This is because the concentration of morphine outside the DepoFoam particles at any given time during its release from the delivery system is subtoxic.

3. DEPOCYT

3.1. Description

DepoCyt® is the first product based on the DepoFoam technology to be approved by the FDA. DepoCyt (cytarabine liposome injection) is a sterile, injectable suspension of the antimetabolite cytarabine (ara-C), encapsulated into multivesicular lipid-based particles. Chemically, cytarabine is 4-amino-1-β-D-arabinofuranosyl-2 (1H)-pyrimidinone, also known as cytosine arabinoside ($C_9H_{13}N_3O_5$; molecular weight, 243.22). DepoCyt is available in 5-mL ready-to-use single-use vials containing 50 mg cytarabine. DepoCyt is formulated as a sterile, nonpyrogenic, white to off-white suspension of cytarabine in sodium chloride 0.9% w/v in water for injection *(34)*. DepoCyt is preservative-free. Cytarabine, the active ingredient, is present at a concentration of 10 mg/mL and is encapsulated in the particles. The DepoCyt particles are approx 10–15 μm in diameter. Inactive ingredients at their respective approximate concentrations are: cholesterol, 4.1 mg/mL; triolein, 1.2 mg/mL; dioleoylphosphatidylcholine (DOPC), 5.7 mg/mL; and dipalmitoylphosphatidylglycerol (DPPG), 1.0 mg/mL. The pH of the product falls within the range of 5.5–8.5. DepoCyt is stable for more than 2 yr at 4 °C.

3.2. Neoplastic Meningitis

DepoCyt was developed for the treatment of neoplastic meningitis. Neoplastic meningitis, a devastating complication of cancer produced by metastasis to leptomeninges surrounding the brain and spinal cord, is ultimately fatal if left untreated. Current standard therapy of neoplastic meningitis consists of radiation therapy to any sites of tumor that are visible on an MRI or CT scan, plus the administration of an anticancer drug 2–3 times per week into the cerebrospinal fluid (CSF) either by lumbar puncture into the lumbar sac, or by injection into a reservoir implanted under the scalp and connected to a catheter positioned in a lateral ventricle of the brain. There are two major problems with current therapy. All three of the agents available for intrathecal administration (cytarabine, methotrexate, and thioTEPA) have relatively short CSF half-lives, and are so rapidly cleared from the CSF that they do not spread evenly throughout the CSF. Even injection of the drug 2–3 times per week does not produce a pharmacologically optimal exposure to the CSF, and the resulting response rates and overall therapeutic success is poor.

The rationale for developing a slow-release formulation of cytarabine (ara-C) is that it is a cell-cycle-specific antimetabolite that kills tumor cells only when they enter the synthesis phase (S phase) of the cell cycle. Thus, its cytotoxicity is a function of both concentration and the duration of exposure. Intracellularly, cytarabine is converted into cytarabine-5′-triphosphate (ara-CTP), which is the active metabolite. The mechanism of action is primarily through inhibition of DNA synthesis. Thus, longer duration exposures permit a larger fraction of the tumor cells in the population to enter the sensitive phase of the cell cycle in which they are at risk to be killed.

When ara-C is injected intravenously, it is rapidly metabolized to the inactive compound ara-U (1-β-D-arabinofuranosyluracil or uracil arabinoside) which is then excreted in the urine. In contrast, when ara-C is injected into the CSF, its conversion to ara-U is negligible because of the very low cytidine deaminase activity in the central nervous system tissues and CSF, and it is cleared primarily by bulk flow at a rate of 0.24 mL/min. Nevertheless, it disappears from the CSF with a half-life of only 3.4 h. Thus, a formulation of ara-C capable of releasing free drug into the CSF at a rate approximating its clearance has the potential of maintaining high free ara-C concentrations in the CSF for prolonged periods of time and producing a more favorable pharmacokinetic profile.

3.3. Preclinical Pharmacokinetics

The distribution, metabolism, and excretion of dioleoylphosphatidylcholine (DOPC), the predominant phospholipid component of DepoCyt, was determined after lumbar intrathecal injection of double-radiolabeled (^{14}C-DOPC, ^{3}H-cytarabine) sustained-release encapsulated cytarabine in rats prepared with chronic spinal catheters (35). Both radiolabels distributed rapidly throughout the neuraxis after injection. Levels of both labels declined in a biphasic manner from CSF and plasma, with an initial rapid decline over the first 96 h, followed by a much slower rate of decline up to 504 h. More than 90% of the drug was excreted in urine. The plasma kinetic profiles of the drug and lipid are similar suggesting that the release of drug is related directly to breakdown of the particles. The lipids enter standard catabolic pathways after breakdown of the DepoCyt particles in the intrathecal space.

The pharmacokinetics of ara-C released from DepoCyt were studied in six rhesus monkeys after intrathecal injection into the lumbar sac (36). Following a single 2-mg dose, the concentration of ara-C associated with DepoCyt particles decreased biexponentially with initial and terminal half-lives of 14.6 and 156 h, respectively. The concentration of the free drug, released from DepoCyt particles, remained above 0.1 μg/mL for more than 672 h. In contrast, the half-life of ara-C following an intrathecal bolus injection of unencapsulated drug in a single animal was 0.74 h.

Following ip injection of unencapsulated ara-C, the amount of ara-C in the peritoneal cavity decreases exponentially with a half-life of 16 min (37,38). Following injection of DepoCyt, the clearance of cytarabine from the peritoneal cavity was markedly reduced with a half-life of approx 21 h. The peritoneal clearance of DepoCyt was further improved by pretreatment with nondrug-containing placebo DepoFoam formulation. In this case, the half-life was 165 h.

The intrathecal half-life of ara-C associated with DepoCyt particles was 148 h, in contrast to the half-life of 2.7 h for an injection of unencapsulated ara-C in a Sprague-Dawley rat model (38).

Subcutaneous administration of DepoCyt to BDF1 mice resulted in slow first-order release from skin, with a half-life of 4 d (37). The half-life was 10 min for unencapsulated cytarabine. A single-dose SC treatment of BDF1 mice, inoculated intravenously with 10^{5} L1210 leukemia cells 24 h previously, resulted in long-term survivors over a wide dose range.

3.4. Clinical Pharmacokinetics

Pharmacokinetic data on DepoCyt were obtained as part of a Phase I trial (19 patients) and two population pharmacokinetic studies, one trial performed in the USA (11 patients) and one in Europe (13 patients). Pharmacokinetic data for different routes

Table 2
Elimination Half-Life ($T_{1/2}$) Values for DepoCyt in Humans as a Function of Dose by
Different Routes of Administration into the CSF and Different Methods of Sampling

Dose (mg)	Elimination Half-Life, $T_{1/2}$ (h)[a]	Route of Administration	Reference
12.5	47±22	Intrathecal	12
25	229±70	Intrathecal	12
37.5	75±16	Intrathecal	12
50	87±15	Intrathecal	12
75	95±16	Intrathecal	12
125	161±75	Intrathecal	12
75	86.4	Intralumbar[b]	46
75	58	Intralumbar[c]	46
75	95	Intraventricular[b]	46
75	149	Intraventricular[c]	46
75	127±33	Intraventricular	41

[a] For intracavitary delivery (intrathecal, intraventricular, intravitreal, and epidural), the pharmacokinetic profile shows an initial distribution and a later elimination phase. Only elimination half-life values are reported here;
[b] Samples were taken by the intralumbar route;
[c] Samples were taken by the intraventricular route.

of administration are summarized in Table 2. The Phase I study was an open-label dose-escalation trial. Nineteen patients with various types of neoplastic meningitis received treatment via intraventricular (IVT) and/or lumbar sac (LP) injection. The dose was escalated from 12.5 to 25, 37.5, 50, 75, and finally, 125 mg. Patients received between two and eight cycles once every 2–4 wk, with an average of 3.9 cycles per patient. CSF and plasma samples were collected from either the ventricle or lumbar sac at various times up to 21 d, and were analyzed for free (unencapsulated) and encapsulated ara-C by HPLC. In addition, DepoFoam particle counts in the CSF were determined microscopically. The AUC of free and encapsulated ara-C after IVT injection of DepoCyt increased linearly with dose. As shown in Fig. 5, as determined in an earlier study (1), the half-life of free ara-C in the CSF following administration of free drug is 3.4 h. In contrast, the ventricular concentration of free ara-C following intraventricular injection of 50 mg of DepoCyt, the dose that was recommended for the subsequent controlled trials, decreased biexponentially with an initial half-life of 9.4 ± 1.6 h and a terminal half-life of 141 ± 23 h. Free ara-C concentrations of 0.02 μg/mL were maintained in both the ventricle and lumbar sac for 14 d in most patients. This concentration of drug is sufficient to kill almost all types of tumor cells when continuous exposure is used. Importantly, injection of DepoCyt into the lumbar sac resulted in therapeutically effective concentrations of ara-C in the lateral ventricles. The levels of free ara-C and its metabolite ara-U were generally below detectable levels in plasma, irrespective of the route of administration. Particle counts demonstrated that, following IVT injection, the count in the ventricle and lumbar sac were the same within 24 h, and that the kinetics of particle disappearance were subsequently identical at both ends of the neuraxis.

Thus, when the patient is dosed every 14 d, there is essentially continuous exposure to concentrations of ara-C that are highly cytotoxic to almost all types of cells. This represents an enormous increase in the "concentration x time" exposure to ara-C over

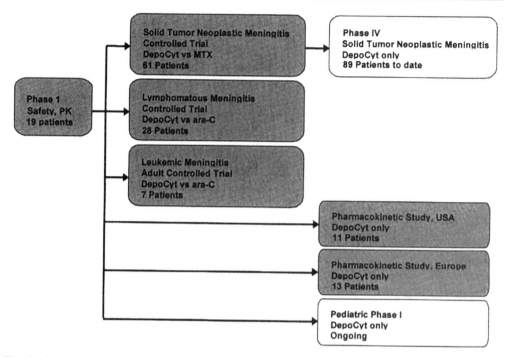

Fig. 5. Schematic diagram of DepoCyt clinical trials. Completed trials are shown as shaded boxes and trials currently underway are shown as unshaded boxes.

what can be attained when ara-C is administered intrathecally in its free form, and over what can be achieved when the drug is administered intravenously. Thus, there is a reasonable basis for the expectation that DepoCyt will be active against both solid tumor neoplastic meningitis and lymphomatous meningitis.

The two population pharmacokinetic trials addressed the question of whether drug exposure was adequate irrespective of whether the DepoCyt was injected via the LP or IVT route. The results of these trials confirmed the findings of the Phase 1 trial. Ara-C concentrations after IVT and LP administration of DepoCyt were maintained at ≥0.02 µg/mL for 2 wk in most patients. Ara-C was generally undetectable in plasma samples and, when detectable, was within the range of 0.3–5 ng/mL. The maximum concentration in the lumbar sac after LP injection was three-fold higher than the maximum concentration in the ventricle after IVT injection.

3.5. Efficacy

Figure 6 presents a schematic diagram of the DepoCyt clinical studies. To date, a total of 237 patients have been entered in these trials; 189 have received DepoCyt (the remaining patients received the control drug in the controlled trials). Patients were scored as having a response if the CSF cytology converted from positive to negative at all sites previously shown to be positive, as has been done in prior published trials. However, additional rigor was added by also requiring that the patient remain neurologically stable at the time the CSF conversion was documented. All studies used a blinded central cytology review.

In a prospective randomized trial, DepoCyt was compared to ara-C for the treatment of patients with lymphomatous meningitis (39). Twenty-eight patients with lymphoma

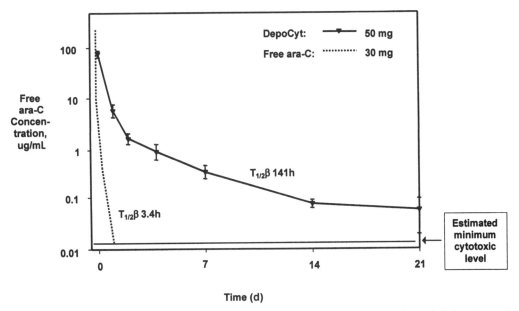

Fig. 6. Free ara-C concentration in ventricular CSF following intraventricular administration of either 30 mg of free ara-C or 50 mg DepoCyt. NB: The curve for free ara-C following administration of 30 mg free ara-C was redrawn from a figure in ref. *47*.

and positive CSF cytology results were randomized to receive either DepoCyt 50 mg once every 2 wk or free ara-C 50 mg twice per week for 1 mo. Patients whose CSF cytology converted from positive to negative and who did not have neurologic progression received an additional 3 mo of consolidation followed by 4 mo of maintenance therapy. All patients received dexamethasone 4 mg orally twice per day on days 1–5 of each 2-wk cycle. The response rate was 71% for DepoCyt and 15% for ara-C on an intent-to-treat basis ($p = 0.006$). All of the patients on the DepoCyt arm, but only 53% of those on the ara-C arm, were able to complete the planned 1-mo induction therapy. Time to neurologic progression and survival trended in favor of DepoCyt (median, 78.5 vs 42 d and 99.5 vs 63 d, respectively; $p > 0.05$). DepoCyt treatment was associated with an improved mean change in Karnofsky Performance Score (KPS) at the end of induction ($p = 0.041$). Thus, DepoCyt injected once every 2 wk produced a higher response rate and a better quality of life as measured by KPS relative to that produced by free ara-C injected twice per week. This is the only randomized trial ever performed in patients with lymphomatous meningitis.

In a second randomized prospective trial, DepoCyt was compared to methotrexate for the treatment of solid tumor neoplastic meningitis *(40)*. Sixty-one patients with histologically proven cancer and positive CSF cytology results were randomized to receive intrathecal DepoCyt (31 patients) or intrathecal methotrexate (30 patients). Patients received up to six 50-mg doses of DepoCyt or up to 16 10-mg doses of methotrexate over 3 mo. Treatment arms were well balanced with respect to demographic and disease-related characteristics. On an intent-to-treat basis, responses occurred in 26% of DepoCyt-treated and 20% of methotrexate-treated patients ($p = 0.76$). Median survival was 105 d in the DepoCyt and 78 d on the methotrexate arm (log rank, $p = 0.15$). The DepoCyt group experienced a greater median time to neurologic progression (58 vs 30 d; log rank, $p = 0.007$) and longer neoplastic meningitis-specific survival (log rank $p = 0.074$; median, 343 vs 98 d). Factors predictive of longer progression-free survival included absence of visible central nervous system disease on neuroimaging studies ($p < 0.001$), longer pretreatment duration of CSF disease ($p < 0.001$), history of intraparenchymal tumor ($p < 0.001$), and treatment with DepoCyt ($p = 0.002$). Thus, in patients with solid tumor neoplastic meningitis, DepoCyt produced a response rate comparable to that of methotrexate, and significantly increased time to neurologic progression, while offering the benefit of a less demanding dose schedule.

The activity of DepoCyt in patients with solid tumor neoplastic meningitis is being explored further in a Phase IV single-arm trial. To date, 89 patients with either a positive CSF cytology result (72 patients) or other findings sufficient to document neoplastic meningitis (17 patients) have been given DepoCyt 50 mg every 2 wk for 1 mo of induction therapy by lumbar puncture or intraventricular injection. Responding patients who did not have neurologic progression received an additional 3 mo of consolidation therapy. All patients received dexamethasone 4 mg orally twice per day on days 1–5 of each cycle. Fifty-eight of the 72 patients with a positive baseline CSF cytology had sufficient repeat CSF sampling to be evaluable for response and 15 (26%) responded. Among the patients who attained a response, 77% did so within two cycles and the remaining did so within four cycles. Median time to neurologic progression was 55 d; median overall survival was 88 d. Among patients with neurologic deficits at baseline, 18% improved after the two induction cycles. This trial confirmed the results of the prior randomized studies indicating that DepoCyt injected once every 2 wk produced a response rate comparable to that attainable with methotrexate given twice per week.

3.6. Safety

Patients with neoplastic meningitis are generally seriously ill, and they suffer a relatively large number of adverse events related to their underlying disease that are not always readily distinguishable from drug-related adverse events. Because most of the adverse events that occurred in these studies were transient, their frequency was examined separately for each cycle of treatment.

The most common adverse events observed in all the trials were headache, nausea, and vomiting, symptoms already known to accompany any form of intrathecal chemotherapy. In the Phase I trial, the dose-limiting toxicity, which occurred at a dose of 125 mg, was encephalopathy *(41)*. In the controlled trials, there were no major differences in the overall frequencies of drug-related adverse events between DepoCyt, ara-C, and methotrexate groups that altered patient management. The majority of adverse events were grade 1 or 2 for all three drugs used in these studies. Of the drug-related adverse events, 75% of those occurring in DepoCyt-treated patients were grade 1 or 2, as were 86% and 78% of those occurring in ara-C and methotrexate-treated patients, respectively. There were very few drug-related grade 4 adverse events, and the rates of occurrence were similar across study drug groups. The adverse events that were scored as drug-related were transient. For example, episodes of headache recorded as discrete events had a median duration of <1 d. The types of events observed with DepoCyt were the same as those observed with ara-C and methotrexate; DepoCyt produced no new types of adverse events. In none of the studies was there any evidence of cumulative toxicity.

One of the major problems with this disease is that infiltration of the meninges by tumor cells causes headache, and many of the patients who entered these studies had

Table 3
Comparison Between Trials of the Percent of Cycles on Which
Drug-Related Headache Occurred

	Controlled Trial Lymphomatous Meningitis		Controlled Trial Solid Tumor Meningitis		Phase IV Trial
	DepoCyt	Ara-C	DepoCyt	MTX	DepoCyt
Number of Cycles	74	44.5	102	69.5	306
Grade 1	9%	0%	7%	4%	4%
Grade 2	12%	2%	6%	1%	6%
Grade 3	5%	0%	4%	1%	3%
All Grades	27%	2%	17%	7%	12%

Table 4
Comparison of the Percent of Cycles on Which Arachnoiditis Occurred Between Trials

	Controlled Trial Lymphomatous Meningitis		Controlled Trial Solid Tumor Meningitis		Phase IV Trial
	DepoCyt	Ara-C	DepoCyt	MTX	DepoCyt
Number of Cycles	74	44.5	102	69.5	306
Arachnoiditis (any grade)	22%	13%	23%	19%	15%
Arachnoiditis (grade 3 or 4)	8%	7%	5%	3%	6%

headache prior to starting treatment. However, headache also occurred during treatment, and this event was analyzed in more detail because it is a recognized toxicity of all forms of intrathecal chemotherapy. Table 3 shows by grade the percentage of cycles at which headache occurred for the two controlled trials and the Phase IV trial. There was a higher frequency of headache on each of the DepoCyt arms, consistent with the desired persistence of drug in the CSF. The incidence of headache was generally lower in the Phase IV trial. It is likely that this is a reflection of the higher degree of compliance to concurrent dexamethasone administration that occurred during the Phase IV trial.

Arachnoiditis was the only medically important complication of intrathecal chemotherapy observed in these studies. A significant fraction of patients in all the studies had arachnoiditis as a result of tumor invasion of the meninges prior to the start of treatment. For example, in the controlled trial of DepoCyt vs methotrexate, disease-related arachnoiditis was already present in 13/29 (45%) of the patients on the DepoCyt arm and 13/30 (43%) of the patients on the methotrexate arm, even before they received any intrathecal drug. Table 4 shows the percent of cycles in which arachnoiditis occurred for each of the three trials. There is no medically significant difference in the per cycle frequency of arachnoiditis for any of the three different drugs used in these trials. When it occurred, arachnoiditis was transient, resolved within several days, and the most severe episodes did not prevent on-schedule administration of additional cycles of treatment for any of the three drugs. There is no evidence that the risk of arachnoiditis increased with increasing cycles of treatment.

4. CONCLUSIONS

DepoFoam is a sustained-release delivery system for water-soluble and water-stable drugs capable of delivering drugs for periods extending from a few days to a few weeks. The duration of release is intermediate to that of microspheres and traditional liposomes. Because their size is larger than that of traditional liposomes, DepoFoam particles encapsulate a higher volume of drug solution per gram of lipid. The encapsulated molecules, particularly macromolecules, maintain full bioactivity and stability. DepoFoam particles are comprised of lipids identical to those occurring naturally within the body, an advantage in terms of toxicity, regulatory approval, and patient acceptance. DepoFoam formulations enhance efficacy, avoid high peak levels of drug that can cause toxicity, and may broaden indications through increased efficacy and safety. Because of the prolonged release of encapsulated molecules, the frequency of injections required is reduced, resulting in a decrease in the cost and inconvenience of treatment and a potential increase in patient compliance. With DepoFoam, nonvascular depot delivery is possible by a number of routes including intrathecal, epidural, sc, im, intraocular, and intraarterial. Although the possibility of targeting specific cell types has not yet been explored, targeting is currently accomplished by local administration.

REFERENCES

1. Spector MS, Zasadzinski JA, Sankaram MB. Topology of multivesicular liposomes, a model biliquid foam. *Langmuir* 1996; 12:4704–4708.
2. Ellena JF, Le M, Cafiso DS, Solis RM, Langston M, Sankaram MB. Distribution of phospholipids and triglycerides in multivesicular lipid particles. *Drug Delivery* 1999; 6:97–106.
3. Kim S, Turker MS, Chi EY, Sela S, Martin GM. Preparation of multivesicular liposomes. *Biochim Biophys Acta* 1983; 728:339–348.
4. Pepper C, Patel M, Hartounian H. cGMP manufacturing scale-up of a multivesicular lipid based drug delivery system. *Pharm Eng Mar./Apr.* 1999; 8–18.
5. Ye Q, Sankaram MB. Modulation of drug loading in multivesicular liposomes. *US Patent* 1999a; 08925532.
6. Ye Q, Sankaram MB. Method for producing liposomes with increased percent of compound encapsulated. *US Patent* 1999b; 5,997,899.
7. Willis RC. Method for utilizing neutral lipids to modify *in vivo* release from multivesicular liposomes. *US Patents* 1999; 5,891,467 and 5,962,016.
8. Sankaram MB, Kim S. Multivesicular liposomes with controlled release of encapsulated biologically active substances. *US Patent* 1998; 5,766,627.
9. Sankaram MB, Kim S. Preparation of multivesicular liposomes for controlled release of encapsulated biologically active substances. *US Patent* 1999; 5,993,850.
10. Kim S. Cyclodextrin liposomes encapsulating pharmacologic compounds and methods for their use. *US Patent* 1998; 5,579,573.
11. Ye Q, Asherman J, Stevenson M, Brownson E, Katre NV. DepoFoam technology: A vehicle for controlled delivery of protein and peptide drugs. *J Controlled Release* 2000, in press.
12. Kim S, Howell SB. Method for treating neurological disorders. *US Patent* 1995; 5,455,044.
13. Kim S, Howell SB. Multivesicular liposomes having a biologically active substance encapsulated therein in the presence of a hydrochloride. *US Patent* 1998; 5,723,147.
14. Assil KK, Weinreb RN. Multivesicular liposomes. Sustained release of the antimetabolite cytarabine in the eye. *Arch Ophthalmol* 1987; 105:400–403.
15. Assil KK, Hartzer M, Weinreb RN, Nehorayan M, Ward T, Blumenkranz M. Liposome suppression of proliferative vitreoretinopathy. Rabbit model using antmetabolite encapsulated liposomes. *Invest Ophthalmol Vis Sci* 1991a; 32:2891–2897.
16. Bonetti A, Chatelut E, Kim S. An extended-release formulation of methotrexate for subcutaneous administration. *Cancer Chemother Pharmacol* 1994; 33:303–306.
17. Chatelut E, Kim T, Kim S. A slow-release methotrexate formulation of intrathecal chemotherapy. *Cancer Chemother Pharmacol* 1993; 32:179–182.

18. Huh J, Chen JC, Furman GM, et al. Local treatment of prosthetic vascular graft infection with multivesicular liposome-encapsulated amikacin. *J Surg Res* 1998; 74:54–58.
19. Roehrborn AA, Hansbrough JF, Gualdoni B, Kim S. Lipid-based slow-release formulation of amikacin sulfate reduces foreign body-associated infections in mice. *Antimicrobial Agents and Chemother* 1995; 39:1752–1755.
20. Grayson LS, Hansbrough JF, Zapata-Sirvent R, Roehrborn AJ, Kim T, Kim S. Soft tissue infection prophylaxis with gentamicin encapsulated in multivesicular liposomes: Results from a prospective, randomized trial. *Critical Care Medicine* 1995; 23:84–91.
21. Roy R, Kim S. Multivesicular liposomes containing bleomycin for subcutaneous administration. *Cancer Chemother Pharmacol* 1991; 28:105–108.
22. Assil KK, Frucht-Perry J, Ziegler E, Schanzlin DJ, Schneiderman T, Weinreb RN. Tobramycin liposomes. Single subconjuctival therapy of pseudomonal keratitis. *Invest Ophthalmol Vis Sci* 1991b; 32:3216–3220.
23. Frucht-Perry J, Assil KK, Ziegler E, et al. Fibrin-enmeshed tobramycin liposomes: single application topical therapy of *Pseudomonas keratitis Cornea* 1992; 11:393–397.
24. Kim T, Kim J, Kim S. Extended-release formulation of morphine for subcutaneous administration. *Cancer Chemother Pharmacol* 1993a; 33:187–190.
25. Kim T, Murdande S, Gruber A, Kim S. Sustained release morphine for epidural analgesia in rats. *Anesthesiology* 1996; 85:331–338.
26. Yaksh TL, Provencher JC, Rathbun ML, Kohn FR. Pharmacokinetics and efficacy of epidurally delivered sustained-release encapsulated morphine in dogs. *Anesthesiology* 1999; 90:1402–1412.
27. Gruber A, Murdande SB, Kim T, Kim S. Epidural administration of therapeutic compounds with sustained rate of release. *US Patent* 1999; 5,931,809.
28. Skuta GL, Assil K, Parrish RK, Folberg R, Weinreb RN. Filtering surgery in owl monkeys treated with the antimetabolite 5-fluorouridine 5′-monophosphate entrapped in multivesicular liposomes. *Am J Ophthalmol* 1987; 103:714–716.
29. Assil KK, Lane J, Weinreb RN. Sustained release of the antimetabolite 5-fluorouridine-5′-monophosphate by multivesicular liposomes. *Ophthal Surg* 1988; 19:408–413.
30. Gariano RF, Assil KK, Wiley CA, Munguia D, Weinreb RN, Freeman WR. Retinal toxicity of the antimetabolite 5-fluorouridine 5′-monophosphate administered intravitreally using multivesicular liposomes. *Retina* 1994; 14:75–80.
31. Shakiba S, Assil KK, Listhaus AD, et al. Evaluation of retinal toxicity and liposome encapsulation of the anti-CHV drug 2′-nor-cyclic GMP. *Invest Ophthalmol Vis Sci* 1993; 34:2903–2910.
32. Bonetti A, Kim S. Pharmacokinetics of an extended-release human interferon alpha-2b formulation. *Cancer Chemother Pharmacol* 1993; 33:258–261.
33. Katre NV, Asherman J, Schaefer H, Hora M. Multivesicular Liposome (DepoFoam) technology for the sustained delivery of insulin-like growth factor-1 (IGF-1). *J Pharm Sci* 1998; 87:1341–1346.
34. DepoCyt (cytarabine liposome injection). Package insert. Chiron Therapeutics. Emeryville, CA, Apr. 1999.
35. Kohn FR, Malkmus SA, Brownson, EA, Rossi SS, Yaksh TL. Fate of the predominant phospholipid component of DepoFoam drug delivery matrix after intrathecal administration of sustained-release encapsulated cytarabine in rats. *Drug Delivery* 1998; 5:143–151.
36. Kim S, Khatibi S, Howell SB, McCully C, Balis, FM, Poplack DG. Prolongation of drug exposure in cerebrospinal fluid by encapsulation into DepoFoam.*Cancer Res* 1993b; 53:1596–1598.
37. Kim S, Kim DJ, Howell SB. Modulation of the peritoneal clearance of liposomal cytosine arabinoside by blank liposomes. *Cancer Chemother Pharmacol* 1987a; 19:307–310.
38. Kim S, Kim DJ, Geyer MA, Howell SB. Multivesicular liposomes containing 1-β-D-arabinofuranosyl-cytosine for slow-release intrathecal therapy. *Cancer Res* 1987b; 47:3935–3937.
39. Glantz MJ, LaFollette S, Jaeckle KA, et al. A randomized trial of a slow-release versus a standard formulation of cytarabine for the intrathecal treatment of lymphomatous meningitis. *J Clin Oncol* 1999a; 17:3110–3116.
40. Glantz M, Jaeckle KA, Chamberlain, MC, et al. A randomized controlled trial comparing intrathecal sustained-release cytarabine (DepoCyt) to intrathecal methotrexate in patients with neoplastic meningitis from solid tumors. *Clin Cancer Res* 1999b; 5:3394–3402.
41. Chamberlain MC, Khatibi S, Kim JC, Howell SB, Chatelut E, Kim S. Treatment of leptomeningeal metastasis with intraventricular administration of depot cytarabine (DTC 101). *Arch Neurol* 1993; 50:261–264.
42. Kim S, Howell SB. Multivesicular liposomes containing cytarabine entrapped in the presence of hydrochloric acid for intracavitary chemotherapy. *Cancer Treat Rep* 1987b; 71:705–711.

43. Kim S, Howell SB. Multivesicular liposomes containing cytarabine for slow-release sc administration. *Cancer Treat Rep* 1987a; 71:447–450.

44. Chatelut E, Suh P, Kim S. Sustained-release methotrexate for intracavitary chemotherapy. *J Pharm Sci* 1994; 83:429–432.

45. Kim S, Scheerer S, Geyer MA, Howell SB. Direct cerebrospinal fluid delivery of an antiretroviral agent using multivesicular liposomes. *J Infect Dis* 1990; 162:750–752.

46. Chamberlain MC, Kormanik P, Howell S, Kim S. Pharmacokinetics of intralumbar DTC-101 for the treatment of leptomeningeal metastases. *Arch Neurol* 1995; 52:912–917.

47. Zimm S, Collins JM, Miser. Cytosine arabinoside cerebrospinal fluid kinetics. *Clin Pharmacol Ther* 1984; 35:826–830.

13 Cancer Vaccines

Susanne Osanto, MD, PhD

1. INTRODUCTION

The concept of vaccination is based on the idea that the patient's immune system is able to recognize antigens expressed by the tumor and that activation of the immune system may result in antitumor immunity. Tumor-associated antigens have been identified for a number of tumors such as melanoma and virus-associated tumors. These antigens have renewed the interest and enthusiasm for the development of cancer vaccines and they provide the basis for antigen-specific vaccines in the form of peptide, protein, or recombinant DNA encoding for such an antigen. At present, the number of relevant tumor-associated antigens against which the patient can be vaccinated is growing, although for the majority of tumors, such tumor-associated antigens are still not identified. Cancer vaccines for these tumors may rely on the use of tumor cells themselves as the source of antigens.

Following the original concept of Burnet *(1)* that tumors arising in vivo are efficiently eliminated by immune surveillance, an increasing body of data indicate that tumor cells may efficiently escape from immune surveillance by several mechanisms. Such mechanisms include the generation of tumor cell variants lacking tumor antigens and HLA antigens, deregulation of antigen processing machinery, and expression of inhibitory molecules that promote tumor cell escape, e.g., Fas ligand and TGF-β. Furthermore, tumors can induce tolerance to their tumor-associated antigens similar to the natural

From: *Drug Delivery Systems in Cancer Therapy*
Edited by: D. M. Brown © Humana Press Inc., Totowa, NJ

mechanism of tolerance induction to self-tissue antigens during ontogeny. Activation of T cells requires antigen-specific signals delivered through the T-cell receptor following binding to the appropriate peptide major histocompatibility complex (MHC) complex, as well as costimulatory signals delivered by antigen-presenting cells (APCs). Engagement of the TCR in the absence of the proper costimulatory signals results in anergy. Vaccination strategies should aim at preventing anergy and overcoming tolerance.

Melanoma serves as paradigm of an immunogenic human tumor. Metastatic lesions are often easily accessible because of their localization in the skin, subcutis, and lymph nodes, which facilitates the collection of tumor material and tumor-infiltrating lymphocytes; most human tumor antigens recognized by MHC class I-restricted cytotoxic T lymphocyte (CTL) that are identified have been isolated from peripheral blood or tumor-infiltrating lymphocytes of melanoma patients. Moreover, early stage melanoma cells have several functions of professional APCs. For instance, they can use the HLA class II route to stimulate T-helper cells, and may express B7 costimulatory molecules and certain cytokines. For these reasons, most novel vaccination strategies have been initiated in metastatic melanoma patients. On the other hand, melanomas often escape from the immune system. Melanoma cells are able to downregulate HLA molecules or $\beta2$-microglobulin and express a cytokine profile similar to Th2 cells, thus skewing the immune response away from a CD8$^+$ cytotoxic T-cell response and expressing Fas ligand.

Vaccines have evolved from nonspecific immune stimulants to much more specific and potent strategies. Phase I and Phase II clinical trials that include peptides, whole protein, recombinant viruses encoding tumor antigens, vaccination with dendritic cells expressing tumor antigens or tumor derived RNA, and/or naked DNA vaccines, are now technically feasible and have already been initiated. A major challenge will be to identify the vaccination strategies that are the most promising. Subsequently, large prospective randomized clinical trials in cancer patients without large tumor burden, i.e., who have minimal residual tumor following cytoreductive conventional chemotherapy, need to be performed to establish the long-term efficacy of the approach in large patient cohorts.

2. RECOGNITION OF TUMOR ANTIGENS BY THE IMMUNE SYSTEM

The immune system has two means of response to antigen: the humoral and the cellular immune response. Antibodies recognize antigens as native, folded protein at the cell surface. T lymphocytes, through their T-cell receptor, recognize antigen as a short fragment of protein complexed with a MHC molecule on the cell surface (2,3). CD8$^+$ T cells recognize the complex of MHC class I and the peptides that are generally 8–10 amino acids in length, whereas CD4$^+$ T cells recognize the complex of MHC class II and the peptides that are 14–25 amino acids long. Some peptides are present abundantly, whereas others exist only in low amounts on the cell surface. MHC molecules are highly polymorphic and the different alleles have distinct peptide-binding specificity. Sequencing of eluted peptides revealed allele-specific motifs, which correspond to critical anchor residues that fit into specific pockets of MHC molecules (4–6). Because all endogenous intracellular proteins can be presented to the immune system in this way, any tumor-specific structure may function as a potential tumor-specific antigen and be recognized by T cells.

APCs are critical for the antigen-specific priming of T lymphocytes. They express costimulatory molecules and high levels of MHC class I and class II molecules that present the processed antigen epitopes to naive and memory T cells to prime for anti-

Table 1
Examples of Human Tumor Antigens That Are
Potential Targets for Vaccination in Cancer Patients

Type of antigen	Type of cancer
Tumor-specific antigens	
MAGE-1, -2, -3	Melanoma, breast, lung cancer
BAGE	Melanoma, breast caner
GAGE-1, -2	Melanoma, breast, lung, bladder cancer
PRAME	Melanoma, lung cancer, head-and-neck cancer
Differentiation antigens	
Tyrosinase	Melanoma
TRP-1	Melanoma
MART-1/Melan-A	Melanoma
gp100	Melanoma
Mucin-1	Gastrointestinal cancer, breast cancer
Prostate-specific antigen	Prostate cancer
Mutated oncogenic or fusion protein	
ras	Gastrointestinal cancer, lung cancer
p53	Colorectal, breast, lung cancer
bcr-abl	Chronic myelogenous leukemia
Overexpressed proteins	
HER-2/*neu*	Breast, ovarian, lung cancer
Viral proteins	
Human papilloma virus E6, E7	Cervical cancer
Epstein-Barr virus	Burkitt's lymphoma, nasopharyngeal cancer
Hepatitis B and C	Hepatocellular carcinoma

gen-specific responses and optimally activate antigen-specific T cells *(7–15)*. APCs capture antigen and migrate to central lymphoid organs where optimal priming of T cells can occur and immune responses are initiated. If peptide is presented by MHC class II molecules in the absence of appropriate co-stimulatory signals, cell death or unresponsiveness of T cells (T cell anergy) may result. Providing the two signals, namely antigen and costimulatory signals, is a particular function of professional antigen-presenting cells. Dendritic cells (DCs) are the most potent stimulatory APCs. DCs constitute heterogeneous populations of cells and can differentiate from bone marrow and peripheral blood precursors.

3. TUMOR ANTIGENS

The rational design of cancer vaccines depends upon the identification of tumor antigens that can be targeted by the immune system, as well as the strategies in antigen presentation to overcome tolerance (Table 1). In the past, to characterize target antigens by serologic methods had been largely unsuccessful. In 1991, the group of Boon reported on the discovery of a gene encoding an antigen recognized by a CTL clone *(16)*. This gene was subsequently named MAGE-1 (melanoma antigen 1). The discovery of the MAGE-1 gene was the result of a huge research effort by Boon et al. This group used cDNA libraries generated from tumor cell-derived mRNA to transfect either recipient COS cells transfected with the appropriate MHC restriction gene or antigen-loss tumor cell variants. They subsequently screened the transfected cells for expression of the tumor-specific antigen by their ability to stimulate T-cell clones. They identified three different categories of tumor-associated antigens recognized by T cells. The first category consists of the shared tumor antigens which are expressed in many tumors, and during development, but not in normal adult tissue with the exception of placenta and testis. For this reason, these antigens are often referred to as cancer testis antigens. The second category consists of differentiation antigens, such as tyrosinase in melanomas, which is expressed by both melanocytes and melanomas. These and other antigens are also normally expressed by the tissue from which the tumor has arisen. A third category consists of unique tumor antigens expressed *exclusively* in the tumor from which they were identified. The latter include mutated antigens specific to an individual tumor. Other categories of tumor-associated antigens that are identified by various investigators include antigens encoded by dominant oncogene or tumor suppressor genes and viral antigens.

3.1. Tumor-Specific Antigens

The first melanoma antigen that was identified (MAGE-1) and the subsequently identified MAGE-2 and -3, were the original family of human melanoma-specific antigens (Table 1; *16,17*). CTL epitopes presented by several HLA class I proteins, including HLA-A1, -A2, and Cw16.01, have been identified *(18–21)*. The MAGE genes are also expressed in carcinomas of breast and lung (Table 1; *22,23*). The function of MAGE has not been yet elucidated. BAGE and GAGE *(24,25)* were identified in melanoma and shown to be expressed in a number of other tumors (Table 1). Using a similar approach with CTLs, another antigen named RAGE was identified in renal cell carcinoma *(26,27)*, and a testis antigen named CAMEL/LAGE-1 was identified in melanoma *(28)*—CAMEL being an antigen derived from an alternative reading frame of LAGE-1. PRAME (preferentially expressed antigen on melanoma) has been cloned by using a CTL clone expressing an NK inhibitory receptor *(29)*. It is expressed in a high percentage of melanomas (95%), as well as in a variety of other tumors, including lung carcinomas (70%), renal carcinomas, head-and-neck squamous cell carcinomas, sarcomas, and breast carcinomas (Table 1).

3.2. Differentiation Antigens

The second group of antigens identified by Boon et al. is specific for melanocytic differentiation and these antigens are shared by melanoma and melanocytes (e.g., tyrosinase, MART-1/Melan-A, gp100; Table 1). The melanoma antigens MART-1/Melan-A, gp100, tyrosinase, tyrosinase-related protein-1 (TRP-1 or gp75), and TRP-2 represent differentiation antigens expressed by normal melanocytes that were shown to be recognized by CTLs derived from melanoma patients *(30–44)*. Tyrosinase is a key enzyme in the melanin synthesis pathway in pigmented cells, the function of the other genes is not known. HLA-A2 is the most frequent MHC class I allele found in Caucasians and appears to be the predominant restriction element for an antimelanoma-directed immune response. The observed immunogenicity of these melanocyte differentiation antigens demonstrates that an immune mechanism against a normal self-antigen with limited tissue distribution can be induced in cancer patients and that it is possible to overcome tolerance to self-antigens.

Other differentiation antigens include carcinoembryonic antigen (CEA) expressed in colorectal and other adenocarcinomas, prostate-specific antigen (PSA) in prostate carcinoma, and MUC-1 (Mucin1, PEM). MUC-1 is a large molecular carbohydrate antigen on the cell surface that is aberrantly glycosylated and upregulated in breast, ovarian, colon, and pancreatic carcinoma. MHC-unrestricted MUC-1 specific CTLs have been isolated from patients with breast, ovarian, and pancreatic cancer *(45,46)*. Studies utilizing tumor-specific CTLs to identify other antigens expressed in breast carcinoma and other epithelial tumors are ongoing *(47)*.

3.3. Unique Tumor Antigens

The third category of antigens are unique antigens resulting from point mutations expressed by the individual patient's tumor (e.g., MUM-1, CDK4, and β-catenin [48–50]). A CTL-epitope encoded by a mutated intron was identified and the gene product resulting from incomplete mRNA splicing was named MUM-1. Other intronic sequences that yield CTL epitopes include p15 and N-acetylglucosaminyltransferase V. Mutated cyclin-dependent kinase 4 (i.e., CDK4, a protein involved in cell cycling) encodes for another CTL epitope. Beta-catenin is involved in cell–cell adhesion.

3.4. Dominant Oncogene and Tumor Suppressor Gene Products

The predominance of oncogene activation in human cancer make the mutated oncogene products attractive candidates for immunotherapy (Table 1; *51,52*). Mutated ras is frequently found in gastrointestinal adenocarcinomas. Mutant ras peptides are therefore candidates for a vaccine for specific immunotherapy in pancreatic and colon carcinoma patients. The p53 tumor suppressor protein represents another potential target *(53,54)* as p53 mutations are found in more than 50% of malignant tumors.

Chromosomal translocations may generate fusion proteins such as the bcr-abl fusion protein in chronic myelogenous leukemia. CTLs specific for bcr-abl peptides that bind to HLA class I molecules can be generated *(56–59)*. Fusion proteins are common in human malignancy and are candidate antigens for vaccine trials.

HER-2/*neu* is an oncogene (a growth factor receptor homologous to epidermal growth factor receptor) that is activated by gene amplification in 15–30% of human adenocarcinomas. The HER-2/*neu* gene amplification results in increased expression of a normal gene product. In patients with overexpression of HER-2/*neu,* both T cells and antibodies reactive to HER-2/*neu* could be demonstrated *(60–63)*, indicating that tolerance to this self-antigen can be overcome. Animal studies indicate that vaccines consisting of subdominant epitopes derived from these self-proteins may elicit an effective immune response *(64)*.

3.5. Virus-Associated Tumor Antigens

Viral antigens associated with tumor pathogenesis include the Epstein-Barr virus (EBV) which is associated with lymphoma and nasopharyngeal cancer, human papilloma virus (HPV) associated with cervical cancer, and HBV/HCC associated with hepatocellular carcinoma (Table 1). A number of HLA-A2-binding peptides encoded by the viral oncogenes E6 and E7 from human papilloma virus type 16 are identified *(65–67)*, although only a small number of patients with HPV16-associated cervical lesions were shown to have a natural CTL response to these peptides *(68)*.

4. CANCER VACCINES

The concept of using tumor cells to treat cancer is far from new. Historically, the initial cancer vaccines were cell-based, using tumor cells themselves as a source of antigen. In order to induce an immune response, it is necessary to use an adjuvant, e.g., Freund's adjuvant, Bacille Calmette-Guerin (BCG), or keyhole limpet hemocyanin (KLH). This is necessary to induce an inflammatory response so that APCs taking up antigen are adequately activated. To trigger the immune system efficiently, factors such as bacterial or viral components, e.g., bacterial DNA, dsRNA, proinflammatory cytokine (e.g., IL-1, TNF-α), or interaction with T helper cells providing stimulation through CD40 and MHC class II proteins, could be of major importance to activate DCs efficiently. It has recently become clear that there are many factors that promote DC maturation. Clearly, the presence of the proper conditions to efficiently maturate DCs may determine the outcome of the vaccination strategy. Throughout the last decades, both autologous and allogeneic cell lines have been used as vaccines. Most of the studies with nonmodified tumor cell vaccines have been performed in melanoma, renal cell, and colorectal carcinoma patients.

4.1. Cell-Specific Vaccines

The approach of a vaccine prepared from tumor cells is designed to stimulate the patient's immune system against a wide spectrum of tumor antigens. As most antigens remain unknown, the advantage of the use of whole cells is that it contains the complete set of relevant antigens. A disadvantage of tumor cell vaccines is that tumor cells have poor expression of MHC and costimulatory molecules and they are poor professional antigen-presenting cells; thus, a drawback of this approach is the development of tolerance.

One approach is the use of autologous tumor cells as vaccine. Vaccines based on autologous tumor cells are labor-intensive. Major disadvantages of autologous tumor cell vaccines is the uncertain outcome of the culture procedure, the time-consuming and laborious process to cultivate tumor cells for each individual patient, and the difficulty of evaluating autologous tumor cell vaccines for antigen expression. An alternative strategy is to use more universally applicable allogeneic cell-based vaccines because many tumor antigens are shared rather than unique. Allogeneic tumor cell vaccines are easy to prepare and standardize with respect to assessment of antigen expression by the vaccine tumor cells. The use of allogeneic tumor cell vaccines is justified in that a high percentage of tumors express common shared tumor antigens, such as in melanoma.

Experimental animal studies using a wide array of tumor models have indicated that the gene transfer of cytokine genes (costimulatory molecules such as B7.1 and B7.2) and foreign MHC molecules may render tumor cells more immunogenic. Vaccination with such transfected tumor cells, or with tumor cells admixed with similarly transfected bystander cells, are able to elicit protective antitumor immune response in naive animals and therapeutic response in tumor-bearing hosts.

Hybrid cell vaccination is a new approach in which vaccines are generated by fusion of the patient's tumor cells with allogeneic MHC class II-expressing cells in order to create an immunogenic cell that combines the tumor's antigenicity with the immunogenicity of allogeneic MCH molecules. The generated hybrid cell will express all antigens of the tumor and be highly immunogenic by the known strong effect of allogeneic MHC class II and costimulatory molecules contributed by the fusion partner cell (69,70). Animal studies have confirmed the strength of this approach, resulting in cure of the animals from transplanted tumors and the generation of long-lasting immunity to subsequent challenge with the same tumor.

4.2. Antigen-Specific Vaccines

Another approach is to design specific vaccines aiming at stimulating the immune response to selected antigens. Directing the immune response toward a selected antigen has the advantage of being more practical for use in clinical studies, as the product can be much more easily standardized. The advantage is that, for most tumors, tumor-associated antigens have not been identified and they may not be the most potent antigen involved in the rejection of a particular tumor. To this purpose, peptide vaccines (single or multivalent peptide vaccine), peptides linked to lipids, administered as liposomes, or peptides pulsed onto antigen-presenting cells may be explored.

Until now, most of the peptide vaccines have used HLA class I-restricted peptides (usually nonamers or decamers). Another approach is to vaccinate with much larger overlapping peptides, whole proteins, proteins linked to lipids, or peptides pulsed onto antigen-presenting cells. Such vaccines will result in vivo in a greater set of relevant peptides against which the immune response can now be directed.

Naked DNA can also induce tumor antigen-specific immunity. Direct injection of DNA into skin or muscle results in the expression of the gene product and can stimulate an immune response. Vaccines containing DNA-encoding tumor antigens, administered by gene gun for intradermal injection or intramuscular injection, or DNA linked to lipids could potentially be used for vaccination. Antigen-presenting cells, transduced with DNA-encoding tumor antigens or a minigene containing multiple CTL epitopes, may be more effective in triggering an immune response. The relative simple technology of DNA-based vaccinations with naked DNA encoding tumor antigen may supersede the more complex technology of other gene therapy protocols.

Recombinant viruses encoding tumor antigens, and/or genes encoding cytokine, costimulatory molecules, or other genes to enhance the immune response, may be used to vaccinate patients against their tumor.

5. TUMOR CELL VACCINES, NONMODIFIED OR GENE MODIFIED

Various clinical trials employing autologous or allogeneic tumor-cell vaccines have been reported (71–80). In some studies, development of antibodies directed against tumor-associated antigens expressed by melanoma correlated with survival, suggesting either a specific effect of vaccination or identification of a subpopulation of patients with more favorable immunobiological characteristics. Morton et al. (74) observed a survival benefit in stage IIIA and IV melanoma patients following vaccination with an allogeneic whole-cell vaccine comprised of three melanoma cell lines, that expressed multiple immunogenic tumor antigens, plus BCG. A large, multicenter, randomized trial with the three melanoma cell line vaccines is ongoing. In 54 melanoma patients with in-transit metastases treated at John Wayne Cancer Institute during the period of 1985–1997 with this melanoma cell vaccine, nine (17%) objective responses were observed, including 13% complete remissions (79). Recently, an adjuvant trial in 412 stage II and stage III colorectal cancer patients (following surgical resection) randomized between observation and autologous tumor cell-BCG vaccine administration; the long-term results failed to demonstrate any survival benefit in the patients who received active specific immunotherapy (ASI) *(80)*. Vermorken et al. *(81)* reported the results of a study in 254 stage II and stage III colorectal cancer patients randomized to receive immunization with autologous tumor vaccine plus BCG or observation. Patients who received ASI appeared to have a reduction in risk of disease in the recurrence-free period (particularly stage II patients).

With the developments in molecular genetics and the cloning of genes encoding immune system regulatory molecules, a new generation of cell-based vaccine strategies has arisen through transduction of tumor cells with genes encoding immunologically active molecules. The use of genetically modified tumor cells to vaccinate against tumor has been extensively studied in animal models. In general, the types of immunologically active genes that have been introduced into tumor cells can be divided into three categories: MHC genes, cytokine genes, and genes encoding membrane associated costimulatory molecules. This may result in increased antitumor responses to both gene modified, as well as nonmodified tumor cells. Genetically modified vaccines aim at converting the tumor cell itself into an effective antigen-presenting cell, which can now stimulate T lymphocytes directly and aim at enhancing cross priming. Owing to the change in tumor cell and microenvironment (resulting in influx of immune cells and enhanced tumor cell degradation), APC progenitors will be attracted to the site of vaccination where they may differentiate to dendritic cells. Following ingestion and processing of released tumor antigen, DCs will migrate to lymph nodes where they may present tumor antigen-derived peptide by their MHC class molecules to activate T cells.

Several investigators reported prevention of tumor and/or rejection of small established tumors following immunization with tumor cells genetically modified with cytokine cDNA encoding IL-2, IL-4, IL-7, IFN-γ, TNF-α, G-CSF, and GM-CSF *(82–93)*. Similar strong antitumor responses were obtained following vaccination with gene-modified tumor cells expressing foreign/allogeneic MHC gene class I or class II molecules or the B7 costimulatory molecule *(94–102)*. We have initiated a clinical study in cancer melanoma patients to evaluate the toxicity and antitumor efficacy of injections of an HLA class I-matched, irradiated allogeneic melanoma cell line, which expresses most of the in melanoma identified tumor antigens, and secretes IL-2 following genetic modification *(103)*. Inflammatory reactions of metastases accompanied by apoptosis and necrosis have been observed, as well as one complete, and one nearly complete, regression of metastases lasting for more than 1 yr. A number of patients experienced mixed responses and stabilization of the disease. An increase in antitumor CTLp frequencies was found in some of the patients. Similar studies employing vaccines with autologous or allogeneic tumor cells engineered to express cytokine, costimulatory molecules or vaccines consisting of nonmodified tumor cells admixed with cytokine-gene-modified autologous fibroblasts have been mainly performed in melanoma patients *(104–107, see also* Chapter 14).

6. PEPTIDE-BASED VACCINES

The advantages of synthetic peptides are that the preparations show chemical consistency from batch to batch and that immunological monitoring of defined T-cell epitope is easier. Another advantage is the relatively simple and inexpensive production of large quantities, and the possibilities of constructing multiepitope vaccines by combining CTL-epitopes derived from different tumor antigens. The limitation of peptide-based vaccines is the limitation of HLA-restriction, necessitating the *a priori* knowledge of the patient's HLA haplotype *(108)* in order to choose appropriate peptides compatible with that particular haplotype. Another limitation is the tumor heterogeneity, as not all tumor cells will express the target T-cell epitope. For a peptide-based vaccine to be widely applicable, it will be necessary to identify multiple peptide epitopes that are presented by all the major MHC class alleles. Persistence of peptide antigen in vivo will be limited by clearance and degradation. The presence of serum peptidases may alter the antigenicity of peptides or rapidly inactivate peptides. To raise the immunogenicity, peptides can be injected in the following ways: with adjuvants, in liposomes, or by direct attachment of lipids *(109)*.

Analysis of more than 4000 peptides eluted from MHC molecules has identified over 100 motifs binding to a wide range of MHC molecules. These motifs can be used to analyze proteins to identify potential T-cell epitopes. Further analysis of the binding properties of potential T-cell epitopes and their ability to stimulate an appropriate T-cell response, may identify subdominant peptides that can now be tested as vaccines in the treatment of cancer patients.

Various peptide-based vaccines studies have been performed in melanoma patients and resulted in clinical responses in some trials. Marchand et al. *(110)* reported significant tumor regressions (one complete remission) in three out of 12 HLA-A1 positive tumor-bearing melanoma patients who were immunized with subcutaneous injections of the synthetic HLA-A1-binding MAGE-3 peptide. Jaeger et al. *(111)* vaccinated six HLA-A$^+$ metastatic melanoma patients intradermally with multiple CTL-epitopes, i.e., peptides derived from MART-1/Melan-A, tyrosinase, and gp100/Pmel17. The influenza matrix peptide was administered as a control. DTH reactions were observed in five of six patients. Generation of peptide-specific CTL was documented against MART-1/Melan-A-derived peptide epitopes, the tyrosinase signal peptide, and the influenza matrix peptide after vaccination. No tumor regressions were observed.

The group of Rosenberg has performed a number of clinical studies with synthetic HLA-A2 binding peptides derived from the melanoma differentiation antigens MART-1/Melan-A and with immunodominant gp100 peptides as well as with modified gp100 peptides *(112,117)*. Because the immunodominant gp100 peptides have relatively low binding affinity to HLA-A2, peptides modified at the HLA-A2-binding anchor positions were selected based on MHC binding affinity *(113)*. Two high-affinity binding peptides containing an amino acid substitution in gp100$_{aa209-217}$ and gp100$_{aa209-289}$ seem to be more immunogenic than the native epitopes. Clinical studies with these modified high-affinity binding peptides, resulted in an increase in vaccine-specific T-cell frequency. Another peptide study was performed in melanoma patients utilizing tyrosinase peptides in combination with GM-CSF *(118)*. Vaccination of cancer patients with mutant *ras* peptide-pulsed antigen-presenting cells from peripheral blood indicated that vaccination of end-stage pancreatic carcinoma patients resulted in a transient *ras*-specific proliferative T-cell response in some patients *(119,120)*. Khleif et al. *(121)* conducted a Phase I trial in which they immunized patients with advanced cancer with 13-*mer* mutated *ras* peptides reflecting codon 12 mutations. Fifteen patients were vaccinated. Tumors from 139 potential patients were screened; tumors from 37 of the 139 patients were found to carry the appropriate mutation. Three of 10 patients generated a mutant *ras*-specific CD4+ and/or CD8+ response; CD8+ CTLs specific for Gly to Val mutation at codon 12 were capable of lysing an HLA-A2-matched tumor cell line carrying the corresponding *ras* mutation.

Vaccination of 12 patients with chronic-phase CML with *bcr-abl* fusion peptides plus QS-21 as immunological stimulant generated peptide-specific T-cell proliferative responses *(122)*. However, no CTL responses could be identified and no clinical remissions were induced.

Interestingly, intradermal immunization of breast and ovarian cancer patients with selected subdominant 15–18 amino acids-long peptides (derived from intracellular and extracellular domain HER-2/*neu* mixed with GM-CSF as an adjuvant) elicited both peptide-specific, as well as protein-specific CD4+ T-cell responses, demonstrating that tolerance for this self-antigen can be broken *(123)*.

Steller et al. *(124)* immunized 12 patients with refractory cervical carcinoma with an HPV-16 E7 lipopeptide. There were no clinical responses or treatment toxicities. T-cell-mediated immune responses against HPV were retained following vaccination in patients who mounted a cellular immune response *before* vaccination. Anti-HPV responses were induced in two of three patients who were nonreactive before vaccination.

MacLean et al. *(125,126)* administered a vaccine containing STn-KLH (STn is a synthetic epitope of a natural mucin) with or without chemotherapy (consisting of low-dose cyclophosphamide) to patients with metastatic adenocarcinoma. Antibodies against mucin-associated sialyl-Tn epitopes correlated with survival, whereas survival was significantly longer in patients with breast cancer receiving the combination of the vaccine and cyclophosphamide than in patients receiving the vaccine only.

7. PROTEIN VACCINES

Several lines of evidence may support the delivery of entire proteins rather than the use of a peptide-based vaccine as following the use of a protein-based vaccine, patients are not excluded based on HLA haplotype restriction. In addition, the protein will provide a wider range of multiple HLA class I and class II epitopes. Therefore, whole proteins may provide T-cell epitopes that have not already been identified in the context of other, common HLA alleles. In a Phase I study, 18 colorectal cancer patients without macroscopic disease were immunized with recombinant human CEA with (*n*=9) or without (*n*=19) GM-CSF as adjuvant *(127)*. Strong anti-CEA responses were particularly seen following immunization with rHuCEA plus GM-CSF. No signs of autoimmune reaction were observed.

Complete molecular remissions were induced in lymphoma patients after vaccination with patient-specific idiotype protein plus GM-CSF *(128)*. Tumor-specific CD4 and cytotoxic CD8 T cells were uniformly found (19 of 20 patients), whereas antibodies were detected. Vaccination was associated with long-term disease-free survival.

8. DENDRITIC CELLS PULSED WITH PEPTIDE, TUMOR LYSATES, OR PROTEIN

Animal models have clearly shown that bone marrow-derived DCs pulsed with tumor-derived peptide or genetically engineered to express costimulatory cytokines may effectively generate antitumor CTLs in vivo. DCs have unique abilities to induce T-cell-dependent immunity, are capable of presenting processed antigen for days, and traffic to lymphoid organs. DCs pulsed with peptides may induce protective immunity against tumor challenge making them potent professional APCs *(129–131)*. These and other experiments generate enormous enthusiasm to clinically apply DCs as cancer vaccines in patients. Various approaches utilizing DCs can be followed. Genetic modification of DCs with cDNA encoding tumor antigen will result in a wealth of tumor peptides already expressed in the proper HLA context of each individual patient. In addition, tumor antigens can be loaded onto DCs' MHC antigen-presenting molecules by pulsing the cells with synthetic peptides, purified proteins, tumor lysates or crude lysates eluded from tumor cells, tumor-derived RNA encoding for tumor antigens, or apoptotic bodies. Also, such tumor antigen-loaded DCs or hybrid fusion cells, generated by fusion between DC and tumor cell, will result in a wide range of tumor-derived peptides against which a T-cell response can now be efficiently generated. Because autologous cells serve as source of antigen, such vaccines are available to all patients, irrespective of HLA type.

DCs have recently become easier to isolate *(132)*. They can be expanded in vitro from CD34+ cells or from peripheral blood monocytes using IL-4 and GM-CSF *(133–135)*. A major disadvantage of preparing DCs is the time consumption and costly procedure to generate mature and functionally active DCs. DCs have been administered in the skin or intravenously. Thus far, DC-based clinical trials have shown promising results in patients with B-cell lymphoma, melanoma, and prostate cancer.

8.1. DCS Pulsed with Peptide or Tumor Lysate

Mukherji et al. *(135)* monitored patients who were immunized with a vaccine consisting of autologous APCs pulsed with MAGE-1 peptide. Autologous tumor and peptide-specific responses were observed following vaccination. Chakraborty et al. *(136)* immunized 17 melanoma patients intradermally with tumor-lysate-pulsed autologous APC. The vaccine was administered monthly in a dose-escalating fashion, from 10^5 to 10^7 cells/injection, during a 4-mo period. Antigen-specific CD8+ T-cell responses could be generated from in vitro expanded vaccine-infiltrating lymphocytes.

Nestle et al. *(137)* reported on the vaccination of 16 melanoma patients with peptide- and tumor-lysate-pulsed DCs. KLH was added as a CD4+ helper antigen and immunological tracer molecule. Five of 16 patients demonstrated objective responses to the DC vaccination, including two complete and three partial responses.

Following vaccination with mature monocyte-derived DC pulsed with MAGE-3 HLA-A2.1-binding peptides and influenza matrix HLA-A2.1-control peptides, as well as the recall antigen tetanus toxoid, antigen-specific CD8+ effector T cells were generated and were detectable in all eight patients in blood directly ex vivo. Regression of individual metastases was observed in 6 of 11 patients. Nonregressing metastases lacked MAGE-3 mRNA expression *(138,139)*.

MacKensen et al. *(140)* performed a Phase I study with DC-pulsed with a pool of peptides that included MAGE-1, MAGE-3 (HLA-A1), Melan-A/MART-1, gp100, and tyrosinase (HLA-A2) in HLA-A1+ or -A2+ melanoma patients. Antitumor responses were observed in two of the 14 immunized patients.

8.2. DCS Pulsed with Protein

B-cell malignancies abundantly express a unique tumor-specific cell surface antigen (immunoglobulin). Each individual lymphoma has a unique idiotype immunoglobulin, and antiidiotype strategies must, therefore, be tailored to individual patients. Four patients with follicular B-cell lymphoma received a series of three or four infusions of antigen-pulsed, i.e., tumor-specific idiotypic protein-pulsed, dendritic cells followed by sc injections of antiidiotype 2 wk later *(141)*. All patients developed antitumor cellular immune responses, whereas two complete and one partial remission were observed. In a follow-up report, Hsu et al. *(142)* reported the results of vaccination with idiotype protein-pulsed dendritic cells in 41 patients with B-cell lymphoma. Fifty percent of the patients experienced a specific immune response against the idiotypes of their tumor immunoglobulin. Of these, two experienced a complete regression of residual disease. The ability to generate an immune response correlated with improved clinical outcome.

Lim et al. *(143)* reported their results of vaccination with dendritic cells pulsed with idiotypic protein and KLH as a control in six multiple myeloma patients. Peripheral blood mononuclear cell proliferative antiidiotype responses in most patients and an increase in CTL precursor frequency against idiotype-pulsed autologous tumor cells in some patients were observed.

8.3. Hybrid Cells

Kugler et al. *(144)* reported on 17 patients with renal carcinoma who were vaccinated subcutaneously in close proximity to inguinal lymph nodes with allogeneic DCs fused to autologous tumor cells. Cells were immediately administered following electrofusion and 200 Gy irradiation of the generated hybrid cells. No serious side effects occurred, and 7 of the 17 patients responded favorably to the hybrid cell vaccination (complete tumor remission, 4; partial remission, 2; mixed response, 1). The vaccination is an example of an individualized immune therapeutic therapy. Given the heterogeneity of tumor cells within one lesion, a strategy aimed at the induction of CTLs directed against multiple different tumor-associated antigens may account for the results obtained in this study. However, the validity of the DC-tumor cell hybrid system is still uncertain as other researchers have not been able to confirm these data.

Trefzer et al. *(145)* reported on the results of their hybrid cell vaccination in metastatic melanoma patients. Results obtained were complete response (1), partial response (1), and stable disease (5), in 16 melanoma patients who were immunized with hybrids of allogeneic peripheral blood mononuclear cells enriched for B cells, and freshly isolated melanoma cells, or melanoma cell lines.

9. RECOMBINANT VIRAL VECTORS

In animal models, it has been shown that immunization with recombinant viruses encoding model tumor antigens elicits a strong specific immune response against the model tumor antigen, whereas the same model antigen presented by tumor cells is not immunogenic *(145)*. Several viruses encoding model tumor antigens have been shown to express antigens within the cytoplasm of infected cells, resulting in the induction of murine immunity. This approach carries a safety risk because the delivery of whole genes encoding tumor antigens that are involved in carcinogenesis may lead to malignant transformation of recombinant virus-infected cells. Viral vector vaccines containing the functional human papilloma virus E6 and HPV E7 oncogenes, mutated oncogenes, or tumor antigens such as MAGE, GAGE, and BAGE (whose function is still unknown) should not be considered safe. In contrast, cloning of the genetic code for one or multiple CTL epitopes *(147,148)* derived from such tumor antigens into viral vectors to use as recombinant viral vaccine may result in T-cell immunity without introducing potential risks.

Several studies investigating the use of recombinant viral vectors engineered to express candidate tumor antigens such as CEA and PSA *(149–155)* have been initiated. In one study, 26 patients with metastatic adenocarcinoma (gastrointestinal, lung, and breast) were immunized with dermal scarification monthly with a recombinant vaccinia virus (rV) containing the self-antigen carcinoembryonic antigen (CEA). No severe toxicity was encountered. Immunological monitoring showed that tolerance can be broken by vaccination with rV-CEA *(149);* CTL responses to a specific CEA epitope could be demonstrated after prolonged in vitro culture of peripheral blood lymphocytes from patients after vaccination and the CTLs were able to lyse tumor cells expressing CEA.

Comparison between intradermal vs sc immunization with rV-CEA administered to 20 metastatic adenocarcinoma patients failed to show a more favorable immune response following intradermal vaccination *(152).*

Immunization with a canary pox vector (ALVAC) containing the gene encoding for CEA resulted in significant increases in CTL precursors specific for CEA in PBMCs after vaccination compared with before the treatment *(153).*

Rosenberg et al. *(154)* used recombinant adenovirus encoding MART-1 or gp100 melanoma antigens, either alone or followed by IL2, to immunize metastatic melanoma patients. One of 16 vaccinated patients receiving only rAd-MART-1 experienced a complete remission, whereas none of the patients receiving rAd-gp100 alone had an antitumor response.

In other studies, a similar approach was taken; men with rising PSA levels after treatment for prostate cancer were immunized with vaccinia viral vectors encoding prostate-specific antigen *(155).* A number of patients had stable disease for 11–25 mo, whereas PSA levels were stable. Immunological studies demonstrated a specific T-cell response to a peptide derived from PSA. Other clinical studies involve the use of viral vectors encoding MUC-1 to immunize patients with adenocarcinoma.

Cervical carcinoma is associated with human papilloma virus (HPV) types. The HPV E6 and HPV E7 genes encode for oncoproteins that are able to deregulate cell growth by inactivating the products of p53 and Rb, respectively. Because E6 and E7 are viral proteins without sequence homology to human cellular proteins, there does not seem to be a risk of inducing an autoimmune response by targeting E6 and E7. Borysiewicz et al. *(156)* vaccinated late-stage HPV-16-positive cervical cancer patients by dermal scarification with a recombinant vaccinia viral construct encoding modified E6 and E7 genes of HPV 16 and 18. All eight patients mounted an antivaccinia antibody response, whereas three patients produced antibodies to HPV. HPV-specific CTLs were detected in one of three evaluated patients.

10. DNA VACCINATION

DNA delivery methods have been shown in animals to be efficient enough to raise immune responses *(157–160).* In the case of naked DNA vaccines, the host cell manufactures the protein and CTL epitope. Plasmids are easy to manipulate and can accommodate large sequences of foreign DNA. These can be produced at a high level of purity and are associated with low immunogenicity.

The "gene gun" gene delivery system *(161–163)* is an effective means of introducing antigen-encoding expression vectors into the epidermis. The immunization of the skin results in the temporal presence of DNA and expression of antigen, but elicits humoral and cellular immune responses and protective immunity. The skin is rich in dendritic cells and ballistic cutaneous genetic immunization may lead to in vivo transfection of skin-derived dendritic cells. Endogenously synthesized antigen can access the MHC class I-restricted pathway of transfected DCs. Following migration to regional lymphoid organs, the DCs can present the tumor antigen to T cells with appropriate costimulatory signals for T-cell activation. DNA immunization can produce long-term humoral and cellular immune responses *(159)*.

Although treatment of B-cell lymphoma patients with antiidiotype antibody has been demonstrated to be successful, analysis of lymphoma cells at the time of relapse has demonstrated that, because of antigenic selection, clonal expansion of lymphoma cells with mutation in the idiotypic variable genes (idiotypic escape) had occurred. Importantly, loss of surface immunoglobulin does not appear to occur. Therefore, a more recent strategy has involved the molecular cloning of the idiotype sequence of both the light chain (V_L) and the heavy chain (V_H). Variable region gene sequences coding for the lymphoma idiotype can be isolated directly from biopsy material by polymerase chain reaction (PCR) amplification, cloned, and DNA sequence analysis of the cloned PCR product performed. Light chain and heavy chain can be assembled with flexible linker sequences to encode a single-chain fusion. If needed, the idiotype sequence can be further subcloned into a vector and idiotype protein produced in a suitable system. A clinical trial has been initiated to test the safety of the genetic approach to personalized idiotypic vaccination with DNA encoding the idiotypic V gene *(164)*.

Nabel et al. *(165)* showed that the introduction of allogeneic HLA-B7 DNA cationic liposome complexes into cutaneous melanoma metastases by direct injection resulted in expression of HLA-B7 protein in the tumor cells near the site of injection. Regression of metastases occurred, suggesting that allogeneic effects may indeed enhance antitumor immune response. In an update on 10 patients, Nabel et al. *(166)* reported that HLA-B7 gene transfer did not markedly alter the frequency of circulating tumor-specific CTL in peripheral blood, whereas T-cell migration into treated lesions was enhanced in the majority of patients. In one patient, subsequent treatment with tumor-infiltrating lymphocytes derived from gene-modified tumor, resulted in a complete regression of the residual disease. Thus, immunological monitoring of lymphocytes from metastatic sites could be more informative than such monitoring of T cells from the peripheral blood compartment.

11. CONCLUSION

Advances in molecular genetics and in tumor immunology enables us to explore the application of genetically modified tumor cell vaccines, tumor peptide and protein or DNA-based tumor antigen vaccines in cancer patients. Until now, cancer vaccines have shown a favorable toxicity and safety profile. Antitumor responses vary in reported studies. The low numbers of patients entered in these studies preclude any statistically meaningful conclusion about the efficacy of the approach. Increasing efforts will be made to explore the value of dendritic cells to initiate an effective immune response and to prevent or break tolerance.

In the coming years, various new approaches including adoptive cellular immunotherapy with DCs loaded with peptides or proteins or genetically modified to express tumor antigens will be explored. Clinical investigation of new adjuvants is required in order to optimize novel vaccination approaches. Decisions regarding type of vaccination strategy should include assessment of tumor antigen and HLA class I expression in the individual patient's tumor. Careful analysis of current trials and direct comparison of different approaches will be necessary to establish vaccination as an effective treatment modality for cancer patients.

Immunological monitoring of clinical vaccination trials is critical to our understanding of the complex events that happen in vivo following administration of a vaccine. Therefore, efforts should be made to further develop and validate assays, such as the ELISPOT- and MHC-tetramer technologies, for efficient monitoring of the state of immunization of cancer patients against tumor antigens. Monitoring of lymphocytes migrating to the sites of metastases could be more relevant than monitoring of circulating blood lymphocytes. Until now in vaccination studies, DTH, T-cell proliferative, or CTL responses have been observed, although not consistently. Various adjuvants have been coadministered in various studies, and their specific contribution to the observed clinical and immunological effect is difficult to assess.

Results from animal studies and human trials of various vaccine types, indicate that active immunization against a patient's preexisting tumor is likely to be effective only when the tumor load is small. Unfortunately, the vast majority of clinical trials have enrolled patients with widespread disease. Once the feasibility and safety of a new protocol has been shown, patients with small tumor volume and minimal residual disease should be selected for vaccination strategies.

REFERENCES

1. Burnet FM. The concept of immunological surveillance. *Prog Exper Tumor Res* 1970; 13:1–27.
2. Brodsky FM, Guagliardi LE. The cell biology of antigen processing and presentation. *Annu Rev Immunol* 1991; 9:707–744.
3. Parham P. Antigen processing. Transporters of delight. *Nature* 1990; 348:674–675.
4. Falk K, Rotzscke O, Stevanovic S, Jung G, Rammensee HG. Allele-specific motifs revealed by sequencing of self-peptides eluted from MHC molecules. *Nature* 1991; 351:290–294.
5. Falk K, Rotzscke O. Consensus motifs and peptide ligands of MHC class I molecules. *Semin Immunol* 1993; 5:81–87.
6. Rammensee HG, Friede T, Stevanovic S. MHC ligands and peptide motifs: first listing. *Immunogenet* 1995; 41:178–228.
7. Steinman RM. The dendritic cell system and its role in immunogenicity. *Annu Rev Immunol* 1991; 9:271–296.
8. Allison JP, Hurwitz AA, Leach DR. Manipulation of co-stimulatory signals to enhance antitumor T-cell responses. *Curr Opin Immunol* 1995; 7:682–686.
9. Rock KL, Rothstein L, Gamble S, Fleischacker C. Presentation of exogenous antigen with class I major histocompatibility complex molecules. *Science* 1990; 249:918–921.
10. Grant EP, Rock KL. MHC class I-restricted presentation of exogenous antigen by thymic antigen-presenting cells in vitro and in vivo. *J Immunol* 1992; 148:13–18.
11. Rock KL, Rothstein L, Gamble S, Fleischacker C. Characterization of antigen-presenting cells that present exogenous antigens in association with class I MHC molecules. *J Immunol* 1993; 150:438–446.
12. Harding CV, Song R. Phagocytic processing of exogenous particulate antigens by macrophages for presentation by class I MHC molecules. *J Immunol* 1994; 153:4925–4933.
13. Kovacsovics-Bankowski M, Rock KL. A phagosome-to-cytosol pathway for exogenous antigens presented on MHC class I molecules. *Science* 1995; 267:243–245.

14. Bevan MJ. Antigen presentation to cytotoxic T lymphocytes in vivo. *J Exp Med* 1995; 182:639–641.
15. Huang AY, Golumbek P, Ahmadzadeh M, Jaffee E, Pardoll D, Levitsky H. Role of bone-marrow-derived cells in presenting MHC class I restricted tumor antigens. *Science* 1994; 264:961–968.
16. Van der Bruggen P, Traversari C, Chomez P, et al. A gene encoding an antigen recognized by cytolytic lymphocytes-T on a human melanoma. *Science* 1991; 254:1643–1647.
17. De Plaen E, Arden K, Traversari C, et al. Structure, chromosomal localization and expression of twelve genes of the MAGE family. *Immunogenetics* 1994; 40:360–369.
18. Traversari C, van der Bruggen P, Luescher IF, et al. A nonapeptide encoded by human gene MAGE-1 is recognized on HLA-A1 by cytolytic T-lymphocytes directed against tumor antigen-MZ2-E. *J Exp Med* 1992; 176:1453–1457.
19. Gaugler B, Van den Eynde B, van der Bruggen P, et al. Human gene MAGE-3 codes for an antigen recognized on a melanoma by autologous cytolytic T lymphocytes. *J Exp Med* 1994; 179:921–930.
20. Van der Bruggen P, Bastin J, Gajewski T, et al. A peptide encoded by human gene MAGE-3 and presented by HLA-A2 induces cytolytic T lymphocytes that recognize tumor cells expressing MAGE-3. *Eur J Immunol* 1994; 24:3038–3043.
21. Van der Bruggen P, Szikora JP, Boel P, et al. Autologous cytolytic T lymphocytes recognize a MAGE-1 nonapeptide on melanomas expressing HLA-Cw*1601. *Eur J Immunol* 1994; 24:2134–2140.
22. Zakut R, Topalian SL, Kawakami Y, Mancini M, Eliyahu S, Rosenberg SA. Differential expression of MAGE-1. -2, -3 messenger RNA in transformed and normal cell lines. *Cancer Res* 1993; 53:54–57.
23. Toso JF, Oei C, Oshidari F, et al. MAGE-1-specific precursor cytotoxic T-lymphocytes present among tumor-infiltrating lymphocytes from a patient with breast cancer: characterization and antigen-specific activation. *Cancer Res* 1996; 56:16–20.
24. Boel P, Wildmann C, Sensi ML, et al. BAGE: a new gene encoding an antigen recognized on human melanomas by cytolytic T lymphocytes. *Immunity* 1995; 2:167–175.
25. Van den Eynde B, Peeters O, De Backer O, Gaugler B, Lucas S, Boon T. A new family of genes coding for an antigen recognized by autologous cytolytic T lymphocytes on a human melanoma. *J Exp Med* 1995; 182:689–698.
26. Brouwenstijn N, Gaugler B, Krüse KM, et al. Renal cell carcinoma-specific lysis by CTL clones isolated from peripheral blood lymphocytes and tumor infiltrating lymphocytes. *Int J Cancer* 1996; 68:177–182.
27. Gaugler B, Brouwenstijn N, Vantomme V, et al. A new gene coding for an antigen recognized by autologous cytolytic T lymphocytes on a human renal carcinoma. *Immunogenetics* 1996; 44:323–330
28. Aarnoudse CA, van den Doel PB, Heemskerk B, Schrier PI. Interleukin-2-induced, melanoma-specific T cells recognize CAMEL, an unexpected translation product of LAGE-1. *Int J Cancer* 1999; 82:442–448.
29. Ikeda H, Lethe B, Lehmann F, et al. Characterization of an antigen that is recognized on a melanoma showing partial loss by CTL expressing an NK inhibitory receptor. *Immunity* 1997; 6:199–208.
30. Bakker ABH, Schreurs MJW, de Boer AJ, et al. Melanocyte lineage-specific antigen gp100 is recognized by melanoma derived tumor infiltrating lymphocytes. *J Exp Med* 1994; 179:1005–1009.
31. Kawakami Y, Eliyahu S, Delgado CH, et al. Cloning of the gene coding for a shared human melanoma antigen recognized by autologous T cell infiltrating into tumor. *Proc Natl Acad Sci USA* 1994; 91:3515–3519.
32. Coulie PG, Brichard V, Van Pel A, et al. A new gene coding for a differentiation antigen recognized by autologous cytolytic T-lymphocytes on HLA-A2 melanomas. *J Exp Med* 1994; 180:35–42.
33. Kawakami Y, Eliyahu S, Sakaguchi K, et al. Identification of the immunodominant peptides of the MART-1 human melanoma antigen recognized by the majority of HLA-A2 restricted tumor infiltrating lymphocytes. *J Exp Med* 1994; 180:347–352.
34. Kawakami Y, Eliyahu S, Jennings C, et al. Recognition of multiple epitopes in the human melanoma antigen gp100 by tumor-infiltrating T lymphocytes associated with in vivo tumor regression. *J Immunol* 1995; 154:3961–3968.
35. Kawakami Y, Eliyahu S, Delgado CH, et al. Identification of a human melanoma antigen recognized by tumor infiltrating lymphocytes associated with in vivo tumor rejection. *Proc Natl Acad Sci USA* 1994; 91:6458–6462.
36. Castelli C, Storkus WJ, Maeurer MJ, et al. Mass spectrometric identification of a naturally processed melanoma peptide recognized by CD8+ cytotoxic T lymphocytes. *J Exp Med* 1995; 181:363–368.
37. Brichard V, Van Pel A, Wölfel T, et al. The tyrosinase gene codes for an antigen recognized by autologous cytolytic T-lymphocytes on HLA-A2 melanomas. *J Exp Med* 1993; 178:489–495.

38. Wölfel T, Van Pel A, Brichard V, et al. Two tyrosinase nonapeptides recognized on HLA-A2 melanomas recognized by autologous cytolytic T lymphocytes. *Eur J Immunol* 1994; 24:759–764.

39. Brichard VG, Herman J, Van Pel A, et al. A tyrosinase nonapeptide presented by HLA-B44 is recognized on a human melanoma by autologous cytolytic T lymphocytes. *Eur J Immunol* 1996; 26:224–230.

40. Kang X-Q, Kawakami Y, El-Gamil M, et al. Identification of a tyrosinase epitope recognized by HLA-A24 restricted tumor-infiltrating lymphocytes. *J Immunol* 1995; 155:1343–1348.

42. Robbins PF, el-Gamil M, Kawakami Y, Stevens E, Yannelli JR, Rosenberg SA. Recognition of tyrosinase by tumor infiltrating lymphocytes from a patient responding to immunotherapy. *Cancer Res* 1994; 54:3124–4125.

43. Topalian SL, Rivoltini L, Mancini M, et al. Human CD4⁺ T cells specifically recognize a shared melanoma associated antigen encoded by the tyrosinase gene. *Proc Natl Acad Sci USA* 1994; 91:9461–9465.

44. Topalian SL, Gonzales MI, Parkhurst M, et al. Melanoma-specific CD4⁺ T cells recognize nonmutated HLA-DR-restricted tyrosinase epitopes. *J Exp Med* 1996; 183:1965–1971.

45. Barnd DL, Lan MS, Metzgar RS, Finn OJ. Specific, major histocompatibility complex-unrestricted recognition of tumor-associated mucins by human cytotoxic T cells. *Proc Natl Acad Sci USA* 1989; 86:7159–7163.

46. Jerome KR, Barnd DL, Bendt KM, et al. Cytotoxic lymphocytes-T derived from patients with breast adenocarcinoma recognize an epitope present on the protein core of a mucin molecule preferentially expressed by malignant cells. *Cancer Res* 1991; 51:2908–2916.

47. Verdegaal EM, Huinink DB, Hoogstraten C, et al. Isolation of broadly reactive, tumor-specific, HLA Class-I restricted CTL from blood lymphocytes of a breast cancer patient. *Hum Immunol* 1999; 60:1195–1206.

48. Coulie PG, Lehmann F, Lethe B, et al. A mutated intron sequence codes for an antigenic peptide recognized by cytolytic T lymphocytes on a human melanoma. *Proc Natl Acad Sci USA* 1995; 92:7976–7980.

49. Wölfel T, Hauer M, Schneider J, et al. A p16INK4a-insensitive CDK4 mutant targeted by cytolytic T lymphocytes in a human melanoma. *Science* 1995; 269:1281–1284.

50. Robbins PF, El-Gamil M, Li YF, et al. A mutated β-catenin gene encodes a melanoma-specific antigen recognized by tumor infiltrating lymphocytes. *J Exp Med* 1996; 183:1185–1192.

51. Qin H, Chen W, Takahashi M, et al. CD4⁺ T cell immunity to mutated ras protein in pancreatic and colon cancer patients. *Cancer Res* 1995; 55:2984–2987.

52. Van Elsas A, Nijman HW, Van der Minne CE, et al. Induction and characterization of cytotoxic T-lymphocytes recognizing a mutated p21 ras peptide presented by HLA-A*0201. *Int J Cancer* 1995; 61:389–396.

53. Yanuck M, Carbone DP, Pendleton CD, et al. A mutant p53 tumor suppressor protein is a target for peptide-induced CD8+ cytotoxic T cells. *Cancer Res* 1993; 53:3257–3261.

54. Tilkin AF, Lubin R, Soussi T, et al. Primary proliferative T cell response to wild-type p53 protein in patients with breast cancer. *Eur J Immunol* 1995; 25:1765–1769.

55. Theobald M, Biggs J, Dittmer D, Levine AJ, Sherman LA. Targeting p53 as a general tumor antigen. *Proc Natl Acad Sci USA* 1995; 92:11,993–11,997.

56. Chen W, Peace DJ, Rovira DK, You SG, Cheever MA. T-cell immunity to the joining region of p210 bcr-abl protein. *Proc Natl Acad Sci USA* 1992; 89:1468–1472.

57. Bocchia M, Wentworth PA, Southwood S, et al. Specific binding of leukemia oncogene fusion protein peptides to HLA class I molecules. *Blood* 1995; 85:2680–2684.

58. Bocchia M, Korontsvit T, Xu Q, et al. Specific human cellular immunity to bcr-abl oncogene-derived peptides. *Blood* 1996; 87:3587–3592.

59. Ten-Bosch GJ, Toornvliet AC, Friede T, Melief CJ, Leeksma OC. Recognition of peptides corresponding to the joining region of p210bcr-abl protein by human T cells. *Leukemia* 1995; 9:1344–1348.

60. Disis ML, Smith JW, Murphy AE, Chen W, Cheever MA. In vitro generation of human cytologic T-cells specific for peptides derived from the HER-2/neu protooncogene protein. *Cancer Res* 1994; 54:1071–1076.

61. Disis ML, Calenoff E, McLaughlin G, et al. Existent T-cell and antibody immunity to HER-2/neu protein in patients with breast cancer. *Cancer Res* 1994; 54:16–20.

62. Fisk B, Blevins TL, Wharton JT. Identification an immunodominant peptide of HER-2/neu protooncogene recognized by ovarian tumor-specific cytotoxic T lymphocytes lines. *J Exp Med* 1995; 181:2109–2117.

63. Peoples GE, Goedegebuure PS, Smith R, Linehan DC, Yoshino I, Eberlein TJ. Breast and ovarian cancer-specific cytotoxic T lymphocytes recognize the same HER-2/neu-derived peptide. *Proc Natl Acad Sci USA* 1995; 432–436.

64. Disis ML, Gralow JR, Bernhard H, Hand SL, Rubin WD, Cheever MA. Peptide-based, but not whole protein, vaccines elicit immunity to HER-2/neu, an oncogenic self-protein. *J Immunol* 1996; 156:3151–3158.

65. Kast WM, Brandt RM, Drijfhout JW, Melief CJ. HLA-A2.1 restricted candidate CTL epitopes of human papillomavirus type 16 E6 and E7 proteins identified by using the processing defective human cell line T2. *J Immunother* 1993; 14:115–120.

66. Kast WM, Barndt RM, Sidney J, et al. Role of HLA-A motifs in identification of potential CTL epitopes in human papillomavirus type 16 E6 and E7 proteins. *J Immunol* 1994; 152:3904–3912.

67. Ressing ME, Sette A, Brandt RM, et al. Human CTL epitopes encoded by HPV16 E6 and E7 identified through in vivo and in vitro immunogenicity studies of HLA-A*0201 binding peptides. *J Immunol* 1995; 154:5934–5943.

68. Ressing ME, van Driel WJ, Celis E, et al. Occasional memory CTL responses of patients with human papillomavirus type 16 positive cervical lesions against a human leukocyte antigen A*0201 restricted E7 encoded epitope. *Cancer Res* 1996; 56:582–588.

69. Guo Y, Wu M, Chen H, et al. Effective tumor vaccine generated by fusion of hepatoma cells with activated B cells. *Science* 1994; 263:518–520.

70. Gong J, Chen D, Kashiwaba M, Kufe D. Induction of antitumor activity by immunisation with fusions of dendritic cells and carcinoma cells. *Nat Med* 1997; 3:558–561.

71. Berd D, Maguire HC, McCue P, Mastrangelo MJ. Treatment of metastatic melanoma with an autologous tumor-cell vaccine: clinical and immunological results in 64 patients. *J Clin Oncol* 1990; 8:1858–1867.

72. McCune CS, O'Donnell RW, Marquis DM, Sahasrabudhe DM. Renal cell carcinoma treated by vaccines for active specific immunotherapy: Correlation of survival with skin testing by autologous tumor cells. *Cancer Immunol Immunother* 1990; 32:62–66.

73. Bystryn JC, Oratz R, Roses D, Harris M, Henn M, Lew R. Relationship between immune response to melanoma vaccine immunization and clinical outcome in stage-II malignant melanoma. *Cancer* 1992; 69:1157–1164.

74. Morton DL, Foshag LJ, Hoon DS, et al. Prolongation of survival in metastatic melanoma after active specific immunotherapy with a new polyvalent melanoma vaccine. *Ann Surg* 1992; 216:463–482.

75. Mitchell MS, Harel W, Kan-Mitchell J, et al. Active specific immunotherapy of melanoma with allogeneic cell lysates: rationale, results, and possible mechanisms of action. *Ann N Y Acad Sci* 1993; 690:147–152.

76. Barth A, Hoon DSB, Foshag LJ, et al. Polyvalent melanoma cell vaccine induces delayed-type hypersensitivity and in vitro cellular immune response. *Cancer Res* 1994; 54:3342–3345.

77. Berd D, Maguire HC, Schuchter LM, et al. Autologous hapten-modified melanoma vaccine as postsurgical adjuvant treatment after resection of nodal metastases. *J Clin Oncol* 1997; 15:2359–2370.

78. Hsueh EC, Gupta RK, Qi K, Morton DL. Correlation of specific immune responses with survival in melanoma patients with distant metastases receiving polyvalent melanoma cell vaccine. *J Clin Oncol* 1998; 16:2913–2920.

79. Hsueh EC, Nathanson L, Foshag LJ, et al. Active specific immunotherapy with polyvalent melanoma cell vaccine for patients with in-transit melanoma metastases. *Cancer* 1999; 85:2160–2169.

80. Harris JE, Ryan L, Hoover HC, et al. Adjuvant active specific immunotherapy for stage II and III colon cancer with an autologous tumor cell vaccine: Eastern Cooperative Oncology Group Study E5283. *J Clin Oncol* 2000; 18:148–157.

81. Vermorken JB, Claessen AM, van Tinteren H, et al. Active specific immunotherapy for stage II and stage III human colon cancer: a randomised trial. *Lancet* 1999; 353:345–350.

82. Bubenik J, Simova J, Jandlova T. Immunotherapy of cancer using local administration of lymphoid cells transformed by IL-2 cDNA and constitutively producing IL-2. *Immunol Lett* 1990; 23:287–292.

83. Tepper RI, Pattengale PK, Leder P. Murine interleukin 4 displays potent antitumor activity in vivo. *Cell* 1989; 57:503–512.

84. Fearon ER, Pardoll DM, Itaya T, et al. Interleukin-2 production by tumor cells bypasses T-helper function in the generation of an antitumor response. *Cell* 1990; 60:397–403.

85. W, Diamantstein T, Blankenstein T. Lack of tumorigenicity of Interleukin 4 autocrine growing cells seems related to the antitumor function of Interleukin 4. *Mol Immunol* 1990; 27:1331–1337.

86. Gansbacher B, Zier K, Daniels B, Cronin K, Bannerji R, Gilboa E. Interleukin 2 gene transfer into tumor cells abrogates tumorigenicity and induces protected immunity. *J Exp Med* 1990; 172:1217–1224.

87. Blankenstein T, Qin Z, Überla K, et al. Tumor suppression after tumor cell-targeted tumor necrosis factor α gene transfer. *J Exp Med* 1991; 173:1047–1052.

88. Colombo MP, Ferrari G, Stoppacciaro A, et al. Granulocyte colony-stimulating factor gene transfer suppresses tumorigenicity of a murine adenocarcinoma in vivo. *J Exp Med* 1991; 173:889–897.

89. Golumbek PT, Lazenby AJ, Levitsky HI, et al. Treatment of established renal cancer by tumor cells engineered to secrete Interleukin-4. *Science* 1991; 254:713–716.

90. Hock H, Dorsch M, Diamantstein T, Blankenstein T. Interleukin-7 induces CD4+ T-Cell-dependent tumor rejection. *J Exp Med* 1991; 174:1291–1298.

91. Dranoff G, Jaffee EM, Lazenby AJ. Vaccination with irradiated tumor cells engineered to secrete granulocyte-macrophage colony-stimulating factor stimulates potent, specific, and long-lasting anti-tumor immunity. *Proc Natl Acad Sci USA* 1993; 90:3539–3543.

92. Abdel-Wahab Z, We-Ping L, Osanto S, et al. Transduction of human melanoma cells with interleukin-2 gene reduces tumorigenicity and enhances antitumor immunity: a nude mouse model. *Cell Immunol* 1994; 159:26–39.

93. Abdel-Wahab Z, Dar M, Osanto S, et al. Eradication of melanoma pulmonary metastases by immunotherapy with tumor cells engineered to secrete interleukin-2 or gamma interferon. *Cancer Gene Ther* 1997; 4:33–41.

94. Fearon ER, Itaya T, Hunt B, Vogelstein B, Frost P. Induction in a murine tumor of immunogenic tumor variants by transfection with a foreign gene. *Cancer Res* 1988; 38:2975–2980.

95. Hui K, Grosveld F, Festenstein H. Rejection of transplantable AKR leukaemia cells following MHC DNA-mediated cell transformation. *Nature* 1984; 311:750–752.

96. Isobe K, Hasegawa Y, Iwamoto T, et al. Induction of antitumor immunity in mice by allo-major histo-compatibility complex class-I gene transfectant with strong antigen expression. *J Natl Cancer Inst* 1989; 81:1823–1828.

97. Hui KM, Sim T, Foo TT, Oei AA. Tumor rejection mediated by transfection with allogeneic class-I histocompatibility gene. *J Immunol* 1989; 143:3835–3843.

98. Gelber C, Plaksin D, Vadai E, Feldman M, Eisenbach L. Abolishment of metastasis formation by murine tumor cells transfected with "foreign" H-2K genes. *Cancer Res* 1989; 49:2366–2373.

99. Ostrand-Rosenberg S, Roby C, Clements VK, Cole GA. Tumor-specific immunity can be enhanced by transfection of tumor cells with syngeneic MHC-class-II genes or allogeneic MHC-class-I genes. *Int J Cancer* 1991; supplement 6:61–68.

100. Chen L, Ashe S, Brady WA, et al. Co-stimulation of antitumor immunity by the B7 counterreceptor for the T lymphocyte molecules CD28 and CTLA-4. *Cell* 1992; 71:1093–1102.

101. Townsend SE, Allison JP. Tumor rejection after direct co-stimulation of CD8+ T-cells by B7-transfected melanoma cells. *Science* 1993; 259:368–370.

102. Chen L, McGowan P, Ashe S, et al. Tumor immunogenicity determines the effect of B7 co-stimulation on T cell-mediated tumor immunity. *J Exp Med* 1994; 179:523–531.

103. Osanto S, Schiphorst PP, Weijl NI, et al. Vaccination of melanoma patients with an allogeneic, genetically modified interleukin 2-producing melanoma cell line. *Hum Gene Ther* 2000; 11:739–750.

104. Arienti F, Sule-Suso J, Melani C, et al. Limited antitumor T cell response in melanoma patients vaccinated with interleukin-2 gene-transduced allogeneic melanoma cells. *Hum Gene Ther* 1996; 7:1955–1963.

105. Soiffer R, Lynch T, Mihm M, et al. Vaccination with irradiated autologous melanoma cells engineered to secrete human granulocyte-macrophage colony-stimulating factor generates potent antitumor immunity in patients with metastatic melanoma. *Proc Natl Acad Sci USA* 1998; 95:13,141–13,146.

106. Schreiber S, Kampgen E, Wagner E, et al. Immunotherapy of metastatic malignant melanoma by a vaccine consisting of autologous interleukin 2-transfected cancer cells: outcome of a phase I study. *Hum Gene Ther* 1999; 10:983–993.

107. Veelken H, Mackensen A, Lahn M, et al. A phase-I clinical study of autologous tumor cells plus interleukin-2-gene-transfected allogeneic fibroblasts as a vaccine in patients with cancer. *Int J Cancer* 1997; 70:269–277.

108. Kubo RT, Sette A, Grey HM, et al. Definition of specific peptide motifs for four major HLA-A alleles. *J Immunol* 1994; 152:3913–3924.

109. Vitiello A, Ishioka G, Grey HM, et al. Development of a lipopeptide-based therapeutic vaccine to treat chronic HBV infection. *J Clin Invest* 1995; 95:341–349.

110. Marchand M, Weynants P, Rankin E, et al. Tumor regression responses in melanoma patients treated with a peptide encoded by the gene MAGE-3. *Int J Cancer* 1995; 63:883–885.

111. Jaeger E, Bernhard H, Romero P, et al. Generation of cytotoxic T-cell responses with synthetic melanoma-associated peptides in vivo: implications for tumor vaccines with melanoma-associated antigens. *Int J Cancer* 1996; 66:162–169.

112. Salgaller ML, Marincola FM, Cormier JN, Rosenberg SA. Immunization against epitopes in the human melanoma antigen gp100 following patient immunization with synthetic peptides. *Cancer Res* 1996; 56:4749–4757.

113. Parkhurst MR, Salgaller ML, Southwood S, et al. Improved induction of melanoma reactive CTL with peptides from melanoma antigen gp100 modified at HLA-A*0201 binding residues. *J Immunol* 1995; 157:2539–2548.

114. Rosenberg SA, Yang JC, Schwartzentruber DJ, et al. Immunologic and therapeutic evaluation of a synthetic peptide vaccine for the treatment of patients with metastatic melanoma. *Nat Med* 1998; 4:321–327.

115. Lee KH, Wang E, Nielsen MB, et al. Increased vaccine-specific T cell frequency after peptide-based vaccination correlates with increased susceptibility to in vitro stimulation but does not lead to tumor regression. *J Immunol* 1999; 163:6292–6300.

116. Rosenberg SA, Yang JC, Schwartzentruber DJ, et al. Impact of cytokine administration on the generation of antitumor reactivity in patients with metastatic melanoma receiving a peptide vaccine. *J Immunol* 1999; 163:1690–1695.

117. Wang F, Bade E, Kuniyoshi C, et al. Phase I trial of a MART-1 peptide vaccine with incomplete Freund's adjuvant for resected high-risk melanoma. *Clin Cancer Res* 1999; 5:256–265.

118. Scheibenbogen C, Schmittel A, Keilholz U, et al. Phase 2 trial of vaccination with tyrosinase peptides and granulocyte-macrophage colony-stimulating factor in patients with metastatic melanoma. *J Immunother* 2000; 23:275–281.

119. Gjertsen MK, Bakka A, Breivik J, et al. Vaccination with mutant ras peptides and induction of T-cell responsiveness in pancreatic carcinoma patients carrying the corresponding ras mutation. *Lancet* 1995; 346:1399–1400.

120. Gjertsen MK, Bakka A, Breivik J, et al. Ex vivo ras peptide vaccination in patients with advanced pancreatic cancer: results of a phase I/II study. *Int J Cancer* 1996; 65:450–453.

121. Khleif SN, Abrams SI, Hamilton JM, et al. A phase I vaccine trial with peptides reflecting ras oncogene mutations of solid tumors. *J Immunother* 1999; 22:155–165.

122. Pinilla-Ibarz J, Cathcart K, Korontsvit T, et al. Vaccination of patients with chronic myelogenous leukemia with bcr-abl oncogene. *Blood* 2000; 95:1781–1787.

123. Disis ML, Grabstein KH, Sleath PR, Cheever MA. Generation of immunity to the HER-2/neu oncogenic protein in patients with breast and ovarian cancer using a peptide-based vaccine. *Clin Cancer Res* 1999; 5:1289–1297.

124. Steller MA, Gurski KJ, Murakami M, et al. Cell-mediated immunological responses in cervical and vaginal cancer patients immunized with a lipidated epitope of human papillomavirus type 16 E7. *Clin Cancer Res* 1998; 4:2103–2109.

125. MacLean GD, Reddish MA, Koganty RR, Longenecker BM. Antibodies against mucin-associated sialyl-Tn epitopes correlate with survival of metastatic adenocarcinoma patients undergoing active specific immunotherapy with synthetic STn vaccine. *J Immunother Emphasis Tumor Immunol* 1996; 19:59–68.

126. MacLean GD, Miles DW, Rubens RD, Reddish MA, Longenecker BM. Enhancing effect of THERATOPE Stn-KLH cancer vaccine in patients with metastatic breast cancer by pretreatment with low-dose intravenous cyclophosphamide. *J Immunother Emphasis Tumor Immunol* 1996; 19:309–316.

127. Samanci A, Qing Y, Fagerberg J, et al. Pharmacological administration of granulocyte/macrophage-colony-stimulating factor is of significant importance for the induction of a strong humoral and cellular response in patients immunized with recombinant carcinoembryonic antigen. *Cancer Immunol Immunother* 1998; 47:131–142.

128. Bendandi M, Gocke CD, Kobrin CB, et al. Complete molecular remissions induced by patient-specific vaccination plus granulocyte-monocyte colony-stimulating factor against lymphoma. *Nat Med* 1999; 5:1171–1177.

129. Mayordomo JI, Zorina T, Storkus WJ, et al. Bone marrow-derived dendritic cells pulsed with synthetic tumour peptides elicit protective and therapeutic antitumour immunity. *Nat Med* 1995; 1:1297–1302.

130. Zitvogel L, Mayordomo JI, Tjandrawan T, et al. Therapy of murine tumors with tumor peptide-pulsed dendritic cells: dependence on T cell, B7 co-stimulation, and T helper cell 1-associated cytokines. *J Exp Med* 1996; 183:87–97.

131. Porgador A, Snyder D, Gilboa E. Induction of antitumor immunity using bone-marrow generated dendritic cells. *J Immunol* 1996; 156:2918–2926.
132. Caux C, Duzetter-Dambuyant C, Schmitt D, Banchereau J. GM-CSF and TNF-α cooperate in the generation of dendritic Langerhans cells. *Nature* 1992; 360:258–260.
133. Sallusto F, Lanzavecchia A. Efficient presentation of soluble antigen by cultured human dendritic cells is maintained by granulocyte/macrophage colony-stimulating factor plus interleukin-4 and downregulated by tumor necrosis factor alpha. *J Exp Med* 1994; 179:1109–1118.
134. Romani N, Runer S, Brang D, et al. Proliferating dendritic cell progenitors in human blood. *J Exp Med* 1994; 180:83–93.
135. Mukherji B, Chakraborty NG, Yamasaki S, et al. Induction of antigen-specific cytolytic T cells in situ in human melanoma by immunization with synthetic peptide-pulsed autologous antigen presenting cells. *Proc Natl Acad Sci USA* 1995; 92:8078–8082.
136. Chakraborty NG, Sporn JR, Tortora AF, et al. Immunization with a tumor-cell-lysate-loaded autologous-antigen-presenting-cell-based vaccine in melanoma. *Cancer Immunol Immunother* 1998; 47:58–64.
137. Nestle FO, Alijagic S, Gilliet M, et al. Vaccination of melanoma patients with peptide- or tumor lysate-pulsed dendritic cells. *Nat Med* 1998; 4:328–332.
138. Schuler-Thurner B, Dieckmann D, Keikavoussi P, et al. Mage-3 and influenza-matrix peptide-specific cytotoxic T cells are inducible in terminal stage HLA-A2.1+ melanoma patients by mature monocyte-derived dendritic cells. *J Immunol* 2000; 165:3492–3496.
139. Thurner B, Haendle I, Roder C, et al. Vaccination with mage-3A1 peptide-pulsed mature, monocyte-derived dendritic cells expands specific cytotoxic T cells and induces regression of some metastases in advanced stage IV melanoma. *J Exp Med* 1999; 190:1669–1678.
140. Mackensen A, Herbst B, Chen JL, et al. Phase I study in melanoma patients of a vaccine with peptide-pulsed dendritic cells generated in vitro from CD34(+) hematopoietic progenitor cells. *Int J Cancer* 2000; 86:385–392.
141. Hsu FJ, Benike C, Fagnoni F, et al. Vaccination of patients with B-cell lymphoma using autologous antigen-pulsed dendritic cells. *Nat Med* 1996; 2:52–58.
142. Hsu FJ, Caspar CB, Czerwinski D, et al. Tumor-specific idiotype vaccines in the treatment of patients with B-cell lymphoma-long-term results of a clinical trial. *Blood* 1997; 89:3129–3135.
143. Lim SH, Bailey-Wood R. Idiotypic protein-pulsed dendritic cell vaccination in multiple myeloma. *Int J Cancer* 1999; 83:215–222.
144. Kugler A, Stuhler G, Walden P, et al. Regression of human metastatic renal cell carcinoma after vaccination with tumor cell-dendritic cell hybrids. *Nat Med* 2000; 6:332–336.
145. Trefzer U, Weingart G, Chen Y, et al. Hybrid cell vaccination for cancer immune therapy: first clinical trial with metastatic melanoma. *Int J Cancer* 2000; 85:618–626.
146. Wang M, Bronte V, Chen PW, et al. Active immunotherapy of cancer with a nonreplicating recombinant fowlpox virus encoding a model tumor-associated antigen. *J Immunol* 1995; 154:4685–4692.
147. Whitton JL, Sheng N, Oldstone MB, McKee TA. A "string-of-beads" vaccine, comprising linked minigenes, confers protection from lethal-dose virus challenge. *J Virol* 1993; 67:348–352.
148. Thomson SA, Khanna R, Gardner J, et al. Minimal epitopes expressed in a recombinant polyepitope protein are processed and presented to CD8+ cytotoxic T-cells: implications for vaccine design. *Proc Natl Acad Sci USA* 1995; 92:5845–5849.
149. Tsang KY, Zaremba S, Nieroda CA, Zhu MZ, Hamilton JM, Schlom J. Generation of human cytotoxic T cells specific for human carcinoembryonic antigen epitopes from patients immunized with recombinant vaccine-CEA vaccine. *J Natl Cancer Inst* 1995; 87:982–990.
150. Conry RM, Khazaeli MB, Saleh MN, et al. Phase I trial of a recombinant vaccinia virus encoding carcinoembryonic antigen administration. *Clin Cancer Res* 1999; 5:2330–2337.
151. Conry RM, Allen KO, Lee S, Moore SE, Shaw DR, LoBuglio AF. Human autoantibodies to carcinoembryonic antigen (CEA) induced by a vaccinia-CEA vaccine. *Clin Cancer Res* 2000; 6:34–41.
152. Conry RM, Khazaeli MB, Saleh MN, et al. Phase I trial of a recombinant vaccinia virus encoding carcinoembryonic antigen in metastatic adenocarcinoma: comparison of intradermal versus subcutaneous administration. *Clin Cancer Res* 1999; 5:2330–2337.
153. Marshall JL, Hawkins MJ, Tsang KY, et al. Phase I study in cancer patients of a replication-defective avipox recombinant vaccine that expresses human carcinoembryonic antigen. *J Clin Oncol* 1999; 17:332–337.
154. Zhu MZ, Marshall J, Cole D, Schlom J, Tsang KY. Specific cytolytic T-cell responses to human CEA from patients immunized with recombinant avipox-CEA vaccine. *Clin Cancer Res* 2000; 6:24–33.

155. Eder JP, Kantoff PW, Roper K, et al. A phase I trial of a recombinant vaccinia virus expressing prostate-specific antigen in advanced prostate cancer. *Clin Cancer Res* 2000; 6:1632–1638.

156. Borysiewicz LK, Fiander A, Nimako M, et al. A recombinant vaccinia virus encoding human papillomavirus types 16 and 18, E6 and E7 proteins as immunotherapy for cervical cancer. *Lancet* 1996; 347:1523–1527.

157. Wolff JA, Malone RW, Williams P, et al. Direct gene transfer into mouse muscle in vitro. *Science* 1990; 247:1465–1468.

158. Tang DC, Devit M, Johnston SA. Genetic immunization is a simple method for eliciting an immune response. *Nature* 1992; 356:152–154.

159. Yankauckas MA, Morrow JE, Parker SE, et al. Long-term antinucleoprotein and humoral immunity is induced by intramuscular injection of plasmid DNA containing NP gene. *DNA & Cell Biol* 1993; 12:771–776.

160. Montgomery DL, Shiver JW, Leander KR, et al. Heterologous and homologous protection against influenza A by DNA vaccination: optimization of DNA vectors. *DNA & Cell Biol* 1993; 12:777–783.

161. Eisenbraun MD, Fuller DH, Haynes JR. Examination of parameters affecting the elicitation of humoral immune responses by particle bombardment-mediated genetic immunization. *DNA & Cell Biol* 1993; 12:791–797.

162. Jiao S, Cheng L, Wolff JA, Yang NS. Particle-bombardment-mediated gene transfer and expression in rat brain tissues. *Biotechnology* 1993; 11:497–502.

163. Fynan EF, Webster RG, Fuller DH, Haynes JR, Santoro JC, Robinson HL. DNA vaccines: Protective immunizations by parenteral, mucosal, and gene-gun inoculations. *Proc Natl Acad Sci USA* 1993; 90:11478–11482.

164. Hawkins RE, Zhu D, Ovecka M, et al. Idiotypic vaccination against human B-cell lymphoma. Rescue of variable region sequences from biopsy material for assembly as single-chain Fv personal vaccines. *Blood* 1994; 83:3279–3288.

165. Nabel GJ, Nabel EG, Yang ZY, et al. Direct gene transfer with DNA-liposome complexes in melanoma: Expression, biologic activity, and lack of toxicity in humans. *Proc Natl Acad Sci USA* 1993; 90:11307–11311.

166. Nabel GJ, Gordon D, Bishop DK, et al. Immune response in human melanoma after transfer of an allogeneic class I major histocompatibility complex gene with DNA-liposome complexes. *Proc Natl Acad Sci USA* 1996; 93:15,388–15,393.

IV   FUTURE DIRECTIONS:
NOVEL CANCER DRUG TARGETS AND DELIVERY SYSTEMS

14   Gene Therapy of Cancer

Susanne Osanto, MD, PhD

CONTENTS

1. INTRODUCTION

Our knowledge of the human genome and the technological development of molecular biology have enabled the development of gene therapy *(1)*. Gene therapy can be defined as the introduction of genetic material into "defective" somatic cells to restore normal function and produce a therapeutic effect. Gene therapy may replace a missing gene, restore a gene function that is altered by mutation, increase the expression of a gene, introduce a new gene, or abrogate the expression of a gene. Somatic gene therapy involves the transfer of genetic material into nongermline cells.

Historically, somatic cell gene therapy has been thought of as a treatment for and potential cure of classical inherited diseases based on single gene defects. This is in contrast to the multifactorial inherited disorders that involve multiple genes and environmental factors. In patients with single gene disorders such as hemophilia, severe combined immunodeficiency (SCID), cystic fibrosis, and Duchenne's muscular dystrophy, gene replacement therapy involving transfer of the normal gene and continued expression of the normal protein is desired. In dominantly inherited disorders where the presence of an abnormal protein interferes with the function and development of organ or tissue, selective mutation of the mutant gene could result in a therapeutic effect.

Critical requirements in gene therapy are efficient gene transfer techniques and gene expression at appropriate levels for therapy. Gene transfer can be achieved by two methods: direct transfer in vivo or ex vivo. The in vitro gene transfer techniques are currently most widely used for clinical trials because these techniques are generally more efficient. Various gene transfer methods, including the use of defective viruses, are currently under development. Each of these defective viruses has specific advantages and disadvantages.

From: *Drug Delivery Systems in Cancer Therapy*
Edited by: D. M. Brown © Humana Press Inc., Totowa, NJ

Table 1

Characteristics of Vectors for Gene Transfer

Virus	Properties	Clinical Applications
Retrovirus 7–10 kb ss RNA	Only 8–9 kb insert Integrates randomly Wide target cell range	Integrates in host genome Long-term expression in dividing cells Suitable for permanent correction
Adenovirus 36-kb ds DNA	15 kb insert Wide target cell range High titre production	Suitable for non-dividing cells Transient transgene expression No chronic administration Immunogenic, inflammatory reactions

AAV
4.7-kb ss DNA
	Limited size insert
	Integrates into chromosome
	   19 of the host genome?
	Wide target range
	Difficult large scale production
	May require adenovirus
	   products for efficient
	   transduction
		No known disease in humans
		Considered a safe vector

HSV-1 152 kb ds DNA	Large genome Easy to manipulate Insert up to 30 kb	Suitable for specific (e.g.,neurologi- cal) diseases Does not integrate into host genome
Vaccinia virus 190 kb ds DNA	Accommodates large inserts	Considered safe
Liposomes	Low transfer efficiency	Transient expression Commercially available Non-toxic Repeated administration possible Fewer safety issues
Naked DNA	Simple production Safe No size limitation	Inefficient entry into cells Not stable Fewer safety issues
Complexed DNA	More efficient uptake than naked DNA Targetable	Inefficient cell entry Not stable Fewer safety issues

2. VECTORS OF GENE THERAPY

For introduction of genes into living cells, a number of methods are available at present. Vehicles that facilitate the transfer of genes into a cell are called vectors. A vector carries the DNA to the desired site, i.e., the nucleus of the cell. Vectors can be divided into viral and nonviral delivery systems. The most commonly used viral vectors are derived from retrovirus and adenovirus. Other viral vectors include vectors derived from adenoassociated virus (AAV), herpes simplex virus type 1 (HSV-1), and vaccinia virus. The characteristics of vectors that have been generated are shown in Table 1. Important features that distinguish the different viral vectors include the size of the gene that can be accommodated, the duration of expression, target cell infectivity, and integration into the genome. Most gene delivery systems are nonintegrating, indicating that the exogenous DNA will remain extra chromosomal in the nucleus and will not be passed on to daughter cells as the cells divide. Integrating vectors insert their genes into chromosomes and will pass the integrated gene to all daughter cells.

Viruses are very efficient at transferring genetic information. They have evolved the mechanism to insert their genetic material into cells of the host so that the host cell machinery can be used to permit the virus to replicate. Viral vectors can be produced by removing some or all of the genes that encode viral proteins, and replacing them with a therapeutic gene. These vectors are produced by cells that also express any protein necessary for producing a viral particle. A risk of viral vectors is that they might recombine to generate replication-competent virus capable of multiple rounds of replication that could cause disease in humans.

Available nonviral vectors include plasmids (circular double-stranded DNA) which can be propagated in bacteria, or oligonucleotides that can be synthesized chemically. Plasmids can transfer a therapeutic gene into a cell, whereas oligonucleotides inhibit the expression of endogenous genes. In contrast to viral vectors, transfer of nonviral vectors into cells is inefficient. The effect is generally transient, but these vectors do not carry the risk of generating (replication-competent) wild-type virus.

2.1. Viral Vectors

2.1.1. RETROVIRAL VECTORS

Retroviruses are lipid-enveloped particles comprised of two copies of a positive single-strand RNA genome of 7–11 kb. All retroviruses have two long terminal repeat (LTR) sequences at their ends. The LTR sequences frame the *gag, pol,* and *env* genes. The *gag* molecule is required to form the viral core and functions in viral RNA incorporation into the core during packaging. *Pol* is the viral reverse transcriptase that converts viral DNA into double-stranded proviral DNA. Integrase, a virus-encoded protein, mediates random integration of the proviral DNA into the host chromosome. *Env* is the viral envelope glycoprotein. Retroviruses contain a membrane envelope containing a virus-encoded glycoprotein that specifies the host range of cell types that can be infected by binding to a cellular receptor. Each virus strain has a particular *env* that determines its infectivity host range. Following entry into target cells, their RNA genome is retrotranscribed into linear double-stranded DNA, which integrates stably into random sites of the host genome by a mechanism involving the virus-encoded enzyme integrase.

Retroviral vectors for gene transfer are defective and have been constructed by replacing the viral protein-coding regions with the cDNA of interest, thus making these vectors replication-defective. The cDNA of interest is flanked by the retroviral LTRs that drive the expression of the inserted gene. In order to produce retroviral particles for gene delivery, recombinant retrovirus vectors are transfected into packaging cell lines that stably produce the *gag, pol,* and *env* proteins. This production system avoids generation of infectious retrovirus beyond the initial retrovirus infection into the host (replication competent virus is not generated).

The most widely used retroviral vectors are derived from the retrovirus Moloney murine leukemia virus (MLV). MLV is capable only of infecting dividing cells, as transfer of the DNA to the nucleus occurs only during disruption of the nuclear membrane during mitosis. Just a fraction of cells pass through mitosis at any given time, and this severely limits the application of retroviral vectors in gene therapy.

Retroviral vectors lack retroviral genes and result in high-level long-term expression owing to their ability to integrate into chromosomes *(2,3)*. Once the vector is integrated, the vector genes become a stable part of the inheritance of that cell, being passed along to all cell progeny during normal cell division. This feature is particularly important for the possibility of permanent cure of genetic diseases. The host range of cells that they infect includes epithelial cells and fibroblasts; cells of lymphoid origin are more resistant. One major disadvantage of MLV-based retroviral vectors for many gene applications is the fact that they only transduce dividing cells. For some applications, such as targeting of proliferating tumor vascular endothelial cells as opposed to quiescent endothelial cells, this may be advantageous. At present, a major obstacle to effective gene transfer by retroviral vectors is the fact that not all tumor cells in a certain tumor are replicating and that not all replicating cells are transduced *(4)*. Also, they integrate randomly and this random integration implies that vector gene expression may vary by each cell and that the integration event could result in activation of an oncogene or inactivation of a tumor suppressor gene. Random vector integration could thus contribute to the malignant transformation of that cell. Other disadvantages are the low production titre, resulting in reduced transduction efficiency into solid tumors. Retroviral vectors are also limited by the size of the transgene that can be inserted. Furthermore, the in vivo use of retroviral vectors is limited resulting from inactivation by complement *(5)*.

2.1.2. LENTIVIRAL VECTORS

Recently developed lentiviral vectors transduce nondividing cells, but there are concerns regarding the safety of these vectors *(6,7)*. Lentiviruses (such as HIV and other immunodeficiency viruses) are retroviruses that, in contrast to other members of the family, can infect both dividing and nondividing cells. Lentiviruses have a more complex genome than other retroviruses: in addition to *gag, pol,* and *env,* they encode two regulatory genes, *tat* and *rev,* essential for expression of the genome, and a variable set of accessory genes. Unlike retroviruses, they rely on active transport of the preinitiation complex through the nucleopore by the nuclear import machinery of the target cell enabling infection of nondividing cells. The latter makes them an attractive vector for gene therapy. The recent development of novel vector packaging systems can significantly facilitate availability, and new self-inactivating lentiviral vectors can allow safer use *(8,9)*.

There is a substantial risk of genetic recombination between infectious HIV and an HIV vector. These combinatorial events could possibly lead to new infectious HIV viruses, rendering HIV vectors unsuitable for clinical use. One possibility to minimize the risk is to include a suicide gene in the vector. This gene confers a selective toxicity to drugs and the transfer of such a vector would result in cellular destruction when the patient is treated with the prodrug.

2.1.3. ADENOVIRAL VECTORS

Adenoviruses are common double-stranded DNA viruses that produce infection of the upper respiratory tracts. Adenovirus has a natural tropism for respiratory epithelium, the cornea, and the gastrointestinal tract. The adenoviral genome is divided into four early regions, E1–E4, which are expressed prior to viral DNA replication, and the late genes L1–L5, which encode primarily viral structural proteins. Current adenoviral vectors are primarily derived from adenovirus type 2 and 5, the most common serotypes to which most adults have been exposed. To improve safety of adenoviral vectors, they have been made replication-deficient by deletion of all or part of their regulatory sequences. The first-generation adenoviral vectors were obtained by substitution of the early E1A and E1b regulatory sequences by the transgene and by deletion of the E3 regions of the genome. The sequences necessary for replication and packaging are provided by the packaging cell line, usually the 293 cell line. Adenoviral vectors are able to transfer genes into most tissues of the body; the major advantage of adenoviral vectors is the high efficiency of gene transfer, not only in dividing but also in nondividing cells *(10–13)*.

Entry of adenoviruses into susceptible cells requires two sequential steps mediated by interaction of two viral capsid proteins with receptors on the surface of the target cell *(14–20)*. The initial binding of the adenovirus to the "coxsackievirus and adenovirus receptor CAR" *(14–16)* occurs via the carboxy-terminal knob domain of the fiber *(17,18)*. The subsequent step involves interaction of Arg-Gly-Asp (RGD) peptide sequences in the penton base of the adenovirus with host cell integrins and internalization by receptor-mediated endocytosis *(19,20)*. After cell entry, the viral particle contains proteins that promote lysis of the endosomes. Thereafter, the vector may enter the nucleus.

Because adenoviruses have larger genomes than retroviruses, more regions can be removed allowing up to 36 kb of DNA to be inserted. Adenoviral vectors are able to transfer genes into most tissues of the body, e.g., liver, lung, brain, muscle, and heart. In contrast to retroviral vectors, adenoviral vectors can be produced at high titres. There are several disadvantages to the use of adenoviral vectors. For instance, the limited (transient) transgene expression as a consequence of nonintegration, suggests that the transferred vector and transgene sequences are not inherited by daughter cells. Thus, with the proliferation of transduced cells, vector sequences are lost, with the consequence of limited duration of transgene expression. Administration of the vector may induce an antiviral immune response that may result in a significant local inflammatory and systemic immune response *(21–25)*. The transient expression is, therefore, primarily caused by the immune response to residual adenoviral genes or the transgene in early generation vectors. This antiviral immune response will limit the effects of repeated administration. Long-term expression, especially in proliferating cells, requires repeated administration of the vector, whereas the immune response will preclude effective repeated administration. In cell types with low proliferative index, the adenoviral vector may result in expression for months.

Adenoviral vectors contain many adenoviral genes, although "gutless" adenoviral vectors in which all viral coding sequences have been deleted but which expresses a transgene and is packaged in a functional adenoviral capsid, have been developed recently *(26)*.

Another major problem for the application in gene therapy of adenoviral vectors has been the presence of replication-competent adenovirus (RCA) in batches of replication-defective adenovirus. RCAs are generated by recombination between sequences in the adenovector and homologous sequences in helper cells, resulting in the acquisition by the vector of early region E1. To prevent the generation of RCA, a new helper cell line named PER was developed. Propagation of matched adenoviral vectors, which lack Ad5 nucleotides 459–3510 in one of the PER clones (PER.C6) does not result in the generation of RCA, thus generating a safe vector for clinical application *(27)*.

2.1.4. AAV Vectors

The AAV vectors lack AAV genes and can transduce nondividing cells *(28–30)*. They have resulted in long-term expression, although it is unclear if, following transduction, they remain episomal or integrate into the chromosome in nondividing cells. Production of large amounts of AAV vector is difficult. AAV vectors have potential risks of insertional mutagenesis, generation of wild-type AAV, and administration of contaminating adenovirus. It is theoretically possible that AAV could activate an oncogene or inactivate a tumor suppressor gene by integrating into the chromosome in vivo. As AAV has not been shown to be pathogenic and is not capable of efficient replication in the absence of helper virus, the possible generation of wild-type AAV may not be a serious concern in human gene therapy. Careful testing of AAV vectors for the presence of contaminating helper virus would reduce the risk of coadministration of adenovirus. It appears that AAV vectors are relatively safe, although long-term studies are necessary.

2.2. Nonviral Vectors

Nonviral vectors include any method of gene transfer that does not involve production of a viral particle. The size of the insert accepted varies considerably among the different nonviral vectors. A major problem of nonviral vectors is the difficulty to efficiently transfer the highly charged DNA molecules into a cell. Larger pieces of DNA are transferred less efficiently than smaller pieces. For ex vivo transfer, genes are usually transferred into the cell by using calcium phosphate coprecipitation, electroporation, cationic lipids, or liposomes. For most cell types, only a minor proportion of the cells can be modified. In vitro, transfected cells can be enriched by the use of a selectable marker present on the section of DNA.

2.2.1. Plasmids

Plasmids are double-stranded circular DNA molecules that contain a bacterial origin of replication. They are easily amplified to a high copy number in bacteria or eukaryotic cells, produced at a high level of purity, and are associated with low immunogenicity. Plasmids are easy to manipulate and can accommodate large sequences of foreign DNA. A major disadvantage of nonviral vectors is the transient and low level of gene expression. Most plasmids remain episomal. However, plasmids can integrate at low frequency into the chromosome, particularly when—in vitro—a procedure is used to select clones exhibiting long-term expression.

2.2.2. Liposomes and Lipids

Efficient in vivo transfer is somewhat more difficult to achieve than ex vivo gene transfer. Many investigators have used liposomes, cationic lipids, or anionic lipids. Liposomes are gene delivery vehicles based on artificially generated lipid vesicles. Liposomes entrap DNA and allow cell membrane fusion through the lipid portion of the molecule. The lipid coating allows for the DNA to survive in vivo, bind to cells, and be endocytosed into the cell. Liposomal vectors are often composed of cationic lipids mixed with cholesterol and dioleoylphosphatidylethanolamine. Liposome/DNA complexes were expected to be less immunogenic than viral vectors, but these vectors can also generate significant inflammatory responses that are probably related to the immunogenicity of bacterial-derived DNA *(31,32)*.

Despite major improvements in the effectiveness of cationic lipids for gene transfer, several limitations still remain including the stability of the lipid:DNA complexes in the systemic circulation, their biodistribution, lack of specificity for relevant target cells, and their inability to mediate sustained expression.

2.2.3. NAKED DNA AND THE GENE GUN

Another method of gene transfer into the cell is direct injection of "naked DNA" (DNA not coated and not bound to lipid, protein, or antibody) into specific tissue or infused through a vascular bed (e.g., liver). Alternatively, microscopic (gold) particles attached to DNA are "shot" into the target cell using a ballistic device referred to as a "gene gun." By this method, a large number of cells can be treated, and it can be used in vivo as well. The DNA gun-gene delivery system is an effective means of introducing gene-encoding expression vectors into the epidermis, resulting in temporal presence of DNA and expression of antigen.

2.2.4. RECEPTOR-MEDIATED ENDOCYTOSIS

Selective delivery of a nonviral vector to a specific organ or cell type would be desirable for some applications and may involve linking of DNA to a targeting ligand, that will bind to a specific cell-surface receptor, inducing internalization and transfer of the DNA into the cells. For example, DNA has been targeted to the asialoglycoprotein receptor of hepatocytes by complexing the DNA with polylysine-conjugated asialoglycoprotein. Similarly, cells expressing a transferrin or folate receptor may be targeted by complexing DNA to the ligand.

A risk of using nonviral vectors for gene therapy is the potential toxicity of the compounds that are used to facilitate the entry of DNA into a cell and the insertional mutagenesis that could activate oncogenes or inactivate tumor suppressor genes if the plasmid integrates.

2.2.5. OLIGONUCLEOTIDES

Oligonucleotides are short nucleotide strands designed to bind specifically to DNA or RNA sequences. Oligonucleotides probably enter the cell via receptor-mediated endocytosis. Oligonucleotides can modulate gene expression in cells by formation of triplex DNA, i.e., three associated deoxynucleotides strands, usually involving binding of oligonucleotide in the major groove of a DNA double helix. The binding can block access of transcription factors, thus, inhibiting transcription of a gene. Oligonucleotides can act as an antisense molecule (33) by inhibiting gene expression through binding to the mRNA counterpart via base pairing, thereby blocking the initiation codon, translational initiation, or resulting in degradation of mRNA by RNAse H (an enzyme that degrades the RNA portion of an RNA–DNA hybrid). Oligonucleotides can also bind to transcription factors, preventing association of the oligonucleotides with endogenous genes.

The major toxicity of oligonucleotides relates to the administration of large doses to achieve the clinical effect. Oligonucleotides are unlikely to have any long-term toxicity as they do not integrate into the chromosome. Their use for gene therapy will be probably limited to diseases where transient expression is sufficient. A potential problem of oligonucleotides may be the rapid degradation in vivo.

3. STRATEGIES TO IMPROVE VECTORS

3.1. Replicative Vector Systems

The major limitation of current gene therapy vectors is the suboptimal tumor transduction of therapeutic genes in vivo. One method to overcome this is to use a replication-competent virus that selectively replicates in tumor but not in normal tissues *(34)*. A replication-competent virus would be used to replicate selectively within infected tumor cells, leaving normal tissues unaffected. Production of progeny virions from the infected tumor cells would then result in infection of surrounding tumor cells. This would increase the number of cells infected with virus and markedly improve tumor transduction efficiency. In addition, the use of viruses that display a lytic life cycle would allow virus-mediated oncolysis. This effect would occur irrespective of the delivered transgene and amplification of the antitumor effect would be achieved. For clinical application of this strategy, both recombinant adenoviruses and herpesviruses have the potential to provide the required properties. Also, hybrid vectors (chimeras) that match elements of established vector systems are being developed.

Mutant adenoviruses have been designed to replicate selectively in cells lacking functional *p53*. E1B 55 kDa-deleted adenovirus, ONYX-015, has recently been shown to replicate selectively in, and lyse, tumor cells lacking functional *p53* both in vitro and in vivo *(35–37)*. The normal function of E1B protein is to bind and inactivate the p53 protein in infected cells. Because these modified viruses lack E1B, they cannot replicate in cells with functional *p53*, because it cannot activate *p53*. Instead, these viruses will replicate in cells with nonfunctional *p53*. Because *p53* is mutated in more than 50% of tumors, the replication of this lytic adenovirus would be selective in many tumors. Based on this concept, clinical trials using this virus are ongoing, and encouraging preliminary results have been obtained. However, studies in a variety of cell lines and animal tumor models have to date failed to confirm the selective properties of the virus to replicate only in *p53* mutant tumors *(38–39)*.

Herpesviruses have also been developed that replicate conditionally in dividing or tumor cells. This selectivity is based on several possible mutations engineered in the viral genome that prevent it from replicating unless the infected cell provides for a substituting molecular activity. Brain tumors, which are surrounded by nonmitotic cells, form an ideal model for testing replication-conditional herpes vectors. Clinical trials using adenovirus and herpesvirus-based replicative vector systems for the treatment of human cancer are ongoing.

3.2. Strategies to Prevent Immunogenicity of Vectors

Gene delivery via adenoviral vectors has been associated in vivo with the induction of characteristically intense inflammatory and immunological responses, and with attenuation of expression of the transferred therapeutic gene due, at least in part, to loss of the vector-transduced cells. To modulate the antiviral immune response recombinant viral vectors can be genetically engineered to delete viral genes encoding highly immunogenic or cytotoxic viral proteins. However, viral vectors with most of their genomes deleted are more difficult to propagate and purify, and transgene expression tends to be unstable. Alternatively, different serotypes and species of adenoviruses are being screened for their ability to elicit an immune response and to use selected adenovirus strains for vectors in order to minimize the stimulus for an immune response.

3.3. Selective and Efficient Gene Delivery

Any approach to cancer gene therapy requires a high level of efficiency of gene transfer specifically to the tumor cells. Viral vectors or retroviral vector-producing cells expressing a toxin gene have been directly injected into localized tumors. The presently available vectors are inadequate for the treatment of metastatic disease. In order to achieve gene delivery to disseminated cancer cells, the vector must be administered intravenously. Limitations of current vectors preclude genetic modification of a high percentage of cells in tumors and specificity of gene delivery to the tumor cells could overcome this limitation.

3.4. Tumor Targeting

Targeted gene therapy for cancer can be accomplished by delivery of a vector that binds selectively to the target cancer cell. Alternatively, the therapeutic gene can be placed under the control of tumor-specific transcriptional regulatory sequences that are activated in tumor cells but not in normal cells and, therefore, target expression selectively to the tumor cell.

Adenoviral vector modifications are being developed to achieve tumor targeting and enhance infectivity. Strategies to alter adenoviral tropism are based on modification of the viral capsid proteins, fiber and penton base, to allow the recognition of alternative cell-specific receptors (40). In contrast to adenoviruses, retroviruses use only one envelope glycoprotein for binding to cellular receptors and the subsequent step of membrane fusion. For this reason, modification of retroviral tropism has proven more difficult (41,42). The envelope protein of retroviral vectors has been modified to include various targeting ligands. For instance, various molecules, including single-chain antibodies, growth factors such as epidermal growth factor, and cytokines, have been genetically incorporated into the retroviral envelope glycoprotein, thus providing novel binding properties to the retroviral particles (43–49). However, the retroviral envelope protein is not only involved in the initial attachment to the cell membrane, but is also involved in production of infectious retroviral particles and in the virion cell fusion process. Therefore, modification of the retroviral envelope carries the risk of abrogating additional functions of successful targeted gene transfer.

3.5. Targeting by Use of Tissue-Specific Promoters

Tumor- or tissue-specific regulatory sequences, e.g., the CEA-, tyrosinase-, prostate-specific antigen (PSA), and α-fetoprotein promoter, have been employed to restrict expression of the transgene or prodrug-converting enzyme specifically to target cancer cells (50–52; see also subheading 4.2.). For example, targeting of adenoviral vector–expressing toxin genes under the control of the tumor-specific α-fetoprotein promoter have been employed in approaches to hepatocellular carcinoma (53), whereas the tyrosinase promotor may be used to target melanoma. A limitation of this approach may be that certain regulatory sequences are too large to be accommodated in currently used vectors.

4. APPROACHES TO GENE THERAPY

In cancer, approaches to gene therapy may include the insertion of a normal copy of a tumor supressor gene into tumors with mutated tumor suppressor genes or lost genes, the inhibition of a dominant oncogene, or down-regulation of an overexpressed growth factor receptor gene. Other strategies involve tumor modification with prodrug-activating enzyme genes, followed by treatment with prodrug (resulting in death of the transduced tumor cells, i.e., suicide), introduction of multidrug resistance genes into bone marrow or stem cells, and immunogene therapy utilizing gene-modified tumor cells as vaccines, or adoptive cellular therapy with gene-modified effector cells. Furthermore, antiangiogenic gene therapy strategies aiming at destruction of tumor vasculature are being currently explored.

4.1. Tumor Suppressor Gene Replacement and Inhibition of Dominant Oncogene Expression

Inactivation of tumor suppressor genes contributes to the neoplastic phenotype by abrogating critical cell cycle checkpoints, DNA repair mechanisms, and proapoptotic controls. Preclinical studies have demonstrated expression of the wild-type protein after gene delivery and reversion of the malignant phenotype. Mutations of several tumor suppressor genes have been described in human cancers. Normal *p53, RB1,* and *BRCA1* are currently being administered in clinical trials as gene replacement therapy for the corresponding mutated gene.

For dominant oncogenes, the goal of therapeutic intervention is to inhibit expression of the dominant oncogene that causes the malignant transformation. Inhibition of oncogenic function can be attempted at different levels. Transcription of the oncogene can be inhibited by triplex-forming oligonucleotides or specific antisense sequences preventing translation of the oncogene messenger RNA into protein or promoting degradation of the complementary message. Oligonucleotides are currently undergoing clinical evaluation.

Human tumors are often heterogeneous with regard to the expression of relevant oncogenes. Thus, therapeutic targeting of a single molecular abnormality may not be effective. Furthermore, corrective gene therapy requires extremely efficient gene transfer vectors to achieve permanent incorporation and expression of the gene of interest.

4.1.1. TUMOR SUPPRESSOR GENE REPLACEMENT OF *P53*

The *p53* gene is the most commonly mutated gene identified in human cancer to date. It is a tumor-suppressor gene that protects the cells from DNA damage by sensing the damage and either stopping cell division to allow for repair or inducing cell death (if damage is too extensive). Loss or damage of *p53* allows cells to accumulate extensive chromosomal damage. Most effort has been put into correcting the effects of *p53* mutations. Retroviral and adenoviral vectors have been used to carry wild-type *p53*. In vitro and experimental animal studies have shown that, following transduction and restoration of *p53* function, the malignant phenotype is reverted and tumor growth is suppressed. Also, restoration of wild-type *p53* function markedly increases the sensitivity to chemotherapeutic agents *(54)*.

4.2. Suicide Gene Therapy

Another approach to the treatment of localized cancer is suicide gene therapy. Suicide gene therapy concerns the transfer of a gene that is not normally expressed in mammalian cells and is directly toxic to the cell or that codes for an enzyme capable of activating an inactive prodrug to a potent cytotoxic drug. Commonly, a nontoxic pro-

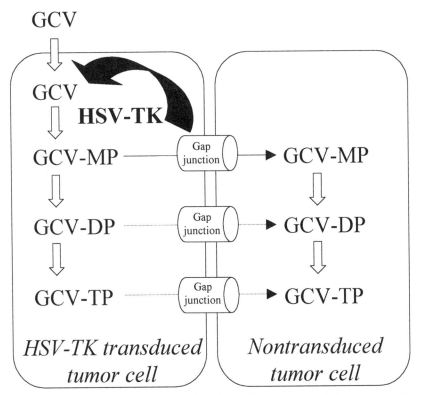

Fig. 1. Mode of action of the herpes simplex virus thymidine kinase ganciclovir system. Ganciclovir (GCV) diffuses into cells. In contrast to nontransduced cells, the transduced HSV-TK-expressing tumor cells are able to phosphorylate GCV efficiently. Phosphorylated GCV does not diffuse across cell membranes, but passes through gap junctions to adjacent tumor cells. This way, phosphorylated GCV is able to mediate the cytotoxic effect to untransduced adjacent cells. Monophosphate (MP); Diphosphate (DP); Triphosphate (TP).

drug is administered that requires activation in genetically modified cells in order to be transformed into a toxic metabolite that ultimately leads to cell death *(55–58)*.

The most widely used system to accomplish cell killing ("cell suicide") has been the herpes simplex virus thymidine kinase *(HSV-TK)* gene given in combination with the prodrug ganciclovir. In contrast to normal mammalian thymidine kinase, *HSV-TK* preferentially converts the normally nontoxic nucleoside analog ganciclovir (GCV) into a form toxic to the cell. Ganciclovir is then further phosphorylated by cellular kinases to produce triphosphates that are incorporated into cellular DNA (Fig. 1). The incorporation of the triphosphate form of ganciclovir causes inhibition of DNA synthesis and of RNA polymerase, leading to cell death. Thus, tumor cells (or any other cell undergoing mitosis) transduced to express the viral thymidine kinase gene have enhanced sensitivity to cell killing after exposure to ganciclovir. Because the *HSV-TK* GCV regimen is most effective against cells in the S-phase, repeated gene therapy cycles may be more effective (similar to chemotherapy cycles). The toxicity and efficacy of the transfer of *HSV-TK* are currently being tested in a large number of human clinical trials, including tumors of the brain, ovary, prostate, and head and neck.

One limitation is the inability to genetically modify 100% of the tumor cells with the toxin gene. In a number of experimental tumor models, it has been shown that not all tumor cells need to contain the *HSV-TK* gene to obtain complete eradication of the tumor. It has been demonstrated that the efficacy of the *HSV-TK*-ganciclovir approach was mediated in part by the so-called bystander effect *(59–61)*. This "bystander effect" seen in suicide gene therapy indicates that not all tumor cells in a solid tumor need to be transduced to achieve efficient killing. Nontransduced *HSV-TK*-negative tumor cells surrounding *HSV-TK*-positive tumor cells can still be killed because of transfer of toxic metabolites from transduced cells to nontransduced cells through gap junctions (Fig. 1). This bystander effect can also be produced by the generation of an immunostimulatory environment in vivo that enhances immune responses against tumors *(62)*.

Several other combinations of enzyme/prodrug have been developed to improve the efficacy of suicide gene therapy *(63–66)*. For example, the gene encoding for the *Escherichia coli* cytosine deaminase enzyme, which converts the nontoxic 5-fluorocytosine prodrug into cytotoxic 5-fluorouracil.

To enhance the therapeutic efficacy of suicide gene therapy the development of new prodrugs with higher affinity for the suicide gene are being explored. Also, combination with other treatment modalities such as chemotherapy and radiotherapy may enhance efficacy of the treatment.

4.3. Immunogene Therapy

One attractive approach to the treatment of disseminated cancer is to enhance the immunogenicity of tumor cells, thus allowing systemic immune-mediated tumor cell kill. Several experimental animal studies have shown that immunization with tumor cells engineered to produce IL-2 or other cytokines, e.g., IL-4, IL-7, IFN-γ, TNF-α, G-CSF, GM-CSF, results in enhanced immunogenicity and decreased tumorigenicity *(67–77)*. Most of these reports indicate that this approach is highly effective to protect animals from subsequent tumorigenic doses of nonmodified tumor cells, whereas few studies indicate that this approach is also effective in eradication of already established tumors *(73,77)*. Similar strong antitumor responses were obtained following vaccination with tumor cells engineered to express foreign MHC genes class I or II or the B7 (costimulatory molecule) cDNA *(78–83)*. The repertoire of effector cells that mediate the observed reduced tumor regression in these animal studies may differ depending on the molecule introduced and have included CD4+ and CD8+ T cells, macrophages, and eosinophils.

The advantage of a genetically modified autologous cell vaccine is that it contains the whole collection of tumor proteins and therefore has the greatest chance to induce an immune response against relevant tumor antigens. However, growing autologous tumor cells in vitro to establish tumor cell lines is labor-intensive and often not successful. Following administration, allogeneic tumor cells that share an HLA class I allele, may in vivo either directly present shared immunodominant tumor peptides to class I restricted CTLs or may first be degraded and processed by professional antigen-presenting cells (APCs). These APCs will process and select the appropriate epitopes, which will enter the class II or even the class I route to stimulate the patient's CD4+ or CD8+ T cells.

Another approach to gene therapy of cancer is the genetic modification of immune effector cells, e.g., blood T lymphocytes or tumor-infiltrating lymphocytes (TILs). The first gene-marking study already demonstrated that such tumor-derived T lymphocytes may home to metastatic melanoma deposits. In subsequent therapeutic studies, T lymphocytes expressing cytokines following transduction, were reinfused into patients. As the systemic administration of TNF has significant side effects, attempts to genetically alter T lymphocytes to deliver high concentrations of TNF directly to the tumor have been made. Also, several groups are now working on gene modified T cells to express tumor-specific TCRs to obtain a more universally applicable product for adoptive cellular immunotherapy.

Genetically modified lymphocytes that are transduced with (retroviral) vectors containing the *HSV-TK* gene can be infused into the patient to decrease morbidity and mortality associated with GVHD following allogeneic bone marrow and stem cell transplantation. Bordignon et al. *(84)* have demonstrated that adoptive cellular immunotherapy with such gene-modified lymphocytes is feasible. Transduced cells were present up to 12 mo after infusion and in the two patients who developed GVHD, transduced cells were eliminated following ganciclovir administration, resulting in regression of hepatic and cutaneous GVHD. Similar protocols to treat GVHD in transplantation patients have been developed.

4.4. Bone Marrow Protection from Chemotherapy

Gene therapy can be used to protect against hematological toxicity produced by chemotherapy used for the treatment of cancer patients. This approach of gene therapy may be accomplished by the insertion of the multiple-drug-resistance type 1 *(MDR-1)* gene into stem cells of bone marrow, thus allowing the administration of higher drug doses without reaching an otherwise limiting myelosuppression *(85–87)*. The use of the MDR gene is of interest because the gene product, a transmembrane molecule that serves as an efflux pump for various drugs, confers resistance to several commonly used chemotherapeutic agents. At present, the low transduction efficiency of the target human hematopoietic cells with retrovirus vectors, the dose-limiting effects determined by other nonhematological toxicities, inadvertent transduction of contaminating cancer cells in the marrow with the drug-resistance gene which could rapidly give rise to clones of treatment-resistant tumor cells, are major limiting factors precluding clinical success. Therefore, autologous peripheral stem cell transplantation provides a more practical solution to support high-dose chemotherapy trials.

4.5. Antiangiogenic Gene Therapy of Cancer

Targeting of tumor vasculature is rapidly developing as a field of research. Tumors are dependent for their growth on the development of a blood vessel network and may trigger angiogenesis by release of specific growth factors such as vascular endothelial growth factor (VEGF). The tumor vasculature is pivotal for the survival of the tumor cells, suggesting that strategies that can compromise the function of the tumor vasculature may have therapeutic potential *(88–92)*. Because vascular endothelial cells are in direct contact with the blood, they are likely to be easier to transduce with systematically administered vectors than tumor cells because the diffusion of vector into the tumor stroma will not be an issue. Moreover, as limited destruction of tumor-associated vasculature may result in massive tumor cell death, even relatively modest gene transfer efficiencies may well have a dramatic effect on tumor growth *(93,94)*. Numerous genes, induced at the sites of angiogenesis, are candidates for use in cancer gene therapy, e.g., the *(flk-1* and *flt-1)* VEGF receptor genes, VEGF itself, angiostatin, thrombospondin, and platelet factor 4 *(95–104)*.

The enhanced proliferation of tumor-associated endothelial cells allows the use of retroviral vectors for this purpose. There is evidence that ganciclovir-mediated antitumor activity observed in experimental brain tumor models following the administration of retroviral packaging cell lines encoding HSV-TK can be attributed to transduction of proliferating tumor-associated vascular endothelial cells.

5. APPROVAL FROM REGULATORY AUTHORITIES TO INITIATE GENE THERAPY TRIALS

The first gene therapy protocol was a gene-marking study using retrovirally transduced tumor-infiltrating lymphocytes (TILs) marked with the neomycin-resistance gene that were infused into metastatic melanoma patients *(105)*. The protocol received NIH Recombinant DNA Advisory Committee (RAC) approval in October 1988 and NIH approval in March 1989. Thereafter, the first gene therapy study was performed in children suffering from SCID, who received retrovirally transduced autologous lymphocytes now expressing the normal ADA gene *(106)*.

The first human gene marking was approved and conducted in the United States, and a series of marrow gene-marking studies followed. The aim of these marking studies was insertion of marker genes using retroviral vectors into the bone marrow of leukemia patients in remission and undergoing autologous, purged bone marrow transplantation. These first studies have identified leukemic relapses that occurred from the gene-marked marrow, although there was no evidence of leukemic cells in the infused marrow at the time of transplantation. Apparently, marrow-purging techniques were not optimal. For these studies retroviral vectors were used that apparently inserted into dividing tumor cells and thereafter—in vivo—the gene was passed to all daughter tumor cells.

Subsequent to the first gene-marking and gene-therapy studies, several gene therapy protocols have been initiated worldwide. The number of gene protocols in the United States received by the Office of Recombinant DNA Activities (ORDA) as of May 1999 was 313 cell-marking studies and 277 therapeutic studies. Of these protocols, 189 protocols concerned cancer therapy.

In the United States, a detailed clinical protocol plus investigator brochure has to be approved by one or more institutional review boards, biosafety committees, the RAC and the Food and Drug Administration (FDA). Compliance with the NIH guidelines for research involving recombinant DNA research is mandatory. Protocols involving human gene transfer are required to be simultaneously submitted to the FDA for Investigational New Drug (IND). Despite intended harmonization, the routing to apply for a permit to perform a clinical gene therapy trial and the number of committees that have to approve still varies from country to country in Europe. The complicated routes necessary to obtain approval from the regulatory authorities are often cumbersome and time consuming for the investigator, whereas the tremendous costs of manufacturing of GMP-approved products for gene-therapy studies preclude rapid progress in the field of gene therapy.

6. CLINICAL TRIALS

6.1. Brain Tumors

Astroglial brain tumors, including the highly malignant glioblastoma multiforme, are the most common primary brain tumors. They have a poor prognosis despite conventional therapy such as surgery and radiotherapy and, therefore, present a target for gene therapy. Brain tumors in general do not metastasize; death usually results from increase in intracerebral pressure. Therefore, local therapy is required and as the patient's brain cells do not divide while the tumor cells are mitotically active, brain tumors are an attractive target for suicide gene therapy as this method will be cytotoxic only to dividing cells.

Retroviral vectors that selectively infect dividing (tumor) cells in the central nervous system are attractive vectors to use in the treatment of brain tumors. However, a major obstacle to the present direct gene therapy is the inability to transduce the majority of cells within the tumor. Furthermore, although theoretically retroviral vectors seem advantageous in brain tumors, even in the most malignant brain tumors the percentage of actively dividing tumor cells is low, precluding 100% transduction efficiency. For this reason, other vectors such as adenoviral vectors may be as efficient as retroviral vectors.

In an early clinical trial, an *HSV-TK* vector-producing murine cell line was injected via an Ommaya reservoir after debulking of recurrent glioblastoma tumor(s), followed 2 wk later by administration of ganciclovir, or was injected following resection of the tumor *(107)*. A large multicenter Phase III study was performed in which patients were randomized to receive surgery plus radiotherapy or surgery, retroviral vector-producing cell-*HSV-TK* suicide gene therapy, and radiotherapy. No significant difference was observed between the two arms of the study. Recently, Ram et al. *(108)* have reported the results of an *HSV-TK* clinical trial in patients with brain tumors. Clinical remissions were obtained in five patients with smaller tumors (1.4 ± 0.5 mL). *In situ* hybridization for *HSV-TK* demonstrated survival of vector-producing cells at 7 d, but indicated limited gene transfer to tumors, suggesting that indirect "bystander" mechanisms provide local antitumor activity.

6.2. Head-and-Neck Cancer

Thirty end-stage patients who had failed conventional treatments for advanced recurrent squamous carcinoma of the head and neck were enrolled in a dose escalation trial *(109);* each of the 30 patients was injected with *Adp53* vector. Seventeen nonresectable patients underwent *Ad-p53* intratumoral injections every other day for 2 wk, were observed for 2 wk, and then repeated the treatment cycle. The remaining 13 patients with resectable tumors received *Ad-p53* every other day for 2 wk, had intraoperative injections 3 d later, during resection, and a last injection 3 d postresection. Vector-related toxicity was minimal. No adverse side effects attributable to the *p53* gene were observed in any of the 30 patients. The 17 nonresectable patients continued treatment cycles until progression. Five of the 17 patients had stable disease and two exhibited partial regression (> 50% reduction in tumor volume). At the time of the report, three of the 13 resectable patients had died of cancer and five displayed a total disappearance of all measurable signs of cancer for more than 6 mo posttherapy. At the time of surgery, one patient demonstrated a complete pathological response to *Ad-p53*.

Clinical trials using selectively replicating E1B-deleted adenoviral vectors such as ONYX-015 virus to target *p53*-deficient tumors seem to be encouraging. In a Phase II trial in 40 patients with recurrent head-and-neck cancer, ONYX-015 was directly injected into the tumor. No serious toxicity was demonstrated. Evidence of antitumor activity was found as 14% of patients had partial to complete regression and 41% had stable disease *(110)*.

6.3. Lung Cancer

The most widely used vector in lung gene therapy has been replication-incompetent recombinant adenovirus. Disadvantages of adenoviruses are that they result in only transient gene expression and that they elicit a prominent local and systemic inflammatory response. This inflammatory response, which initially involves cytokine release and subsequently results in the generation of neutralizing antiadenoviral antibodies and cytotoxic T lymphocytes, has been the primary source of adenoviral vector toxicity and has limited the amount of vector that can be delivered.

One of the most common genetic abnormalities in nonsmall-cell lung cancer is mutation of the tumor suppressor gene *p53*. Phase I clinical trials in humans using gene transfer of *p53* have been reported. Viral vectors encoding wild-type *p53* were injected into the tumors of patients with nonsmall-cell lung cancer by means of a bronchoscope or percutaneous computed tomography (CT) guided needles. In the first trial, a retroviral vector was used in nine patients who failed conventional treatment *(111)*. The treatments were well tolerated, with minimal side effects. Some evidence of gene transfer was noted in patients given higher doses (highest dose 5×10^8 CFU). Three patients showed evidence of regression of the injected tumors and the tumor growth of three other patients stabilized. No effects on noninjected tumors were noted.

Swisher et al. *(112)* used up to six monthly intratumoral injections of an adenovirus *p53* vector in conjunction with administration of cisplatin in 28 patients. No dose-limiting toxicity was observed and treatment was well tolerated. Although the repeated administration of the adenoviral vector induced antiadenoviral antibodies, gene transfer was detected in these patients. Apoptosis and areas of tumor necrosis were observed following treatment. No change was observed in inflammatory cells infiltrating the tumor. Therapeutic activity was observed in some patients, including two (8%) of the 25 evaluable patients showing a partial remission and 16 (84%) showing stabilization of disease.

Sterman et al. *(113)* conducted a Phase I clinical trial of adenoviral vector encoding *HSV-TK* that was delivered intrapleurally to 21 patients with pleural mesothelioma followed by ganciclovir therapy. Side effects were minimal and dose-related gene transfer was confirmed in 11 of 20 evaluable patients. However, strong antiadenoviral immune responses, including high titres of neutralizing antibody and proliferative T-cell responses, were induced by the administration of the adenoviral vector. Patients who received the higher doses of vector partial tumor regressions were observed. Transduction efficiency in mesothelioma may improve by multiple administrations of vector in combination with surgical tumor debulking.

6.4. Hematological Malignancies

BCL-2 antisense therapy was explored in patients with non-Hodgkin lymphoma *(114)*. Daily subcutaneous (sc) infusions were administered for 2 wk to nine patients with *BCL-2*+ relapsed non-Hodgkin lymphoma. Antisense therapy led to an improvement in symptoms, objective biochemical and radiological evidence of tumor response, and downregulation of the BCL-2 protein in some patients.

In a Phase I study, *p53* antisense oligonucleotide was administered to 16 patients with hematological malignancies (six with refractory acute myelogenous leukemia and 10 with advanced myelodysplastic syndrome). No specific toxicity was related to the *p53* oligonucleotide administration *(115)*.

6.5. Melanoma

Thirty-one metastatic melanoma patients received three injections of a IL-2 gene modified, allogeneic melanoma cell line, which shared one or more HLA class I alleles with the patient, and expressed all of the known melanoma antigens identified at that time. Patients were evaluated for toxicity and antitumor efficacy *(116)*. No severe side effects were observed. Interestingly, vaccination induced inflammatory reactions in distant metastases containing necrosis and apoptosis, along with T-cell infiltration. Apoptosis occurred only in *BCL*-2 negative areas, but not in *BCL*-2 expressing parts of the metastases. One complete remission lasting for more than 1 yr, one almost complete remission, and several minor responses were observed following administration of the gene-modified melanoma cells. Seven of the 33 patients had disease stabilization for a period of several months to more than 4 yr. Vaccination induced a change in the number of antivaccine cytotoxic T lymphocytes in peripheral blood. In two of five patients, the frequency of antiautologous tumor CTL was significantly higher than before vaccination. In some of the other reported human gene therapy trials employing a similar approach with either allogeneic or autologous tumor cells engineered to express costimulatory molecules or to secrete cytokines for the treatment of patients with cancer *(117–119)*, enhancement of the immune response against the autologous tumor of the patients was shown. Metastatic lesions resected after vaccination with GM-CSF gene-modified autologous melanoma cells were shown to be densely infiltrated with lymphocytes and plasma cells, and showed extensive tumor destruction *(118)*.

Another approach is to enhance the anti-tumor immune response by in vivo injection of a foreign *HLA* class I gene, i.e., *HLA* B7, by DNA liposome complexes directly into tumor deposits. Nabel et al. *(120)* showed that following the direct injection of a gene coding for (allogeneic) HLA-B7 protein into cutaneous melanoma metastases, HLA-B7 protein was expressed in the tumor cells near the site of injection and its corresponding transferred plasmid DNA (detected by PCR). No systemic toxicity was observed and regression of a distant lung metastasis occurred in one of the five reported patients. In all five patients, antitumor (autologous) and anti-HLA-B7 (allogeneic) cytotoxic lymphocyte immune responses were detected. In one patient, two injected nodules regressed completely, as well as other distant noninjected metastatic lung lesions. In an update on 10 patients, Nabel et al. *(121)* reported that T-cell migration into treated lesions was enhanced in the majority of patients and tumor-infiltrating frequency of lymphocyte reactivity was enhanced in the two patients studied. In one patient, subsequent treatment with tumor-infiltrating lymphocytes derived from gene-modified tumors resulted in a complete regression of the residual disease. On the basis of this study, other Phase I *HLA*-B7 gene therapy clinical trials were initiated using *HLA*-B7 DNA-cationic lipid vector in *HLA*-B7-negative patients with melanoma *(122)*, renal cell carcinoma, and colon carcinoma. In most posttreatment biopsies, the plasmid DNA and *HLA*-B7 protein could be detected. Moreover, most patients developed a lymphocyte-proliferative response to *HLA*-B7, indicating that immunization against the foreign HLA protein was successful. Clinical responses were seen in metastatic melanoma patients.

A Phase I study was conducted in patients with accessible *p*53-aberrant breast or melanoma skin lesions *(123)*. Following intratumoral injection of adenoviral wild-type *p*53, vector-specific wild-type *p*53 RNA sequences could be detected after the lowest and highest dose of viral particles in five of the six patients (dose range 2×10^7 to $5 \times$

10^8 pfu per patient). Immune responses to the adenoviral component of the vector, indicating effective biological delivery of the vector, were also documented.

6.6. Ovarian Cancer

A Phase I trial using the *BRCA1* breast cancer gene in chemoresistant recurrent or persistent ovarian cancer, patients received daily intraabdominal infusions of *BRCA1* retroviral vectors through a catheter for four consecutive days *(124)*. Side effects were minimal. Three of twelve patients experienced an immune reaction resulting in severe but transient abdominal pain. The *BRCA1* gene and its expression were detected in cancer cells. Tumor reduction was observed in three of 12 patients. In a subsequent Phase II study in which ovarian cancer patients with less-extensive disease received vector infusions via surgically implanted catheters, vector instability, rapid antibody development, but no clinical responses, were observed *(125)*.

6.7. Prostate Cancer

Prostate cancer is particularly suitable to study the use of gene therapy. Prostate cancer is the most common cancer and the second leading cause of death in males. The prostate gland produces products such as PSA and prostate acid phosphatase that are relatively unique to the prostate. Each protein may be exploited for vector targeting or vaccine immunization. Gene expression can be confined to the prostate by incorporating prostate-specific promoters into vectors to direct the prostate-specific expression of the gene of interest. Also, the prostate is an ideal target for gene therapy because it is easily accessible by transurethral, transperineal, and transrectal approaches for the intratumoral administration of gene therapy, and the effects of treatment can be easily evaluated by ultrasound, digital rectal examination, MRI, and CT scan. Because prostate cancer has generally a low proliferation index, (retroviral) vectors that require cell division are not suitable for the treatment of prostate cancer.

Various ongoing clinical trials are investigating the effects of suicide gene therapy in recurrent prostate cancer or as neoadjuvant treatment before cytoreductive surgery. In contrast to, for instance, brain tumors, there is no need to distinguish normal prostate tissue from cancerous prostate tissue, because the prostate gland does not have a critical function. Herman et al. *(126)* reported a Phase I dose-escalating study in which they injected increasing concentrations of replication-deficient adenovirus containing *HSV-TK* intraprostatic under ultrasound guidance. In three of the 18 patients treated, a fall of more than 50% in PSA, sustained for 6 wk to 1 yr, was observed. Other trials include vaccination with gene-modified prostate cancer cells secreting cytokines such as IL-2 or IL-12, aiming at an immunological response against the patient's own tumor.

7. CONCLUSION

Although the field of gene therapy is still in its infancy, genes have been safely and successfully transferred into animals and patients. Until now, early Phase I and II clinical gene therapy trials have been conducted often at submaximal doses in a limited number of cancer patients who generally had large tumor burdens. Further technological advances are required to improve inefficient and transient gene delivery and inappropriate regulation of gene expression before successful gene therapy can become a reality. The major challenge is posed by inefficient gene delivery. Even more important will be optimization of existing vectors (such as "gutless" adenoviral vectors that express no endogenous viral genes, or improved liposomal preparations) or development of new vectors that induce minimal inflammatory responses and permit repeated administration. Improved vectors will have enhanced specificity for a single target cell type. By employing genetic methods viral vectors can be engineered to redirect the tropism of viral vectors away from the natural cellular receptor and toward surface proteins that are highly expressed on target cells.

Another approach in cancer gene therapy may be the development of replicating viral vectors that can kill tumors by primary viral lysis or enhanced delivery of therapeutic genes to cancer cells. Some tumor cell specificity has been achieved with replicating vectors. Clinical trials currently underway are using modified adenoviruses that lack the *E1B* gene (a deletion that allows the virus to replicate selectively in tumor cells) or have tumor-selective promoters driving key viral genes, such as *E1A*.

Significant barriers to the success of gene therapy in cancer remain the insufficient efficiency and accuracy of gene delivery. The identification of genes and the unraveling of the human genome is occurring much faster than the development of in vivo gene delivery methods. Therefore, further technical advances to optimize gene delivery and regulation of gene expression are critically needed before gene therapy can be widely and successfully applied in the 21st century.

REFERENCES

1. Anderson WF. Human gene therapy. *Science* 1992; 256:808–813.
2. Eglitis MA, Kantoff P, Gilboa E, Anderson WF. Gene expression in mice after high efficiency retroviral-mediated gene transfer. *Science* 1985; 230:1395–1398.
3. Engelhardt JF, Ye X, Doranz B, Wilson JM. Ablation of EA2 in recombinant retroviruses improves transgene persistence and decreases inflammatory response in mouse liver. *Proc Natl Acad Sci USA* 1994; 91:6196–6200.
4. Miller DG, Adam MA, Miller AD. Gene transfer by retrovirus vectors occurs only in cells that are actively replicating at time of infection. *Mol Cell Biol* 1990; 10:4239–4242.
5. Takeuchi Y, Cosset FL, Lachmann PJ, Okada H, Weiss RA, Collins MKL. Type C retrovirus inactivation by human complement is determined by both the viral genome and producer cell. *J Virol* 1993; 68:8001–8007.
6. Naldini L, Blömer U, Gage FH, Trono D, Verma IM. Efficient transfer, integration, and sustained long term expression of the transgene in adult rat brains injected with a lentiviral vector. *Proc Natl Acad Sci USA* 1996; 93:11,382–11,388.
7. Naldini L, Blömer U, Gallay P, et al. In vivo gene delivery and stable transduction of nondividing cells by a lentiviral vector. *Science* 1996; 272:263–267.
8. Miyoshi H, Blomer U, Takahashi M, Gage FH, Verma IM. Development of a self-inactivating lentivirus vector. *J Virol* 1998; 72:8150–8157.
9. Zufferey R, Dull T, Mandel RJ, et al. Self-inactivating lentivirus vector for safe and efficient in vivo gene delivery. *J Virol* 1998; 72:9873–9880.
10. Jaffe HA, Danel C, Longenecker G, et al. Stratford-Perricaudet LD, Perricaudet M, Pavirani A, Lecocq J-P, Crystal RG. Adenovirus-mediated in vivo gene transfer and expression in normal rat liver. *Nat Genet* 1992; 1:372–378.
11. Yeh P, Perricaudet M. Advances in adenoviral vectors: from genetic engineering to their biology. *FASEB J* 1997; 11:615–623.
12. Zhang WW. Development and application of adenoviral vectors for gene therapy of cancer. *Cancer Gene Ther* 1999; 6:113–138.
13. Schiedner G, Morral N, Parks RJ, et al. Genomic DNA transfer with a high-capacity adenovirus vector results in improved in vivo gene expression and decreased toxicity. *Nat Genet* 1998; 18:180–183.
14. Bergelson JM, Cunningham JA, Droguett G, et al. Isolation of a common receptor for Coxsackie B viruses and adenoviruses 2 and 5. *Science* 1997; 275:1320–1323.

15. Tomko RP, Xu R, Philipso L. HCAR and MCAR: the human and mouse cellular receptors for subgroup C adenoviruses and group B coxsackieviruses. *Proc Nat Acad Sci USA* 1997; 94:3352–3356.
16. Dmitriev I, Krasnykh V, Miller CR, et al. An adenovirus vector with genetically modified fibers demonstrates expanded tropism via utilization of a coxsackievirus and adenovirus receptor-independent cell entry mechanism. *J Virol* 1998; 72:9706–9713.
17. Henry LJ, Xia D, Wilke ME, Deisenhofer J, Gerard RD, Characterization of the knob domain of the adenovirus type 5 fiber protein expressed in Escherichia coli. *J Virol* 1994; 68:5239–5246.
18. Louis N, Fender P, Barge A, Kitts P, Chroboczek J. Cell-binding domain of adenovirus serotype 2 fiber. *J Virol* 1994; 68:4104–4106.
19. Wickham TJ, Mathias P, Cheresh DA, Nemerow GR. Integrins alpha v beta 3 and alpha v beta 5 promote adenovirus internalization but not virus attachment. *Cell* 1993; 73:309–319.
20. Bai M, Harfe B, Freimuth P. Mutations that alter an Arg-Gly-Asp (RGD) sequence in the adenovirus type 2 penton base protein abolish its cell-rounding activity and delay virus reproduction in flat cells. *J Virol* 1993; 67:5198–5205.
21. Yang Y, Nunes FA, Berencsi K, Furth EE, Gönczöl E, Wilson JM. Cellular immunity to viral antigens limits E1-deleted adenoviruses for gene therapy. *Proc Natl Acad Sci USA* 1994; 91:4407–4411.
22. Worgall S, Wolff G, Falck-Pedersen E, Crystal RG. Innate immune mechanisms dominate elimination of adenoviral vectors following in vivo administration. *Hum Gene Ther* 1997; 8:37–44.
23. Wold WS, Doronin K, Toth K, Kuppuswamy M, Lichtenstein DL, Tollefson AE. Immune responses to adenoviruses: viral evasion mechanisms and their implications for the clinic. *Curr Opin Immunol* 1999; 11:380–386.
24. Gahéry-Segard H, Farace F, Godfrin D, et al. Immune response to recombinant capsid proteins of adenovirus in humans: antifiber and anti-penton base antibodies have a synergistic effect on neutralizing activity. *J Virol* 1998; 72:2388–2397.
25. Worgall S, Wolff G, Falck-Pedersen E, Crystal RG. Innate immune mechanisms dominate elimination of adenoviral vectors following in vivo administration. *Human Gene Ther* 1997; 8:37–44.
26. Chen H, Mack LM, Kelly R, Ontell M, Kochanek S, Clemens PR. Persistence in muscle of an adenoviral vector that lacks all viral genes. *Proc Natl Acad Sci USA* 1997; 94:1645–1650.
27. Fallaux FJ, Bout A, van der Velde I, et al. New helper cells and matched early region 1-deleted adenovirus vectors prevent generation of replication-competent adenoviruses. *Human Gene Ther* 1998; 9:1909–1917.
28. Halbert CL, Alexander IE, Wolgamot GM, Miller AD. Adeno-associated virus vectors transduce primary cells much less efficiently than immortalized cells. *J Virol* 1995; 69:1473–1479.
29. Ferrari FK, Samulski T, Shenk T, Samulski RJ. Second-strand synthesis is a rate-limiting step for efficient transduction by recombinant adeno-associated virus vectors. *J Virol* 1996; 70:3227–3234.
30. Ferrari FK, Xiao X, McCarty D, Samulski RJ. New developments in the generation of Ad-free, high-titer rAAV gene therapy vectors. *Nat Med* 1997; 3:1295–1297.
31. Scheule RK, St George JA, Bagley RG, et al. Basis of pulmonary toxicity associated with cationic lipid-mediated gene transfer to the mammalian lung. *Hum Gene Ther* 1997; 8:686–707.
32. Yew NS, Wang KX, Przybylska M, et al. Contribution of plasmid DNA to inflammation in the lung after administration of cationic lipid:pDNA complexes. *Hum Gene Ther* 1999; 10:223–234.
33. Mukhopadhyay T, Tainsky M, Cavender AC, Roth JA. Specific inhibition of K-ras expression and tumorigenicity of lung cancer cells by antisense RNA. *Cancer Res* 1991; 51:1744–1748.
34. Russell SJ. Replicating vectors for gene therapy of cancer: risks, limitations and prospects. *Eur J Cancer* 1994; 30A:1165–1171.
35. Bischoff JR, Kirn DH, Williams A, et al. An adenovirus mutant that replicates selectively in p53-deficient human tumor cells. *Science* 1996; 274:373–376.
36. Rodriguez R, Schuur ER, Lim HY, Henderson GA, Simons JW, Henderson DR. Prostate attenuated replication competent adenovirus (ARCA) CN706: a selective cytotoxic for prostate-specific antigen-positive prostate cancer cells. *Cancer Res* 1997; 57:2559–2563.
37. Heise C, Sampson-Johannes A, Williams A, McCormick F, Von Hoff DD, Kirn DH. ONYX-015, an E1B gene-attenuated adenovirus, causes tumor-specific cytolysis and antitumoral efficacy that can be augmented by standard chemotherapeutic agents. *Nat Med* 1997; 3:639–645.
38. Rothmann T, Hengstermann A, Whitaker NJ, Scheffner M, zur Hausen H. Replication of ONYX-015, a potential anticancer adenovirus, is independent of p53 status in tumor cells. *J Virol* 1998; 72:9470–9478.
39. Goodrum FD, Ornelles DA. p53 status does not determine outcome of E1B 55-kilodalton mutant adenovirus lytic infection. *J Virol* 1998; 72:9479–9490.

40. Douglas JT, Rogers BE, Rosenfeld ME, Michael SI, Feng M, Curiel DT. Targeted gene delivery by tropism-modified adenoviral vectors. *Nature Biotechnol* 1996; 14:1574–1578.
41. Kasahara N, Dozy AM, Kan YW. Tissue-specific targeting of retroviral vectors through ligand-receptor interaction. *Science* 1994; 266:1373–1376.
42. Cosset F-L, Russell SJ. Targeting retrovirus entry. *Gene Ther* 1996; 3:946–956.
43. Somia NV, Zoppe M, Verma IM. Generation of targeted retroviral vectors by using single-chain variable fragment: an approach to in vivo gene delivery. *Proc Natl Acad Sci USA* 1995; 92:7570–7574.
44. Chu TT-H, Martinez I, Sheary WC, Dornburg R. Cell targeting with retroviral vector particles containing antibody-envelope fusion proteins. *Gene Ther* 1994; 1:292–299.
45. Cosset F-L, Morling FJ, Takeuchi Y, Weiss RA, Collins MKL, Russell SJ. Retroviral retargeting by envelopes expressing an N-terminal binding domain. *J Virol* 1995; 69:6314–6322.
46. Valsesia-Wittmann S, Morling FJ, Nilson BH, Takeuchi Y, Russel SJ, Cosset FL. Improvement of retroviral retargeting by using amino acid spacers between an additional binding domain and the N terminus of Moloney murine leukemia virus SU. *J Virol* 1996; 70:2059–2064.
47. Chu TT-H, Dornburg R. Retroviral vector particles displaying the antigen-binding site of an antibody enable cell-type-specific gene transfer. *J Virol* 1995; 69:2659–2663.
48. Schnierle BS, Moritz D, Jeschke M, Groner B. Expression of chimeric envelope proteins in helper cell lines and integration into Moloney murine leukemia virus particles. *Gene Ther* 1996; 3:334–342.
49. Valsesia-Wittmann S, Drynda A, Deleage G, et al. Modifications in the binding domain of avian retrovirus envelope protein to redirect the host range of retroviral vectors. *J Virol* 1994; 68:4609–4619.
50. Vile RG, Diaz RM, Miller N, Mitchell S, Russell SJ. Tissue-specific gene expression from Mo-MLV retroviral vectors with hybrid LTRs containing the murine tyrosinase enhancer/promoter. *Virology* 1995; 214:307–313.
51. Chen L, Chen D, Manome Y, Dong Y, Fine HA, Kufe DW. Breast cancer selective gene expression and therapy mediated by recombinant adenoviruses containing the DF3/MUC1 promoter. *J Clin Invest* 1995; 96:2775–2782.
52. Lee C-H, Liu M, Sie KL, Lee M-S. Prostate-specific antigen promoter driven gene therapy targeting DNA polymerase-a and topoisomerase IIa in prostate cancer. *Anticancer Res* 1996; 16:1805–1812.
53. Su H, Chang JC, Xu SM, Kan YW. Selective killing of AFP-positive hepatocellular carcinoma cells by adeno-associated virus transfer of the herpes simplex virus thymidine kinase gene. *Human Gene Ther* 1996; 74:463–470.
54. Fujiwara T, Grimm EA, Mukhopadhyay T, Zhang WW, Owen-Schaub LB, Roth JA. Induction of chemosensitivity in human lung cancer cells in vivo by adenovirus-mediated transfer of the wild-type p53 gene. *Cancer Res* 1994; 54:2287–2291.
55. Moolten FL. Drug sensitivity ("suicide") genes for selective cancer therapy. *Cancer Gene Ther* 1994; 1:279–287.
56. Takamiya Y, Short MP, Ezzeddine ZD, Moolten FL, Breakefield XO, Martuza RL. Gene therapy of malignant brain tumors: a rat glioma line bearing the herpes simplex virus type 1-thymidine kinase gene and wild type retrovirus kills other tumor cells. *J Neurosciences Res* 1992; 33:493–503.
57. Rosenfeld ME, Feng M, Michael SI, Siegal GP, Alvarez RD, Curiel DT. Adenoviral-mediated delivery of the herpes simplex virus thymidine kinase gene selectively sensitizes human ovarian carcinoma cells to ganciclovir. *Clin Cancer Res* 1995; 1:1571–1580.
58. Yee D, McGuire SE, Brunner N, et al. Adenovirus-mediated gene transfer of herpes simplex virus thymidine kinase in an ascites model of human breast cancer. *Human Gene Ther* 1996; 7:1251–1257.
59. Freeman SM, Abboud CN, Whartenby KA, et al. The bystander effect: tumor regression when a fraction of the tumor mass is genetically modified. *Cancer Res* 1993; 3:5274–5283.
60. Elshami AA, Saavedra A, Zhang H, et al. Gap junctions play a role in the "bystander effect" of the Herpes Simplex virus thymidine kinase/ganciclovir system in vitro. *Gene Ther* 1996; 3:85–92.
61. Pope IM, Poston GJ, Kinsella AR. The role of the bystander effect in suicide gene therapy. *Eur J Cancer* 1997; 33:1005–1016.
62. Freeman SM, Ramesh R, Marrogi AJ. Immune system in suicide-gene therapy. *Lancet* 1997; 349:2–3.
63. Aghi M, Kramm CM, Chou TC, Breakefield XO, Chiocca EA. Synergistic anticancer effects of ganciclovir/thymidine kinase and 5-fluorocytosine/cytosine deaminase gene therapies. *J Nat Cancer Inst* 1998; 90:370–380.
64. Bridgewater JA, Springer CJ, Knox RJ, Minton NP, Michael NP, Collins MK. Expression of the bacterial nitroreductase enzyme in mammalian cells renders them sensitive to killing by the prodrug CB1954. *Eur J Cancer* 1995; 31A:2362–2370.

65. Chen L, Waxman DJ. Intratumoral activation and enhanced chemotherapeutic effect of oxazaphos-phorine following cytochrome P-450 gene transfer: development of a combined chemotherapy/cancer gene therapy strategy. *Cancer Res* 1995; 55:581–589.

66. Kanai F, Lan KH, Shiratori Y, et al. In vivo gene therapy for alpha-fetoprotein-producing hepatocellu-lar carcinoma by adenovirus-mediated transfer of cytosine deaminase gene. *Cancer Res* 1997; 57:461–465.

67. Bubenik J, Simova J, Jandlova T. Immunotherapy of cancer using local administration of lymphoid cells transformed by IL-2 cDNA and constitutively producing IL-2. *Immunol Lett* 1990; 23:287–292.

68. Tepper RI, Pattengale PK, Leder P. Murine interleukin 4 displays potent anti-tumor activity in vivo. *Cell* 1989; 57:503–512.

69. Fearon ER, Pardoll DM, Itaya T, et al. Interleukin-2 production by tumor cells bypasses T-helper function in the generation of an antitumor response. *Cell* 1990; 60:397–403.

70. Diamantstein WT, Blankenstein T. Lack of tumorigenicity of Interleukin 4 autocrine growing cells seems related to the anti-tumor function of Interleukin 4. *Mol Immunol* 1990; 27:1331–1337.

71. Blankenstein T, Qin Z, Überla K, et al. Tumor suppression after tumor cell-targeted tumor necrosis factor α gene transfer. *J Exp Med* 1991; 173:1047–1052.

72. Colombo MP, Ferrari G, Stoppacciaro A, et al. Granulocyte colony-stimulating factor gene transfer suppresses tumorigenicity of a murine adenocarcinoma in vivo. *J Exp Med* 1991; 173:889–897.

73. Golumbek PT, Lazenby AJ, Levitsky HI, et al. Treatment of established renal cancer by tumor cells engineered to secrete Interleukin-4. *Science* 1991; 254:713–716.

74. Hock H, Dorsch M, Diamantstein T, Blankenstein T. Interleukin-7 induces CD4+ T-Cell-dependent tumor rejection. *J Exp Med* 1991; 174:1291–1298.

75. Dranoff G, Jaffee EM, Lazenby AJ. Vaccination with irradiated tumor cells engineered to secrete granulocyte-macrophage colony-stimulating factor stimulates potent, specific, and long-lasting anti-tumor immunity. *Proc Natl Acad Sci USA* 1993; 90:3539–3543.

76. Abdel-Wahab Z, We-Ping L, Osanto S, et al. Transduction of human melanoma cells with inter-leukin-2 gene reduces tumorigenicity and enhances anti-tumor immunity: a nude mouse model. *Cel-lular Immunol* 1994; 159:26–39.

77. Abdel-Wahab Z, Dar M, Osanto S, et al. Eradication of melanoma pulmonary metastases by immunotherapy with tumor cells engineered to secrete interleukin-2 or gamma interferon. *Cancer Gene Ther* 1997; 4:33–41.

78. Fearon ER, Itaya T, Hunt B, Vogelstein B, Frost P. Induction in a murine tumor of immunogenic tumor variants by transfection with a foreign gene. *Cancer Res* 1988; 38:2975–2980.

79. Hui KM, Sim T, Foo TT, Oei AA. Tumor Rejection Mediated by Transfection with Allogeneic Class-I Histocompatibility Gene. *J Immunol* 1989; 143:3835–3843.

80. Ostrand-Rosenberg S, Roby C, Clements VK, Cole GA. Tumor-specific immunity can be enhanced by transfection of tumor cells with syngeneic MHC-class-II genes or allogeneic MHC-class-I genes. *Int J Cancer* 1991; supplement 6:61–68.

81. Chen L, Ashe S, Brady WA, Hellstrom I, Hellstrom KE, Ledbetter JA, McGowan P, Linsley PS. Co-stimulation of antitumor immunity by the B7 counterreceptor for the T lymphocyte molecules CD28 and CTLA-4. *Cell* 1992; 71:1093–1102.

82. Townsend SE, Allison JP. Tumor rejection after direct co-stimulation of CD8+ T-cells by B7-trans-fected melanoma cells. *Science* 1993; 259:368–370.

83. Chen L, McGowan P, Ashe S, et al. Tumor immunogenicity determines the effect of B7 co-stimula-tion on T cell-mediated tumor immunity. *J Exp Med* 1994; 179:523–531.

84. Bonini C, Ferrari G, Verzeletti S, et al. HSV-TK gene transfer into donor lymphocytes for control of allogeneic graft-versus-leukemia. *Science* 1997; 276:1719–1724.

85. McLachlin JR, Eglitis MA, Ueda K, et al. Expression of a human complementary DNA for the mul-tidrug resistance gene in murine hematopoietic precursor cells with the use of retroviral gene transfer. *J Natl Cancer Inst* 1990; 82:1260–1263.

86. Sorrentino BP, Brandt SJ, Bodine D, et al. Selection of drug-resistant bone marrow cells in vivo after retroviral transfer of human MDR1. *Science* 1992; 257:99–103.

87. Spencer HT, Sleep SE, Rehg JE, Blakley RL, Sorrentino BP. A gene transfer strategy for making bone-marrow cells resistant to trimetrexate. *Blood* 1996; 87:2579–2587.

88. Bicknell R. Vascular targeting and the inhibition of angiogenesis. *Ann Oncol* 1994; 5 Suppl. 4:45–50.

89. Burrows FJ, Thorpe PE. Vascular targeting—a new approach to the therapy of solid tumors. *Pharma-cology and Therapeutics* 1994; 64:155–174.

90. Boehm T, Folkman J, Browder T, O'Reilly MS. Antiangiogenic therapy of experimental cancer does not induce acquired drug resistance. *Nature* 1997; 390:404–407.

91. Kakeji Y, Teicher BA. Preclinical studies of the combination of angiogenic inhibitors with cytotoxic agents. *Investigational New Drugs* 1997; 15:39–48.

92. Gradishar WJ. An overview of clinical trials involving inhibitors of angiogenesis and their mechanism of action. *Investigational New Drugs* 1997; 15:49–59.

93. Folkman J. Antiangiogenic gene therapy. *Proc Nat Acad Sci USA* 1998; 95:9064–9066.

94. Kong HL, Crystal RG. Gene therapy strategies for tumor antiangiogenesis. *J Nat Cancer Inst* 1998; 90:273–286.

95. Millauer B, Shawver LK, Plate KH, Risau W, Ullrich A. Glioblastoma growth inhibited in vivo by a dominant-negative Flk-1 mutant. *Nature* 1994; 367:576–579.

96. Goldman CK, Kendall RL, Cabrera G, et al. Paracrine expression of a native soluble vascular endothelial growth factor receptor inhibits tumor growth, metastasis, and mortality rate. *Proc Nat Acad Sci USA* 1998; 95:8795–8800.

97. Kong HL, Hecht D, Song W, et al. Regional suppression of tumor growth by in vivo transfer of a cDNA encoding a secreted form of the extracellular domain of the flt-1 vascular endothelial growth factor receptor. *Human Gene Ther* 1998; 9:823–833.

98. Lin P, Buxton JA, Acheson A, et al. Antiangiogenic gene therapy targeting the endothelium-specific receptor tyrosine kinase Tie2. *Proc Natl Acad Sci USA* 1998; 95:8829–8834.

99. Saleh M, Stacker SA, Wilks AF. Inhibition of growth of C6 glioma cells in vivo by expression of antisense vascular endothelial growth factor sequence. *Cancer Res* 1996; 56:393–401.

100. Cheng SY, Huang HJ, Nagane M, et al. Suppression of glioblastoma angiogenicity and tumorigenicity by inhibition of endogenous expression of vascular endothelial growth factor. *Proc Natl Acad Sci USA* 1996; 93:8502–8507.

101. Tanaka T, Cao Y, Folkman J, Fine HA. Viral vector-targeted antiangiogenic gene therapy utilizing an angiostatin complementary DNA. *Cancer Res* 1998; 58:3362–3369.

102. Griscelli F, Li H, Bennaceur-Griscelli A, et al. Angiostatin gene transfer: inhibition of tumor growth in vivo by blockage of endothelial cell proliferation associated with a mitosis arrest. *Proc Nat Acad Sci USA* 1998; 95:6367–6372.

103. Weinstat-Saslow DL, Zabrenetzky VS, VanHoutte K, et al. Transfection of thrombospondin 1 complementary DNA into a human breast carcinoma cell line reduces primary tumor growth, metastatic potential, and angiogenesis. *Cancer Res* 1994; 54:6504–6511.

104. Tanaka T, Manome Y, Wen P, Kufe DW, Fine HA. Viral vector-mediated transduction of a modified platelet factor 4 cDNA inhibits angiogenesis and tumor growth. *Nature Med* 1997; 3:437–442.

105. Rosenberg SA, Aebersold P, Cornetta K, et al. Gene transfer into humans-immunotherapy of patients with advanced melanoma, using tumor-infiltrating lymphocytes modified by retroviral gene transduction. *New Engl J Med* 1990; 323:570–578.

106. Blaese RM, Culver KW, Miller AD, et al. T lymphocyte-directed gene therapy for ADA- SCID: initial trial results after 4 years. *Science* 1995; 270:475–480.

107. Stockhammer G, Brotchi J, Leblanc R, et al. Gene therapy for glioblastoma multiform: in vivo tumor transduction with the herpes simplex thymidine kinase gene followed by ganciclovir. *J Mol Med* 1997; 75:300–304.

108. Ram Z, Culver KW, Oshiro EM, et al. Therapy of malignant brain tumors by intratumoral implantation of retroviral vector-producing cells. *Nat Med* 1997; 3:1354–1361.

109. Clayman GL, el-Naggar AK, Lippman SM, et al. Adenovirus-mediated p53 gene transfer in patients with advanced recurrent head and neck squamous cell carcinoma. *J Clin Oncol* 1998; 16:2221–2232.

110. Nemunaitis J, Khuri F, Ganly I, et al. Phase II trial of intratumoral administration of ONYX-015, a replication-selective adenovirus, in patients with refractory head and neck cancer. *J Clin Oncol* 2001; 19:289–298.

111. Roth JA, Nguyen D, Lawrence DD, et al. Retrovirus-mediated wild-type p53 gene transfer to tumors of patients with lung cancer. *Nat Med* 1996; 2:985–991.

112. Swisher SG, Roth JA, Nemunaitis J, et al. Adenovirus-mediated p53 gene transfer in advanced non-small-cell lung cancer. *J Natl Cancer Inst* 1999; 91:763–771.

113. Sterman DH, Treat J, Litzky LA, et al. Adenovirus-mediated herpes simplex virus thymidine kinase/ganciclovir gene therapy in patients with localized malignancy: results of a phase I clinical trial in malignant mesothelioma. *Hum Gene Ther* 1998; 9:1083–1092.

114. Webb A, Cunningham D, Cotter F, et al. BCL-2 antisense therapy in patients with non-Hodgkin lymphoma. *Lancet* 1997; 349:1137–1141.

115. Bishop MR, Iversen PL, Bayever E, et al. Phase I trial of an antisense oligonucleotide OL(1)p53 in hematologic malignancies. *J Clin Oncol* 1996; 14:1320–1326.

116. Osanto S, Schiphorst PP, Weijl NI, et al. Vaccination of melanoma patients with an allogeneic, genetically modified interleukin 2-producing melanoma cell line. *Hum Gene Ther* 2000; 11:739–750.

117. Arienti F, Sule-Suso J, Melani C, et al. Limited antitumor T cell response in melanoma patients vaccinated with interleukin-2 gene-transduced allogeneic melanoma cells. *Hum Gene Ther* 1996; 7:1955–1963.

118. Soiffer R, Lynch T, Mihm M, et al. Vaccination with irradiated autologous melanoma cells engineered to secrete human granulocyte-macrophage colony-stimulating factor generates potent antitumor immunity in patients with metastatic melanoma. *Proc Natl Acad Sci USA* 1998; 95:13,141–13,146.

119. Schreiber S, Kampgen E, Wagner E, et al. Immunotherapy of metastatic malignant melanoma by a vaccine consisting of autologous interleukin 2-transfected cancer cells: outcome of a phase I study. *Hum Gene Ther* 1999; 10:983–993.

120. Nabel GJ, Nabel EG, Yang ZY, et al. Direct gene transfer with DNA-liposome complexes in melanoma: expression, biologic activity, and lack of toxicity. *Proc Natl Acad Sci USA* 1993; 90:11,307–11,311.

121. Nabel GJ, Gordon D, Bishop DK, et al. Immune response in human melanoma after transfer of an allogeneic class I major histocompatibility complex gene with DNA-liposome complexes. *Proc Natl Acad Sci USA* 1996; 93:15,388–15,393.

122. Stopeck AT, Hersh EM, Apkoriaye ET, et al. Phase I study of direct gene transfer of an allogeneic histocompatibility antigen, HLA-B7, in patients with metastatic melanoma. *J Clin Oncol* 1997; 15:341–349.

123. Dummer R, Bergh J, Karlsson Y, et al. Biological activity and safety of adenoviral vector-expressed wild-type p53 after intratumoral injection in melanoma and breast cancer patients with p53-overexpressing tumors. *Cancer Gene Ther* 2000; 7:1069–1076.

124. Tait DL, Obermiller PS, Redlin-Frazier S, et al. A phase I trial of retroviral BRCA1sv gene therapy in ovarian cancer. *Clin Cancer Res* 1997; 3:1959–1968.

125. Tait DL, Obermiller PS, Hatmaker AR, Redlin-Frazier S, Holt JT. Ovarian cancer BRCA1 gene therapy: Phase I and II trial differences in immune response and vector stability. *Clin Cancer Res* 1999; 5:1708–1714.

126. Herman JR, Adler HL, Aguilar-Cordova E, et al. In situ gene therapy for adenocarcinoma of the prostate: a phase I clinical trial. *Hum Gene Ther* 1999; 10:1239–1249.

15 Progress in Antisense Technology

Stanley T. Crooke, MD, PhD

CONTENTS

1. INTRODUCTION

With the recent FDA approval of Vitravene™, the first drug based on antisense technology to be commercialized, the new technology has achieved an important milestone. Although the basic questions have been addressed, there are still many unanswered questions.

This chapter will provide an overview of the progress in converting the antisense concept into broad therapeutic reality, and provide advice concerning appropriate experimental design and interpretation of data with regard to the therapeutic potential of the technology.

2. PROOF OF MECHANISM

2.1. Factors That May Influence Experimental Interpretations

Clearly, the ultimate biological effect of an oligonucleotide will be influenced by the local concentration of the oligonucleotide at the target RNA, the concentration of the RNA, the rates of synthesis and degradation of the RNA, type of terminating mechanism, and the rates of the events that result in termination of the activity of the RNA. At present, we understand essentially nothing about the interplay of these factors.

2.1.1. OLIGONUCLEOTIDE PURITY

Currently, phosphorothioate oligonucleotides can be prepared consistently and with excellent purity *(1)*. However, this has only been the case for the past three to four years. Prior to that time, synthetic methods were evolving and analytical methods were inadequate. In fact, our laboratory reported that different synthetic and purification procedures resulted in oligonucleotides that varied in cellular toxicity *(2)*, and that potency varied

From: *Drug Delivery Systems in Cancer Therapy*
Edited by: D. M. Brown © Humana Press Inc., Totowa, NJ

from batch to batch. Although there are no longer synthetic problems with phosphorothioates, they undoubtedly complicated earlier studies. More importantly, with each new analog class, new synthetic, purification, and analytical challenges are encountered.

2.1.2. OLIGONUCLEOTIDE STRUCTURE

Antisense oligonucleotides are designed to be single stranded. We now understand that certain sequences, e.g., stretches of guanosine residues, are prone to adopt more complex structures (3). The potential to form secondary and tertiary structures also varies as a function of chemical class. For example, higher affinity 2′-modified oligonucleotides have a greater tendency to self-hybridize, resulting in more stable oligonucleotide duplexes than would be expected based on rules derived from oligodeoxynucleotides (Freier, unpublished results).

2.1.3. RNA STRUCTURE

RNA is structured. The structure of the RNA has a profound influence on the affinity of the oligonucleotide and on the rate of binding of the oligonucleotide to its RNA target (4,5). Moreover, RNA structure produces asymmetrical binding sites that then result in very divergent affinity constants, depending on the position of oligonucleotide in that structure (5–7). This, in turn, influences the optimal length of an oligonucleotide needed to achieve maximal affinity. We understand very little about how RNA structure and RNA protein interactions influence antisense drug action.

2.1.4. VARIATIONS IN IN VITRO CELLULAR UPTAKE AND DISTRIBUTION

Studies in several laboratories have clearly demonstrated that cells in tissue culture may take up phosphorothioate oligonucleotides via an active process, and that the uptake of these oligonucleotides is highly variable depending on many conditions (2,8). Cell type has a dramatic effect on total uptake, kinetics of uptake, and pattern of subcellular distribution. At present, there is no unifying hypothesis to explain these differences. Tissue culture conditions, such as the type of medium, degree of confluence, and the presence of serum, can have enormous effects on uptake (8). Oligonucleotide chemical class obviously influences the characteristics of uptake as well as the mechanism of uptake. Within the phosphorothioate class of oligonucleotides, uptake varies as a function of length, but not linearly. Uptake varies as a function of sequence, and stability in cells is also influenced by sequence (8,9).

Given the foregoing, it is obvious that conclusions about in vitro uptake must be very carefully made and generalizations are virtually impossible. Thus, before an oligonucleotide could be said to be inactive in vitro, it should be studied in several cell lines. Furthermore, although it may be correct that receptor-mediated endocytosis is a mechanism of uptake of phosphorothioate oligonucleotides (10), it is obvious that the generalization that all phosphorothioates are taken up by all cells in vitro primarily by receptor-mediated endocytosis is unwarranted.

Finally, extrapolations from in vitro uptake studies to predictions about in vivo pharmacokinetic behavior are entirely inappropriate and, in fact, there are now several lines of evidence in humans and animals that, even after careful consideration of all in vitro uptake data, one cannot predict in vivo pharmacokinetics of the compounds (8,11–13).

2.1.5. EFFECTS OF BINDING TO NONNUCLEIC ACID TARGETS

Phosphorothioate oligonucleotides tend to bind to many proteins and those interactions are influenced by many factors. The effects of binding can influence cell uptake, distribution, metabolism, and excretion. They may induce nonantisense effects that can be mistakenly interpreted as antisense or complicate the identification of an antisense mechanism. By inhibiting RNase H, protein binding may inhibit the antisense activity of some oligonucleotides. Finally, binding to proteins can certainly have toxicological consequences.

In addition to proteins, oligonucleotides may interact with other biological molecules, such as lipids or carbohydrates, and such interactions like those with proteins will be influenced by the chemical class of oligonucleotide studied. Unfortunately, little or no data bearing on such interactions are currently available.

A complicated experimental situation is encountered in many in vitro antiviral assays: high concentrations of drugs, viruses, and cells are often coincubated. The sensitivity of each virus to nonantisense effects of oligonucleotides varies depending on the nature of the virion proteins and the characteristics of the oligonucleotides (14,15). This has resulted in considerable confusion. In particular for HIV, herpes simplex viruses, cytomegaloviruses, and influenza virus, the nonantisense effects have been so dominant that identifying oligonucleotides that work via an antisense mechanism has been difficult. Given the artificial character of such assays, it is difficult to know whether non-antisense mechanisms would be as dominant in vivo or result in antiviral activity.

2.1.6. TERMINATING MECHANISMS

It has been amply demonstrated that oligonucleotides may employ several terminating mechanisms. The dominant terminating mechanism is influenced by RNA receptor site, oligonucleotide chemical class, cell type, and probably many other factors (16). Obviously, as variations in terminating mechanism may result in significant changes in antisense potency, and studies have shown significant variations from cell type to cell type in vitro, it is essential that the terminating mechanism be well understood. Unfortunately, at present, our understanding of terminating mechanisms remains rudimentary.

2.1.7. EFFECTS OF "CONTROL OLIGONUCLEOTIDES"

A number of types of control oligonucleotides have been used, including randomized oligonucleotides. Unfortunately, we know little about the potential biological effects of such "controls," and the more complicated the biological system and test, the more likely that "control" oligonucleotides may have activities that complicate our interpretations. Thus, when a control oligonucleotide displays a surprising activity, the mechanism of that activity should be explored carefully before concluding that the effects of the control oligonucleotide prove that the activity of the putative antisense oligonucleotide is not caused by an antisense mechanism.

2.1.8. KINETICS OF EFFECTS

Many rate constants may affect the activities of antisense oligonucleotides, e.g., the rate of synthesis and degradation of the target RNA and its protein, the rates of uptake into cells, the rates of distribution, extrusion, and metabolism of an oligonucleotide in human cells and similar pharmacokinetic considerations in animals. Despite this, relatively few time-courses have been reported, and in vitro studies have ranged from a few hours to several days. In animals, we have a growing body of information in pharmacokinetics, but in most studies reported to date, the doses and schedules were chosen arbitrarily and little information on duration of effect and onset of action has been presented.

Clearly, more careful kinetic studies with rational in vitro and in vivo dose schedules are required.

2.2. Recommendations

2.2.1. POSITIVE DEMONSTRATION OF ANTISENSE MECHANISM AND SPECIFICITY

Until more is understood about how antisense drugs work, it is essential to positively demonstrate effects consistent with an antisense mechanism. For RNase H-activating oligonucleotides, Northern blot analysis showing selective loss of the target RNA is the best choice, and many laboratories are publishing reports in vitro and in vivo of such activities (17–20). Ideally, a demonstration that closely related isotypes are unaffected should be included.

More recently, in our laboratories we have used RNA protection assays and DNA chip assays. These assays provide a great deal of information about the levels of various RNA species. Coupled to careful kinetic analysis, such approaches can help assure that the primary mechanism of action of the drug is antisense, and identify events that are secondary to antisense inhibition of a specific target. This can then support the assignment of a target to a particular pathway, and the analysis of the roles of a particular target and the factors that regulate its activity. We have adapted all these methods for use in animals, and we will determine their utility in clinical trials.

For proof of mechanism, the following steps are recommended.

- Perform careful dose response curves in vitro using several cell lines and methods of in vitro delivery.
- Correlate the rank order potency in vivo with that observed in vitro after thorough dose response curves are generated in vivo.
- Perform careful "gene walks" for all RNA species and oligonucleotide chemical classes.
- Perform careful time courses before drawing conclusions about potency.
- Demonstrate the proposed mechanism of action by measuring the target RNA and/or protein.
- Evaluate specificity and therapeutic indices via studies on closely related isotypes and with appropriate toxicological studies.
- Perform sufficient pharmacokinetics to define rational dosing schedules for pharmacological studies.
- Determine the mechanisms involved when control oligonucleotides display surprising activities.

3. MOLECULAR MECHANISMS OF ANTISENSE DRUGS

3.1. Occupancy-Only Mediated Mechanisms

Classic competitive antagonists are thought to alter biological activities because they bind to receptors preventing natural agonists from binding the inducing normal biological processes. Binding of oligonucleotides to specific sequences may inhibit the interaction of the RNA with proteins, other nucleic acids, or other factors required for essential steps in the intermediary metabolism of the RNA or its utilization by the cell.

3.1.1. INHIBITION OF SPLICING

A key step in the intermediary metabolism of most messenger RNA (mRNA) molecules is the excision of introns. These splicing reactions are sequence specific and require the concerted action of spliceosomes. Consequently, oligonucleotides that bind to sequences required for splicing may prevent binding of necessary factors or physically prevent the required cleavage reactions. This, then, would result in inhibition of the production of the mature mRNA. Although there are several examples of oligonu-cleotides directed to splice junctions, none of the studies present data showing inhibi-tion of RNA processing, accumulation of splicing intermediates, or a reduction in mature mRNA. Nor are there published data in which the structure of the RNA at the splice junction was probed and the oligonucleotides demonstrated to hybridize to the sequences for which they were designed *(21–24)*. Activities have been reported for anti-c-*myc* and antiviral oligonucleotides with phosphodiester, methylphosphonate, and phosphorothioate backbones. Very recently, an oligonucleotide was reported to induce alternative splicing in a cell-free splicing system and, in that system, RNA analyses confirmed the putative mechanism *(25)*.

In our laboratory, we have attempted to characterize the factors that determine whether splicing inhibition is effected by an antisense drug *(26)*. To this end, a number of luciferase-reporter plasmids containing various introns were constructed and trans-fected into HeLa cells. Then the effects of antisense drugs designed to bind to various sites were characterized. The effects of RNase H-competent oligonucleotides were compared to those of oligonucleotides that do not serve as RNase H substrates. The major conclusions from this study were: First, that most of the earlier studies in which splicing inhibition was reported were probably due to nonspecific effects. Second, less effectively spliced introns are better targets than those with strong consensus splicing signals. Third, the 3'-splice site and branchpoint are usually the best sites to which to target the oligonucleotide to inhibit splicing. Fourth, RNase H-competent oligonu-cleotides are usually more potent than the higher affinity oligonucleotides that inhibit by occupancy only.

3.1.2. TRANSLATIONAL ARREST

One mechanism for which the many oligonucleotides have been designed is to arrest translation of targeted protein by binding to the translation initiation codon. The posi-tioning of the complementary initiation codon within the area of the oligonucleotide and the length of the oligonucleotide used have varied considerably. Only in relatively few studies have the oligonucleotides, in fact, been shown to bind to the sites for which they were designed, and data that directly support translation arrest as the mechanism have been lacking.

Target RNA species that have been reported to be inhibited by a translational arrest mechanism include HIV, vesicular stomatitis virus (VSV), n-*myc,* and a number of nor-mal cellular genes *(27–33)*. In our laboratories, we have shown that a significant num-ber of targets may be inhibited by binding to translation initiation codons. For example, ISIS 1082 hybridizes to the AUG codon for the UL13 gene of herpes virus types 1 and 2. RNase H studies confirmed that it binds selectively in this area. In vitro protein syn-thesis studies confirmed that it inhibited the synthesis of the UL13 protein, and studies in HeLa cells showed that it inhibited the growth of herpes type 1 and type 2 with IC_{50} of 200–400 ηM by translation arrest *(34)*. Similarly, ISIS 1753, a 30-mer phosphoroth-ioate complementary to the translation initiation codon and surrounding sequences of the *E2* gene of bovine papilloma virus, was highly effective and its activity was shown to be a result of translation arrest. ISIS 2105, a 20-mer phosphorothioate complemen-tary to the same region in human papilloma virus, was shown to be a very potent inhibitor. Compounds complementary to the translation initiation codon of the *E2* gene were the most potent of the more than 50 compounds studied complementary to other regions in the RNA *(35)*. We have shown inhibition of translation of a number of other mRNA species by compounds designed to bind to the translation codon as well.

In conclusion, translation arrest represents an important mechanism of action for antisense drugs. A number of examples purporting to employ this mechanism have been reported, and recent studies on several compounds have provided data that unambiguously demonstrate that this mechanism can result in potent antisense drugs. However, little is understood about the precise events that lead to translation arrest.

3.1.3. DISRUPTION OF NECESSARY RNA STRUCTURE

RNA adopts a variety of three-dimensional (3D) structures induced by intramolecular hybridization, the most common of which is the stem loop. These 3D structures play crucial roles in a variety of functions. They are used to provide additional stability for RNA and as recognition motifs for a number of proteins, nucleic acids, and ribonucleoproteins that participate in the intermediary metabolism and other activities of RNA species. Given the potential general activity of the mechanism, it is surprising that occupancy-based disruption RNA has not been more extensively exploited.

As an example, we designed a series of oligonucleotides that bind to the important stem-loop present in all RNA species in HIV, i.e., the transactivator response (TAR) element. We synthesized a number of oligonucleotides designed to disrupt TAR, and then demonstrated that several bound to TAR, disrupted the structure, and inhibited the TAR-mediated production of a reporter gene *(36)*. Furthermore, general rules useful in disrupting stem-loop structures were developed as well *(7)*.

Although designed to induce relatively nonspecific cytotoxic effects, two other examples are noteworthy. Oligonucleotides designed to bind to a 17-nucleotide loop in Xenopus 28 S RNA, required for ribosome stability and protein synthesis, inhibited protein synthesis when injected into Xenopus oocytes *(37)*. Similarly, oligonucleotides designed to bind to highly conserved sequences in 5.8 S RNA inhibited protein synthesis in both rabbit reticulocyte and wheat germ systems *(38)*.

3.2. Occupancy-Activated Destabilization

RNA molecules regulate their own metabolism. A number of structural features of RNA are known to influence stability, various processing events, subcellular distribution, and transport. It is likely that, as RNA intermediary metabolism is better understood, many other regulatory features and mechanisms will be identified.

3.2.1. 5′-CAPPING

A key early step in RNA processing is 5′-capping. This stabilizes pre-mRNA and is important for the stability of mature mRNA. It also is important in binding to the nuclear matrix and transport of mRNA out of the nucleus. As the unique structure of the cap is understood, it presents an interesting target.

Several oligonucleotides that bind near the cap site have been shown to be active, presumably by inhibiting the binding of proteins required to cap the RNA. For example, the synthesis of SV40 T antigen was reported to be most sensitive to an oligonucleotide linked to polylysine and targeted to the 5′-cap site of RNA *(39)*. Again, in no published study has this putative mechanism been rigorously demonstrated. In fact, in no published study have the oligonucleotides been shown to bind to the sequences for which they were designed.

In our laboratory, we have designed oligonucleotides to bind to 5′-cap structures and reagents to specifically cleave the unique 5′-cap structure *(40)*. These studies demonstrate that 5′-cap targeted oligonucleotides were capable of inhibiting the binding of the translation initiation factor eIF-4a *(41)*.

3.2.2. INHIBITION OF 3′-POLYADENYLATION

In the 3′-untranslated region of pre-mRNA molecules are sequences that result in the posttranscriptional addition of long tracts of polyadenylate that consist of hundreds of nucleotides. Polyadenylation stabilizes mRNA and may play other roles in the intermediary metabolism of RNA species. Theoretically, interactions in the 3′-terminal region of pre-mRNA could inhibit polyadenylation and destabilize the RNA species. Although there are a number of oligonucleotides that interact in the 3′-untranslated region and display antisense activities, to date, no study has reported evidence for alterations in polyadenylation *(17)*.

3.3. Other Mechanisms

In addition to 5′-capping and 3′-adenylation, there are clearly other sequences in the 5′-and 3′-untranslated regions of mRNA that affect the stability of the molecules. Again, there are a number of antisense drugs that may work by these mechanisms.

Zamecnik and Stephenson reported that 13 mer targeted to untranslated 3′- and 5′-terminal sequences in Rous sarcoma viruses was active *(42)*. Oligonucleotides conjugated to an acridine derivative and targeted to a 3′-terminal sequence in type A influenza viruses were reported to be active. Against several RNA targets, studies in our laboratories have shown that sequences in the 3′-untranslated region of RNA molecules are often the most sensitive *(43–45)*. For example, ISIS 1939, a 20-mer phosphorothioate that binds to and appears to disrupt a predicted stem-loop structure in the 3′-untranslated region of the mRNA for the intercellular adhesion molecule (ICAM) is a potent antisense inhibitor. However, inasmuch as a 2′-methoxy analog of ISIS 1939 was much less active, it is likely that, in addition to destabilization to cellular nucleolytic activity, activation of RNase H is also involved in the activity of ISIS 1939 *(17)*.

3.4. Activation of RNase H

RNase H is a ubiquitous enzyme that degrades the RNA strand of an RNA-DNA duplex. It has been identified in organisms as diverse as viruses and human cells *(46)*. At least two classes of RNase H have been identified in eukaryotic cells. Multiple enzymes with RNase H activity have been observed in prokaryotes *(46)*.

Although RNase H is involved in DNA replication, it is found in the cytoplasm as well as the nucleus and may play other roles in the cell *(47)*. However, the concentration of the enzyme in the nucleus is thought to be greater and some of the enzyme found in cytoplasmic preparations may be because of nuclear leakage.

RNase H activity is quite variable in cells. It is absent or minimal in rabbit reticulocytes but present in wheat germ extracts *(46,48)*. In HL-60 cells, for example, the level of activity in undifferentiated cells is greatest, relatively high in DMSO and vitamin D-differentiated cells and much lower in PMA-differentiated cells (Hoke, unpublished data).

The precise recognition elements for RNase H are not known. However, it has been shown that oligonucleotides with DNA-like properties as short as tetramers can activate RNase H *(49)*. Changes in the sugar influence RNase H activation, as sugar modifications that result in RNA-like oligonucleotides, e.g., 2′-fluoro or 2′-methoxy, do not appear to serve as substrates for RNase H *(50,51)*. Alterations in the orientation of the sugar to the base can also affect RNase H activation as α-oligonucleotides are unable to induce RNase H or may require parallel annealing *(52,53)*. Additionally, backbone modifications influence the ability of oligonucleotides to activate RNase H. Methylphosphonates do not activate RNase H *(54,55)*. In contrast, phosphorothioates are excellent substrates *(34,56,57)*. In addition, chimeric molecules have been studied as oligonucleotides that bind to RNA and activate RNase H *(58,59)*. For example, oligonucleotides comprised of wings of 2′-methoxy phosphonates and a five-base gap of deoxyoligonucleotides bind to their target RNA and activate RNase H *(58,59)*. Furthermore, a single ribonucleotide in a sequence of deoxyribonucleotides was shown to be sufficient to serve as a substrate for RNase H when bound to its complementary deoxyoligonucleotide *(60)*.

That it is possible to take advantage of chimeric oligonucleotides designed to activate RNase H and have greater affinity for their RNA receptors and to enhance specificity has also been demonstrated *(61,62)*. In a recent study, RNase H-mediated cleavage of target transcript was much more selective when deoxyoligonucleotides comprised of methylphosphonate deoxyoligonucleotide wings and phosphodiester gaps were compared to full phosphodiester oligonucleotides *(62)*.

Despite the accumulating information about RNase H and the evidence that many oligonucleotides may activate RNase H in lysate and purified enzyme assays, relatively little is known about the role of structural features in RNA targets in activating RNase H *(63–65)*. In fact, direct proof that RNase H activation is the mechanism of action of oligonucleotides in cells is largely lacking.

Recent studies in our laboratories provide additional, albeit indirect, insights into these questions. ISIS 1939 is a 20-mer phosphorothioate complementary to a sequence in the 3′-untranslated region of ICAM-1 RNA *(17)*. It inhibits ICAM production in human umbilical vein endothelial cells, and Northern blots demonstrate that ICAM-1 mRNA is rapidly degraded. A 2′-methoxy analog of ISIS 1939 displays higher affinity for the RNA than the phosphorothioate, is stable in cells, but inhibits ICAM-1 protein production much less potently than ISIS 1939. It is likely that ISIS 1939 destabilizes the RNA and activates RNase H. In contrast, ISIS 1570, an 18-mer phosphorothioate that is complementary to the translation initiation codon of the ICAM-1 message, inhibited production of the protein, but caused no degradation of the RNA. Thus, two oligonucleotides that are capable of activating RNase H had different effects depending on the site in the mRNA at which they bound *(17)*.

A more direct demonstration that RNase H is likely a key factor in the activity of many antisense oligonucleotides was provided by studies in which reverse-ligation PCR was used to identify cleavage products from *bcr-abl* mRNA in cells treated with phosphorothioate oligonucleotides *(66)*.

Given the emerging role of chimeric oligonucleotides with modifications in the 3′- and 5′-wings designed to enhance affinity for the target RNA and nuclease stability and a DNA-type gap to serve as a substrate for RNase H, studies focused on understanding the effects of various modifications on the efficiency of the enzyme(s) are of considerable importance. In one such study on *Escherichia coli* RNase H, we reported that the enzyme displays minimal sequence specificity. When a chimeric oligonucleotide with 2′-modified sugars in the wings was hybridized to the RNA, the initial site of cleavage was the nucleotide adjacent to the methoxy-deoxy junction closest to the 3′-end of the RNA substrate. The initial rate of cleavage increased as the size of the DNA gap increased, and the efficiency of the enzyme was considerably less against an RNA target duplexed with a chimeric antisense oligonucleotide than against a full DNA-type oligonucleotide *(67)*.

In subsequent studies, we evaluated in more detail the interactions of antisense oligonucleotides with structured and unstructured targets, and the impacts of these interactions on RNase H *(68)*. Using a series of noncleavable substrates and michaelis-monten analyses, we were able to evaluate both binding and cleavage. We demonstrated that, in fact, *E. coli* RNase H1 is a double-strand RNA-binding protein. The K_d for our RNA duplex was 1.6 μ*M*, the K_d for a DNA duplex was 176 μ*M*, and the K_d for single-strand DNA was 942 μ*M*. In contrast, the enzyme could only cleave RNA in an RNA-DNA duplex. Any 2′ modification in the antisense drug at the cleavage site inhibited cleavage, but significant charge reduction and 2′ modifications were tolerated at the binding site. Finally, placing a positive charge (e.g., 2′ propoxyamine) in the antisense drug reduced affinity and cleavage.

We have also examined the effects of antisense oligonucleotide-induced RNA structures on the activity of *E. coli* RNase H1 *(69)*. Any structure in the duplex substrate was found to have a significant negative effect on the cleavage rate. Further, cleavage of selected sites was inhibited entirely, and this was explained by sterric hindrance imposed by the RNA loop traversing either the minor or major grooves of the hetroduplex.

Recently, we succeeded in cloning, expressing, and characterizing a human RNase H that is homologous to *E. coli* RNase H1 and has properties comparable to the type 2 enzyme *(70)*. Additionally, we have cloned and expressed a second RNase H homologous to *E. coli* RNase H2 (Wu and Crooke, unpublished observations). Given these steps, we are now able to evaluate the roles of each of these enzymes in cellular activities and antisense pharmacology. We are also characterizing these proteins and their enzymological properties.

3.5. Activation of Double-Strand RNase

By using phosphorothioate oligonucleotides with 2′ modified wings and a ribonucleotide center, we have shown that mammalian cells contain enzymes that can cleave double-strand RNAs *(70)*. This is an important step forward because it adds to the repertoire of intracellular enzymes that may be used to cleave target RNAs and because the 2′ modified wings of chimeric oligonucleotides and the gaps of chimeric oligoribonucleotides have higher affinity for RNA targets than chimeras with oligodeoxynucleotide gaps.

3.6. Selection of an Optimal RNA Binding Site

It has been amply demonstrated that a significant fraction of every RNA species is not accessible to phosphorothioate oligodeoxynucleotides in a fashion that permits antisense effects *(71)*. Thus, substantial efforts have been directed to the development of methods that might predict optimal sites for binding within RNA species. Although a number of screening methods have been proposed *(72–75)*, in our experience the correlation between these antisense effects in cells is insufficient to warrant their use (Wyatt, unpublished results).

Consequently, we have developed rapid throughput systems that use a 96-well format and 96-channel oligonucleotide synthesizer coupled to an automated RT-PCR instrument. This provides rapid screening of up to 80 sites in an RNA species for two chemistries under consistent highly controlled experimental conditions. We are hopeful that, based on such a system (evaluating two genes per week), we will be able to develop improved methods that predict optimal sites.

4. CHARACTERISTICS OF PHOSPHOROTHIOATE OLIGODEOXYNUCLEOTIDES

4.1. Introduction

In the first-generation oligonucleotide analogs, the class that has resulted in the broadest range of activities and about which the most is known, is the phosphorothioate class. Phosphorothioate oligonucleotides were first synthesized in 1969 when a poly rI-rC phosphorothioate was synthesized (76). This modification clearly achieves the objective of increased nuclease stability. In this class of oligonucleotides, one of the oxygen atoms in the phosphate group is replaced with a sulfur atom. The resulting compound is negatively charged, is chiral at each phosphorothioate phosphodiester, and much more resistant to nucleases than the parent phosphorothioate (77).

4.2. Hybridization

The hybridization of phosphorothioate oligonucleotides to DNA and RNA has been thoroughly characterized (1,78–80). The T_m of a phosphorothioate oligodeoxynucleotide for RNA is approx 0.5°C less per nucleotide than for a corresponding phosphodiester oligodeoxynucleotide. This reduction in T_m per nucleotide is virtually independent of the number of phosphorothioate units substituted for phosphodiesters. However, sequence context has some influence as the ΔT_m can vary from –0.3–1.0°C depending on sequence. Compared with RNA and RNA duplex formation, a phosphorothioate oligodeoxynucleotide has a T_m approx –2.2°C lower per unit (4). This means that to be effective in vitro, phosphorothioate oligodeoxynucleotides must typically be 17–20 mer in length and that invasion of double-stranded regions in RNA is difficult (6,36,61,81).

Association rates of phosphorothioate oligodeoxynucleotide to unstructured RNA targets are typically 10^6–$10^7 M^{-1}S^{-1}$ independent of oligonucleotide length or sequence (4,6). Association rates to structured RNA targets can vary from 10^2–$10^8 M^{-1}S^{-1}$ depending on the structure of the RNA, site of binding in the structure, and other factors (4). In other words, association rates for oligonucleotides that display acceptable affinity constants are sufficient to support biological activity at therapeutically achievable concentrations. A recent study using phosphodiester oligonucleotides coupled with fluoroscein, showed that hybridization was detectable within 15 min after microinjection into K562 cells (82).

The specificity of hybridization of phosphorothioate oligonucleotides is, in general, slightly greater than phosphodiester analogs. For example, a T-C mismatch results in a 7.7 or 12.8°C reduction in T_m, respectively, for a phosphodiester or phosphorothioate oligodeoxynucleotide 18 nucleotides in length, with the mismatch centered (4). Thus, from this perspective, the phosphorothioate modification is quite attractive.

4.3. Interactions with Proteins

Phosphorothioate oligonucleotides bind to proteins. The interactions with proteins can be divided into nonspecific, sequence-specific, and structure-specific binding events—each of which may have different characteristics and effects. Nonspecific binding to a wide variety of proteins has been demonstrated. Exemplary of this type of binding is the interaction of phosphorothioate oligonucleotides with serum albumin. The affinity of such interactions is low. The K_d for albumin is approx 200 μM and, thus, in a similar range with aspirin or penicillin (83,84). Furthermore, in this study, no competition was observed between phosphorothioate oligonucleotides and several drugs that bind to bovine serum albumin (BSA). In this study, binding and competition were determined in an assay in which electrospray mass spectrometry was used. In contrast, in a study in which an equilibrium dissociation constant was derived from an assay using albumin loaded on a CH-Sephadex column, the K_m ranged from 1–5×10^{-5} M for BSA and 2–3×10^{-4} M for human serum albumin. Moreover, warfarin and indomethacin were reported to compete for binding to serum albumin (85). Clearly, much more work is required before definitive conclusions can be drawn.

Phosphorothioate oligonucleotides can interact with nucleic acid-binding proteins such as transcription factors and single-strand nucleic acid-binding proteins. However, little is known about these binding events. Additionally, it has been reported that phosphorothioates bind to an 80-K_d membrane protein that was thought to be involved in cellular uptake processes (10). However, little is known about the affinities, sequence, or structure specificities of these putative interactions. More recently, interactions with 30 K_d and 46 K_d are surface proteins in T15 mouse fibroblasts were reported (86).

Phosphorothioates interact with nucleases and DNA polymerases. These compounds are slowly metabolized by both endo- and exonucleases and inhibit these enzymes (78,87). The inhibition of these enzymes appears to be competitive, and this may account for some early data suggesting that phosphorothioates are almost infinitely stable to nucleases. In these studies, the oligonucleotide-to-enzyme ratio was very high and the enzyme was inhibited. Phosphorothioates also bind to RNase H when in an RNA-DNA duplex and the duplex serves as a substrate for RNase H (88). At higher concentrations, presumably by binding as a single strand to RNase H, phosphorothioates inhibit the enzyme (67,78). Again, the oligonucleotides appear to be competitive antagonists for the DNA-RNA substrate.

Phosphorothioates have been shown to be competitive inhibitors of DNA polymerase α and β with respect to the DNA template, and noncompetitive inhibitors of DNA polymerases γ and Δ (88). Despite this inhibition, several studies have suggested that phosphorothioates might serve as primers for polymerases and be extended (9,56,89). In our laboratories, we have shown extensions of only 2–3 nucleotides. At present, a full explanation as to why longer extensions are not observed is not available.

It has been reported that phosphorothioate oligonucleotides are competitive inhibitors for HIV-reverse transcriptase and that they inhibit RT-associated RNase H activity (90,91). They have been reported to bind to the cell surface protein, CD4, and to protein kinase C (92). Various viral polymerases have also been shown to be inhibited by phosphorothioates (56). Additionally, we have shown potent, nonsequence-specific inhibition of RNA splicing by phosphorothioates (26).

Like other oligonucleotides, phosphorothioates can adopt a variety of secondary structures. As a general rule, self-complementary oligonucleotides are avoided, if possible, to prevent duplex formation between oligonucleotides. However, other structures that are less well understood can also form. For example, oligonucleotides containing runs of guanosines can form tetrameric structures called G-quartets, and these appear to interact with a number of proteins with relatively greater affinity than unstructured oligonucleotides *(3)*.

In conclusion, phosphorothioate oligonucleotides may interact with a wide range of proteins via several types of mechanisms. These interactions may influence the pharmacokinetic, pharmacologic, and toxicologic properties of these molecules. They may also complicate studies on the mechanism of action of these drugs, and may obscure an antisense activity. For example, phosphorothioate oligonucleotides were reported to enhance lipopolysacchoride-stimulated synthesis or tumor necrosis factor *(93)*. This would obviously obscure antisense effects on this target.

4.4. Pharmacokinetic Properties

To study the pharmacokinetics of phosphorothioate oligonucleotides, a variety of labeling techniques have been used. In some cases, 3'- or 5 ^{32}P end-labeled or fluorescently labeled oligonucleotides have been used for in vitro or in vivo studies. These are probably less satisfactory than internally labeled compounds because terminal phosphates are rapidly removed by phosphatases, and fluorescently labeled oligonucleotides have physicochemical properties that differ from the unmodified oligonucleotides. Consequently, either uniformly *(35)*. S-labeled or base-labeled phosphorothioates are preferable for pharmacokinetic studies. In our laboratories, a tritium exchange method that labels a slowly exchanging proton at the C-8 position in purines was developed and proved to be quite useful *(94)*. Recently, a method that added radioactive methyl groups via S-adenosyl methionine has also been successfully used *(95)*. Finally, advances in extraction, separation, and detection have resulted in methods that provide excellent pharmacokinetic analyses without radiolabeling *(83)*.

4.4.1. NUCLEASE STABILITY

The principle metabolic pathway for oligonucleotides is cleavage via endo- and exonucleases. Phosphorothioate oligonucleotides, while quite stable to various nucleases, are competitive inhibitors of nucleases *(16,88,96–98)*. Consequently, the stability of phosphorothioate oligonucleotides to nucleases is probably a bit less than initially thought, as high concentrations of oligonucleotides that inhibited nucleases were employed in the early studies. Similarly, phosphorothioate oligonucleotides are degraded slowly by cells in tissue culture with a half-life of 12–24 h and are slowly metabolized in animals *(11,16,96)*. The pattern of metabolites suggests primarily exonuclease activity with, perhaps, modest contributions by endonucleases. However, a number of lines of evidence suggest that, in many cells and tissues, endonucleases play an important role in the metabolism of oligonucleotides. For example, 3'- and 5'-modified oligonucleotides with phosphodiester backbones have been shown to be relatively rapidly degraded in cells and after administration to animals *(13,99)*. Thus, strategies in which oligonucleotides are modified at only the 3'- and 5'-terminus as a means of enhancing stability have not proven to be successful.

4.4.2. IN VITRO CELLULAR UPTAKE

Phosphorothioate oligonucleotides are taken up by a wide range of cells in vitro *(2,16,88,100,101)*. In fact, uptake of phosphorothioate oligonucleotides into a prokaryote, Vibrio parahaemoyticus, has been reported, as has uptake into Schistosoma mansoni *(102,103)*. Uptake is time and temperature dependent. It is also influenced by cell type, cell-culture conditions, media and sequence, and length of the oligonucleotide *(16)*. No obvious correlation between uptake and the lineage of cells—whether the cells are transformed or whether the cells are virally infected—has been identified *(16)*. Nor are the factors understood that result in differences in uptake of different sequences of oligonucleotide. Although several studies have suggested that receptor-mediated endocytosis may be a significant mechanism of cellular uptake, the data are not yet compelling enough to conclude that receptor-mediated endocytosis accounts for a significant portion of the uptake in most cells *(10)*.

Numerous studies have shown that phosphorothioate oligonucleotides, once taken up, distribute broadly in most cells *(16,79)*. Again, however, significant differences in subcellular distribution between various types of cells have been noted.

Cationic lipids and other approaches have been used to enhance uptake of phosphorothioate oligonucleotides in cells that take up little oligonucleotide in vitro *(104–106)*. Again, there are substantial variations from cell type to cell type. Other approaches to enhanced intracellular uptake in vitro have included treatment of cells by streptolysin D, and the use of dextran sulfate and other liposome formulations, as well as physical means such as microinjections *(16,66,107)*.

4.4.3. IN VIVO PHARMACOKINETICS

Phosphorothioate oligonucleotides bind to serum albumin and α-2 macroglobulin. The apparent affinity for albumin is low (200–400 μM) and comparable to the low affinity binding observed for a number of drugs, e.g., aspirin, penicillin *(83–85)*. Serum protein binding, therefore, provides a repository for these drugs and prevents rapid renal excretion. As serum protein binding is saturable at higher doses, intact oligomer may be found in urine *(89,108)*. Studies in our laboratory suggest that, in rats, oligonucleotides administered intravenously at doses of 15–20 mg/kg saturate the serum protein binding capacity (Leeds, unpublished data).

Phosphorothioate oligonucleotides are rapidly and extensively absorbed after parenteral administration. For example, in rats, after an intradermal dose 3.6 mg/kg of ^{14}C-ISIS 2105 (a 20-mer phosphorothioate), approx 70% of the dose was absorbed within 4 h and total systemic bioavailability was in excess of 90% *(12)*. After intradermal injection in humans, absorption of ISIS 2105 was similar to that observed in rats *(8)*. Subcutaneous administration to rats and monkeys results in somewhat lower bioavailability and greater distribution to lymph as would be expected (Leeds, unpublished observations).

Distribution of phosphorothioate oligonucleotides from blood after absorption or intravenous (iv) administration is extremely rapid. We have reported distribution half-lives of less than 1 h, and similar data have been reported by others *(11,12,89,108)*. Blood and plasma clearance is multiexponential, with a terminal elimination half-life from 40–60 h in all species except humans. The terminal elimination half-life may be somewhat longer in humans *(8)*.

Phosphorothioates distribute broadly to all peripheral tissues. Liver, kidney, bone marrow, skeletal muscle, and skin accumulate the highest percentage of a dose, but other tissues display small quantities of drug *(11,12)*. No evidence of significant penetration of the blood-brain barrier has been reported. The rates of incorporation and clearance from tissues vary as a function of the organ studied: liver accumulates drug most rapidly (20% of a dose within 1–2 h) and other tissues accumulate drug more slowly. Similarly, elimination of drug is more rapid from liver than any other tissue, e.g., terminal half-life in liver, 62 h; in renal medulla, 156 h. The distribution into the kidney has been studied more extensively; drug has been shown to be present in Bowman's capsule, the proximal convoluted tubule, the bush border membrane, and within renal tubular epithelial cells (109). The data suggested that the oligonucleotides are filtered by the glomerulus, then reabsorbed by the proximal convoluted tubule epithelial cells. Moreover, the authors suggested that reabsorption might be mediated by interactions with specific proteins in the bush border membranes.

At relatively low doses, clearance of phosphorothioate oligonucleotides is primarily caused by metabolism (11,12,108). Metabolism is mediated by exo- and endonucleases that result in shorter oligonucleotides and, ultimately, nucleosides that are degraded by normal metabolic pathways. Although no direct evidence of base excision or modification has been reported, these are theoretical possibilities that may occur. In one study, radioactive material of larger molecular weight was observed in urine, but was not fully characterized (89). Clearly, the potential for conjugation reactions and extension of oligonucleotides via these drugs serving as primers for polymerases must be explored in more detail. In a thorough study, 20 nucleotide phosphodiester and phosphorothioate oligonucleotides were administered intravenously at a dose of 6 mg/kg to mice. The oligonucleotides were internally labeled with ^{3}H-CH$_3$ by methylation of an internal deoxycytidine residue using *HhaI* methylase and S-(^{3}H) adenosyl methionine (95). The observations for the phosphorothioate oligonucleotide were entirely consistent with those made in our studies. Additionally, in this study, autoradiographic analyses showed drug in renal cortical cells (95).

One study of prolonged infusions of a phosphorothioate oligonucleotide in humans has been reported (110). In this study, five patients with leukemia were given 10-d iv infusions at a dose of 0.05 mg/kg/h. Elimination half-lives reportedly varied from 5.9–14.7 d. Urinary recovery of radioactivity was reported to be 30–60% of the total dose, with 30% of the radioactivity being intact drug. Metabolites in urine included both higher and lower molecular weight compounds. In contrast, when GEM-91 (a 25-mer phosphorothioate oligodeoxynucleotide) was administered to humans as a 2-h iv infusion at a dose of 0.1 mg/kg, a peak plasma concentration of 295.8 mg/mL was observed at the cessation of the infusion. Plasma clearance of total radioactivity was biexponential with initial and terminal eliminations half-lives of 0.18 and 26.71 h, respectively. However, degradation was extensive and intact drug pharmacokinetic models were not presented. Nearly 50% of the administered radioactivity was recovered in urine, but most of the radioactivity represented degradates. In fact, no intact drug was found in the urine at any time (111).

In a more recent study in which the level of intact drug was carefully evaluated using capillary gel electrophoresis, the pharmacokinetics of ISIS 2302 (a 20-mer phosphorothioate oligodeoxynucleotide) after a 2-h infusion were determined. Doses from 0.06 mg/kg to 2.0 mg/kg were studied; the peak plasma concentrations were shown to increase linearly with dose, with the 2 mg/kg dose resulting in peak plasma concentrations of intact drug of approx 9.5 µg/mL. Clearance from plasma, however, was dose dependent, with the 2 mg/kg dose having a clearance of 1.28 mL min^{-1}kg^{-1}, whereas that of 0.5 mg/kg was 2.07 mL min^{-1}kg^{-1}. Essentially, no intact drug was found in urine.

Clearly, the two most recent studies differ from the initial report in several facets. Although a number of factors may explain the discrepancies, the most likely explanation is related to the evolution of assay methodology, not difference between compounds. Overall, the behavior of phosphorothioates in the plasma of humans appears to be similar to that in other species.

In addition to the pharmacological effects that have been observed after phosphorothioate oligonucleotides have been administered to animals (and humans), a number of other lines of evidence show that these drugs enter cells in organs. Autoradiographic, fluorescent, and immunohistochemical approaches have shown that these drugs are localized in endopromal convoluted tubular cells, various bone marrow cells, and cells in the skin and liver (109,112,113).

Perhaps more compelling and of more long-term value are studies recently reported showing the distribution of phosphorothioate oligonucleotides in the liver of rats treated intravenously with these drugs at various doses (114). This study showed that the kinetics and extent of the accumulation into Kuppfer, endothelial, and hepatocyte cell population varied and that, as doses were increased, the distribution changed. Moreover, the study showed that subcellular distribution also varied.

We have also performed oral bioavailability experiments in rodents treated with an H_2 receptor antagonist to avoid acid-mediated depurination or precipitation. In these studies, very limited (<5%) bioavailability was observed (Crooke, unpublished observations). However, it seems likely that a principal limiting factor in the oral bioavailability of phosphorothioates may be degradation in the gut rather than absorption. Studies using everted rat jejunum sacs demonstrated passive transport across the intestinal epithelium (115). Further, studies using more stable 2′-methoxy phosphorothioate oligonucleotides showed a significant increase in oral bioavailability that appeared to be associated with the improved stability of the analogs (116).

In summary, pharmacokinetic studies of several phosphorothioates demonstrate that these are well absorbed from parenteral sites, distribute broadly to all peripheral tissues, do not cross the blood-brain barrier, and are eliminated primarily by slow metabolism. Thus, once a day or every other day, systemic dosing should be feasible. Although the similarities between oligonucleotides of different sequences are far greater than the differences, additional studies are required before determining whether there are subtle effects of sequence on the pharmacokinetic profile of this class of drugs.

4.5. Pharmacological Properties

4.5.1. MOLECULAR PHARMACOLOGY

Antisense oligonucleotides are designed to bind to RNA targets via Watson-Crick hybridization.

As RNA can adopt a variety of secondary structures via Watson-Crick hybridization, one useful way to think of antisense oligonucleotides is as competitive antagonists for self-complementary regions of the target RNA. Obviously, creating oligonucleotides with the highest affinity per nucleotide unit is pharmacologically important, and a comparison of the affinity of the oligonucleotide to a complementary RNA oligonucleotide is the most sensible comparison. In this context, phosphorothioate oligodeoxynucleotides are relatively competitively disadvantaged, as the affinity per nucleotide unit of oligomer is less than RNA (> −2.0°C T_m per unit) (117). This results in a requirement of at least 15–17 nucleotides in order to have sufficient affinity to produce biological activity (81).

Although multiple mechanisms are possible by which an oligonucleotide may terminate the activity of an RNA species to which it binds, examples of biological activity have been reported for only three of these mechanisms. Antisense oligonucleotides have been reported to inhibit RNA splicing, effect translation of mRNA, and induce degradation of RNA by RNase H *(17,22,27)*. Without question, the mechanism that has resulted in the most potent compounds and is best understood is RNase H activation. To serve as a substrate for RNase H, a duplex between RNA and a "DNA-like" oligonucleotide is required. Specifically, a sugar moiety in the oligonucleotide that induces a duplex conformation equivalent to that of a DNA-RNA duplex and a charged phosphate are required *(118)*. Thus, phosphorothioate oligodeoxynucleotides are expected to induce RNase H-mediated cleavage of the RNA when bound. As will be discussed later, many chemical approaches that enhance the affinity of an oligonucleotide for RNA result in duplexes that are no longer substrates for RNase H.

Selection of sites at which optimal antisense activity may be induced in a RNA molecule is complex, dependent on the terminating mechanism and influenced by the chemical class of the oligonucleotide. Each RNA appears to display unique patterns of sites of sensitivity. Within the phosphorothioate oligodeoxynucleotide chemical class, studies in our laboratory have shown antisense activity can vary from undetectable to 100% by shifting an oligonucleotide by just a few bases in the RNA target *(17,78,119)*. Although significant progress has been made in developing general rules that help define potentially optimal sites in RNA species, to a large extent, this remains an empirical process that must be performed for each RNA target and every new chemical class of oligonucleotides.

Phosphorothioates have also been shown to have effects inconsistent with the antisense mechanism for which they were designed. Some of these effects are caused by sequence or are structure specific. Others are a result of nonspecific interactions with proteins. These effects are particularly prominent in in vitro tests for antiviral activity as, often, high concentrations of cells, viruses, and oligonucleotides are coincubated *(15,120)*. Human immune deficiency virus (HIV) is particularly problematic as many oligonucleotides bind to the gp120 protein *(3)*. However, the potential for confusion arising from the misinterpretation of an activity as being caused by an antisense mechanism when, in fact, it is owing to nonantisense effects is certainly not limited to antiviral or in vitro tests *(121–123)*. These data urge caution and argue for careful dose response curves, direct analyses of target protein or RNA, and inclusion of appropriate controls before drawing conclusions concerning the mechanisms of action of oligonucleotide-based drugs. In addition to protein interactions, other factors, such as overrepresented sequences of RNA and unusual structures that may be adopted by oligonucleotides, can contribute to unexpected results *(3)*.

Given the variability in cellular uptake of oligonucleotides, the variability in potency as a function of binding site in an RNA target, and potential nonantisense activities of oligonucleotides, careful evaluation of dose-response curves and clear demonstration of the antisense mechanism are required before drawing conclusions from in vitro experiments. Nevertheless, numerous well-controlled studies have been reported in which antisense activity was conclusively demonstrated. As many of these studies have been reviewed previously, we believe that antisense effects of phosphorothioate oligodeoxynucleotides against a variety of targets are well documented *(1,9,56,78,124)*.

4.5.2. In Vivo Pharmacological Activities

A relatively large number of reports of in vivo activities of phosphorothioate oligonucleotides have appeared, documenting activities after both local and systemic administration *(125)*. However, only a few of these reports include sufficient studies to draw relatively firm conclusions concerning the mechanism of action. Consequently, I will review in some detail only a few reports that provide sufficient data. Local effects have been reported for phosphorothioate and methylphosphonate oligonucleotides. A locally applied phosphorothioate oligonucleotide designed to inhibit *c-myb* production was shown to inhibit intimal accumulation in the rat carotid artery *(126)*. In this study, a Northern blot analysis demonstrated a significant reduction in *c-myb* RNA in animals treated with the antisense compound, but showed no effect by a control oligonucleotide. In a recent study, the effects of the oligonucleotide were suggested to be caused by a nonantisense mechanism *(122)*. However, only one dose level was studied. Similar effects were reported for phosphorothioate oligodeoxynucleotides designed to inhibit cyclin-dependent kinases (CDC-2 and CDK-2). Again, the antisense oligonucleotide inhibited intimal thickening and cyclin-dependent kinase activity, whereas a control oligonucleotide had no effect *(127)*. Additionally, local administration of a phosphorothioate oligonucleotide designed to inhibit N-*myc* resulted in reduction in N-*myc* expression and slower growth of a subcutaneously transplanted human tumor in nude mice *(128)*.

Antisense oligonucleotides administered intraventricularly have been reported to induce a variety of effects in the central nervous system. Intraventricular injection of antisense oligonucleotides to neuropeptide-y-y1 receptors reduced the density of the receptors and resulted in behavioral signs of anxiety *(129)*. Similarly, an antisense oligonucleotide designed to bind to NMDA-R1 receptor channel RNA inhibited the synthesis of these channels and reduced the volume of focal ischemia produced by occlusion of the middle cerebral artery in rats *(129)*.

In a series of well-controlled studies, antisense oligonucleotides administered intraventricularly selectively inhibited dopamine type-2 receptor expression, dopamine type-2 receptor RNA levels, and behavioral effects in animals with chemical lesions. Controls included randomized oligonucleotides and the observation that no effects were observed on dopamine type-1 receptor or RNA levels *(130–132)*. This laboratory also reported the selective reduction of dopamine type 1 receptor and RNA levels with the appropriate oligonucleotide *(133)*.

Similar observations were reported in studies on AT-1 angiotensin receptors and tryptophan hydroxylase. In studies in rats, direct observations of AT-1 and AT-2 receptor densities in various sites in the brain after administration of different doses of phosphorothioate antisense, sense, and scrambled oligonucleotides were reported *(134)*. Again, in rats, intraventricular administration of phosphorothioate antisense oligonucleotide resulted in a decrease in tryptophan hydroxylase levels in the brain, whereas a scrambled control did not *(135)*.

Injection of antisense oligonucleotides to synaptosomal-associated protein-25 into the vitreous body of rat embryos reduced the expression of the protein and inhibited neurite elongation by rat cortical neurons *(136)*.

Aerosol administration to rabbits of an antisense phosphorothioate oligodeoxynucleotide designed to inhibit the production of antisense A_1 receptor has been reported to reduce receptor numbers in the airway smooth muscle and to inhibit adenosine, house dust mite allergen, and histamine-induced bronchoconstriction *(137)*. Neither control or oligonucleotide complementary to bradykinin B_2 receptors reduced the density of adenosine A_1 receptors, although the oligonucleotides complementary to bradykin in B_2 receptor mRNA reduced the density of these receptors.

In addition to local and regional effects of antisense oligonucleotides, a growing number of well-controlled studies have demonstrated systemic effects of phosphorothioate oligodeoxynucleotides. Expression of interleukin-1 in mice was inhibited by systemic administration of antisense oligonucleotides *(138)*. Oligonucleotides to the NF-κB p65 subunit administered intraperitoneally at 40 mg/kg every 3 d slowed tumor growth in mice transgenic for the human T-cell leukemia viruses *(139)*. Similar results with other antisense oligonucleotides were shown in another in vivo tumor model after either prolonged subcutaneous infusion or intermittent subcutaneous injection *(140)*.

Several recent reports further extend the studies of phosphorothioate oligonucleotides as antitumor agents in mice. In one study, a phosphorothioate oligonucleotide directed to inhibition of the *bcr-abl* oncogene was administered intravenously at a dose of 1 mg/day for 9 d intravenously to immunodeficient mice injected with human leukemic cells. The drug was shown to inhibit the development of leukemic colonies in the mice and to selectively reduce *bcr-abl* RNA levels in peripheral blood lymphocytes, spleen, bone marrow, liver, lungs, and brain *(19)*. However, it is possible that the effects on the RNA levels were secondary to effects on the growth of various cell types. In the second study, a phosphorothioate oligonucleotide antisense to the protooncogene *myb,* inhibited the growth of human melanoma in mice. Again, *myb* mRNA levels appeared to be selectively reduced *(141)*.

A number of studies from our laboratories have been completed that directly examined target RNA levels, target protein levels and pharmacological effects using a wide range of control oligonucleotides, and the effects on closely-related isotypes. Single and chronic daily administration of a phosphorothioate oligonucleotide designed to inhibit mouse protein kinase C-α, (PKC-α), selectively inhibited expression of protein kinase C PKC-α RNA in mouse liver without effects on any other isotype. The effects lasted at least 24 h postdose, and a clear dose response curve was observed with an ip dose of 10–15 mg/kg, reducing PKC-α RNA levels in liver by 50% 24 h postdose *(18)*.

A phosphorothioate oligonucleotide designed to inhibit human PKC-α expression selectively inhibited expression of PKC-α RNA and PKC-α protein in human tumor cell lines implanted subcutaneously in nude mice after iv administration *(142)*. In these studies, effects on RNA and protein levels were highly specific and observed at doses lower than 6 mg/kg. A large number of control oligonucleotides failed to show activity.

In a similar series of studies, Monia et al. demonstrated highly specific loss of human c-*raf* kinase RNA in human tumor xenografts and antitumor activity that correlated with the loss of RNA *(143,144)*.

Finally, a single injection of a phosphorothioate oligonucleotide designed to inhibit cAMP-dependent protein kinase type 1 was reported to selectively reduce RNA and protein levels in human tumor xenografts and to reduce tumor growth *(145)*.

Thus, there is a growing body of evidence that phosphorothioate oligonucleotides can induce potent systemic and local effects in vivo. More importantly, there are now a number of studies with sufficient controls and direct observation of target RNA and protein levels that suggest highly specific effects that are difficult to explain by any mechanism other than antisense. As would be expected, the potency of these effects varies depending on the target, the organ, and the endpoint measured, as well as the route of administration and the postdose time point when the effect is measured.

In conclusion, although it is of obvious importance to interpret in vivo activity data cautiously, and it is clearly necessary to include a range of controls and to evaluate the effects on target RNA and protein levels and control RNA and protein levels directly, it is difficult to argue with the conclusion that some effects have been observed in animals that are likely primarily caused by an antisense mechanism.

Additionally, in studies on patients with cytomegalovirus-induced retinitis, local injections of ISIS 2922 have resulted in impressive efficacy, although it is obviously impossible to prove the mechanism of action is antisense in these studies *(146)*. This drug has now been approved for commercialization by the FDA. Recently, ISIS 2302, an ICAM-1 inhibitor, was reported to result in statistically significant reductions in steroid doses and prolonged remissions in a small group of steroid-dependent patients with Crohn's disease. As this study was randomized, double-blinded, and included serial colonoscopies, it may be considered the first study in humans to demonstrate the therapeutic activity of an antisense drug after systemic administration *(147)*. Finally, ISIS 5132 has been shown to reduce c-*raf* kinase message levels in peripheral blood mononuclear cells of patients with cancer after iv dosing *(148)*.

4.6. Toxicological Properties

4.6.1. In Vitro

In our laboratory, we have evaluated the toxicities of scores of phosphorothioate oligodeoxynucleotides in a significant number of cell lines in tissue culture. As a general rule, no significant cytotoxicity is induced at concentrations below 100 μM oligonucleotide. With a few exceptions, no significant effect on macromolecular synthesis is observed at concentrations below 100 μM *(79,100)*.

Polynucleotides and other polyanions have been shown to cause release of cytokines *(149)*. Also, bacterial DNA species have been reported to be mitogenic for lymphocytes in vitro *(150)*. Furthermore, oligodeoxynucleotides (30–45 nucleotides in length) were reported to induce interferons and enhance natural killer cell activity *(151)*. In the latter study, the oligonucleotides that displayed natural killer cell (NK)-stimulating activity contained specific palindromic sequences and tended to be guanosine rich. Collectively, these observations indicate that nucleic acids may have broad immunostimulatory activity.

It has been shown that phosphorothioate oligonucleotides stimulate B lymphocyte proliferation in a mouse splenocyte preparation (analogous to bacterial DNA), and the response may underlie the observations of lymphoid hyperplasia in the spleen and lymph nodes of rodents caused by repeated administration of these compounds *(152)*. We also have evidence of enhanced cytokine release by immunocompetent cells when exposed to phosphorothioates in vitro *(153)*. In this study, both human keratinocytes and an in vitro model of human skin released interleukin 1-α when treated with 250 μM–1 mm of phosphorothioate oligonucleotides. The effects appeared to be dependent on the phosphorothioate backbone and independent of sequence or 2′-modification. In a study in which murine B lymphocytes were treated with phosphodiester oligonucleotides, B-cell activation was induced by oligonucleotides with unmethylated CpG dinucleotides *(154)*. This has been extrapolated to suggest that the CpG motif may be required for immune stimulation of oligonucleotide analogs such as phosphorothioates. This clearly is not the case regarding release of IL-1α from keratinocytes *(153)*. Nor is it the case regarding in vivo immune stimulation.

4.6.2. Genotoxicity

As with any new chemical class of therapeutic agents, concerns about genotoxicity cannot be dismissed, as little in vitro testing has been performed and no data from long-term studies of oligonucleotides are available. Clearly, given the limitations in our understanding about the basic mechanisms that might be involved, empirical data must be generated. We have performed mutagenicity studies on two phosphorothioate oligonucleotides, i.e., ISIS 2105 and ISIS 2922, and found them to be nonmutagenic at all concentrations studied (8).

Two mechanisms of genotoxicity that may be unique to oligonucleotides have been considered. One possible mechanism is that an oligonucleotide analog could be integrated into the genome and produce mutagenic events. Although integration of an oligonucleotide into the genome is conceivable, it is likely to be extremely rare. For most viruses, viral DNA integration is itself a rare event and, of course, viruses have evolved specialized enzyme-mediated mechanisms to achieve integration. Moreover, preliminary studies in our laboratory have shown that phosphorothioate oligodeoxynucleotides are generally poor substrates for DNA polymerases, and it is unlikely that enzymes such as integrases, gyrases, and topoisomerases (that have obligate DNA cleavage as intermediate steps in their enzymatic processes) will accept these compounds as substrates. Consequently, it would seem that the risk of genotoxicity caused by genomic integration is no greater, and probably less, than that of other potential mechanisms, for example, alteration of the activity of growth factors, cytokine release, nonspecific effects on membranes that might trigger arachidonic acid release, or inappropriate intracellular signaling. Presumably, new analogs that deviate significantly more from natural DNA would be even less likely to be integrated.

A second possible mechanism is the risk that oligonucleotides might be degraded to toxic or carcinogenic metabolites. However, metabolism of phosphorothioate oligodeoxynucleotides by base excision would release normal bases, which presumably would be nongenotoxic. Similarly, oxidation of the phosphorothioate backbone to the natural phosphodiester structure would also yield nonmutagenic (and probably nontoxic) metabolites. Finally, it is possible that phosphorothioate bonds could be hydrolyzed slowly, releasing nucleoside phosphorothioates that presumably would be rapidly oxidized to natural (nontoxic) nucleoside phosphates. However, oligonucleotides with modified bases and/or backbones may pose different risks.

4.6.3. IN VIVO

The acute LD_{50} in mice of all phosphorothioate oligonucleotides tested to date is in excess of 500 mg/kg (Kornbrust, unpublished observations). In rodents, we have had the opportunity to evaluate the acute and chronic toxicities of multiple phosphorothioate oligonucleotides administered by multiple routes (155,156). The consistent dose-limiting toxicity was immune stimulation manifested by lymphoid hyperplasia, spelnomegaly, and a multiorgan monocellular infiltrate. These effects were dose-dependent and occurred only with chronic dosing at doses >20 mg/kg. The liver and kidney were the organs most prominently affected by monocellular infiltrates. All of these effects appeared to be reversible and chronic intradermal administration appeared to be the most toxic route, probably because of high local concentrations of the drugs resulting in local cytokine release and initiation of a cytokine cascade. There were no obvious effects of sequence. Minor increases in liver enzyme levels and mild thrombocytopenia were observed at doses ≥100 mg/kg.

In monkeys, the toxicological profile of phosphorothioate oligonucleotides is quite different. The most prominent dose-limiting side effect is sporadic reductions in blood pressure associated with bradycardia. When these events are observed, they are often associated with activation of C-5 complement, and they are dose related and peak plasma concentration related; this appears to be related to the activation of the alternative pathway *(157)*. All phosphorothioate oligonucleotides tested to date appear to induce these effects through there may be slight variations in potency as a function of sequence and/or length *(156,158,159)*.

A second prominent toxicologic effect in monkeys is the prolongation of activated partial thromboplastin time. At higher doses, evidence of clotting abnormalities is observed. Again, these effects are dose and peak plasma-concentration dependent *(156,159)*. Although no evidence of sequence dependence has been observed, there appears to be a linear correlation between number of phosphorothioate linkages and potency between 18–25 nucleotides (Nicklin, P., unpublished observations). The mechanisms responsible for these effects are likely very complex, but preliminary data suggest that direct interactions with thrombin may be at least partially responsible for the effects observed *(160)*.

The toxicological profile differs in humans. When ISIS 2922 is administered intravitreally to patients with cytomegalovirus retinitis, the most common adverse event is anterior chamber inflammation that is easily managed with steroids. A relatively rare and dose-related adverse event is morphological changes in the retina associated with loss in peripheral vision *(146)*.

ISIS 2105 (a 20-mer phosphorothioate designed to inhibit the replication of human papilloma viruses that cause genital warts) is administered intradermally at doses as high as 3 mg/wart per wk for 3 wk; essentially no toxicities have been observed, including (remarkably) a complete absence of local inflammation (Grillone L., unpublished results).

Administration of 2-h intravenous infusions on every second day of ISIS 2302 at doses as high as 2 mg/kg resulted in no significant toxicities, including no evidence of immune stimulation and no hypotension. A slight, subclinical increase in APTT was observed at the 2 mg/kg dose *(161)*.

4.7. Therapeutic Index

Putting toxicities and their dose response relationships in a therapeutic context is particularly important, as considerable confusion has arisen concerning the potential utility of phosphorothioate oligonucleotides for selected therapeutic purposes deriving from unsophisticated interpretation of toxicological data. The immune stimulation induced by these compounds appears to be particularly prominent in rodents and unlikely to be dose-limiting in humans. We have not, to date, observed hypotensive events in humans. Thus, this toxicity appears to occur at lower doses in monkeys than in humans and certainly is not dose limiting in the latter.

We believe that the dose-limiting toxicity in man will be clotting abnormalities and this will be associated with peak plasma concentrations well in excess of 10 µg/mL. In animals, pharmacological activities have been observed with iv bolus doses from 0.006 mg/kg to 10–15 mg/kg depending on the target, the end point, the organ studied, and the postdose time-point when the effect is measured. Thus, it would appear that phosphorothioate oligonucleotides have a therapeutic index that supports their evaluation for a number of therapeutic indications.

4.8. Conclusions

Phosphorothioate oligonucleotides have outperformed many expectations. They display attractive parenteral pharmacokinetic properties. They have produced potent systemic effects in a number of animal models and, in many experiments, the antisense mechanism has been directly demonstrated as the hoped-for selectivity. Further, these compounds appear to display satisfactory therapeutic indices for many indications.

Nevertheless, phosphorothioates clearly have significant limits. Pharmacodynamically, they have relatively low affinity per nucleotide unit. This means that longer oligonucleotides are required for biological activity and that invasion of many RNA structures may not be possible. At higher concentrations, these compounds inhibit RNase H as well. Thus, the higher end of the pharmacologic dose response curve is lost. Pharmacokinetically, phosphorothioates do not cross the blood-brain barrier, are not significantly orally bioavailable and may display dose-dependent pharmacokinetics. Toxicologically, the release of cytokines, activation of complement, and interference with clotting will pose dose limits if they are encountered in the clinical setting.

As several clinical trials are in progress with phosphorothioates and other trials will be initiated shortly, we shall soon have more definitive information about the activities, toxicities, and value of this class of antisense drugs in humans.

5. THE MEDICINAL CHEMISTRY OF OLIGONUCLEOTIDES

5.1. Introduction

The core of any rational drug discovery program is medicinal chemistry. Although the synthesis of modified nucleic acids has been a subject of interest for some time, the intense focus on the medicinal chemistry of oligonucleotides dates, perhaps, to no more than 5–7 yr prior to this chapter. Consequently, the scope of medicinal chemistry has recently expanded enormously, but the biological data to support conclusions about synthetic strategies are only beginning to emerge.

Modifications in the base, sugar, and phosphate moieties of oligonucleotides have been reported. The subjects of medicinal chemical programs include approaches to create enhanced affinity and more selective affinity for RNA or duplex structures; the ability to cleave nucleic acid targets; enhanced nuclease stability, cellular uptake, and distribution; and in vivo tissue distribution, metabolism, and clearance.

5.2. Heterocycle Modifications

5.2.1. PYRIMIDINE MODIFICATIONS

A relatively large number of modified pyrimidines have been synthesized, incorporated into oligonucleotides, and evaluated. The principle sites of modification are C-2, C-4, C-5, and C-6. These and other nucleoside analogs have been thoroughly reviewed *(162)*. A brief summary of the analogs that displayed interesting properties follow.

Inasmuch as the C-2 position is involved in Watson-Crick hybridization C-2 modified pyrimidine containing oligonucleotides have shown unattractive hybridization properties. An oligonucleotide containing 2-thiothymidine was found to hybridize well to DNA and, in fact, even better to RNA ΔT_m 1.5°C modification (Swayze et al., unpublished results).

In contrast, several modifications in the 4-position that have interesting properties have been reported. 4-Thiopyrimidines have been incorporated into oligonucleotides with no significant negative effect on hybridization *(163)*. A bicyclic and an N4-methoxy analog of cytosine were shown to hybridize with both purine bases in DNA with T_m values approx equal to natural base pairs *(164)*. Additionally, a fluorescent base has been incorporated into oligonucleotides and shown to enhance DNA-DNA duplex stability *(165)*.

A large number of modifications at the C-5 position have also been reported, including halogenated nucleosides. Although the stability of duplexes may be enhanced by incorporating 5-halogenated nucleosides, the occasional mispairing with G and the potential that the oligonucleotide might degrade and release toxic nucleosides analogs cause concern *(162)*.

Furthermore, oligonucleotides containing 5-propynylpyrimidine modifications have been shown to enhance the duplex stability ΔT_m 1.6°C/modification, and support the RNase H activity. The 5-heteroarylpyrimidines were also shown to influence the stability of duplexes *(120,166)*. A more dramatic influence was reported for the tricyclic 2'-deoxycytidine analogs, exhibiting an enhancement of 2–5°C/modification depending on the positioning of the modified bases *(167)*. It is believed that the enhanced binding properties of these analogs are a result of extended stacking and increased hydrophobic interactions.

In general, modifications in the C-6 position of pyrimidines are highly duplex destabilizing *(168)*. Oligonucleotides containing 6-aza pyrimidines have been shown to reduce T_m by 1–2°C per modification, but to enhance the nuclease stability of oligonucleotides and to support RNase H-induced degradation of RNA targets *(162)*.

5.2.2. PURINE MODIFICATIONS

Although numerous purine analogs have been synthesized, when incorporated into oligonucleotides, they usually have resulted in destabilization of duplexes. However, there are a few exceptions where a purine modification had a stabilizing effect. A brief summary of some of these analogs is discussed later.

Generally, N1 modifications of purine moiety has resulted in destabilization of the duplex *(169)*, as have C-2 modifications. However, 2–6-diaminopurine has been reported to enhance hybridization by approx 1 °C per modification when paired with T *(170)*. Of the 3-position substituted bases reported to date, only the 3-deaza adenosine analog has been shown to have no negative effective on hybridization.

Modifications at the C-6 and C-7 positions have likewise resulted in only a few interesting bases from the point of view of hybridization. Inosine has been shown to have little effect on duplex stability, but because it can pair and stack with all four normal DNA bases, it behaves as a universal base and creates an ambiguous position in an oligonucleotide *(171)*. Incorporation of 7-deaza inosine into oligonucleotides was destabilizing, and this was considered to be caused by its relatively hydrophobic nature *(172)*. 7-Deaza guanine was similarly destabilizing, but when 8-aza-7-deaza guanine was incorporated into oligonucleotides, it enhanced hybridizations *(173)*. Thus, on occasion, introduction of more than one modification in a nucleobase may compensate for destabilizing effects of some modifications. 7-Iodo 7-deazaguanine residue was recently incorporated into oligonucleotides and shown to enhance the binding affinity dramatically (ΔT_m 10.0°C/modification when compared with 7-deazaguanine) *(174)*. The increase in T_m value was attributed to the hydrophobic nature of the modification, increased stacking interaction, and favorable pKa of the base.

In contrast, some C-8 substituted bases have yielded improved nuclease resistance when incorporated in oligonucleotides, but also seem to be somewhat destabilizing *(162)*.

5.2.3. OLIGONUCLEOTIDE CONJUGATES

Although conjugation of various functionalities to oligonucleotides has been reported to achieve a number of important objectives, the data supporting some of the claims are limited. Generalizations are not possible based on the data presently available.

5.2.3.1. Nuclease Stability. Numerous 3′-modifications have been reported to enhance the stability of oligonucleotides in serum *(169)*. Both neutral and charged substituents have been reported to stabilize oligonucleotides in serum and, as a general rule, the stability of a conjugated oligonucleotide tends to be greater as bulkier substituents are added. Inasmuch as the principle nuclease in serum is a 3′-exonuclease, it is not surprising that 5′-modifications have resulted in significantly less stabilization. Internal modifications of base, sugar, and backbone have also been reported to enhance nuclease stability at or near the modified nucleoside *(169)*. In a recent study, thiono triester (e.g., adamantyl, cholesteryl) modified oligonucleotides have shown improved nuclease stability, cellular association, and binding affinity *(175)*.

The demonstration that modifications may induce nuclease stability sufficient to enhance activity in cells in tissue culture and in animals has proven to be much more complicated because of the presence of 5′-exonucleases and endonucleases. In our laboratory, 3′-modifications and internal point modifications have not provided sufficient nuclease stability to demonstrate pharmacological activity in cells *(96)*. In fact, even a 5-nucleotide long phosphodiester gap in the middle of a phosphorothioate oligonucleotide resulted in sufficient loss of nuclease resistance to cause complete loss of pharmacological activity *(81)*.

In mice, neither a 5′-cholesterol nor 5′-C-18 amine conjugate altered the metabolic rate of a phosphorothioate oligodeoxynucleotide in liver, kidney, or plasma *(83)*. Furthermore, blocking the 3′- and 5′-termini of a phosphodiester oligonucleotide did not markedly enhance the nuclease stability of the parent compound in mice *(13)*. However, 3′-modification of a phosphorothioate oligonucleotide was reported to enhance its stability in mice relative to the parent phosphorothioate *(176)*. Moreover, a phosphorothioate oligonucleotide with a 3′-hairpin loop was reported to be more stable in rats than its parent *(175)*. Thus, 3′-modifications may enhance the stability of the relatively stable phosphorothioates sufficiently to be of value.

5.2.3.2. Enhanced Cellular Uptake. Although oligonucleotides have been shown to be taken up by a number of cell lines in tissue culture, with perhaps the most compelling data relating to phosphorothioate oligonucleotides, a clear objective has been to improve cellular uptake of oligonucleotides *(2,8)*. Inasmuch as the mechanisms of cellular uptake of oligonucleotides are still poorly understood, the medicinal chemistry approaches have been largely empirical and based on many unproven assumptions.

Because phosphodiester and phosphorothioate oligonucleotides are water soluble, the conjugation of lipophilic substituents to enhance membrane permeability has been a subject of considerable interest. Unfortunately, studies in this area have not been systematic and, at present, there is little information about the changes in physicochemical properties of oligonucleotides actually affected by specific lipid conjugates. Phospholipids, cholesterol and cholesterol derivatives, cholic acid, and simple alkyl chains have been conjugated to oligonucleotides at various sites in the oligonucleotide. The effects of these modifications on cellular uptake have been assessed using fluorescent or radiolabeled oligonucleotides, or by measuring pharmacological activities. From the perspective of medicinal chemistry, very few systematic studies have been performed. The activities of short alkyl chains, e.g., adamantine, daunomycin, fluorescein, cholesterol, and porphyrin-conjugated oligonucleotides, were compared in one study *(177)*. A cholesterol modification was reported to be more effective at enhancing uptake than the other substituents. It also seems likely that the effects of various conjugates on cellular uptake may be affected by the cell type and target studied. For example, we have studied cholic acid conjugates of phosphorothioate deoxyoligonucleotides or phosphorothioate 2′-methoxy oligonucleotides, and we observed enhanced activity against HIV and no effect on the activity of ICAM-directed oligonucleotides.

Additionally, polycationic substitutions and various groups designed to bind to cellular carrier systems have been synthesized. Although many compounds have been synthesized, the data reported to date are insufficient to draw firm conclusions about the value of these approaches or their structure-activity relationships *(169)*.

5.2.3.3. RNA Cleaving Groups. Oligonucleotide conjugates were recently reported to act as artificial ribonucleases, albeit in low efficiencies *(178)*. Conjugation of chemically reactive groups such as alkylating agents, photoinduced azides, prophine, and psoralene have been utilized extensively to effect a crosslinking of oligonucleotide and the target RNA. In principle, this treatment may lead to translation arrest. In addition, lanthanides and their complexes have been reported to cleave RNA by means of a hydrolytic pathway. Recently, a novel europium complex was covalently linked to an oligonucleotide and shown to cleave 88% of the complementary RNA at physiological pH *(179)*.

5.2.3.4. In Vivo Effects. To date, relatively few studies have been reported in vivo. The properties of a 5′-cholesterol and 5′-C-18 amine conjugates of a 20-mer phosphorothioate oligodeoxynucleotide have been determined in mice. Both compounds increased the fraction of an iv bolus dose found in the liver. The cholesterol conjugate, in fact, resulted in more than 80% of the dose accumulating in the liver. Neither conjugate enhanced stability in plasma, liver, or kidney *(83)*. Interestingly, the only significant change in the toxicity profile was a slight increase in effects on serum transamineses and the histopathological changes indicative of slight liver toxicity associated with the cholesterol conjugate *(180)*. A 5′-cholesterol phosphorothioate conjugate was also recently reported to have a longer elimination half-life, more potency, and the ability to induce greater liver toxicity in rats *(181)*.

5.2.4. SUGAR MODIFICATIONS

The focus of second-generation oligonucleotide modifications has centered on the sugar moiety. In oligonucleotides, the pentofuranose sugar ring occupies a central connecting manifold that also positions the nucleobases for effective stacking. A symposium series has been published on the carbohydrate modifications in antisense research that covers this topic in great detail *(182)*. Therefore, the content of the following discussion is restricted to a summary.

A growing number of oligonucleotides in which the pentofuranose ring is modified or replaced have been reported *(183)*. Uniform modifications at the 2'-position have been shown to enhance hybridization to RNA and, in some cases, to enhance nuclease resistance *(183)*. Chimeric oligonucleotides containing 2'-deoxyoligonucleotide gaps with 2'-modified wings have been shown to be more potent than parent molecules *(61)*.

Other sugar modifications include α-oligonucleotides, carbocyclic oligonucleotides, and hexapyranosyl oligonucleotides *(183)*. Of these, α-oligonucleotides have been the most extensively studied. These hybridize in parallel fashion to single-stranded DNA and RNA and are nuclease resistant. However, they have been reported to be oligonucleotides designed to inhibit Harvey ras (Ha-*ras*) expression. All these oligonucleotides support RNase H and, as can be seen, a direct correlation between affinity and potency exists.

A growing number of oligonucleotides in which the C-2'-position of the sugar ring is modified have been reported *(169,178)*. These modifications include lipophilic alkyl groups, intercalators, amphipathic amino-alkyl tethers, positively charged polyamines, highly electronegative fluoro or fluoro alkyl moities, and sterically bulky methylthio derivatives. The beneficial effects of a C-2'-substitution on the antisense oligonucleotide cellular uptake, nuclease resistance, and binding affinity have been well documented in the literature. In addition, excellent review articles have appeared in the last few years on the synthesis and properties of C-2'-modified oligonucleotides *(178,184–186)*.

Other modifications of the sugar moiety have also been studied including other sites as well as more substantial modifications. However, much less is known about the antisense effects of these modifications *(16)*.

2'-Methoxy-substituted phosphorothioate oligonucleotides have recently been reported to display enhanced oral bioavailability and to be more stable in mice than their parent compounds *(116,175)*. The analogs displayed tissue distribution similar to that of the parent phosphorothioate.

Similarly, we have compared the pharmacokinetics of 2'-propoxy modified phosphodiester and phosphorothioate deoxynucleotides *(83)*. As expected, the 2'-propoxy modification increased lipophilicity and nuclease resistance, and the 2'-propoxy phosphorothioate was too stable in murine liver or kidney to measure an elimination half-life.

Interestingly, the 2'-propoxy phosphodiester was less stable than the parent phosphorothioate in all organs—except the kidney in which the 2'-propoxy phosphodiester was remarkably stable. The 2'-propoxy phosphodiester did not bind to albumin significantly, whereas the affinity of the phosphorothioate for albumin was enhanced. The only difference in toxicity between the analogs was a slight increase in renal toxicity associated with the 2'-propoxy phosphodiester analog *(180)*.

Incorporation of the 2'-methoxyethyoxy group into oligonucleotides increased the T_m by 1.1°C per modification when hybridized to the complement RNA. In a similar manner, several other 2'-O-alkoxy modifications have been reported to enhance the affinity *(187)*. The increase in affinity with these modifications was attributed to the favorable gauche effect of the side chain and additional solvation of the alkoxy substituent in water.

More substantial carbohydrate modifications have also been studied. Hexose-containing oligonucleotides were created and found to have very low affinity for RNA *(188)*. Also, the 4'-oxygen has been replaced with sulfur. Although a single substitution of a 4'-thio-modified nucleoside resulted in destabilization of a duplex, incorporation of two 4′-thio-modified nucleosides increased the affinity of the duplex *(189)*. Finally, bicyclic sugars have been synthesized with the hope that preorganization into more rigid structures would enhance hybridization. Several of these modifications have been reported to enhance hybridization *(182)*.

5.2.5. BACKBONE MODIFICATIONS

Substantial progress in creating new backbones for oligonucleotides that replace the phosphate or the sugar-phosphate unit has been made. The objectives of these programs are to improve hybridization by removing the negative charge, enhance stability, and potentially improve pharmacokinetics.

Numerous modifications *(16,182)* have been made that replace phosphate, retain hybridization, alter charge, and enhance stability. Since these modifications are now being evaluated in vitro and in vivo, a preliminary assessment should be possible shortly.

Replacement of the entire sugar-phosphate unit has also been accomplished and the oligonucleotides produced have displayed very interesting characteristics. Peptide nucleic acid (PNA) oligonucleotides have been shown to bind to single-stranded DNA and RNA with extraordinary affinity and high sequence specificity. They have been shown to be capable of invading some double-stranded nucleic acid structures. PNA oligonucleotides can form triple-stranded structures with DNA or RNA.

PNA oligonucleotides were shown to be able to act as antisense and transcriptional inhibitors when microinjected in cells *(190)*. PNA oligonucleotides appear to be quite stable to nucleases and peptidases as well.

In the past 5–7 yr, enormous advances in the medicinal chemistry of oligonucleotides have been reported. Modifications at nearly every position in oligonucleotides have been attempted and numerous potentially interesting analogs have been identified. Although it is too early to determine which of the modifications may be most useful for particular purposes, it is clear that a wealth of new chemicals is available for systematic evaluation and that these studies should provide important insights into the SAR of oligonucleotide analogs.

5.3. Conclusions

Although many questions about antisense remain to be answered, progress has continued to be gratifying. As more is learned, we will understand more of the factors that determine whether an oligonucleotide actually works via antisense mechanisms. We should also have the opportunity to learn a great deal more about this class of drugs as additional studies are completed in humans.

ACKNOWLEDGMENTS

The author wishes to thank Donna Musacchia for excellent typographic and administrative assistance.

REFERENCES

1. Crooke ST, Mirabelli, CK. *Antisense Research and Applications.* CRC Boca Raton, FL, 1993, p 579.
2. Crooke RM. In vitro toxicology and pharmacokinetics of antisense oligonucleotides. *Anti-Cancer Drug Design* 1991; 6(6):609–646.
3. Wyatt JR, Vickers TA, Roberson JL, et al. Combinatorially selected guanosine-quartet structure is a potent inhibitor of human immunodeficiency virus envelope-mediated cell fusion. *Proc Natl Acad Sci USA* 1994; 91(4):1356–1360.

4. Freier SM. Hybridization considerations affecting antisense drugs, in *Antisense Research and Applications* (Crooke ST, Lebleu B, eds). CRC, Boca Raton, FL, 1993, pp 67–82.

5. Ecker DJ. Strategies for invasion of RNA secondary structure, in *Antisense Research and Applications* (Crooke ST, Lebleu R, eds). CRC, Boca Raton, FL, 1993, pp 387–400.

6. Lima WF, Monia BP, Ecker DJ, Freier SM. Implication of RNA structure on antisense oligonucleotide hybridization kinetics. *Biochemistry* 1992; 31(48):12,055–12,061.

7. Ecker DJ, Vickers TA, Bruice TW, Freier SM, Jenison RD, Manoharan M, Zounes M. Pseudo-half-knot formation with RNA. *Science* (Washington, D.C., 1883-), 1992; 257(5072):958–961.

8. Crooke ST, Grillone LR, Tendolkar A. et al. A pharmacokinetic evaluation of ^{14}C-labeled afovirsen sodium in patients with genital warts. *Clin Pharmacol Ther* 1994; 56:641–646.

9. Crooke ST, Oligonucleotide therapeutics, in *Burger's Medicinal Chemistry and Drug Discovery* Vol. 1, M.E. Wolff, ed). Wiley, New York, 1995; pp 863–900.

10. Loke SL, Stein CA, Zhang XH, et al. Characterization of oligonucleotide transport into living cells, *Proc Natl Acad Sci USA* 1989; 86:3474–3478.

11. Cossum PA, Sasmor H, Dellinger D, et al. Disposition of the 14C-labeled phosphorothioate oligonucleotide ISIS 2105 after intravenous administration to rats. *J Pharmacol Exp Ther* 1993; 267(3):1181–1190.

12. Cossum PA, Truong L, Owens SR, Markham PM, Shea JP, Crooke ST. Pharmacokinetics of a 14C-labeled phosphorotioate oligonucleotide, ISIS 2105, after intradermal administration to rats. *J Pharmacol Exp Ther* 1994; 269(1):89–94.

13. Sands H, Gorey-Feret LJ, Ho SP, et al. Biodistribution and metabolism of internally 3H-labeled oligonucleotides. II. 3′,5—blocked oligonucleotides. *Molec Pharmacol* 1995; 47:636–646.

14. Cowsert LM. Antiviral activities of antisense oligonucleotides, in *Antisense Research and Applications* (Crooke ST, Lebleu B, eds). CRC Boca Raton, FL, 1993, pp 521–533.

15. Azad RF, Driver VB, Tanaka K, Crooke RM, Anderson KP. Antiviral activity of a phosphorothioate oligonucleotide complementary to RNA of the human cytomegalovirus major immediate-early region. *Antimicrob Agents Chemother* 1993; 37(9):1945–1954.

16. Crooke ST. *Therapeutic Applications of Oligonucleotides* Landes, RG. Austin, TX 1995, p 138.

17. Chiang MY, Chan H, Zounes, MA, Freier SM, Lima WF, Bennett CF. Antisense oligonucleotides inhibit intercellular adhesion molecule 1 expression by two distinct mechanisms. *Journal of Biological Chemistry* 1991; 266(27):18162–18171.

18. Dean NM, McKay R. Inhibition of protein kinase C-.alpha. expression in mice after systemic administration of phosphorothioate antisense oligodeoxynucleotides. *Proc Natl Acad Sci USA* 1994; 91(24):11,762–11,766.

19. Skorski T, Nieborowska-Skorska M, Nicolaides NC, et al. Suppression of Philadelphia leukemia cell growth in mice by *BCR-ABL* antisense oligodeoxynucleotide. *Proc Natl Acad Sci USA* 1994; 91:4504–4508.

20. Hijiya N, Zhang J, Ratajczak MZ, et al. Biologic and therapeutic significance of MYB expression in human melanoma. *Proc Natl Acad Sci USA* 1994; 91(10):4499–4503.

21. McManaway ME, Neckers LM, Loke SL, et al. Tumour-specific inhibition of lymphoma growth by an antisense oligodeoxynucleotide. *Lancet* 1990; 335:808–811.

22. Kulka M, Smith CC, Aurelian L, et al. Site specificity of the inhibitory effects of oligo(nucleoside methylphosphonate)s complementary to the acceptor splice junction of herpes simplex virus type 1 immediate early mRNA 4. *Proc Natl Acad Sci USA* 1989; 86:6868–6872.

23. Zamecnik PC, Goodchild J, Taguchi Y, Sarin PS. Inhibition of replication and expression of human T-cell lymphotropic virus type III in cultured cells by exogenous synthetic oligonucleotides complementary to viral RNA. *Proc Natl Acad Sci USA* 1986; 83:4143–4146.

24. Smith CC, Aurelian L, Reddy MP, Miller PS, Ts'o POP. Antiviral effect of an oligo(nucleoside methylphosphonate) complementary to the splice junction of herpes simplex virus type 1 immediate early pre-mRNAs 4 and 5. *Proc Natl Acad Sci USA* 1986; 83:2787–2791.

25. Dominski Z, Kole R. Restoration of correct splicing in thalassemic pre-mRNA by antisense oligonucleotides. *Proc Natl Acad Sci USA* 1993; 90:8673–8677.

26. Hodges D, Crooke ST. Inhibition of splicing of wild-type and mutated luciferase-adenovirus pre-mRNAs by antisense oligonucleotides. *Mol Pharmacol* 1995; 48(5):905–918.

27. Agrawal S, Goodchild J, Civeira MP, Thornton AH, Sarin PS, Zamecnik PC. Oligodeoxynucleoside phosphoramidates and phosphorothioates as inhibitors of human immunodeficiency virus [published erratum appears in Proc Natl Acad Sci U S A 1989 Mar;86(5):1504]. *Proc Natl Acad Sci USA* 1988; 85(19):7079–7083.

28. Lemaitre M, Bayard B, Lebleu B. Specific antiviral activity of a poly(L-lysine)-conjugated oligodeoxyribonucleotide sequence complementary to vesicular stomatitis virus N protein mRNA initiation site. *Proc Natl Acad Sci USA* 1987; 84(3):648–652.

29. Rosolen A, Whitesell L, Ikegaki N, Kennett RH, Neckers LM. Antisense inhibition of single copy N-*myc* expression results in decreased cell growth without reduction of c-myc protein in a neuroepithelioma cell line. *Cancer Res* 1990; 50(19):6316–6322.

30. Vasanthakumar G, Ahmed NK. Modulation of drug resistance in a daunorubicin resistant subline with oligonucleoside methylphosphonates [published erratum appears in Cancer Commun 1990;2(8):295]. *Cancer Commun* 1989; 1(4):225–232.

31. Sburlati AR, Manrow RE, Berger SL. Prothymosin alpha antisense oligomers inhibit myeloma cell division. *Proc Natl Acad Sci USA* 1991; 88:253–257.

32. Zheng H, Sahai BM, Kilgannon P, Fotedar A, Green DR. Specific inhibition of cell-surface T-cell receptor expression by antisense oligodeoxynucleotides and its effect on the production of an antigen-specific regulatory T-cell factor. *Proc Natl Acad Sci USA* 1989; 86(10):3758–3762.

33. Maier JA, Voulalas P, Roeder D, Maciag T. Extension of the life-span of human endothelial cells by an interleukin-1 alpha antisense oligomer. *Science* 1990; 249(4976):1570–1574.

34. Mirabelli CK, Bennett CF, Anderson K, Crooke ST. In vitro and in vivo pharmacologic activities of antisense oligonucleotides. *Anti-Cancer Drug Design* 1991; 6(6):647–661.

35. Cowsert LM, Fox MC, Zon G, Mirabelli CK. In vitro evaluation of phosphorothioate oligonucleotides targeted to the E2 mRNA of papillomavirus: potential treatment for genital warts. *Antimicrob Agents Chemother* 1993; 37(2):171–177.

36. Vickers T, Baker BF, Cook PD, et al. Inhibition of HIV-LTR gene expression by oligonucleotides targeted to the TAR element. *Nucl Acids Res* 1991; 19(12):3359–3368.

37. Saxena SK, Ackerman EJ. Microinjected oligonucleotides complementary to the α-sarcin loop of 28 S RNA abolish protein synthesis in *Xenopus* oocytes. *J Biol Chem* 1990; 265:3263–3269.

38. Walker K, Elela SA, Nazar RN. Inhibition of protein synthesis by Anti-5.8 S rRNA oligodeoxyribonucleotides. *J Biol Chem* 1990; 265:2428–2430.

39. Westermann P, Gross B, Hoinkis G. Inhibition of expression of SV40 virus large T-antigen by antisense oligodeoxyribonucleotides. *Biomed Biochim Acta* 1989; 48(1):85–93.

40. Baker BF. Decapitation of a 5′-capped oligoribonucleotide by o-phenanthroline:copper(II). *J Am Chem Soc* 1993; 115(8):3378–3379.

41. Baker BF, Miraglia L, Hagedorn CH. Modulation of eukaryotic initiation factor-4E binding to 5′-capped oligoribonucleotides by modified anti-sense oligonucleotides. *J Biol Chem* 1992; 267(16): 11,495–11,499.

42. Zamecnik PC, Stephenson ML. Inhibition of Rous sarcoma virus replication and cell transformation by a specific oligodeoxynbucleotide. *Proc Natl Acad Sci USA* 1978; 75:289–294.

43. Zerial A, Thuong NT, Helene C. Selective inhibition of the cytopathic effect of type A influenza viruses by oligodeoxynucleotides covalently linked to an intercalating agent. *Nucl Acids Res* 1987; 15(23):9909–9919.

44. Thuong NT, Asseline U, Monteney-Garestier T. Oligodeoxynucleotides covalently linked to intercalating and reactive substances: synthesis, characterization and physicochemical studies, in *Oligodeoxynucleotides: Antisense Inhibitors of Gene Expression* CRC, Boca Raton, FL, 1989, pp 25.

45. Helene C, Toulme J-J. Control of gene expression by oligonucleotides covalently linked to intercalating agents and nucleic acid-cleaving reagents, in *Oligonucleotides: Antisense Inhibitors of Gene Expression* (Cohen JS, ed). CRC, Boca Raton, FL, 1989, pp 137–172.

46. Crouch RJ, Dirksen M-L. Ribonucleases H, in *Nucleases* (Linn SM, Roberts RJ, eds). Cold Spring Harbor Laboratory Press, Cold Spring Harbor, NY, 1985, pp 211–241.

47. Crum C, Johnson JD, Nelson A, Roth D. Complementary oligodeoxynucleotide mediated inhibition of tobacco mosaic virus RNA translation in vitro. *Nucl Acids Res* 1988; 16(10):4569–4581.

48. Haeuptle MT, Frank R, Dobberstein B. Translation arrest by oligodeoxynucleotides complementary to mRNA coding sequences yields polypeptides of predetermined length. *Nucl Acids Res* 1986; 14(3):1427–1448.

49. Donis-Keller H. Site specific enzymatic cleavage of RNA. *Nucl Acids Res* 1979; 7.

50. Kawasaki AM, Casper MD, Freier SM, et al. Uniformly modified 2′-deoxy-2′-fluoro-phosphorothioate oligonucleotides as nuclease-resistant antisense compounds with high affinity and specificity for RNA targets *J Med Chem* 1993; 36(7):831–841.

51. Sproat BS, Lamond AI, Beijer B, Neuner P, Ryder U. Highly efficient chemical synthesis of 2′-O-methyloligoribonucleotides and tetrabiotinylated derivatives; novel probes that are resistant to degradation by RNA or DNA specific nucleases. *Nucl Acids Res* 1989; 17:3373–3386.

52. Morvan F, Rayner B, Imbach JL. Alpha-oligonucleotides: a unique class of modified chimeric nucleic acids. *Anticancer Drug Des* 1991; 6(6):521–529.

53. Gagnor C, Rayner B, Leonetti JP, Imbach JL, Lebleu B. Alpha-DNA.IX: Parallel annealing of alpha-anomeric oligodeoxyribonucleotides to natural mRNA is required for interference in RNase H mediated hydrolysis and reverse transcription. *Nucl Acids Res* 1989; 17(13):5107–5114.

54. Maher LJ III, Wold B, Dervan PB. Inhibition of DNA binding proteins by oligonucleotide-directed triple helix formation. *Science* 1989; 245:725–730.

55. Miller PS. Non-ionic antisense oligonucleotides, in *Oligodeoxynucleotides: Antisense Inhibitors of Gene Expression* (Cohen JS, ed). CRC, Boca Raton, FL, 1989, p 79.

56. Stein CA, Cheng Y-C. Antisense oligonucleotides as therapeutic agents-Is the bullet really magical? *Science* 1993; 261:1004–1012.

57. Cazenave C, Stein CA, Loreau N, et al. Comparative inhibition of rabbit globin mRNA translation by modified antisense oligodeoxynucleotides. *Nucl Acids Res* 1989; 17:4255–4273.

58. Quartin RS, Brakel CL, Wetmur JG. Number and distribution of methylphosphonate linkages in oligodeoxynucleotides affect exo- and endonuclease sensitivity and ability to form RNase H substrates. *Nucl Acids Res* 1989; 17:7253–7262.

59. Furdon PJ, Dominski Z, Kole R. RNase H cleavage of RNA hybridized to oligonucleotides containing methylphosphonate, phosphorothioate and phosphodiester bonds. *Nucl Acids Res* 1989; 17:9193–9204.

60. Eder PS, Walder JA. Ribonuclease H from K562 human erythroleukemia cells. *J Biol Chem* 1991; 266:6472–6479.

61. Monia BP, Lesnik EA, Gonzalez C, et al. Evaluation of 2'-modified oligonucleotides containing 2'-deoxy gaps as antisense inhibitors of gene expression. *J Biol Chem* 1993; 268(19):14,514–14,522.

62. Giles RV, Tidd DM. Increased specificity for antisense oligodeoxynucleotide targeting of RNA cleavage by RNase H using chimeric methylphosphonodiester/phosph odiester structures. *Nucl Acids Res* 1992; 20:763–770.

63. Walder RY, Walder JA. Role of RNase H in hybrid-arrested translation by antisense oligonucleotides. *Proc Natl Acad Sci USA* 1988; 85:5011–5015.

64. Minshull J, Hunt T. The use of single-stranded DNA and RNase H to promote quantitative 'Hybrid Arrest of Translation' of mRNA/DNA hybrids in reticulocyte lysate cell-free translations. *Nucl Acids Res* 1986; 14:6433–6451.

65. Gagnor C, Bertrand JR, Thenet S, et al. alpha-DNA. VI: Comparative study of alpha- and beta-anomeric oligodeoxyribonucleotides in hybridization to mRNA and in cell free translation inhibition. *Nucl Acids Res* 1987; 15(24):10,419–10,436.

66. Giles RV, Spiller DG, Tidd DM. Detection of ribonuclease H-generated mRNA fragments in human leukemia cells following reversible membrane permeabilization in the presence of antisense oligodeoxynucleotides. *Antisense Res Develop* 1995; 5:23–31.

67. Crooke ST, Lemonidis KM, Neilson L, Griffey R, Lesnik EA, Monia BP. Kinetic characteristics of Escherichia coli RNase H1: Cleavage of various antisense oligonucleotide-RNA duplexes. *Biochem J* 1995; 312(2):599–608.

68. Lima WF, Crooke ST. Binding affinity and specificity of Escherichia coli RNase H1: Impact on the kinetics of catalysis of antisense oligonucleotide-RNA hybrids. *Biochemistry* 1997; 36(2):390–398.

69. Lima WF, Venkatraman M, Crooke ST. The influence of antisense oligonucleotide-induced RNA structure on E. coli RNase H1 activity. *J Biol Chem* 1997; 272(29):18,191–18,199.

70. Wu H, Lima WF, Crooke ST. Molecular cloning and expression of cDNA for human RNase H. *Antisense Nucl Acid Drug Dev* 1998; 8(1):53–61.

71. Crooke ST. Progress toward oligonucleotide therapeutics: Pharmacodynamic properties. *FASEB J* 1993; 7(6):533–539.

72. Bruice TW, Lima WF. Control of complexity constraints on combinatorial screening for preferred oligonucleotide hybridization sites on structured RNA. *Biochemistry* 1997; 36(16):5004–5019.

73. Matveeva O, Felden B, Audlin S, Gesteland RF, Atkins JF. A rapid in vitro method for obtaining RNA accessibility patterns for complementary DNA probes: correlation with an intracellular pattern and known RNA structures. *Nucl Acids Res* 1997; 25(24):5010–5016.

74. Southern EM. *Ciba Foundation* Wiley, London, UK, 1977.

75. Ho SP, Bao Y, Lesher T, et al. Mapping of RNA accessible sites for antisense experiments with oligonucleotide libraries. *Nat Biotechnol* 1998; 16(1):59–63.

76. De Clercq E, Eckstein F, Merigan TC. Interferon induction increased through chemical modification of synthetic polyribonucleotide. *Science* 1969; 165:1137–1140.

77. Cohen JS. Phosphorothioate oligodeoxynucleotides, in *Antisense Research and Applications* (Crooke ST, Lebleu B, eds). CRC, Boca Raton, FL, 1993, pp 205–222.

78. Crooke ST. Therapeutic applications of oligonucleotides. *Bio/Technology* 1992; 10(8):882–886.

79. Crooke RM. Cellular uptake, distribution and metabolism of phosphorothioate, phosphodiester, and methylphosphonate oligonucleotides, in *Antisense Research and Applications* (Crooke ST, Lebleu B, eds). CRC, Boca Raton, FL, 1993, pp 427–449.

80. Crooke ST. Therapeutic applications of oligonucleotides. *Ann Rev Pharmacol Toxicol* 1992; 32:329–376.

81. Monia BP, Johnston JF, Ecker DJ, Zounes MA, Lima WF, Freier SM. Selective inhibition of mutant Ha-ras mRNA expression by antisense oligonucleotides. *J Biolog Chem* 1992; 267(28):19,954–19,962.

82. Sokol DL, Zhang X, Lu P, Gewirtz AM. Real time detection of DNA.cntdot.RNA hybridization in living cells. *Proc Natl Acad Sci USA* 1998; 95(20):11,538–11,543.

83. Crooke ST, Graham MJ, Zuckerman JE, et al. Pharmacokinetic properties of several novel oligonucleotide analogs in mice. *J Pharmacol Exp Ther* 1996; 277(2):923–937.

84. Joos RW, Hall WH. Determination of binding constants of serum albumin for penicillin. *J Pharmacol Exp Ther* 1969; 166:113.

85. Srinivasan SK, Tewary HK, Iversen PL. Characterization of binding sites, extent of binding, and drug interactions of oligonucleotides with albumin. *Antisense Res Dev* 1995; 5(2):131–139.

86. Hawley P, Gibson I. Interaction of oligodeoxynucleotides with mammilian cells. *Antisense Nucl Drug Dev* 1996; 6:185–195.

87. Crooke RM, Graham MJ, Cooke ME, Crooke ST. In vitro pharmacokinetics of phosphorothioate antisense oligonucleotides. *J Pharmacol Exp Ther* 1995; 275(1):462–473.

88. Gao W-Y, Han F-S, Storm C, Egan W, Cheng Y-C. Phosphorothioate oligonucleotides are inhibitors of human DNA polymerases and RNase H: Implications for antisense technology. *Mol Pharmacol* 1992; 41:223–229.

89. Agrawal S, Temsamani J, Tang JY. Pharmacokinetics, biodistribution, and stability of oligodeoxynucleotide phosphorothioates in mice. *Proc Natl Acad Sci USA* 1991; 88:7595–7599.

90. Majumdar C, Stein CA, Cohen JS, Broder S, Wilson SH. Stepwise mechanism of HIV Reverse transcriptase: primer function of phosphorothioate oligodeoxynucleotide. *Biochemistry* 1989; 28:1340–1346.

91. Cheng Y, Gao W, Han F. Phosphorothioate oligonucleotides as potential antiviral compounds against human immunodeficiency virus and herpes viruses. *Nucleosides and Nucleotides* 1991; 10:155–166.

92. Stein CA, Neckers M, Nair BC, Mumbauer S, Hoke G, Pal R. Phosphorothioate Oligodeoxycytidine Interferes with Binding of HIV-1 gp120 to CD4. *J Acquired Immune Defic Synd* 1991; 4:686–693.

93. Hartmann G, Krug A, Waller-Fontaine K, Endres S. Oligodeoxynucleotides enhance lipopolysaccharide-stimulated synthesis of tumor necrosis factor: dependence on phosphorothioate modification and reversal by Heparin. *Mol Med* 1996; 2(4):429–438.

94. Graham MJ, Freier SM, Crooke RM, Ecker DJ, Maslova RN, Lesnik EA. Tritium labeling of antisense oligonucleotides by exchange with tritiated water. *Nucl Acids Res* 1993; 21(16):3737–3743.

95. Sands H, Gorey-Feret LJ, Cocuzza AJ, Hobbs FW, Chidester D, Trainor GL. Biodistribution and metabolism of internally ^{3}H-labeled oligonucleotides. I. Comparison of a phosphodiester and a phosphorothioate. *Molec Pharmacol* 1994; 45:932–943.

96. Hoke GD, Draper K, Freier SM, et al. Effects of phosphorothioate capping on antisense oligonucleotide stability, hybridization and antiviral efficacy versus herpes simplex virus infection. *Nucl Acids Res* 1991; 19(20):5743–5748.

97. Wickstrom E. Oligodeoxynucleotide stability in subcellular extracts and culture media. *J Biochem Biophys Meth* 1986; 13:97–102.

98. Campbell JM, Bacon TA, Wickstrom E. Oligodeoxynucleoside phosphorothioate stability in subcellular extracts, culture media, sera and cerebrospinal fluid. *J Biochem Biophys Meth* 1990; 20:259–267.

99. Miyao T, Takakura Y, Akiyama T, Yoneda F, Sezaki H, Hashida M. Stability and pharmacokinetic characteristics of oligonucleotides modified at terminal linkages in mice. *Antisense Res Dev* 1995; 5(2):115–121.

100. Crooke RM. In vitro and in vivo toxicology of first generation analogs, in *Antisense Research and Applications* (Crooke ST, Lebleu B, eds). CRC, Boca Raton, FL, 1993, pp 471–492.

101. Neckers LM. Cellular internalization of oligodeoxynucleotides, in *Antisense Research and Applications* (Crooke ST, Lebleu B, eds). CRC, Boca Raton, FL, 1993, pp 451–460.

102. Chrisey LA, Walz SE, Pazirandeh M, Campbell JR. Internalization of oligodeoxyribonucleotides by *Vibrio parahaemolyticus*. *Antisense Res Dev* 1993; 3(4):367–381.

103. Tao LF, Marx KA, Wongwit W, Jiang Z, Agarwal S, Coleman RM. Uptake, intracellular distribution, and stability of oligodeoxynucleotide phosphorothioate by Schistosoma mansoni. *Antisense Res Dev* 1995; 5(2):123–129.
104. Bennett CF, Chiang MY, Chan H, Grimm S. Use of cationic lipids to enhance the biological activity of antisense oligonucleotides. *J Liposome Res* 1993; 3(1):85–102.
105. Bennett CF, Chiang MY, Chan H, Shoemaker JEE, Mirabelli CK. Cationic lipids enhance cellular uptake and activity of phosphorothioate antisense oligonucleotides. *Molec Pharmacol* 1992; 41(6):1023–1033.
106. Quattrone A, Papucci L, Schiavone N, Mini E, Capaccioli S. Intracellular enhancement of intact antisense oligonucleotide steady-state levels by cationic lipids. *Anti-Cancer Drug Design* 1994; 9:549–553.
107. Wang S, Lee RJ, Cauchon G, Gorenstein DG, Low PS. Delivery of antisense oligodeoxyribonucleotides against the human epidermal growth factor receptor into cultured KB cells with liposomes conjugated to folate via polyethylene glycol. *Proc Natl Acad Sci USA* 1995; 92:3318–3322.
108. Iversen P. In vivo studies with phosphorothioate oligonucleotides: pharmacokinetics prologue. *Anticancer Drug Des* 1991; 6(6):531–538.
109. Rappaport J, Hanss B, Kopp JB, et al. Transport of phosphorothioate oligonucleotides in kidney: Implications for molecular therapy. *Kidney Int* 1995; 47:1462–1469.
110. Bayever E, Iversen PL, Bishop MR, et al. Systemic administration of a phosphorothioate oligonucleotide with a sequence complementary to p53 for acute myelogenous leukemia and myelodysplastic syndrome: initial results of a phase I trial. *Antisense Res Dev* 1993; 3(4):383–390.
111. Zhang R, Yan J, Shahinian H, et al. Pharmacokinetics of an anti-human immunodeficiency virus antisense oligodeoxynucleotide phosphorothioate (GEM 91) in HIV-infected subjects. *Clin Pharmacol Ther* 1995; 58:44–53.
112. Takakura Y, Mahato RI, Yoshida M, Kanamaru T, Hashida M. Uptake characteristics of oligonucleotides in the isolated rat liver perfusion system. *Antisense Nucl Acid Drug Del* 1996; 6:177–183.
113. Butler M, Stecker K, Bennett CF. Cellular distribution of phosphorothioate oligodeoxynucleotides in normal rodent tissues. *Lab Invest* 1997; 77(4):379–388.
114. Graham MJ, Crooke ST, Monteith DK, et al. In vivo distribution and metabolism of a phosphorothioate oligonucleotide within rat liver after intravenous administration. *J Pharmacol Exp Ther* 1998; 286(1):447–458.
115. Hughes JA, Avrutskaya AV, Brouwer KLR, Wickstrom E, Juliano RL. Radiolabeling of methylphosphonate and phosphorothioate oligonucleotides and evaluation of their transport in everted rat jejunum sacs. *Pharmaceut Res* 1995; 12:817–824.
116. Agrawal S, Zhang X, Lu Z, et al. Absorption, tissue distribution and in vivo stability in rats of a hybrid antisense oligonucleotide following oral administration. *Biochem Pharmacol* 1995; 50(4):571–576.
117. Cook PD. Medicinal chemistry strategies for antisense research, in *Antisense Research and Applications* (Crooke ST, Lebleu B, eds). CRC, Boca Raton, FL, 1993, pp 149–187.
118. Mirabelli CK, Crooke ST. Antisense oligonucleotides in the context of modern molecular drug discovery and development, in *Antisense Research and Applications* (Crooke ST, Lebleu B, eds). CRC, Boca Raton, FL, 1993, pp 7–35.
119. Bennett CF, Crooke ST. Oligonucleotide-based inhibitors of cytokine expression and function. *Ther Modulation Cytokines* (Henderson BB, Mark W, ed). CRC, Boca Raton, FL, 1996, pp 171–193.
120. Wagner RW, Matteucci MD, Lewis JG, Gutierrez AG, Moulds C, Froehler BC. Antisense gene inhibition by oligonucleotides containing C-5 propyne pyrimidines. *Science* 1993; 260:1510–1513.
121. Barton CM, Lemoine NR. Antisense oligonucleotides directed against p53 have antiproliferative effects unrelated to effects on p53 expression. *Br J Cancer* 1995; 71:429–437.
122. Burgess TL, Fisher EF, Ross SL, et al. The antiproliferative activity of c-myb and c-myc antisense oligonucleotides in smooth muscle cells is caused by a nonantisense mechanism. *Proc Natl Acad Sci USA* 1995; 92:4051–4055.
123. Hertl M, Neckers LM, Katz SI. Inhibition of interferon-gamma-induced intercellular adhesion molecule-1 expression on human keratinocytes by phosphorothioate antisense oligodeoxynucleotides is the consequence of antisense-specific and antisense-non-specific effects. *J Invest Dermatol* 1995; 104:813–818.
124. Nagel KM, Holstad SG, Isenberg KE. Oligonucleotide pharmacotherapy: an antigene strategy. *Pharmacotherapy* 1993; 13(3):177–188.
125. Crooke ST, ed. *Antisense Research and Application.* [In: Handb. Exp. Pharmacol., 1998; 131] Springer, Berlin, Germany, 1998, p 630.

126. Simons M, Edelman ER, DeKeyser J-L, Langer R, Rosenberg RD. Antisense c-myb oligonucleotides inhibit arterial smooth muscle cell accumulation in vivo. *Nature* 1992; 359:67–70.

127. Abe J, Zhou W, Taguchi J, et al. Suppression of neointimal smooth muscle cell accumulation in vivo by antisense CDC2 and CDK2 oligonucleotides in rat carotid artery. *Biochem Biophys Res Commun* 1994; 198:16–24.

128. Whitesell L, Rosolen A, Neckers LM. In vivo modulation of N-myc expression by continous perfusion with an antisense oligonucleotide. *Antisense Res Develop* 1991; 1:343–350.

129. Wahlestedt C, Pich EM, Koob GF, Yee F, Heilig M. Modulation of anxiety and neuropeptide Y-Y1 receptors by antisense oligodeoxynucleotides. *Science* 1993; 259:528–531.

130. Weiss B, Zhou L-W, Zhang S-P, Qin Z-H. Antisense oligodeoxynucleotide inhibits D_2 dopamine receptor-mediated behavior and D_2 messenger RNA. *Neuroscience* 1993; 55:607–612.

131. Zhou L-W, Zhang S-P, Qin Z-H, Weiss B. In vivo administration of an oligodeoxynucleotide antisense to the D_2 dopamine receptor messenger RNA inhibits D_2 dopamine receptor-mediated behavior and the expression of D_2 dopamine receptors in mouse striatum. *J Pharmacol Exp Ther* 1994; 268:1015–1023.

132. Qin ZH, Zhou LW, Zhang SP, Wang Y, Weiss B. D2 dopamine receptor antisense oligodeoxynucleotide inhibits the synthesis of a functional pool of D2 dopamine receptors. *Mol Pharmacol* 1995; 48:730–737.

133. Zhang S-P, Zhou L-W, Weiss B. Oligodeoxynucleotide antisense to the D_1 dopamine receptor mRNA inhibits D_1 dopamine receptor-mediated behaviors in normal mice and in mice lesioned with 6-hydroxydopamine, *J Pharmacol Exp Ther* 1994; 271:1462–1470.

134. Ambuhl P, Gyurko R, Phillips MI. A decrease in angiotensin receptor binding in rat brain nuclei by antisense oligonucleotides to the angiotensin AT1 receptor. *Reg Pept* 1995; 59(2):171–182.

135. McCarthy MM, Nielsen DA, Goldman D. Antisense oligonucleotide inhibition of tryptophan hydroxylase activity in mouse brain, *Reg Pept* 1995; 59(2):163–170.

136. Osen-Sand A, Catsicas M, Staple JK, et al. Inhibition of axonal growth by SNAP-25 antisense oligonucleotides in vitro and in vivo. *Nature* 1993; 364:445–448.

137. Nyce JW, Metzger WJ. DNA antisense therapy for asthma in an animal model. *Nature* 1997; 385(6618):721–725.

138. Burch RM, Mahan LC. Oligonucleotides antisense to the interleukin 1 receptor mRNA block the effects of interleukin 1 in cultured murine and human fibroblasts and in mice. *J Clin Invest* 1991; 88:1190–1196.

139. Kitajima I, Shinohara T, Bilakovics J, Brown DA, Xiao X, Nerenberg M. Ablation of transplanted HTLV-1 tax-transformed tumors in mice by antisense inhibition of NF-KB. *Science* 1992; 258:1792–1795.

140. Higgins KA, Perez JR, Coleman TA, et al. Antisense inhibition of the p65 subunit of NF-kappaB blocks tumorigenicity and causes tumor regression. *Proc Natl Acad Sci USA* 1993; 90:9901–9905.

141. Hijiya N, Zhang J, Ratajczak MZ, et al. Biologic and therapeutic significance of *MYB* expression in human melanoma. *Proc Natl Acad Sci USA* 1994; 91:4499–4503.

142. Dean N, McKay R, Miraglia L, et al. Inhibition of growth of human tumor cell lines in nude mice by an antisense oligonucleotide inhibitor of protein kinase C-.alpha. expression. *Cancer Res* 1996; 56(15):3499–3507.

143. Monia BP, Johnston JF, Geiger T, Muller M, Fabbro D. Antitumor activity of a phosphorothioate oligodeoxynucleotide targeted against C-*raf* kinase. *Nature Med* 1995; 2(6):668–675.

144. Monia BP, Johnston JF, Sasmor H, Cummins LL. Nuclease resistance and antisense activity of modified oligonucleotides targeted to Ha-ras. *J Biol Chem* 1996; 271(24):14,533–14,540.

145. Nesterova M, Cho-Chung YS. A single-injection protein kinase A-directed antisense treatment to inhibit tumor growth. *Nature Med* 1995; 1:528–533.

146. Hutcherson SL, Palestine AG, Cantrill HL, Lieberman RM, Holland GN, Anderson KP. Antisense oligonucleotide safety and efficacy for CMV retinitis in AIDS patients. *35th ICAAC* 1995; 204.

147. Yacyshyn BR, Bowen-Yacyshyn MB, Jewell L, et al. A placebo-controlled trial of ICAM-1 antisense oligonucleotide in the treatment of Crohn's disease. *Gastroenterology* 1998; 114(6):1133–1142.

148. O'Dwyer PJ, Stevenson JP, Gallagher M, et al. Phase I/phamracokinetic/pharmacodynamic trial of *raf*-1 antisense ODN (ISIS 5132, CGP 69846A), in 34th *Ann Meeting of the Am Soc Clin Oncol* 1998, Los Angeles, CA.

149. Colby CJ. The induction of interferon by natural and synthetic polynucleotides. *Prog Nucl Acid Res Mol Biol* 1971; 11:1–32.

150. Messina JP, Gilkeson GS, Pisetsky DS. Stimulation of in vitro murine lymphocyte proliferation by bacterial DNA. *J Immunol* 1991; 147(6):1759–1764.

151. Kuramoto E, Yano O, Kimura Y, et al. Oligonucleotide sequences required for natural killer cell acti-vation. *Jpn J Cancer Res* 1992; 83(11):1128–1131.
152. Pisetsky DS, Reich CF. Stimulation of murine lymphocyte proliferation by a phosphorothioate oligonucleotide with antisense activity for herpes simplex virus. *Life Sci* 1994; 54:101–107.
153. Crooke RM, Crooke ST, Graham MJ, Cooke ME. Effect of antisense oligonucleotides on cytokine release from human keratinocytes in an in vitro model of skin. *Toxicol Appl Pharmacol* 1996; 140(1):85–93.
154. Krieg AM, Yi A-K, Matson S, et al. CpG motifs in bacterial DNA trigger direct B-cell activation. *Nature* 1995; 374:546–549.
155. Henry SP, Grillone LR, Orr JL, Brunner RH, Kornbrust DJ. Comparison of the toxicity profiles of ISIS 1082 and ISIS 2105, phosphorothioate oligonucleotides, following subacute intradermal admin-istration in Sprague-Dawley rats. *Toxicology* 1997; 116(1–3):77–88.
156. Henry SP, Taylor J, Midgley L, Levin AA, Kornbrust DJ. Evaluation of the toxicity profile of ISIS 2302, a phosphorothioate oligonucleotide in a 4-week study in CD-1 mice. *Antisense Nucl Acid Drug Dev* 1997; 7(5):473–481.
157. Henry SP, Giclas PC, Leeds J, et al. Activation of the alternative pathway of complement by a phos-phorothioate oligonucleotide: Potential mechansim of action. *J Pharmacol Exp Ther* 1997; 281:810–816.
158. Cornish KG, Iversen P, Smith L, Arneson M, Bayever E. Cardiovascular effects of a phosphorothioate oligonucleotide to p53 in the conscious rhesus monkey. *Pharmacol Comm* 1993; 3:239–247.
159. Galbraith WM, Hobson WC, Giclas PC, Schechter PJ, Agrawal S. Complement activation and hemo-dynamic changes following intravenous administration of phosphorothioate oligonucleotides in the monkey. *Antisense Res Dev* 1994; 4(3):201–206.
160. Henry SP, Novotny W, Leeds J, Auletta C, Kornbrust DJ. Inhibition of coagulation by a phosphoroth-ioate oligonucleotide. *Antisense Nucl Acid Drug Dev* 1997; 7(5):503–510.
161. Glover JM, Leeds JM, Mant TGK, et al. Phase I safety and pharmacokinetic profile of an intercellular adhesion molecule-1 antisense oligodeoxynucleotide (ISIS 2302), *J Pharmacol Exp Ther* 1997; 282(3):1173–1180.
162. Sanghvi YS. Heterocyclic base modifications in nucleic acids and their applications in antisense oligonucleotides, in *Antisense Research and Applications* (Crooke ST, Lebleu B, eds). CRC, Boca Raton, FL, 1993, pp 273–288.
163. Nikiforov TT, Connolly BA. The synthesis of oligodeoxynucleotides containing 4-thiothymidine residues. *Tetrahedron Lett* 1991; 32(31):3851–3854.
164. Lin PKT, Brown DM. Synthesis and duplex stability of oligonucleotides containing cytosine-thymine analogues. *Nucl Acids Res* 1989; 17:10,373–10,383.
165. Inoue H, Imura A, Ohtsuka E. Synthesis and hybridization of dodecadeoxyribonucleotides containing a fluorescent pyridopyrimidine deoxynucleoside. *Nucl Acids Res* 1985; 13(19):7119–7128.
166. Gutierrez AJ, Terhorst TJ, Matteucci MD, Froehler BC. 5-Heteroaryl-2'-deoxyuridine Analogs. Synthe-sis and incorporation into high-affinity oligonucleotides. *J Am Chem Soc* 1994; 116(13):5540–5544.
167. Lin K-Y, Jones RJ, Matteucci M. Tricyclic-2'-deoxycytidine analogs: Synthesis and incorporation into oligodeoxynucleotides which have endhanced binding to complementary RNA *J Am Chem Soc* 1995; 117:3873–3874.
168. Sanghvi YS, Hoke GD, Freier SM, et al. Antisense oligodeoxynucleotides: Synthesis, biophysical and biological evaluation of oligodeoxynucleotides containing modified pyrimidines. *Nucl Acids Res* 1993; 21(14):3197–3203.
169. Manoharan M. Designer antisense oligonucleotides: Conjugation chemistry and functionality place-ment, in *Antisense Research and Applications* (Crooke ST, Lebleu B, eds). CRC, Boca Raton, FL, 1993, pp 303–349.
170. Sproat BS, Iribarren AM, Garcia RG, Beijer B. New synthetic routes to synthons suitable for 2'-0-allyloligoribonucleotide assembly. *Nucl Acids Res* 1991; 19(4):733–738.
171. Martin FH, Castro MM, Aboul-ela F, Tinoco IJ. Base pairing involving deoxyinosine: implications for probe. *Nucl Acids Res* 1985; 13:8927–8938.
172. SantaLucia J Jr, Kierzek R, Turner DH. Functional group substitutions as probes of hydrogen bond-ing between GA mismatches in RNA internal loops. *J Am Chem Soc* 1991; 113(11):4313–4322.
173. Seela F, Kaiser K, Bindig U. 2'-Deoxy-.beta.-D-ribofuranosides of N6-methylated 7-deazaadenine and 8-aza-7-deazaadenine: solid-phase synthesis of oligodeoxyribonucleotides and properties of self-complementary duplexes. *Helv Chim Acta* 1989; 72(5):868–881.

174. Seela F, Ramzaeva N, Chen Y. Oligonucleotide duplex stability controlled by the 7-substituents of 7-deazaguanine bases. *Bioorgan Med Chem Lett* 1995; 5(24):3049–3052.

175. Zhang R, Lu Z, Zhang X, et al. In vivo stability and disposition of a self-stabilized oligodeoxynucleotide phosphorothioate in rats. *Clin Chem* 1995; 41(6, Pt. 1):836–843.

176. Temsamani J, Tang J, Padmapriya A, Kubert M, Agarwal S. Pharmacokinetics, biodistribution, and stability of capped oligodeoxynucleotide phosphorothioates in mice. *Antisense Res Develop* 1993; 3:277–284.

177. Boutorine A, Huet C, Saison T. Cell penetration studies of oligonucleotide derivatized with cholesterol and porphyrins, in *Nucleic Acid Therapeutics* 1991.

178. De Mesmaeker A, Haener R, Martin P, Moser HE. Antisense Oligonucleotides. *Acc Chem Res* 1995; 28(9):366–374.

179. Hall J, Hüsken D, Pieles U, Moser HE, Haner R. Efficient sequence-specific cleavage of RNA using novel europium complexes conjugated to oligonucleotides. *Chemistry & Biology* 1994; 1(3):185–190.

180. Henry SP, Zuckerman JE, Rojko J, et al. Toxicological properties of several novel oligonucleotide analogs in mice, *Anti-Cancer Drug Des* 1997; 12(1):1–14.

181. Desjardins J, Mata J, Brown T, Graham D, Zon G, Iversen P. Cholesteryl-conjugated phosphorothioate oligodeoxynucleotides modulate CYP2B1 expression in vivo. *J Drug Targeting* 1995; 2:477–485.

182. Sanghvi YS, Cook PD. Carbohydrate Modifications in Antisense Research. ACS Symp Series No. 580(Ed) (1994) Washington, D.C.: *Am Chem Soc* p 232.

183. Breslauer KJ, Frank R, Blocker H, Marky LA. Predicting DNA duplex stability from base sequence. *Proc Natl Acad Sci USA* 1986; 83:3746–3750.

184. Lamond AI, Sproat BS. Antisense oligonucleotides made of 2′-O-alkylRNA: Their properties and applications in RNA biochemistry. *FEBS Lett* 1993; 325:123–127.

185. Sproat BS, Lamond AI. 2′-O-alkyloligoribonucleotides, in *Antisense Research and Applications* (Crooke ST, Lebleu B, eds). CRC, Boca Raton, FL, 1993, pp 351–362.

186. Parmentier G, Schmitt G, Dolle F, Luu B. A convergent synthesis of 2′-O-methyl uridine. *Tetrahedron* 1994; 50(18):5361–5368.

187. Martin P. Ein neuer zugang zu 2′-O-alkylribonucleosiden und eigenschaften deren oligonucleotide. *Helv Chim Acta* 1995; 78:486–489.

188. Pitsch S, Krishnamurthy R, Bolli M, et. al. Pyranosyl-RNA ('p-RNA'): base-pairing selectivity and potential to replicate. *Helv Chim Acta* 1995; 78(7):1621–1635.

189. Bellon L, Leydier C, Barascut JL. 4-Thio RNA: A novel class of sugar-modified B-RNA., in *Carbohydrate Modifications in Antisense Research* (Sanghvi YS, Cook PD, eds). American Chemical Society: Washington, DC, 1994, pp 68–79.

190. Hanvey JC, Peffer NC, Bisi JE, et al. Antisense and antigene properties of peptide nucleic acids. *Science* 1992; 258:1481–1485.

16   Tumor Vaccines

Francesco M. Marincola, MD

CONTENTS

1. SUMMARY

Recent advances in the understanding of the molecular basis governing the interactions between the immune system and tumor cells in humans occurred mainly by studying patients with metastatic melanoma. Several melanoma-associated antigens (MA) and their epitopes recognized by HLA class I-restricted cytotoxic T cells (CTL) have been identified *(1,2)*. Most of these MA were noted to be nonmutated molecules expressed by most melanoma cell lines *(3)*. The demonstration that MA expression is shared by tumors from different patients stimulated interest in the development of MA-specific vaccines suitable for broad patient populations. Repeated in vitro stimulation of peripheral blood mononuclear cells (PBMC) with MA-derived epitopes demonstrated a high frequency of MA-reactive T cells in patients with melanoma *(4,5)*. The same epitopes could be utilized to enhance MA-specific T-cell reactivity in vivo when administered in combination with Incomplete Freund's Adjuvant (IFA) *(6,7)*. Epitope-based vaccinations however, have not shown strong clinical effectiveness unless combined with the administration of interleukin 2 (IL-2) *(8)*. Thus, paradoxically, it is possible to detect immunization against cancer but this does not seem to correspond to regression of tumors. In this chapter, we will discuss in detail some examples of clinical trials in which cancer vaccines have successfully induced immunization and critically evaluate the possible mechanisms that allowed tumors to escape immune destruction in the context of these studies.

2. INTRODUCTION AND HISTORICAL BACKGROUND

The immune response against pathogens is composed of a humural and a cellular arm. Although the former is directed toward extracellular pathogens, the latter is directed toward proteins produced by infectious agents replicating within permissive cells. Intracellular proteins produced by infectious agents are enzymatically degraded

From: *Drug Delivery Systems in Cancer Therapy*
Edited by: D. M. Brown © Humana Press Inc., Totowa, NJ

into short peptides (9–11 amino acids in length) and presented on the surface of infected cells in association with major histocompatibility complex (MHC) class I molecules. The complex of peptide and the MHC molecule (epitope) is what is required for triggering of T cells. Vaccines aimed at prevention of disease might be particularly effective because they can arm the host with neutralizing antibodies against subsequent infections, which may dramatically reduce the number of pathogens reaching the host's cells. After the pathogen is hidden in cells, the immune system relies predominantly on T-cell function *(9)*. Most known tumor antigens are intracellular molecules and it is, therefore, likely that the cellular response is the prevalent immunological defense of the organism against tumors *(10)*. Furthermore, experimental models suggest that the cellular rather than the humoral arm of the immune response plays a major role in the elimination of cancer *(11)*.

With the identification of the human T-cell growth factor, IL-2, stable human T-cell lines were expanded that could specifically recognize autologous tumor cells *(12)*. Because the 5-yr survival of patients with metastatic melanoma is less than 2%, and chemotherapy is not effective in improving it *(13)*, alternative approaches were attempted including the administration of IL-2 *(14)*. Administration of high-dose IL-2 resulted in 7% complete and 10% partial tumor regressions in patients with metastatic melanoma *(15)*. IL-2 does not have direct activity on cancer cells but works through stimulation of the immune system *(16)*. IL-2 could also be utilized to expand in vitro lymphokine-activated killer (LAK) cells generated by culturing PBMC *(17)* or tumor-infiltrating lymphocytes (TIL) expanded from single-cell suspensions of tumor *(18)*. Although able to kill tumor targets in vitro, LAK cells did not prove useful in randomized clinical trials for the treatment of patients with metastatic melanoma and renal cancer *(17)*. The adoptive transfer of ex vivo expanded TIL suggested, on the other hand, an additional advantage over the administration of IL-2 alone. Treatment of 86 patients with metastatic melanoma using TIL plus IL-2 resulted in 34% objective response rates in patients that included those who had previously failed treatment with high-dose IL-2 alone *(15)*. Because of the ease with which tumor-specific TIL could be obtained from melanoma patients, and their potential therapeutic relevance, melanoma has served as the prototype model for human tumor immunology.

2.1. The Identification of MA

Interest in the TIL phenomenon brought to the identification of MA *(12,18,19)*. Kawakami et al. had shown that the majority of TIL recognized "shared" antigens because they could kill melanoma cell lines from different patients that expressed the relevant MHC (HLA in humans) molecule *(20)*. This observation encouraged efforts to identify them with the assumption that they could be broadly used for antimelanoma immunization.

The identification of MA was done on the basis of their HLA restriction. The region encoding for the *HLA* class I molecules is located in chromosome 6 in humans and includes three genes termed *HLA-A, -B,* and *-C.* Each of the *HLA* genes is extremely polymorphic *(21)*. Thus, most individuals are heterozygous for each *HLA* gene and express six different *HLA* alleles on the cell surface. Most of the *HLA* polymorphism is clustered within the peptide-binding or T-cell receptor (TCR)-interacting domains of the HLA molecule *(22)*. Thus, HLA alleles are very stringent with respect to ligand specificity and the stringency of the requirements for TCR/HLA interaction is referred to as "HLA restriction." HLA-restricted recognition of MA was formally proved by transduction of the appropriate HLA allele (restriction element) for a particular TIL into melanoma cells which did not express such alleles. Recognition of the transfected tumor cell (but not the wild type) by the TIL constituted a formal proof of the HLA-restricted recognition of shared MA (20). For the identification of MA, a cDNA library from a melanoma cell line was established. Genes from the library were transfected into nonmelanoma cells. The transfected target cells were then tested for recognition by TIL specific for the melanoma from which the cDNA library was generated. The cDNA clones that caused recognition upon transfection were then isolated and sequenced for identification of the antigen (15,23).

Two major categories of MA were identified. The first category includes Tumor Differentiation Antigens (TDA) such as MART-1/MelanA, gp100/Pmel17, tyrosinase and TRP-1, and TRP-2. TDA are expressed by melanoma cells as well as normal melanocytes (24–27) but not other malignancies and normal tissues (28). Tumor-specific antigens (TSA) represent another large family of MA. TSA are not expressed by normal melanocytes, but are found in testes (cancer-testis antigens) and in a subset of patients with melanoma or other malignancies. TSA include the MAGE, BAGE, and GAGE families, and NY-ESO-1 (29). Although the identification of the first MA occurred in association with HLA-A*0101 (23), owing to the prevalence of HLA-A*0201 in the melanoma population (30,31) a significant number of MA were subsequently identified in association with this allele. These include MART-1/Melan A (32,33), gp100/Pmel 17 (34), tyrosinase (35), MAGE-3 (36), N-Acetylglucosaminyltransferase V (37), and NY-ESO-1 (38). Among them, MART-1 has received particular attention because of its "immunodominance" in the context of HLA-A*0201 (32). Approximately 90% of TIL originated from HLA-A*0201 patients recognize MART-1_{27-35} (39). The second MA most commonly recognized by TIL is gp100. Analysis of 217 fresh metastatic melanoma specimens showed heterogeneous expression of MART-1 and gp100 in vivo (26). However, the majority of lesions expressed these MA in at least 50–75% of their cells. Because of the frequency of their expression in tissues and their immunodominance in HLA-A*0201 patients, these two MA have been the main focus of vaccination efforts.

2.2. Peptide-Based Vaccines

Among multiple peptides, only MART-1_{27-35} was found to be consistently recognized by MART-specific, tumor-recognizing T cells (4). At least five HLA-A*0201-restricted peptides could be identified for the larger gp100 molecule that could be used in vitro to generate melanoma specific CTL (40). However, gp100 epitopes were not as efficient as MART-1_{27-35} for in vitro induction of anti-gp100 CTL. Thus, to enhance their immunogenicity, single amino acid substitutions were made to increase their binding affinity to HLA-A*0201. A peptide was identified (G9–209–2M: IMDQVPFSV, natural sequence: ITDQVPFSV), which had increased immunogenic reactivity in vitro and in vivo (7,41). Thus, MART-1_{27-35} or G9–209–2 have been mostly used for vaccination at National Institutes of Health.

Because HLA-A*0201 is the predominant allele in the melanoma population (30), peptide-based vaccinations restricted to HLA-A*0201 patients were initiated by subcutaneously administering MART-1_{27-35} emulsified in IFA. Comparison of in vitro-elicited reactivity of PBMC obtained before and after vaccination demonstrated strong enhancement of immune-competence toward MART-1 by the vaccination *(6)*. In a second trial, melanoma patients were treated with g209–2M alone or in combination with high-dose iv IL-2. Successful immunization could be documented in patients immunized with g209–2M; however, in spite of strong CTL responses, no clinical responses were observed unless IL-2 treatment was added *(8)*.

2.3. Dendritic Cell (DC)-Based Vaccines

Preclinical studies suggest that the administration of peptide alone for the treatment of cancer is not as efficient *(42)* as the addition of an appropriate adjuvant. Among adjuvants, DCs play a critical role because they are highly specialized antigen presenting cells (APC) with unique immunostimulatory properties. DCs can induce primary cellular immune responses *(43)*. Activated DCs are capable of migration from areas of antigen capture in the peripheral tissues to areas infiltrated with naïve T cells such as those of lymphoid organs. The key role of DCs in the initiation of immune responses has focused the attention of many investigators on the potential efficacy of these cells in tumor immunotherapy. Several groups have shown that DCs can be an efficient adjuvant for MHC class I-restricted antitumor sensitization in vivo *(44–50)*. Importantly, peptide-pulsed DCs appeared more efficient in inducing antitumor immunity than immunization with peptide alone *(45,48)* or emulsified in IFA *(49)*. The successes of TAA-pulsed DCs in murine models supported the use of autologous, peptide-pulsed DCs in recent clinical trials *(51,52)*.

DCs can be expanded from CD34+ hematopoietic progenitor cells in the presence of granulocyte/macrophage-colony-stimulating factor (GM-CSF) and matured to functional DCs with TNF-α *(53,54)*. DCs can be also generated from PBMC by culture of adherent cells for 5–7 d in medium containing GM-CSF and IL-4 *(55–58)*. A significant difference between the two methods of preparation is that, although CD34+ derived DCs can actively proliferate ex vivo, DCs derived from PBMC do not proliferate. Therefore, the number of DCs obtainable with the latter method is a constant fraction (~approx 10–20%) of the starting PBMC number *(59)*.

DCs cultured in IL-4 and GM-CSF could sensitize in vitro PBMC from melanoma patients against HLA-A*0201 restricted epitopes including MART-1$_{27-35}$ and g9-209-2M by a single exposure of responder cells to the relevant MA *(60)*. These findings stimulated a Phase I clinical trial in which patients with metastatic melanoma were immunized with DCs pulsed with MART-1 and gp100 epitopes. The MART-1$_{27-35}$ or the g9-209-2M peptides were separately pulsed onto the surface of autologous DCs, which were then delivered to patients within the same day in separate aliquots. Previously reported clinical studies had generally used minimal numbers of DCs, compared with the potential yield of DCs from a standard leukapheresis, and had applied different routes of administration *(51,52)*. A first cohort of patients (*n*=3) was treated with 6×10^7 DCs and a second cohort (*n*=5) with 2×10^8 DCs (both regimens, half of the DCs pulsed with MART-1$_{27-35}$ and half with gp-100-209-2M). In a final cohort under accrual (*n*=2), the latter dose of DC was administered in combination with IL-2 (720,000 IU/kg every 8 h). DCs could be safely administered without serious toxicity. Because of the minimal toxicity noted, it was concluded that the iv administration of DCs could safely be performed on an outpatient basis. One patient experienced a temporary partial response to DC treatment with regression of sc and pulmonary metastases; however, the duration of the response was short and correlated with loss of gp100 and MART-1 expression in the recurring metastases *(26)*. Monitoring of the systemic T-cell response pre-, postsecond, and postfourth vaccination could not identify strong immune reactivity compared with treatment with peptide alone.

Nestle et al. reported high rates of tumor regression in response to the intralymphatic administration of a small number of DCs prepared with methods similar to the those used in the NCI study and pulsed either with MAderived peptides or with tumor preparations *(51)*. It is possible that the different routes of administration used in the two studies could account for the differences noted in clinical outcome.

2.4. Whole Antigen Vaccines

Usage of MA-derived peptides requires knowledge of the amino acid sequence of the epitopic determinant specific for each HLA allomorph *(61)*. Various strategies have been reported to obviate this problem. The use of unfractionated acid-eluted tumor-derived peptides *(47)* has been proposed. Other strategies have taken advantage of the ability of APC to incorporate exogenous particles or messenger-RNA and present them to T cells in an MHC class I restricted fashion *(62,63)*. Bhardwaj et al. *(64)* demonstrated that DCs can be infected efficiently by influenza virus and they are permissive for the expression of viral products. We infected DCs with viral constructs encoding for MA to be used as immunogen in an autologous human system *(60,65)*. Using this model, we could show that DCs are permissive to pox virus-driven expression of MA. Virally induced MA into DCs were naturally processed through the endogenous pathway, presented as relevant epitopes bound to the appropriate HLA class I restriction element *(65)*, and efficiently induced MA-specific T cells *(60)*.

With virally infected DCs, we have extensively analyzed the stringent allele/epitope requirement characteristics of MART-1 immunodominance in the context of HLA-A*0201 *(66)*. Those studies demonstrated that autologous induction of MART-1 CTL by whole antigen processing and presentation by virally infected DC is restricted to a unique allele/ligand combination and is excluded by minimal changes in HLA structure. Thus, the use of whole antigen as an immunization strategy aimed at utilizing multiple epitopes associated with multiple restriction elements may not be useful for small molecular size proteins. Contrary to MART-1, DCs infected with rVV-gp 100 (five- to six-fold larger than MART-1) could elicit CTL against more than one epitope recognized in the context of HLA-A*0201 *(66)* or other HLA alleles *(67)*. Furthermore, multiple epitopes could be identified for tyrosinase in association with various HLA alleles using similar strategies *(68)*. Thus, future clinical studies should consider the use of whole antigen vaccines.

Adenoviral vectors have been tested in a Phase I clinical trial in which 54 patients received escalating doses of virus encoding either MART-1 or gp100 *(69)*. These recombinant vectors were administered either alone or in combination with iv IL-2. One of 16 patients receiving adeno-MART-1 experienced a complete response. Other objective responses (two complete and two partial responses) occurred in patients receiving IL-2 simultaneously. No consistent evidence of immunization to MART-1 or gp-100 could be demonstrated in contrast with the results described for peptide vaccines. Possibly, neutralizing antibodies generated by exposure to the virus eliminated the vector before it could generate antigen for immunization *(69)*.

3. ESCAPE FROM VACCINE-INDUCED IMMUNE RESPONSES

A remarkable breakthrough in the understanding of human tumor immunology resulted when studies demonstrated that the host can mount immune responses against antigens expressed by autologous cancer cells *(1,2,70)*. It was previously believed that the immune system could control tumor growth by recognizing as foreign "new" molecules expressed by tumor cells *(71,72)*. Obviously, self/nonself-discrimination does not apply broadly to tumor immunology because most identifiable immune responses against cancer are directed against self-molecules *(1,2,70)*.

MA-specific vaccination studies have shown that immunization induces detectable MA-specific CTL responses *(6–8)* but does not yield the clinical responses predicted by murine models. Human treatments deal with the polymorphic nature of tumors and the human immune system. Furthermore, the extreme heterogeneity of cancer cells has to be acknowledged and, therefore, tumor escape mechanisms may play a bigger role in human disease than in prefabricated olygo-clonal murine models. Immune escape and immune tolerance are general terms that include a variety of mechanisms. Inadequate immune responses in patients with cancer and other chronic illness have been attributed to decreased T-cell receptor (TCR) signaling capacity *(73,74)*. However, there is no convincing evidence that cancer patients are immune compromised. Flu-specific CTL reactivity is not different between healthy controls and patients with melanoma *(5)*. Furthermore, MA-specific CTL reactivity is easier to induce in patients with melanoma than in nontumor-bearing individuals *(5,75)*. Deletion of T cells by excessive stimulation has been implicated in the induction of systemic, epitope-specific immune tolerance *(76–81)*. However, because MA-specific T cells can be activated and expanded in vivo by antigen-specific vaccines *(6–8)*, deletion of tumor reactive clones may not play a significant role in human cancers *(76,79,82–84)*.

Localization of MA-specific CTL at the tumor site is expected for their effector function. Adoptive transfer of [111]Indium-labeled TIL has shown that their localization is necessary for a clinical response to occur *(85)*. However, in some cases, although TIL home (i.e., localize) within the tumor, no regression is observed, suggesting that other factors within the tumor microenvironment may influence the status of T-cell activation or the sensitivity of tumor cells to them.

Paradoxically, TIL can be routinely expanded ex vivo from growing melanoma metastases and shown to be able to effectively kill in vitro tumor cells. Thus, TIL/tumor cell interactions observed in vitro do not explain in vivo phenomena. This discrepancy may reflect lack of sufficient stimulation in vivo as the expansion ex vivo of TIL requires incubation not only with tumor cells but also with IL-2. Matzinger's "danger model" *(86,87)* proposes an explanation for the coexistence of effector and target cells in tissues without the development of tumor rejection suggesting that the default interaction between tumor cells and host immune system is absent or minimal. This model suggests that immune responses start when tissue distress (danger; "signal one") is detected which provides a second signal bearer of the environmental conditions in which the immune interaction is occurring *(88,89)*. The second signal can be provided either by cytokines ("help") or by costimulatory molecules expressed by APC *(90)* during tissue distress. Cancer cells do not constitutively express costimulatory molecules and do not secrete immune stimulatory cytokines. Thus, by offering only signal one, tumors might induce tolerance because the interaction of antigen-specific T cells with signal one in the absence of the second signal causes their deletion *(87)*.

Expression of MHC class I molecules is necessary for tumor recognition by CTL *(91–93)*. Thus, complete loss of expression of either MA or HLA has, as an undisputed consequence, loss of recognition by MA-specific CTL. It is, however, still controversial whether decreased expression of MA and/or HLA affects significantly tumor/host interactions in vivo. An extensive description of MA and HLA loss or downregulation has recently been prepared *(94)*. In humans, MA expression is quite heterogeneous. TSA are variably expressed in tumors *(23)* in correlation with a genome-wide demethylation process associated with tumor progression *(95–97)*. Treatment with demethylating agents such as 5-Aza-2′-deoxycytidine can induce expression of TSA and sensitize cell lines to lysis by TAA-specific CTL *(95,98,99)*. The ability of demethylating agents to restore recognition of tumor cells by CTL has not been exploited in clinical grounds because of the widespread effects that these agents have on normal cells *(95,98)*. TDA are more commonly expressed than TSA. Earlier studies detected MART-1/MelanA mRNA in all cell lines and melanoma lesions tested *(33)*. These studies, however, might have underestimated the heterogeneity of TDA protein expression. IHC analysis with mAb specific for gp100/Pmel17, MART-1/MelanA, and tyrosinase revealed that their expression is not as ubiquitous as suggested by molecular methods *(24,25,34,35,100–106)*. Furthermore, contrary to TSA, the frequency of TDA expression decreases with disease progression *(26,107–110)* probably because TSA are not related to neoplastic transformation. In particular, gp100/Pmel17 is less frequently expressed than MART-1/MelanA, which is less frequently expressed than tyrosinase *(24,26,27,109,110)*.

About 25% of synchronous metastases of patients with melanoma display significant differences in the percent of tumor cells expressing a given MA *(26,109,110)*. In addition, IHC of metastatic lesions has shown heterogeneity not only in the percentage of tumor cells expressing a MA but also in the level of MA expression by demonstrating differences in intensity of staining *(24,26,107)*. These findings have been corroborated in cell lines by analysis of TDA by FACS analysis *(111)* and by quantitative RT-PCR *(109)*. In vitro studies have also shown a correlation between variability of expression of MA and recognition of tumor cells by CTL *(25,111–113)*. Variation in the level of MA expression may explain the coexistence of MA-specific TIL in tissues expressing the target MA. Decreased expression of MA and/or HLA class I molecules has been noted in residual tumors following immunotherapy *(26,109,110,114)*. A recent analysis of pooled metastases from HLA-A*0201 melanoma patients showed a significant increase in frequency of gp100 negative lesions (29% of 155 lesions) after immunization compared with metastases analyzed before immunization (18% of 175) *(109)*. Another study has shown a reduced expression of the *ErbB-2* protooncogene in *HLA-A2*-expressing breast cancer lesions compared with *HLA-A2*-negative lesions *(115)*. Because this antigen has a well-defined *HLA-A2*-associated epitope, this finding suggests that lesions expressing HLA alleles other than *HLA-A2* may experience reduced immune pressure.

Within the tumor environment, immunological mediators—particularly cytokines *(116)*—may control host defenses. Wojtowicz-Praga suggested a predominant role of transforming growth factor-β (TGF-β) as a cause of "tumor-induced immune suppression" *(74)*. *In situ* expression of various isoforms of TGF (TGF-β1 –β2 and –β3) is common in tumors and correlates with progression of melanoma *(117–119)* and other skin tumors *(120)*. In murine models, TGF-β modulates melanoma growth by inducing immunosuppression of the host *(121,122)*. It is not clear, however, whether the immunosuppressive effects of TGF-β produced by tumor cells are limited to the tumor microenvironment or can affect the entire host immune system. In patients with melanoma, a correlation exists between plasma levels of TGF-β and disease progression *(74)*. This association, however, may simply reflect the higher tumor burden in patients with progressive disease. TGF-β has been shown to act synergistically to IL-10 to induce immune privilege *(123)*. It is not known whether IL-10 produced by melanoma cells plays a similar role by turning tumors into immune privileged sites.

Interactions between the vascular endothelium and tumor cells may also affect the outcome of the antitumor immune response *(124,125)*. By selectively recognizing a target tissue, CTL may trigger *in situ* an inflammatory cascade by producing TNF-α, IFN-γ, and other cytokines. Some tumors might be more sensitive than others to these inflammatory signals. As TNF-α is one of the cytokines secreted by activated CTL, it is reasonable to postulate that factors modulating its antitumor effects could play a significant role in determining the sensitivity of a tumor to T-cell attack. Recently, Wu et al. have shown that melanoma cell lines produce a cytokine called Endothelial-Monocyte-Activating Polypeptide II (EMAPII), which increases sensitivity of endothelial cells to TNF-α *(126)*. Melanoma cell lines secreting higher amounts of EMAPII are more sensitive in vivo to the antineoplastic effects of TNF-α.

Fas ligand *(FasL)* has been reported to be expressed in melanoma lesions *(127)* suggesting a novel mechanism of tumor escape through interaction with *Fas* on the surface of TIL. This model, however, is not supported by the available experimental data. Rivoltini et al. reported that TIL are insensitive to *FasL* *(128)* and, in murine models, the implantation of *FasL* transduced tumors does not abrogate antitumor immune responses *(129,130)*. Furthermore, a recent analysis of a large panel of melanoma cell lines found no evidence of *FasL* in melanoma *(131,132)*. Thus, the available information indicates that the expression of *FasL* in malignant lesions is minimal and its role in inducing immune escape is limited, as recognized by the same group which had originally proposed this theory *(133)*.

4. SUMMARY

The identification of MA and their respective CTL epitopes has raised interest in peptide-based vaccinations *(1)* as clinical studies have shown that MA-specific vaccines can powerfully enhance MA-specific CTL reactivity *(6–8)*. However, systemic CTL responses to the vaccines most often do not correspond to clinical regression leaving investigators with the paradoxical observation of identifiable CTL reactivity that is not capable of destroying the targeted tissues. Among the questions raised by this paradox stands the enigma of whether tumors resist immunotherapy because the immune response elicited is insufficient *(87)* or because tumor cells rapidly adapt to immune pressure by switching into less immunogenic phenotypes *(94)*. It is possible that a balance between subliminal immune responses and fading immunogenicity of tumors governs the fine equilibrium, allowing tumor survival in the immune competent host.

Antigen-specific vaccination protocols for the immunotherapy of melanoma, although disappointing in their clinical results, have given us the unique opportunity of comparing systemic T-cell responses with localization and status of activation of the same T cells in the target organ. At the same time an accurate analysis of the molecules targeted by the vaccination can be performed. Prospective analyses of large cohorts of patients undergoing these "immunologically simplified" treatments may allow, in the near future, an expedited understanding of the immune biology governing cancer rejection by the host.

REFERENCES

1. Rosenberg SA. Cancer vaccines based on the identification of genes encoding cancer regression antigens. *Immunol Today* 1997; 18:175–182.
2. Boon T, Coulie PG, Van den Eynde B. Tumor antigens recognized by T cells. *Immunol Today* 1997; 18:267–268.
3. Kawakami Y, Rosenberg SA. T-cell recognition of self peptides as tumor rejection antigens. *Immunol Res* 1996; 15:179–190.
4. Rivoltini L, Kawakami Y, Sakaguchi K, et al. Induction of tumor reactive CTL from peripheral blood and tumor infiltrating lymphocytes of melanoma patients by in vitro stimulation with an immunodominant peptide of the human melanoma antigen MART-1. *J Immunol* 1995; 154:2257–2265.
5. Marincola FM, Rivoltini L, Salgaller ML, Player M, Rosenberg SA. Differential anti-MART-1/MelanA CTL activity in peripheral blood of HLA-A2 melanoma patients in comparison to healthy donors: evidence for in vivo priming by tumor cells. *J Immunother* 1996; 19:266–277.
6. Cormier JN, Salgaller ML, Prevette T, et al. Enhancement of cellular immunity in melanoma patients immunized with a peptide from MART-1/Melan A [see comments]. *Cancer J Sci Am* 1997; 3:37–44.
7. Salgaller ML, Marincola FM, Cormier JN, Rosenberg SA. Immunization against epitopes in the human melanoma antigen gp100 following patient immunization with synthetic peptides. *Cancer Res* 1996; 56:4749–4757.
8. Rosenberg SA, Yang JC, Schwartzentruber D, et al. Immunologic and therapeutic evaluation of a synthetic tumor associated peptide vaccine for the treatment of patients with metastatic melanoma. *Nat Med* 1998; 4:321–327.
9. Zinkernagel RM. Immunology taught by viruses. *Science* 1996; 271:173–178.
10. Yewdell JW, Bennink JR. The binary logic of antigen processing and presentation to T cells. *Cell* 1990; 62:203–206.
11. Restifo, NP, Wunderlich JR. Principles of tumor immunity: biology of cellular immune responses, in *Biologic Therapy of Cancer.* 1st ed. (DeVita VT, Hellman S, Rosenberg SA, eds.) J.B. Lippincott, Philadelphia, PA, 1996 pp. 3–21.
12. Knuth A, Danowski B, Oettgen HF, Old LJ. T-cell-mediated cytotoxicity against autologous malignant melanoma: analysis with interleukin 2-dependent T-cell cultures. *Proc Natl Acad Sci USA* 1984; 81:3511–3515.
13. Mc CE, Mc CM. Systemic chemotherapy for the treatment of metastatic melanoma. *Semin Oncol* 1996; 23:744–753.
14. Marincola FM, Rosenberg SA. Biologic therapy with Interleukin-2. Clinical applications-melanoma, in *Biologic Therapy of Cancer.* 2 ed. (DeVita VT, Hellman S, Rosenberg SA, eds.) J.B. Lippincott, Philadelphia, PA, 1995, pp. 250–262.
15. Rosenberg SA. Keynote address: perspective on the use of Interleukin-2 in cancer treatment. *Cancer J Sci Am* 1997; 3:S2–S6.
16. Lotze MT. Interleukin-2: Basic principles, in *Biologic Therapy of Cancer.* 1 ed. (DeVita VT, Hellman S, Rosenberg SA, eds.) J.B.Lippincott, Philadelphia, 1991, pp. 123–141.
17. Rosenberg SA, Lotze MT, Yang JC, et al. Prospective randomized trial of high-dose interleukin-2 alone or in conjunction with lymphokine-activated killer cells for the treatment of patients with advanced cancer. *J Natl Cancer Inst* 1993; 85:622–632.
18. Rosenberg SA, Spiess P, Lafreniere R. A new approach to the adoptive immunotherapy of cancer with tumor-infiltrating lymphocytes. *Science* 1986; 233:1318–1321.
19. Itoh K, Tilden AB, Balch CM. Interleukin 2 activation of cytotoxic T-lymphocytes infiltrating into human metastatic melanomas. *Cancer Res* 1986; 46:3011–3017.
20. Kawakami Y, Zakut R, Topalian SL, Stotter H, Rosenberg SA. Shared human melanoma antigens. Recognition by tumor- infiltrating lymphocytes in HLA-A2.1-transfected melanomas. *J Immunol* 1992; 148:638–643.
21. Zemmour J, Parham P. HLA Class I nucleotide sequences, 1992. *Immunobiology* 1993; 187:70–101.

22. Bjorkman PJ, Parham P. Structure, function, and diversity of class I major histocompatibility complex molecules. *Annu Rev Biochem* 1990; 59:253–288.

23. van der Bruggen P, Traversari C, Chomez P, et al. A gene encoding an antigen recognized by cytolytic T lymphocytes on a human melanoma. *Science* 1991; 254:1643–1647.

24. Chen Y-T, Stockert E, Tsang S, Coplan KE, Old LJ. Immunophenotyping of melanomas for tyrosinase: implications for vaccine development. *Proc Natl Acad Sci USA* 1995; 92:8125–8129.

25. Marincola FM, Hijazi YM, Fetsch P, et al. Analysis of expression of the melanoma associated antigens MART-1 and gp100 in metastatic melanoma cell lines and in in situ lesions. *J Immunother* 1996; 19:192–205.

26. Cormier JN, Hijazi YM, Abati A, et al. Heterogeneous expression of melanoma-associated antigens (MAA) and HLA-A2 in metastatic melanoma in vivo. *Int J Cancer* 1998; 75:517–524.

27. Cormier JN, Abati A, Fetsch P, et al. Comparative analysis of the in vivo expression of tyrosinase, MART-1/Melan-A, and gp100 in metastatic melanoma lesions: implications for immunotherapy. *J Immunother* 1998; 21:27–31.

28. Fetsch PA, Kleiner D, Marincola FM, Abati A. Analysis of melanoma associated antigen MART-1 in normal tissues and in selected non-melanomatous neoplasms. *Modern Path* 1997; 10:43.

29. Chen YT, Scanlan MJ, Sahin U, et al. A testicular antigen aberrantly expressed in human cancers detected by autologous antibody screening. *Proc Natl Acad Sci USA* 1997; 94:1914–1918.

30. Marincola FM, Shamamian P, Rivoltini L, et al. HLA associations in the anti-tumor response against malignant melanoma. *J Immunother* 1996; 18:242–252.

31. Player MA, Barracchini KC, Simonis TB, et al. Differences in frequency distribution of HLA-A2 sub-types between American and Italian Caucasian melanoma patients: relevance for epitope specific vaccination protocols. *J Immunother* 1996; 19:357–363.

32. Kawakami Y, Eliyahu S, Delgado CH, et al. Cloning of the gene coding for a shared human melanoma antigen recognized by autologous T cells infiltrating into tumor. *Proc Natl Acad Sci USA* 1994; 91:3515–3519.

33. Coulie PG, Brichard V, Van Pel A, et al. A new gene coding for a differentiation antigen recognized by autologous cytolytic T lymphocytes on HLA-A2 melanomas [see comments]. *J Exp Med* 1994; 180:35–42.

34. Kawakami Y, Eliyahu S, Delgado CH, et al. Identification of a human melanoma antigen recognized by tumor-infiltrating lymphocytes associated with in vivo tumor rejection. *Proc Natl Acad Sci USA* 1994; 91:6458–6462.

35. Wolfel T, Van Pel A, Brichard V, et al. Two tyrosinase nonapeptides recognized on HLA-A2 melanomas by autologous cytolytic T lymphocytes. *Eur J Immunol* 1994; 24:759–764.

36. van der Bruggen P, Bastin J, Gajewski T, et al. A peptide encoded by human gene MAGE-3 and presented by HLA-A2 induces cytolytic T lymphocytes that recognize tumor cells expressing MAGE-3. *Eur J Immunol* 1994; 24:3038–3043.

37. Guilloux Y, Lucas S, Brichard VG, et al. A peptide recognized by human cytolytic T lymphocytes on HLA-A2 melanomas is encoded by an intron sequence of the N- acetylglucosaminyltransferase V gene. *J Exp Med* 1996; 183:1173–1183.

38. Jager E, Chen YT, Drijfhout JW, et al. Simultaneous humoral and cellular immune response against Cancer-Testis antigen NY-ESO-1: definition of human histocompatibility leukocyte antigen (HLA)-A2-binding peptide epitopes. *J Exp Med* 1998; 187:265–275.

39. Kawakami Y, Eliyahu S, Sakaguchi K, et al. Identification of the immunodominant peptides of the MART-1 human melanoma antigen recognized by the majority of HLA-A2- restricted tumor infiltrating lymphocytes. *J Exp Med* 1994; 180:347–352.

40. Salgaller ML, Afshar A, Marincola FM, Rivoltini L, Kawakami Y, Rosenberg SA. Recognition of multiple epitopes in the human melanoma antigen gp 100 by peripheral blood lymphocytes stimulated in vitro with synthetic peptides. *Cancer Res* 1995; 55:4972–4979.

41. Parkhurst MR, Salgaller ML, Southwood S, et al. Improved induction of melanoma reactive CTL with peptides from the melanoma antigen gp100 modified at HLA-A*0201 binding residues. *J Immunol* 1996; 157:2539–2548.

42. Vitiello A, Ishioka G, Grey HM, et al. Development of a lipopeptide-based therapeutic vaccine to treat chronic HBV infection. I. Induction of a primary cytotoxic T lymphocyte response in humans. *J Clin Invest* 1995; 95:341–349.

43. Steinman RM. The dendritic cell system and its role in immunogenicity. *Annu Rev Immunol* 1991; 9:271.

44. Porgador A, Snyder D, Gilboa E. Induction of antitumor immunity using bone marrow-generated dendritic cells. *J Immunol* 1996; 156:2918–2926.

45. Celluzzi CM, Mayordomo JI, Storkus WJ, Lotze MT, Falo LD Jr. Peptide-pulsed dendritic cells induce antigen-specific CTL- mediated protective tumor immunity. *J Exp Med* 1996; 183:283–287.

46. Young JW, Inaba K. Dendritic cells as adjuvants for class I major histocompatibility complex-restricted antitumor immunity. *J Exp Med* 1996; 183:7–11.

47. Zitvogel L, Mayordomo JI, Tjandrawan T, et al. Therapy of murine tumors with tumor peptide-pulsed dendritic cells: dependence on T cells, B7 costimulation, and T helper cell 1-associated cytokines [see comments]. *J Exp Med* 1996; 183:87–97.

48. Paglia P, Chiodoni C, Rodolfo M, Colombo MP. Murine dendritic cells loaded in vitro with soluble protein prime cytotoxic T lymphocytes against tumor antigen in vivo. *J Exp Med* 1996; 183:317–322.

49. Mayordomo JI, Zorina T, Storkus WJ, et al. Bone marrow-derived dendritic cells pulsed with synthetic tumour peptides elicit protective and therapeutic antitumour immunity. *Nat Med* 1995; 1:1297–1302.

50. Fields RC, Shimizu K, Mule JJ. Murine dendritic cells pulsed with whole tumor lysates mediate potent antitumor immune responses in vitro and in vivo. *Proc Natl Acad Sci USA* 1998; 95:9482–9487.

51. Nestle FO, Alijagic S, Gilliet M, et al. Vaccination of melanoma patients with peptide- or tumor lysate-pulsed dendritic cells. *Nat Med* 1998; 4:328–332.

52. Hsu FJ, Benike C, Fagnoni F, et al. Vaccination of patients with B-cell lymphoma using autologous antigen-pulsed dendritic cells. *Nat Med* 1996; 2:52–58.

53. Inaba K, Inaba M, Romani N, et al. Generation of large numbers of dendritic cells from mouse bone marrow cultures supplemented with granulocyte/macrophage colony-stimulating factor. *J Exp Med* 1992; 176:1693–1702.

54. Inaba K, Steinman RM, Pack MW, et al. Identification of proliferating dendritic cell precursors in mouse blood. *J Exp Med* 1992; 175:1157–1167.

55. Sallusto F, Lanzavecchia A. Efficient presentation of soluble antigen by cultured human dendritic cells is maintained by granulocyte/macrophage colony- stimulating factor plus interleukin 4 and downregulated by tumor necrosis factor alpha. *J Exp Med* 1994; 179:1109–1118.

56. Bender A, Sapp M, Schuler G, Steinman RM, Bhardwaj N. Improved methods for the generation of dendritic cells from nonproliferating progenitors in human blood. *J Immunol Methods* 1996; 196:121–135.

57. Kiertscher SM, Roth MD. Human CD14+ leukocytes acquire the phenotype and function of antigen-presenting dendritic cells when cultured in GM-CSF and IL-4. *J Leukoc Biol* 1996; 59:208–218.

58. Xu H. Dendritic cells differentiated from human monocytes through a combination of IL-4, GM-CSF and IFN-gamma exhibit phenotype and function of blood dendritic cells. *Adv Exp Med Biol* 1995; 378:75–78.

59. Panelli MC, Wunderlich J, Jeffries J, et al. Phase I study in patients with metastatic melanoma of immunization with dendritic cells presenting epitopes derived from the melanoma associated antigens MART-1 and gp100. *J Immunother* 1999; 23:487–498.

60. Kim CJ, Prevette T, Cormier JN, et al. Dendritic cells infected with poxviruses encoding MART-1/MelanA sensitize T lymphocytes in vitro. *J Immunother* 1997; 20:276–286.

61. van der Burg SH, Visseren MJ, Brandt RM, Kast WM, Melief JM. Immunogenicity of peptide bound to MHC class I molecules depends on the MHC-peptide complex stability. *J Immunol* 1996; 156:3308–3314.

62. Huang AY, Golumbek P, Ahmadzadeh M, Jaffee E, Pardoll D, Levitsky H. Role of bone marrow-derived cells in presenting MHC class I- restricted tumor antigens. *Science* 1994; 264:961–965.

63. Boczkowski D, Nair SK, Snyder D, Gilboa E. Dentritic cells pulsed with RNA are potent antigen-presenting cells in vitro and in vivo. *J Exp Med* 1996; 184:465–472.

64. Bhardwaj N, Bender A, Gonzalez N, Bui LK, Garrett MC, Steinman RM. Influenza virus-infected dendritic cells stimulate strong proliferative and cytolytic responses from human CD8+ T cells. *J Clin Invest* 1994; 94:797–807.

65. Kim CJ, Cormier JN, Roden M, et al. Use of recombinant poxviruses to stimulate anti-melanoma T cell reactivity. *Ann Surg Oncol* 1998; 5:64–76.

66. Bettinotti M, Kim CJ, Lee K-H, et al. Stringent allele/epitope requirements for MART-1/Melan A immunodominance: implications for peptide-based immunotherapy. *J Immunol* 1998; 161:877–889.

67. Skipper JC, Kittlesen DJ, Hendrickson RC, et al. Shared epitopes for HLA-A3-restricted melanoma-reactive human CTL include a naturally processed epitope from Pmel-17/gp100. *J Immunol* 1996; 157:5027–5033.

68. Yee C, Gilbert MJ, Riddell SR, et al. Isolation of tyrosinase-specific CD8+ and CD4+ T cell clones from the peripheral blood of melanoma patients following in vitro stimulation with recombinant vaccinia virus. *J Immunol* 1996; 157:4079–4086.

69. Rosenberg SA, Zhai Y, Yang JC, et al. 1-1-1. Immunization of patients with metastatic melanoma using recombinant adenoviruses encoding the MART-1 or gp100 melanoma antigens. *J Natl Cancer Inst* 90:1894–1899.

70. Old LJ, Chen YT. New paths in human cancer serology. *J Exp Med* 1998; 187:1163–1167.

71. Thomas L. *Cellular and Humoral Aspects of the Hypesensitive State* Hoeber, New York, 1959, pp. 529–552.

72. Burnet FM. The concept of immunological surveillance. *Prog Exp Tumor Res* 1970; 13:1–27.

73. Zea AH, Curti BD, Longo DL, et al. Alterations in T cell receptor and signal transduction molecules in melanoma patients. *Clin Cancer Res* 1995; 1:1327–1335.

74. Wojtowicz-Praga S. Reversal of tumor-induced immunosuppression: a new approach to cancer therapy [see comments]. *J Immunother* 1997; 20:165–177.

75. D'Souza S, Rimoldi D, Lienard D, Lejeune F, Cerottini JC, Romero P. Circulating Melan-A/Mart-1 specific cytolytic T lymphocyte precursors in HLA-A2+ melanoma patients have a memory phenotype. *Int J Cancer* 1998; 78:699–706.

76. Lauritzsen GF, Hofgaard PO, Schenck K, Bogen B. Clonal deletion of thymocytes as a tumor escape mechanism. *Int J Cancer* 1998; 78:216–222.

77. Toes RE, Blom RJ, Offringa R, Kast WM, Melief CJ. Enhanced tumor outgrowth after peptide vaccination. Functional deletion of tumor-specific CTL induced by peptide vaccination can lead to the inability to reject tumors. *J Immunol* 1996; 156:3911–3918.

78. Van Parijs L, Abbas AK. Homeostasis and self-tolerance in the immune system: turning lymphocytes off. *Science* 1998; 280:243–248.

79. Moskophidis D, Lechner F, Pircher HP, Zinkernagel RM. Virus persistence in acutely infected immunocompetent mice by exhaustion of antiviral cytotoxic effector T cells. *Nature* 1993; 362:758–761.

80. Alexander-Miller MA, Leggatt GR, Sarin A, Berzofsky JA. Role of antigen, CD8, and cytotoxic T lymphocyte (CTL) avidity in high dose antigen induction of apoptosis of effector CTL. *J Exp Med* 1996; 184:485–492.

81. Toes RE, Schoenberger SP, van der Voort EI, et al. Activation or frustration of anti-tumor responses by T-cell-based immune modulation. *Semin Immunol* 1997; 9:323–327.

82. Effros RB, Pawelec G. Replicative senescence of T cells: does the Hayflick Limit lead to immune exhaustion? *Immunol Today* 1997; 18:450–454.

83. Effros RB, Allsopp R, Chiu CP, et al. Shortened telomeres in the expanded CD28-CD8+ cell subset in HIV disease implicate replicative senescence in HIV pathogenesis. *AIDS* 1996; 10:F17–F22.

84. Toes RE, Offringa R, Blom RJ, Melief CJ, Kast WM. Peptide vaccination can lead to enhanced tumor growth through specific T-cell tolerance induction. *Proc Natl Acad Sci USA* 1996; 93:7855–7860.

85. Pockaj BA, Sherry RM, Wei JP, et al. Localization of 111indium-labeled tumor infiltrating lymphocytes to tumor in patients receiving adoptive immunotherapy. Augmentation with cyclophosphamide and correlation with response. *Cancer* 1994; 73:1731–1737.

86. Fuchs EJ, Matzinger P. Is cancer dangerous to the immune system? *Semin Immunol* 1996; 8:271–280.

87. Matzinger P. An innate sense of danger. *Semin Immunol* 1998; 10:399–415.

88. Schwartz RH. A cell culture model for T lymphocyte clonal anergy. *Science* 1990; 248:1349–1356.

89. Matzinger P. Tolerance, danger, and the extended family. *Annu Rev Immunol* 1994; 12:991–1045.

90. Jenkins MK, Schwartz RH. Antigen presentation by chemically modified splenocytes induces antigen-specific T cell unresponsiveness in vitro and in vivo. *J Exp Med* 1987; 165:302–319.

91. Wolfel T, Klehmann E, Muller C, Schutt KH, Meyer zum Buschenfelde KH, Knuth A. Lysis of human melanoma cells by autologous cytolytic T cell clones. Identification of human histocompatibility leukocyte antigen A2 as a restriction element for three different antigens. *J Exp Med* 1989; 170:797–810.

92. Crowley NJ, Darrow TL, Quinn-Allen MA, Seigler HF. MHC-restricted recognition of autologous melanoma by tumor- specific cytotoxic T cells. Evidence for restriction by a dominant HLA-A allele. *J Immunol* 1991; 146:1692–1699.

93. Rosenberg SA, Packard BS, Aebersold PM, et al. Use of tumor-infiltrating lymphocytes and interleukin-2 in the immunotherapy of patients with metastatic melanoma. A preliminary report. *N Engl J Med* 1988; 319:1676–1680.

94. Marincola FM, Jaffe EM, Hicklin DJ, Ferrone S. Escape of human solid tumors from T cell recognition: molecular mechanisms and functional significance. *Adv Immunol* 1999; 74:181–273.

95. De Smet C, De Backer O, Faraoni I, Lurquin C, Brasseur F, Boon T. The activation of human gene MAGE-1 in tumor cells is correlated with genome-wide demethylation. *Proc Natl Acad Sci USA* 1996; 93:7149–7153.

96. Bedford MT, van Helden PD. Hypomethylation of DNA in pathological conditions of the human prostate. *Cancer Res* 1987; 47:5274–5276.

97. Liteplo RG, Kerbel RS. Reduced levels of DNA 5-methylcytosine in metastatic variants of the human melanoma cell line MeWo. *Cancer Res* 1987; 47:2264–2267.

98. Weber J, Salgaller M, Samid D, et al. Expression of the MAGE-1 tumor antigen is up-regulated by the demethylating agent 5-aza-2′-deoxycytidine. *Cancer Res* 1994; 54:1766–1771.

99. Lee L, Wang RF, Wang X, et al. NY-ESO-1 may be a potential target for lung cancer immunotherapy. *Cancer J Sci Am* 1999; 5:20–25

100. Vennegoor C, Hageman P, Van Nouhuijs H, et al. A monoclonal antibody specific for cells of the melanocyte lineage. *Am J Pathol* 1988; 130:179–192.

101. Vennegoor C, Calafat J, Hageman P, et al. Biochemical characterization and cellular localization of a formalin-resistant melanoma-associated antigen reacting with monoclonal antibody NKI/C-3. *Int J Cancer* 1985; 35:287–295.

102. Kang X, Kawakami Y, el-Gamil M, et al. Identification of a tyrosinase epitope recognized by HLA-A24- restricted, tumor-infiltrating lymphocytes. *J Immunol* 1995; 155:1343–1348.

103. Brichard VG, Herman J, Van Pel A, et al. A tyrosinase nonapeptide presented by HLA-B44 is recognized on a human melanoma by autologous cytolytic T lymphocytes. *Eur J Immunol* 1996; 26:224–230.

104. Kawakami Y, Battles JK, Kobayashi T, et al. Production of recombinant MART-1 proteins and specific antiMART- 1 polyclonal and monoclonal antibodies: use in the characterization of the human melanoma antigen MART-1. *J Immunol Meth* 1997; 202:13–25.

105. Scott-Coombes DM, Whawell SA, Vipond MN, Crnojevic L, Thompson JN. Fibrinolytic activity of ascites caused by alcoholic cirrhosis and peritoneal malignancy. *Gut* 1993; 34:1120–1122.

106. Busam KJ, Iversen K, Coplan KA, et al. Immunoreactivity for A103, an antibody to melan-A (Mart-1), in adrenocortical and other steroid tumors. *Am J Surg Pathol* 1998; 22:57–63.

107. de Vries TJ, Fourkour A, Wobbes T, Verkroost G, Ruiter DJ, van Muijen GN. Heterogeneous expression of immunotherapy candidate proteins gp100, MART-1, and tyrosinase in human melanoma cell lines and in human melanocytic lesions. *Cancer Res* 1997; 57:3223–3229.

108. Busam KJ, Chen YT, Old LJ, et al. Expression of melan-A (MART1) in benign melanocytic nevi and primary cutaneous malignant melanoma. *Am J Surg Pathol* 1998; 22:976–982.

109. Riker A, Kammula US, Panelli MC, et al. Immune selection following antigen specific immunotherapy of melanoma. *Surgery* 1999; 126:112–120.

110. Scheibenbogen C, Weyers I, Ruiter D, Willhauck M, Bittinger A, Keilholz U. Expression of gp100 in melanoma metastases resected before or after treatment with IFN alpha and IL-2. *J Immunother* 1996; 19:375–380.

111. Cormier JN, Panelli MC, Hackett JA, et al. Natural variation of the expression of HLA and endogenous antigen modulates CTL recognition in an *in vitro* melanoma model. *Int J Cancer* 1999; 80:781–790.

112. Yoshino I, Peoples GE, Goedegebuure PS, Maziarz R, Eberlein TJ. Association of HER2/neu expression with sensitivity to tumor- specific CTL in human ovarian cancer. *J Immunol* 1994; 152:2393–2400.

113. Caux C, Massacrier C, Dezutter-Dambuyant C, et al. Human dendritic Langerhans cells generated in vitro from CD34+ progenitors can prime naive CD4+ T cells and process soluble antigen. *J Immunol* 1995; 155:5427–5435.

114. Jager E, Ringhoffer M, Karbach J, Arand M, Oesch F, Knuth A. Inverse relationship of melanocyte differentiation antigen expression in melanoma tissues and CD8+ cytotoxic-T-cell responses: evidence for immunoselection of antigen-loss variants in vivo. *Int J Cancer* 1996; 66:470–476.

115. Nistico' P, Moulese M, Mammi C, et al. Low frequency of ErbB-2 proto-oncogene overexpression in human leukocyte antigen A2 positive breast cancer patients. *J Natl Cancer Inst* 1997; 89:319–321.

116. Chouaib S, Asselin-Paturel C, Mami-Chouaib F, Caignard A, Blay JY. The host-tumor immune conflict: from immunosuppression to resistance and destruction. *Immunol Today* 1997; 18:493–497.

117. Van Belle P, Rodeck U, Nuamah I, Halpern AC, Elder DE. Melanoma-associated expression of transforming growth factor-beta isoforms. *Am J Pathol* 1996; 148:1887–1894.

118. Schmid P, Itin P, Rufli T. In situ analysis of transforming growth factor-beta s (TGF-beta 1, TGF-beta 2, TGF-beta 3), and TGF-beta type II receptor expression in malignant melanoma. *Carcinogenesis* 1995; 16:1499–1503.

119. Moretti S, Pinzi C, Berti E, et al. In situ expression of transforming growth factor beta is associated with melanoma progression and correlates with Ki67, HLA-DR and beta 3 integrin expression. *Melanoma Res* 1997; 7:313–321.

120. Schmid P, Itin P, Rufli T. In situ analysis of transforming growth factors-beta (TGF-beta 1, TGF-beta 2, TGF-beta 3) and TGF-beta type II receptor expression in basal cell carcinomas. *Br J Dermatol* 1996; 134:1044–1051.
121. Wojtowicz-Praga S, Verma UN, Wakefield L, et al. Modulation of B16 melanoma growth and metastasis by anti-transforming growth factor beta antibody and interleukin-2. *J Immunother* 1996; 19:169–175.
122. Park JA, Wang E, Kurt RA, Schluter SF, Hersh EM, Akporiaye ET. Expression of an antisense transforming growth factor-beta1 transgene reduces tumorigenicity of EMT6 mammary tumor cells. *Cancer Gene Ther* 1997; 4:42–50.
123. D'Orazio TJ, Niederkorn JY. A novel role for TGF-beta and IL-10 in the induction of immune privilege. *J Immunol* 1998; 160:2089–2098.
124. Herlyn M. Endhotelial cells as targets for tumor therapy. *J Immunother* 1999; 22(3), 185–185.
125. Desai SB, Libutti SK. Tumor angiogenesis and endothelial cell modulatory factors. *J Immunother* 5-1-1999; 22(3), 186–211.
126. Wu PC, Alexander HR, Huang J, et al. *In vivo* sensititivy of human melanoma to tumor necrosis factor (TNF)-α is determined by tumor production of the novel cytokine endothelial-monocyte activating polypeptide II (EMAII). *Cancer Res* 1999; 59:205–212.
127. Hahne M, Rimoldi D, Schroter M, et al. Melanoma cell expression of Fas (Apo-1/CD95) ligand: Implications for tumor immune escape. *Science* 1996; 274:1363–1366.
128. Rivoltini L, Radrizzani M, Accornero P, et al. Human melanoma-reactive CD4+ and CD8+ CTL clones resist Fas ligand-induced apoptosis and use Fas/Fas ligand-independent mechanisms for tumor killing. *J Immunol* 1998; 161:1220–1230.
129. Arai H, Gordon D, Nabel EG, Nabel GJ. Gene transfer of Fas ligand induces tumor regression in vivo. *Proc Natl Acad Sci USA* 1997; 94:13,862–13,867.
130. Seino K, Kayagaki N, Okumura K, Yagita H. Antitumor effect of locally produced CD95 ligand. *Nat Med* 1997; 3:165–170.
131. Shiraki K, Tsuji N, Shioda T, Isselbacher KJ, Takahashi H. Expression of Fas ligand in liver metastases of human colonic adenocarcinomas. *Proc Natl Acad Sci USA* 1997; 94:6420–6425.
132. Chappell DB, Zaks TZ, Rosenberg SA, Restifo NP. Human melanoma cells do not express Fas (Apo-1/Cd95) ligand. *Cancer Res* 1999; 59:59–62.
133. Rimoldi D, Muehlethaler K, Romero P, et al. Limited involvement of the Fas/FasL pathway in melanoma-induced apoptosis of tumor-specific T cells. *Proc Cancer Vacc Week* 1998; 1:3–82.

17

Diagnosis and Treatment of Human Disease Using Telomerase As a Novel Target

Lynne W. Elmore, PhD
and Shawn E. Holt, PhD

CONTENTS

1. INTRODUCTION

Telomerase has been associated with almost 90% of all malignant human cancers, making it the most prominent molecular marker known to date. Because of its association with malignancy, telomerase is also regarded as a novel diagnostic marker and a specific target for gene therapy or chemotherapy. This chapter provides a general overview of the telomerase field, its relationship to telomere biology, and the potential roles of telomeres and telomerase in human cancer diagnosis and treatment, as well as in treatment of age-associated disorders.

Normal human somatic cells have a limited replicative lifespan in culture, followed by a process known as cellular senescence or the Hayflick limit *(1)*. Unique structures at the end of the chromosomes (telomeres) are necessary for chromosomal integrity and overall genomic stability *(2)*. Vertebrate telomeres are composed of a hexameric sequence (TTAGGG) repeated for many kilobases *(3)*. Telomeres continuously shorten with successive cell divisions owing to the inability of normal DNA polymerases to replicate the ends of linear molecules. This "end replication problem" occurs on the lagging strand during DNA synthesis, leaving a gap between the final priming event and the end of the chromosome *(4,5)*. Without appropriate mechanisms to offset telom-

From: *Drug Delivery Systems in Cancer Therapy*
Edited by: D. M. Brown © Humana Press Inc., Totowa, NJ

ere shortening, normal human cells proliferate for a certain number of divisions, or population doublings (PDs), followed by growth arrest or cellular senescence (6–8).

The decline in proliferative capacity correlates with progressive telomere shortening in aging cells. This shortening is counterbalanced in specific germ-line cells, stem cells, and most immortal cells through the telomere lengthening activity of telomerase. The ribonucleoprotein, telomerase, provides the necessary enzymatic activity to restore telomere length (9). Telomerase utilizes its associated RNA component as a template for catalyzing DNA addition at the telomere (10,11). Telomerase is a reverse transcriptase that restores telomeres by adding G-rich repeats (TTAGGG for vertebrates) to the 3' single-stranded overhang at the end of the chromosomes. In humans, at least two components of telomerase are required for the synthesis of telomeric DNA: a protein catalytic subunit (hTERT) and an integral RNA template (hTR). hTERT is the limiting component for reconstituting telomerase activity in normal cells. This protein contains multiple reverse transcriptase motifs essential for enzymatic activity that are conserved among similar genes in diverse organisms such as *Saccharomyces cerevisiae* Est2 and *Euplotes aediculatus* p123. Because most normal cells that undergo senescence experience telomere shortening, telomere attrition has been proposed as a primary cause of cellular aging or senescence (12,13).

In the absence of telomerase, normal human cells in culture have a finite lifespan and undergo cellular senescence typically after 40 to 70 PDs. This stage of the cellular life cycle has become known as Mortality stage 1 (M1). The functions of normal tumor suppressor proteins, such as p53 and pRb, are required for the M1 block to cell division (13). The onset of M1 is thought to be primarily caused by shortened telomeres, which are recognized as damaged DNA. The ensuing DNA damage response involves the mechanistic action of p53 and pRb, along with a host of other cellular proteins. Viral oncoproteins like human papillomavirus type 16 E6 and E7 can block the progression to senescence (block M1) leading to an extended lifespan until affected cells reach Mortality stage 2 (M2) (14,15). M2 may be caused by extreme telomere shortening, where there exists a natural balance between cell division and cell death. For cells to become immortal, they must overcome the normal block to cell proliferation (M1), acquire additional mutations in the extended lifespan, and bypass crisis (M2) (13). The process of immortalization almost always requires the activation of telomerase to maintain structural integrity at the ends of the chromosomes (16).

The creation of the PCR-based telomerase assay (TRAP assay) has allowed for assessment of telomerase activity in a wide variety of immortal and tumor-derived cell lines as well as human tumors (16,17). Telomerase activity has been detected in 85–90% of a wide variety of malignant human tumors tested to date (reviewed in 18) (Table 1). Thus, detection of telomerase activity may be a potentially important and novel method for cancer diagnostics. Moreover, because telomerase activity is required for continuous tumor cell proliferation, it is also an attractive anticancer target. Loss of heterozygosity at chromosome 3 correlates tightly with telomerase activation (19), and repression of telomerase in immortal cell lines results in telomere shortening followed by the eventual restoration of cellular senescence (20–22). Thus, the study of the regulation of the telomerase holoenzyme is critical to further understand the cellular factors involved in controlling telomerase activity and for developing novel diagnostic and therapeutic strategies.

Table 1
Prevalence of Telomerase in a Variety of Tissues and Tumor Types[a]

Pathology	Normal	Benign/Premalignant	Malignant
Breast	0%	15%	88%
Lung	3%	54%	81%
Prostate	0%	9%	87%
Bladder	0%	40%	92%
Kidney	nd[b]	nd[b]	83%
Liver	0%	29%	86%
Endometrium	0%	0%	100%

[a] Summarized from ref. *18*
[b] nd – not determined

2. TELOMERE SHORTENING AND SENESCENCE

With the cloning of the gene corresponding to the catalytic subunit of telomerase *(23–26)*, telomerase activity was exogenously expressed in a cell-free system and in cultured normal human cells *(27–31)*. Using an in vitro transcription/translation system, both the RNA component (hTR) and the protein subunit (hTERT) were expressed in vitro and reconstituted activity with properties similar to native telomerase *(27,30)*. Because normal diploid cells express hTR without detectable telomerase activity, transient transfection of the hTERT cDNA into primary cells resulted in expression of telomerase activity *(27,29)*. These results indicate that hTERT is the catalytic subunit of telomerase, that hTERT and hTR are required to reconstitute telomerase activity, and that hTERT is the limiting factor for the activation of telomerase in normal human diploid cells *(27)*.

To determine if telomere shortening contributed to cellular senescence, we and others have taken advantage of the results obtained with the transiently transfected primary cells to directly test whether telomerase activity would result in extension of cellular lifespan *(28,31)*. Although ectopic hTERT allows expression of telomerase activity in normal cells, the most important criteria for assessing the role of telomeres in cellular senescence was to directly determine if this activity was fully functional, resulting in maintenance of telomere lengths and an increase in cellular lifespan. Stable clones expressing telomerase activity were found to be capable of maintaining or even elongating telomeres, resulting in prevention of cellular senescence and, ultimately, an extension of in vitro cellular lifespan. Currently, these clones have more than quadrupled their proliferative capacity without signs of cancer-associated changes *(31,32)*, suggesting that telomerase is not responsible for malignant transformation and is, therefore, not oncogenic. Together, these results provide direct experimental evidence that telomere erosion in normal diploid cells is one of the primary causes of cellular senescence. It may even be the molecular clock that controls the number of cell divisions prior to senescence. Although telomerase activation on its own may confer cellular immortality, many additional genetic alterations affecting cell cycle controls, invasiveness, and metastasis are likely required for a cell to become tumorigenic or malignant. Nevertheless, telomerase activation is linked to cancer, with approx 90% of human malignant cancers testing positive for telomerase activity, suggesting that maintenance of telomere length is required for the sustained growth of tumor cells.

Table 2
Telomerase Expression as a Potential Therapy for Age-Related Diseases

Problem	Cause	Possible Future Outcome
Aging Diseases	Blindness	Reverse aging in retinal cells
	Heart disease	Eliminate senescence in cells of blood vessels and decrease plaque formation
Replacement	Bone marrow transplants	Regenerate bone marrow cells from healthy donors
	Burn victims	Replace burns with healthy skin cells
	AIDS	Rejuvenate immune cells not infected with HIV
Basic Science	Produce permanent cell lines without a cancer phenotype	Production of human vaccines and reduction of normal cell procurement

3. POTENTIAL TREATMENT AND UTILITY OF TELOMERASE EXPRESSION IN THE PREMATURE AGING OF CELLS

Ectopic expression of telomerase in normal somatic cells maintains telomeres and leads to an extended lifespan, establishing an experimental model for preventing aging in a tissue culture system. This has far-reaching implications for the treatment of many types of human diseases (Table 2) *(34)*, including heart disease and blindness, as well as replacement therapy for patients with severe burns and those receiving bone marrow transplants. Data on allogenic bone marrow transplants indicate that the donor cells, when transplanted to the recipient, shorten their telomeres nearly 1000 base pairs over the course of bone marrow regeneration within the first year *(35–38)*. This may be the reason for the aged-related problems that occur 5–10 yr after the transplant, which include several different forms of leukemia.

In addition, the cells of certain accelerated aging syndromes, such as Hutchison-Guilford Progeria, have significantly shorter telomeres than age-matched controls *(12)*, which may be responsible for the increase in age-related medical problems, which include heart disease and thinning of the skin. Introduction of telomerase into some of the affected cells may allow for increased cell proliferation and elimination of aging for the treated cells. One excellent target for telomerase-mediated therapy would be for cardiovascular disease, where aging of the vascular endothelial cells is thought to prevent the uptake of cholesterol and induce the formation of plaques. If telomerase can be targeted to these cells specifically, one may be able to prevent premature senescence in the endothelial, allowing for increased cholesterol uptake and metabolism and decreased plaque formation. Clearly, prevention of aging in many cell types will be useful for the treatment of age-related disease, and the use of telomerase to prevent telomere shortening may be a critical tool for accomplishing that task.

4. CANCER DIAGNOSTICS AND TELOMERASE

Being associated with the vast majority of human cancers, telomerase is a leading candidate for molecular diagnostic strategies. Yet, there are currently no diagnostic tests that have been approved for general clinical use. It is also very important to note that detection of telomerase activity in tumor biopsies or resections does not always indicate malignancy, especially considering the number of normal cells that express telomerase activity (including lymphocytes, stem cells of the intestine and skin, germ cells, and so on) *(39–41)*. Although the current best method for cancer diagnosis is conventional pathology, even pathologists are looking for less qualitative and more reliable quantitative measures for assessing malignancy in order to reduce the number of false negatives (as well as false positives).

Clearly, the use of the TRAP assay will be critical for validation of diagnostic studies; however, molecular diagnosticians are more interested in nucleic acid-based strategies rather than those assays that rely on protein or enzymatic activity. Therefore, the conversion of protein-based assays into nucleic acid methodology will be highly desirable. Because hTERT is such a low abundant molecule (on the order of 10 copies of mRNA per cancer cell) (Kim N.W., personal communication), amplification techniques, such as reverse-transcriplase polymerase chain reaction (RT-PCR), will be necessary. To realistically be considered as a feasible molecular diagnostic assay, an RT-PCR-based telomerase approach should have high throughput potential and accurate quantification capabilities, as well as controls for false-negative assessment of PCR inhibition (use of an internal control). However, because hTERT is alternatively spliced with multiple variants expressed in most immortalized and cancer cells and some of these variants have the capacity to induce dominant-negative effects on telomerase *(42,43)*, appropriate steps will be required to control for assessment of wild-type hTERT expression.

For instance, appropriate primers will have to be designed to assess only those hTERT mRNA molecules that would express active enzyme. To ensure that wild-type hTERT is amplified, primer sequences should be used that would occur for the most common splice variants, including α, β, and α/β deletions *(48,49)*.

One can envision techniques that utilize fluorescent-based amplification of the targets (in this case, hTERT and hTR) as a multiplex RT-PCR strategy in a 96-well plate, while compensating for the alternatively spliced forms of the genes with appropriately engineered primers. For instance, one method may involve the amplification of hTERT (with a fluorescein tag) and hTR (with a Texas Red label) simultaneously in a single tube using real-time measurement, followed by a comparison of the ratio of hTERT and hTR amplification with overall telomerase activity as measured by the TRAP assay. Because hTR is ubiquitously expressed, it can serve as an appropriate quantitative internal control. At least initially, telomerase activity levels will have to assessed in order to determine the feasibility of the test, but subsequent RT-PCR assays may be useful for estimating the relative telomerase activity levels based solely on the amplification profile of the hTERT and hTR components. Importantly, it has been shown that hTERT levels correlate with activity in most cancer cases *(44–47)*.

Because it is desirable to convert this assay to a fluorescent-based, real-time assay, differentiation of spliced vs wild-type hTERT based on size would not be appropriate. Converting the standard telomerase activity assay into a nucleic acid-based molecular diagnostic assay may not be applicable for every type of cancer, but it will certainly be capable of assisting pathologists in the diagnosis of some human cancers.

Detection of telomerase in benign or preneoplastic conditions may also be useful for determining malignant potential or severity of disease. Currently many "benign" tumors are pathologically classified as being of very low malignant potential, yet some have detectable telomerase activity, which may suggest that these tumors may have significant proliferative and progressive potential. It may also indicate that these presumably benign lesions harbor malignant cells with the capacity to form a neoplasm. In addition, high levels of telomerase activity have routinely been associated with increased tumor grade, decreased prognosis, and reduced sampling error. Although there are some examples of this in the literature *(50,51)*, the more likely reason for elevated telomerase levels is caused by increased tumor homogeneity. Many tumors are sampled from frozen gross specimens, which contain a significant amount of normal tissue, as well as interspersed cancer. Because telomerase extraction typically utilizes homogenization and lysis of the entire tumor section rather than microdissection of only malignant tissue, the contribution of telomerase-negative normal cells will be significantly more in those lower-graded lesions that contain fewer cancer cells. During progression, increased tumor homogeneity results, and more cancer cells (and fewer normal cells) will be sampled, which will result in the detection of increased telomerase activity. Thus, while telomerase activity levels appear to be elevated as tumors increase their overall grade, it is more likely that telomerase activity on a per-cell basis is less variable.

In addition to using telomerase as an early screening marker for malignant potential, it may also be useful for detecting recurrence of malignant disease and monitoring treatment response. The fact that telomerase activity is specifically detected in the urine of patients with bladder cancer *(52)* provides an attractive, noninvasive means to monitor tumor recurrence as well as response to therapy. The ability to detect telomerase activity in upper tract urothelial *(53)* and intestinal lavage solutions *(54)* could also assist in the diagnosis and management of individuals with renal and colorectal cancers, respectively.

In the vast majority of cases, endstage malignancy is not caused by primary cancers but by secondary tumors that develop and cause problems associated with tumor invasion and metastasis. During removal of the primary tumor, it is critical for surgeons to obtain cleared margins; that is, the area of normal tissue surrounding the malignancy should be free of tumor cells. Pathologists typically analyze frozen specimens while the patient is on the operating table, but because they are virtually searching for a "needle in a haystack," these micrometastatic cells go undetected. The use of telomerase to assess the level of occult micrometastasis may be advantageous in that only the tumor cells (telomerase-positive) would be detected in the TRAP assay, whereas the surrounding normal tissue is expected to be telomerase-negative. Obviously, a critical control for this experiment is testing the primary tumor for telomerase activity. If it turns out to be one of the rare telomerase-negative tumors, this would not be a useful diagnostic test. Yet most malignancies (approx 90%) have telomerase activity, making this type of approach potentially quite useful. One other caveat is that the current telomerase detection protocols are quite time-consuming. As previously stated, it will be necessary to improve the efficiency of the telomerase assay by making it quantitative and reliable, eliminating the radioactivity and gel running steps, and decreasing the overall time required for analysis. Current experimentation indicates that the overall protocol can be streamlined into approx 4 h from sample preparation to real-time analysis of telomerase activity *(55)*, which still remains too long for patients to wait during surgery. However, additional methods for quantitative telomerase activity are currently being explored which, in addition to traditional pathology, may be extremely useful for cancer diagnostics, especially for those cases that are difficult to differentiate as benign or malignant.

5. TELOMERES AND TELOMERASE AS TARGETS
FOR CANCER THERAPY

Tumor development is initiated by multiple genetic events that ultimately result in either a block in terminal differentiation/senescence or activation of an inappropriate growth stimulatory pathway, the net result being the clonal expansion of a subset of cells with infinite proliferative potential. As cells approach senescence, telomere erosion is one of the obstacles that has to be overcome in order to proliferate indefinitely. Those cells with uninterrupted growth continue to shorten their telomeres, and the rare cell that does immortalize/transform almost always activates telomerase to maintain telomere lengths. There are some reports of telomerase-independent modes of immortalization (termed ALT for alternative lengthening of telomeres) in in vitro culture *(56),* yet most advanced human cancers—conservatively estimated at 95%—have detectable telomerase *(18)*, suggesting that the ALT pathway may play only a minor role in immortalization and tumor formation. Still, there is some concern that inhibition of telomerase as a means of cancer therapy might trigger this ALT pathway and result in a more aggressive tumor. However, the studies to date suggest that blocking telomerase in tumor-derived cells results either in the reappearance of the senescence pathway *(22)*, activation of an apoptosis pathway *(57–61)*, or a more differentiated state *(59)*. Therefore, it seems that although the ALT pathway is a viable alternative for cellular immortalization during in vitro culture, it appears to be less relevant when discussing telomerase inhibition and cancer therapy. This suggests that those cells that are committed to a telomerase-dependent immortalization pathway remain as such, and that conversion to the ALT pathway does not occur.

So, what influences the fate of a cancer cell following telomerase inhibition? Certainly, it will likely be dependent on a variety of factors including, but not limited to, overall telomere length within the tumor, the levels of telomerase activity, the status of *p53,* and so on. Telomere length in the tumor is most certainly a critical component that will determine the pathway a cell will take after telomere/telomerase inhibition. Those tumors harboring short telomeres may be more likely to undergo programmed cell death or apoptosis, while those with much longer telomeres may follow a senescence pathway *(62).*

There are a number of potential therapeutic agents directed at both the telomerase enzyme and the telomere. Because telomerase is a reverse transcriptase, traditional reverse transcriptase inhibitors may be applicable for cancer therapy. Compounds, such as dideoxyguanosine (ddG) and azidothymidine (AZT), exist that specifically block the activity of retroviral reverse transcriptases. Telomerase-positive cell lines have previously been subjected to treatment with these inhibitors to determine the effect on telomerase activity and telomere length in cells in culture *(63).* Indeed, both ddG and AZT inhibit telomerase activity, but the telomeres in these cells were highly unstable and did not appear to differ in length from the untreated controls. Because of the use of high concentrations of these compounds, deleterious effects on cellular polymerases, such as mitochondria RNA and DNA polymerases, may be contributing to the observed decline in proliferation under these conditions. Thus, it is likely that RT-inhibitors will lack specificity for telomerase inhibition, resulting in a host of additional nonspecific problems for normal cells, as well as side effects for patients.

Antisense expression of either RNA complementary hTR *(11,64)* or RNA complementary to telomeric sequences *(64)* in human cell lines results in repression of telomerase activity, telomere shortening, and eventual cellular crisis. Others have used more
stable oligonucleotide analogs to enhance the specificity and affinity of directed inhibition of telomerase, using hTR as a target. Norton et al. *(65)* inhibited telomerase activity using peptide nucleic acids (PNAs) complementary to the template region of hTR
with inhibitory concentrations (IC_{50}) of 1–5 nM. Others have followed this example
with similar results using antisense hTR sequences within the framework of stable
inhibitory oligonucleotides *(59,66,67)*. Hammerhead ribozymes used to cleave hTR
have been shown to inhibit telomerase activity in vitro and in cell culture systems *(68)*.
In this system, ribozymes designed to cleave hTR near the templating region were
more effective at reducing telomerase activity in cultured cells than ribozymes that
cleave elsewhere in hTR.

Additional gene modulation directed at the hTERT subunit has been shown to
induce a programmed cell death (apoptosis) response in a variety of cell lines expressing telomerase. This dominant-negative approach utilizes expression of a mutated
hTERT sequence in tumor-derived cell lines that causes a dramatic decline in telomerase activity. The dominant-negative hTERT cells undergo growth arrest and eventually apoptosis, dependent on the length of the telomere—the shorter the telomere, the
more profound the effect of hTERT blockage. Most of these gene-directed approaches
may be useful for studying the effects of telomerase inhibition on cells, but may not be
practical for therapeutic treatment of actual cancer patients.

Numerous chemotherapeutic compounds are capable of inducing terminal differentiation or an exit from the cell cycle (quiescence). Many of the pathways for telomerase
regulation and repression are summarized in Fig. 1. Presumably, nondividing nonreplicating cells would not require a telomere maintenance function, as they do not shorten
their telomeres, resulting in a downregulation of telomerase activity. In fact, activation
of differentiation pathways causes a gradual decline in telomerase activity, an event
that is irreversible *(69–72)*. In addition, cells that undergo a quiescent state, either by
removal of critical growth factors or by elimination of mitogen stimulation, also downregulate telomerase activity, but in a reversible manner. That is, if stimulated to enter
the cell cycle and undergo cell division, telomerase will be upregulated *(70,73)*. Cells
treated with chemotherapeutic drugs, such as adriamycin or 5–fluorouracil, undergo a
growth arrested state as well *(74)*. Treatment of wild-type *p53* breast tumor cells,
MCF-7, with clinically relevant, acute doses of adriamycin results in growth arrest and
downregulation of telomerase, similar to previous results using induction of quiescence
(75). What makes this an extremely novel finding is that these adriamycin-treated
MCF-7 cells repress hTERT transcription within the first 24 h of treatment and undergo
a prolonged growth arrest indicative of cellular senescence as a result of telomere dysfunction *(75a)*. Interestingly, after 14–21 d, some cells start dividing and recover their
telomerase activity *(75a)*. Breast tumor cell lines with mutated *p53* treated with adriamycin growth arrest as well, and eventually undergo a delayed apoptosis without an
immediate decline in telomerase activity or hTERT transcription. Current evidence
also suggests that *p53* interacts with the *Sp1*, and perhaps *Sp3*, transcription factors to
downregulate hTERT transcription *(76,77)*, while c-*myc*, either directly or indirectly,
activates transcription of the hTERT promoter *(78)*. Taken together, these data suggest
that adriamycin treatment of cells with mutated *p53* are more inclined toward apoptosis

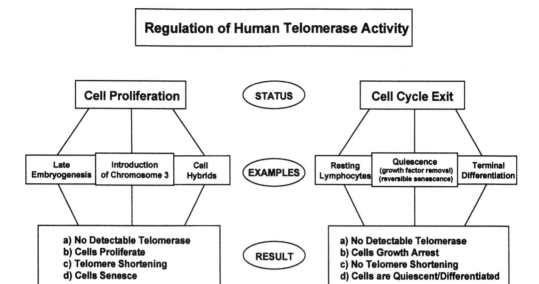

Fig. 1. Regulation of human telomerase. Current evidence suggests multiple avenues for telomerase-positive cells to regulate the activity of telomerase. Telomerase can either be repressed in cells that continue to divide (Cell Proliferation) or as a consequence of growth arrest (Cell Cycle Exit). During late embryogenesis, after introduction of a normal human chromosome 3, and following fusion of normal cells to telomerase-positive cancer cells, all result in repression of telomerase, followed by telomere shortening, and eventually cellular senescence. In some cases, introduction of exogenous genes (including a dominant-negative hTERT) causes induction of apoptosis rather than senescence, perhaps because of the lack of wild-type *p53* or their critically short telomeres *(57)*. Cell Cycle Exit results in nonmitotic cells and indirectly causes the repression of telomerase in multiple cell systems. Resting, quiescent lymphocytes contain little or no active telomerase, whereas their activated counterparts have robust telomerase activity levels. Cells can be induced to either terminally differentiate by addition of differentiating agents or undergo a quiescent state after growth factor removal, contact inhibition, or activation of reversible senescence *(70)*. Together, both the proliferative and cell cycle exit pathways are viable alternatives for inhibiting telomerase activity as a means of cancer treatment.

rather than senescence in breast tumor cells and that *p53* may play a role in hTERT transcriptional silencing. Importantly, our results indicate that the mechanism of adriamycin-induced senescence in breast tumor cells is dependent upon *p53* and telomere dysfunction *(75a)*.

G-quartet stabilizers are another potential telomere-targeting agent. After adding each telomeric repeat, telomerase pauses and repositions its integral RNA template component (hTR) prior to synthesizing the next repeat. During this translocation step, telomerase dissociates from the telomere and realigns itself for the next round of elongation. This step is facilitated by telomeric secondary structures in the form of a tetraplex, which is held together by the G-quartet structures *(79,80)*. This structure needs to be dissociated in order for telomerase to function properly and add telomeric tracts to the ends of the chromosomes. Thus, G-quartet stabilizing molecules, including porphyrins and anthraquinones, interact with the G4-quadruplex and functionally stabilize the structure *(81,82)*. This stabilization results in prevention of the telomerase-telomere association and inactivates the overall telomerase function by preventing the enzyme from using the telomere as a substrate *(62)*. However, as is the case for the RT-inhibitors, G-quartet stabilizers have proven ineffective at low concentrations and only high levels are capable of blocking telomerase activity.

Another potential target for telomerase inhibition is the interaction of molecular chaperones, specifically the hsp90 chaperone complex, with telomerase. The hTERT component functionally interacts with both hsp90 and p23, an acidic phosphoprotein *(83)*. Hsp90 and p23 directly participate in the assembly of the enzyme complex and may be associated with functional enzyme. The benzoquinone ansamycin, geldanamycin, specifically blocks the binding of p23 to hsp90 by associating in the ATP binding pocket and preventing ATP hydrolysis. In vitro reconstitution of telomerase activity is blocked by the addition of geldanamycin to the assembly reaction. Treatment of quiescent tumor-derived cells with serum (to progress them into the cell cycle) and low concentrations of geldanamycin (to block hsp90/telomerase function) results in entry of the cells into the cell cycle but repression of telomerase activity *(83)*. Recent evidence indicates that malignant cells have substantially more hsp90, p23, and hsp70 than normal or benign tissues *(84)*, suggesting that the use of geldanamycin for chaperone inhibition therapy may be a plausible treatment. However, one of the caveats for a chaperone-based cancer treatment is the lack of specificity. Hsp90 is a ubiquitously expressed chaperone that is required for numerous cellular functions independent of telomerase activity, including hormone receptor activation. Thus, the use of antichaperone treatment as a cancer therapy would likely be as detrimental to normal proliferating cells as cancer cells.

Telomerase inhibitors, if specific, would certainly be a novel and effective therapeutic strategy. However, inhibition of telomerase should not be considered as the first line of defense. For most solid tumors, surgical resection is critical for reducing tumor burden. After the tumor is removed, treatments should be designed to eliminate the recurrence of more aggressive disease. Often either local radiation and/or chemotherapy are used as adjuvant treatments. However, specifically inhibiting telomerase in micrometastatic cells that were not surgically removed with the original tumor could be a more precise and effective therapy to prevent recurring cancer. As suggested by Kondo *(60)*, inhibition of telomerase increases the sensitivity of cancer cells to cisplatin-induced apoptosis, suggesting that telomerase inhibition may also represent a new chemosensitization for tumors resistant to conventional chemotherapeutics. One other consideration when discussing telomerase inhibitors is the effect on the "normal" cells in the body that express telomerase activity, such as lymphocytes, germ cells, and stem cells *(39–41,85–88)*. The effects on such cells using antitelomerase treatments would be expected to produce cellular toxicity for significantly prolonged regimens. It is critical to note that while the vast majority of tumors have considerably shorter telomeres and higher proliferation rates, progenitor and germ cells with telomerase have much longer, more stable telomere lengths, and divide only rarely. Thus, treatment should only be necessary for short periods of time; that is, long enough to shorten cancer cell telomeres to a senescent or apoptotic length without adversely affecting the viability of immune, germ, or stem cells during therapy.

6. TUMOR SUPPRESSION USING TELOMERASE?

In this chapter, there are two paradoxical issues that have yet to be addressed, namely, that telomerase is associated with over 90% of malignant human cancer and that telomerase expression can prevent cellular aging. If telomerase and cancer go

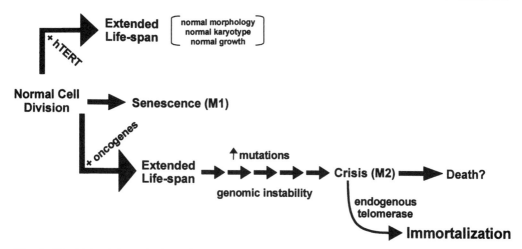

Fig. 2. The M1/M2 hypothesis revisited. Three differing fates of normal cells: First, cells can proceed normally with telomere shortening to senescence (M1). Second, oncogenes can be introduced prior to senescence to inactivate *p53* and pRB, bypass senescence, and allow for continued telomere shortening, increased genomic instability and mutation, and progression to crisis (M2). At this point, cell death and cell division are balanced, and the rare cell that immortalizes almost always reactivates telomerase. These cells are then considered functionally immortal. Third, expression of hTERT in normal cells prior to senescence provides telomere maintenance and an extended lifespan without the changes typically associated with immortalization. Senescence has been prevented, rather than bypassed, with cells exhibiting normal morphology, karyotype, and tumor suppressor function. Therefore, these cells should be considered either extended lifespan cells *(89)* or telomerized cells *(34)*, rather than immortal.

hand-in-hand, why don't normal cells with ectopically expressed telomerase also become tumorigenic? Although this is a very relevant question, the generalized answer is quite simple. As cells progress past senescence and crisis, toward immortality, genomic instability is enhanced, which results in increased frequencies of mutation and, ultimately, the eventual immortalization process. As has been previously discussed *(89)*, introduction of telomerase into normal cells prior to the onset of senescence may prevent much of the genomic instability and increased mutation frequency that would typically occur if viral oncoproteins were expressed. Because telomerase-expressing normal cells have not bypassed senescence, they should be considered as extended lifespan rather than immortalized, which by definition requires numerous mutations, an atmosphere of genomic instability, and reactivation of endogenous telomerase (Fig. 2). With the extended lifespan or "telomerized" cells, none of these things have taken place, yet the cells continuously divide in a normal fashion without changes in karyotype, growth characteristics, or tumor suppressor function *(32,33)*. The difference between the telomerase-expressing extended lifespan cells and the oncogene-induced extension of lifespan cells is that the latter have bypassed senescence, whereas the telomerized cells prevent the senescence process altogether.

The classic definition of immortalization has always been continuous growth beyond a certain number of population doublings (i.e., beyond the Hayflick limit), usually more than 100 doublings, depending on the cell type. However, we are compelled to rethink this classic usage of "immortality" as the current definition has progressed into a more global meaning with more relevance to cancer. Immortalization is currently deemed as cells that have bypassed crisis and have undergone the functional and morphological changes typical of a cell prone to transformation. Immortalization appears to be the requisite step in the process of tumor cell conversion to a malignant state and almost exclusively involves the reactivation of endogenous telomerase. If telomerase is expressed prior to the changes in genomic integrity, senescence, and perhaps progression toward immortalization, are prevented. However, if telomerase is expressed after oncogene expression, it is likely that telomerase would not be capable of overcoming or correcting the instability/mutations that would normally occur upon oncoprotein expression.

The telomere maintenance function of telomerase provides cells with the ability to continuously proliferate in the absence of cell cycle or karyotypic changes. In fact, current evidence indicates that telomerase expression results in the prevention of p16 methylation *(90)*, a functional step required for mammary epithelial cells to spontaneously inactivate the pRB arm of cellular senescence, a stage known as M0 *(91)*. Recent findings suggest that telomerase and its telomere maintenance function may also prevent some of the karyotypic changes associated with age and/or oncogene expression *(32,33)*. In fact, we have recently found that expression of telomerase in human cells prone to spontaneous crisis and immortalization provides for maintenance of telomere function and extension of lifespan without the karyotypic abnormalities associated with the spontaneous event *(92)*. Thus, it seems likely that telomerase expression in normal cells may allow for increased genetic and genomic stability, not only preventing senescence and aging, but blocking immortalization and progression to a tumorigenic state as well.

7. FINAL THOUGHTS

Although not found in normal somatic cells, telomerase is associated with approx 90% of all human malignancies, making it the most prominent molecular cancer marker known to date. Because it is found in almost all cancers, telomerase is an obvious candidate for improved diagnostic and therapeutic strategies. Understanding its functional role in tumor cells is critically important for determining how to inhibit telomerase as a means of cancer treatment.

Because progression from normal cells to cancer is a multistep process involving many genetic changes, the activation of telomerase is quite often one of the final, rate-limiting occurrences in the in vitro model of immortalization. With that in mind, data are accumulating to indicate that expression of telomerase in normal somatic cells prevents cellular aging and may protect cells from cancer-associated changes. Therefore, telomerase may be useful for prevention and early detection, as well as being an important chemotherapeutic target. Thus, the goals of prevention, detection, and treatment of human cancer are all relevant to telomerase: 1) use telomerase to prevent both cellular aging and progression to cancer; 2) if there is detectable cancer, find it early using telomerase as a screen and increase the chances for a full, cancer-free recovery; and 3) if the cancer has progressed, use a novel anti-telomerase adjuvant therapy (together with tumor resection or conventional therapies) to specifically and effectively inhibit tumor growth and prevent recurrence with minimal side effects.

The prospects of the current studies and the ability to translate the findings of basic research into a clinically practical setting makes telomeres and telomerase an extremely novel set of diagnostic and therapeutic targets. It is an exciting time in the field of cancer biology, and telomerase research will surely serve to more rapidly advance this discipline in the areas of prevention, diagnosis, and treatment.

REFERENCES

1. Hayflick L, Moorhead PS. The serial cultivation of human diploid cells strains. *Exp Cell Res* 1961; 25:585–621.
2. de Lange T, Shiue L, Meyers RM, et al. Structure and variability of human chromosome ends. *Mol Cell Biol* 1990; 10:518–527.
3. Moyzis RK, Buckingham JM, Cram S, et al. A highly conserved repetitive DNA sequence, (TTAGGG)n, present at the telomeres of human chromosomes. *Proc Natl Acad Sci USA* 1988; 85:6622–6626.
4. Olovnikov AM. Principle of marginotomy in template synthesis of polynucleotides. *Doklady Biochem* 1971; 201:394–397.
5. Watson JD. Origin of concatameric T4 DNA. *Nat New Biol* 1972; 239:197–201.
6. Harley CB, Futcher AB, Greider CW. Telomeres shorten with aging. *Nature* 1990; 345:458–460.
7. Hastie ND, Dempster M, Dunlop MG, Thompson AM, Green DK, Allshire RC. Telomere reduction in human colorectal carcinoma and with ageing. *Nature* 1990; 346:866–868.
8. Lindsey J, McGill N, Lindsey L, Green D, Cooke H. In vivo loss of telomeric repeats with age in humans. *Mutat Res* 1991; 256:45–48.
9. Greider CW, Blackburn EH. Identification of a specific telomere terminal transferase activity in Tetrahymena extracts. *Cell* 1985; 43:405–413.
10. Blackburn EH. Telomerases. *Ann Rev Biochem* 1992; 61:113–129.
11. Feng J, Funk WD, Wang S-S, et al. The RNA component of human telomerase. *Science* 1995; 269:1236–1241.
12. Allsopp RC, Vaziri H, Patterson C, et al. Telomere length predicts replicative capacity of human fibroblasts. *Proc Natl Acad Sci USA* 1992; 89:10,114–10,118.
13. Wright WE, Shay JW. The two-stage mechanism controlling cellular senescence and immortalization. *Exp Geron* 1992; 27:383–389.
14. Wright WE, Pereira-Smith OM, Shay JW. Reversible cellular senescence: implications for immortalization of normal human diploid fibroblasts. *Mol Cell Biol* 1989; 9:3088–3092.
15. Shay JW, Pereira-Smith OM, Wright WE. A role for both RB and p53 in the regulation of human cellular senescence. *Exp Cell Res* 1991; 196:33–39.
16. Kim NW, Piatyszek MA, Prowse KR, et al. Specific association of human telomerase activity with immortal cells and cancer. *Science* 1994; 266:2011–2015.
17. Piatyszek MA, Kim NW, Weinrich SL, et al. Detection of telomerase activity in human cells and tumors by a telomeric repeat amplification protocol (TRAP). *Meth Cell Sci* 1995; 17:1–15.
18. Shay JW, Bacchetti S. A survey of telomerase activity in human cancer. *Europ J Cancer* 1997; 33:787–791.
19. Mehle C, Lindblom A, Ljungberg B, Stenling R, Roos G. Loss of heterozygosity at chromosome 3p correlates with telomerase activity in renal cell carcinoma. *Int J Cancer* 1998; 13:289–295.
20. Horikawa I, Oshimura M, Barrett JC. Repression of the telomerase catalytic subunit by a gene on human chromosome 3 that induces cellular senescence. *Molec Carcin* 1998; 22:65–72.
21. Tanaka H, Shimuzu M, Horikawa I, Kugoh H, Yokota J, Barrett JC, Oshimura M. Evidence for a putative telomerase repressor in the 3p14.2-p21.1 region. *Genes Chrom Cancer* 1998; 23:123–133.
22. Ohmura H, Tahara H, Suzuki M, et al. Restoration of the cellular senescence program and repression of telomerase by human chromosome 3. *Jpn J Cancer Res* 1995; 86:899–904.
23. Lingner J, Hughes TR, Shevchenko A, Mann M, Lundblad V, Cech TR. Reverse transcriptase motifs in the catalytic subunit of telomerase. *Science* 1997; 276:561–567.
24. Nakamura TM, Morin GB, Chapman B, et al. Telomerase catalytic subunit homologs from fission yeast and human. *Science* 1997; 277:955–959.
25. Meyerson M, Counter CM, Eaton EN, et al. hEST2, the putative human telomerase catalytic subunit gene, is up-regulated in tumor cells and during immortalization. *Cell* 1997; 90:785–795.
26. Harrington L, Zhou W, McPhail T, et al. Human telomerase contains evolutionarily conserved catalytic and structural subunits. *Genes Devel* 1997; 11:3109–3115.
27. Weinrich SL, Pruzan R, Ma L, et al. Reconstitution of human telomerase with the template RNA component hTR and the catalytic protein subnit hTRT. *Nat Genet* 1997; 17:498–502.
28. Bodnar AG, Ouellette M, Frolkis M, et al. Extension of lifespan by introduction of telomerase into normal human cells. *Science* 1998; 279:349–352.
29. Counter CM, Meyerson M, Eaton EN, et al. Telomerase activity is restored in human cells by ectopic expression of hTERT (hEST2), the catalytic subunit of telomerase. *Oncogene* 1998; 16:1217–1222.

30. Beattie TL, Zhou W, Robinson M, Harrington L. Reconstitution of telomerase activity in vitro. *Curr Biol* 1998; 8:177–180.

31. Vaziri H, Benchimol S. Reconstitution of telomerase activity in normal human cells leads to elongation of telomeres and extended replicative life span. *Curr Biol* 1998; 8:279–282.

32. Morales CP, Holt SE, Ouellette M, et al. Absence of cancer-associated changes in human fibroblasts immortalized with telomerase. *Nat Gen* 1999; 21:55–58.

33. Jiang Z-R, Jimenez G, Chang E, et al. Telomerase expression in human somatic cells does not induce changes associated with a transformed phenotype. *Nat Genet* 1999; 21:111–114.

34. Shay JW, Wright WE. The use of telomerized cells for tissue engineering. *Nat Biotech* 2000; 18:22–23.

35. Chui C-P, Dragowska W, Kim NW, et al. Differential expression of telomerase activity in hematopoietic progenitors from adult human bone marrow. *Stem Cells* 1996; 14:239–248.

36. Curtis RE, Rowlings PA, Deeg HJ, et al. Solid cancers after bone marrow transplantation. *New Engl J Med* 1997; 336:897–905.

37. Notaro R, Cimmino A, Tabarini D, Rotoli B, Luzzatto L. In vivo dynamics of human hematopoietic stem cells. *Proc Natl Acad Sci USA* 1997; 94:13,782–13,785.

38. Weng RF, Cross MA, Hatton C, et al. Accelerated telomere shortening in young recipients of allogeneic bone marrow transplants. *Lancet* 1997; 351:178–181.

39. Ramirez RD, Wright WE, Shay JW, Taylor RS. Telomerase activity concentrated in the mitotically active segments of human hair follicles. *J Invest Dermatol* 1997; 108:113–117.

40. Harle-Bachor C, Boukamp P. Telomerase activity in the regenerative basal layer of the epidermis in human skin and in immortal and carcinoma-derived skin keratinocytes. *Proc Natl Acad Sci USA* 1996; 93:6476–6481.

41. Yasmoto S, Kunimura C, Kikuchi K, et al. Telomerase activity in normal human epithelial cells. *Oncogene* 1996; 13:433–439.

42. Yi X, White DM, Aisner DL, Baur JA, Wright WE, Shay JW. An alternate splicing variant of the human telomerase catalytic subunit inhibits telomerase activity. *Neoplasia* 2000; 2:433–440.

43. Yi X, Shay JW, Wright WE. Quantitation of telomerase components and hTERT mRNA splicing patterns in immortal human cells. *Nucl Acids Res* 2001; 29:4818–4825.

44. Ito H, Kyo S, Kanaya T, Takakura M, Koshida K, Namiki M, Inoue M. Detection of human telomerase reverse transcriptase messenger RNA in voided urine samples as a useful diagnostic tool for bladder cancer. *Clin Cancer Res* 1998; 4:2807–2810.

45. Kanaya T, Kyo S, Takakura M, Ito H, Namiki M, Inoue M. hTERT is a critical determinant of telomerase activity in renal-cell carcinoma. *Int J Can* 1988; 78:539–543.

46. Kyo S, Kanaya T, Takakura M, Tanaka M, Inoue M. Human telomerase reverse transcriptase as a critical determinant of telomerase activity in normal and malignant endometrial tissues. *Int J Cancer* 1999; 80:60–63.

47. Wu A, Ichihashi M, Ueda M. Correlation of the expression of human telomerase subunits with telomerase activity in normal skin and skin tumors. *Cancer* 1999; 86:2038–2044.

48. Kilian A, Bowtell DDL, Abud HE, et al. Isolation of a candidate human telomerase catalytic subunit gene, which reveals complex splicing patterns in different cell types. *Hum Molec Genet* 1997; 6:2011–2019.

49. Ulaner GA, Hu JF, Vu TH, Giudice LC, Hoffman AR. Telomerase activity in human development is regulated by human telomerase reverse transcriptase (hTERT) transcription and by alternate splicing of hTERT transcripts. *Cancer Res* 1998; 58:4168–4172.

50. Clark GM, Osborne CK, Levitt D, Wu F, Kim NW. Telomerase activity and survival of patients with node-positive breast cancer. *J Natl Cancer Inst* 1997; 89:1874–1881.

51. Poremba C, Willenbring H, Hero B, et al. Telomerase activity distinguishes between neuroblastoma with good and poor prognosis. *Ann Oncol* 1999; 10:715–721.

52. Kinoshita H, Ogawa O, Kakehi Y, et al. Detection of telomerase activity in exfoliated cells in urine from patients with bladder cancer. *J Natl Cancer Inst* 1997; 89:724–730.

53. Wu W, Liu L, Huang C, Huang C, Chang L. The clinical implications of telomerase activity in upper tract urothelial cancer and washings. *BJU Int* 2000; 86:213–219.

54. Ishibashi K, Hirose K, Kato H, Ogawa K, Haga S. Determining the telomerase activity of exfoliated cells in intestinal lavage solution to detect colorectal carcinoma. *Anticancer Res* 1999; 19(4B): 2831–2836.

55. Elmore LW, Forsythe HL, Ferreira-Gonzalez A, Garrett CT, Clark GM, Holt SE. Real-time quantitative analysis of telomerase activity in breast tumor specimens using a highly specific and sensitive fluorescent-based assay. *Diag Mol Pathol* 2002a; 11:177–185.

56. Bryan TM, Englezou A, Dalla-Pozza L, Dunhan MA, Reddel RR. Evidence for an alternative mechanism for maintaining telomere length in human tumors and tumor-derived cell lines. *Nat Med* 1997; 3:1271–1274.

57. Hahn WC, Stewart SA, Brooks MW, et al. Inhibition of telomerase limits the growth of human cancer cells. *Nat Med* 1999; 5:1164–1170.

58. Zhang X, Mar V, Zhou W, Harrington L, Robinson MO. Telomere shortening and apoptosis in telomerase-inhibited human tumor cells. *Genes Dev* 1999; 13:2388–2399.

59. Kondo S, Tanaka Y, Kondo Y, et al. Anti-sense telomerase treatment: induction of 2 distinct pathways, apoptosis and differentiation. *FASEB J* 1998a; 12:801–811.

60. Kondo S, Kondo Y, Li G, Silverman RH, Cowell JK. Targeted therapy of human malignant glioma in a mouse model by 2–5A antisense directed against telomerase RNA. *Oncogene* 1998b; 16:3323–3330.

61. Herbert B, Pitts AE, Baker SI, et al. Inhibition of human telomerase in immortal human cells leads to progressive telomere shortening and cell death. *Proc Natl Acad Sci USA* 1999; 96:14,276–14,281.

62. Lichtsteiner SP, Lebkowski JS, Vasserot AP. Telomerase, a target for anticancer therapy. *Ann NY Acad Sci* 1999; 886:1–11.

63. Strahl C, Blackburn EH. Effects of reverse transcriptase inhibitors on telomere length and telomerase activity in two immortalized human cell lines. *Mol Cell Biol* 1996; 16:53–65.

64. Bisoffi M, Chakerian AE, Fore ML, et al. Inhibition of human telomerase by a retrovirus expressing telomeric antisense RNA. *Europ J Cancer* 1998; 34:1242–1249.

65. Norton JC, Piatyszek MA, Wright WE, Shay JW, Corey DR. Inhibition of human telomerase activity by peptide nucleic acids. *Nature Biotech* 1996; 14:615–619.

66. Kondo Y, Koga S, Komata T, Kondo S. Treatment of prostate cancer in vitro and in vivo with 2-5A-anti-telomerase RNA component. *Oncogene* 2000; 19:2205–2211.

67. Pitts A, Corey DR. Inhibition of human telomerase by 2′-O-methyl-RNA. *Proc Natl Acad Sci USA* 1998; 95:11,549–11,554.

68. Yokoyama Y, Takahashi Y, Shinohara A, et al. Attenuation of telomerase activity by a hammerhead ribozyme targeting the template region of telomerase RNA in endometrial carcinoma cells. *Cancer Res* 1998; 58:5406–5410.

69. Sharma HW, Sokoloski JA, Perez JR, et al. Differentiation of immortal cells inhibits telomerase activity. *Proc Natl Acad Sci USA* 1995; 92:12,343–12,346.

70. Holt SE, Wright WE, Shay JW. Regulation of telomerase activity in immortal cell lines. *Mol Cell Biol* 1996; 16:2932–2939.

71. Bestilny LJ, Brown CB, Miura Y, Robertson LD, Riabowol KT. Selective inhibition of telomerase activity during terminal differentiation of immortal cell lines. *Cancer Res* 1996; 56:3796–3802.

72. Albanell J, Han W, Mellado B, et al. Telomerase activity is repressed during differentiation of maturation-sensitive but not resistant human tumor cell lines. *Cancer Res,* 1996; 56:1503–1508.

73. Buchkovich KJ, Greider CW. Telomerase regulation during entry into the cell cycle in normal human T cells. *Mol Biol Cell* 1996; 7:1443–1454.

74. Holt SE, Aisner DL, Shay JW, Wright WE. Lack of cell cycle regulation of telomerase activity in human cells. *Proc Natl Acad Sci USA* 1997; 94:10,687–10,692.

75. Elmore LW, Rehder CW, Di X, et al. Adriamycin-induced replicative senescence in tumor cells requires functional p53 and telomere dysfunction. *J Biol Chem* 2002; 277:35,509–35,515.

75a. Elmore LW, Rehder CW, Di M, et al. Adriamycin-induced replicative senescence in tumor cells requires functional p53 and telomere dysfunction. *J Biol Chem* 2002; 277:35,509–35,515.

76. Kanaya T, Kyo S, Hamada K, et al. Adenoviral expression of p53 represses telomerase activity through down-regulation of human telomerase reverse transcriptase transcription. *Clin Cancer Res* 2002; 6:1239–1247.

77. Won J, Yim J, Tae Kook Kim TK. Sp1 and Sp3 recruit histone deacetylase to repress transcription of human telomerase reverse transcriptase (hTERT) promoter in normal human somatic cells. *J Biol Chem.* 2002; 277:38,230–38,238.

78. Wang J, Xie LY, Allan S, Beach D, Hannon GJ. Myc activates telomerase. *Genes Devel* 1998; 12:1769–1774.

79. Fang G, Cech TR. Characterization of a G-quartet formation reaction promoted by the beta-subunit of the Oxytricha telomere-binding protein. *Biochem* 1993; 32:11,646–11,657.

80. Zahler AM, Williamson JR, Cech TR, Prescott DM. Inhibition of telomerase by G-quartet DNA structures. *Nature* 1991; 350:718–720.

81. Wheelhouse RT, Sun D, Han H, Han FX, Hurley LH. Cationic porphyrins as telomerase inhibitors: the interaction of tetra-(n-methyl-4-pyridyl)porphine with quadraplex DNA. *J Am Chem Soc* 1998; 120:3261–3262.

82. Sun D, Thompson B, Cathers BE, et al. Inhibition of human telomerase by a G-quadruplex-interactive compound. *J Med Chem* 1997; 40:2113–2116.

83. Holt SE, Aisner DL, Baur J, et al. Functional requirement of p23 and hsp90 in telomerase complexes. *Genes Develop* 1999; 13:817–826.

84. Akalin A, Elmore LW, Forsythe HL, et al. A novel mechanism for chaperone-mediated telomerase regulation during prostate cancer progression. *Cancer Res* 2001; 61:4791–4796.

85. Zhang W, Piatyszek MA, Kobayashi T, et al. Telomerase activity in human acute myelogenous leukemia: inhibition of telomerase activity by differentiation-inducing agents. *Clin Cancer Res* 1996; 2:799–803.

86. Broccoli D, Young JW, de Lange T. Telomerase activity in normal and malignant hematopoietic cells. *Proc Natl Acad Sci USA* 1995; 92:9082–9086.

87. Counter CM, Gupta J, Harley CB, Leber B, Bacchetti S. Telomerase activity in normal leukocytes and in hematological malignancies. *Blood* 1995; 85:2315–2320.

88. Hiyama K, Hirai Y, Kyoizumi S, et al. Activation of telomerase in human lymphocytes and hematopoietic progenitor cells. *J Immunol* 1995; 155:3711–3715.

89. Elmore LW, Holt SE. Telomerase and telomere stability: A new class of tumor suppressor? *Mol Carcin* 2000; 28:1–4.

90. Kiyono T, Foster SA, Koop JI, McDougall JK, Galloway DA, Klingelhutz AJ. Both Rb/p16ink4a inactivation and telomerase activity are required to immortalize human epithelial cells. *Nature* 1998; 396:84–88.

91. Foster SA, Galloway DA. Human papillomavirus type 16 E7 alleviates a proliferation block in early passage human mammary epithelial cells. *Oncogene* 1996; 12:1773–1779.

92. Elmore LW, Turner KC, Gollahon LS, Landon MR, Jackson-Cook CK, Holt SE. Telomerase protects cancer-prone cells from chromosomal instability and spontaneous immortalization. *Cancer Biol Ther* 2002b; 1:395–401.

INDEX

f: figure;
t: table